P.M. Pour · Y. Konishi · G. Klöppel
D.S. Longnecker (Eds.)

Atlas of Exocrine Pancreatic Tumors

Morphology, Biology, and Diagnosis with an International Guide for Tumor Classification

A Publication of the International Pancreatic Cancer Study Group (IPCSG)

With 363 Illustrations, 41 in Full Color

Springer-Verlag
Tokyo Berlin Heidelberg New York
London Paris Hong Kong
Barcelona Budapest

Parviz M. Pour, M.D.
The Eppley Institute for Research in Cancer; Department of Pathology and Microbiology, University of Nebraska Medical Center, Omaha, NE 68198-6805, USA

Yoichi Konishi, M.D.
Department of Oncological Pathology, Cancer Center, Nara Medical College, Kashihara, Nara, 634 Japan

Günter Klöppel, M.D.
Department of Pathology, Academy Hospital Jette, Free University of Brussels, 1090 Brussels, Belgium

Daniel S. Longnecker, M.D.
Department of Pathology, Dartmouth Medical School, Hanover, NH 03756, USA

ISBN 4-431-70129-X Springer-Verlag Tokyo Berlin Heidelberg New York
ISBN 3-540-70129-X Springer-Verlag Berlin Heidelberg New York Tokyo
ISBN 0-387-70129-X Springer-Verlag New York Berlin Heidelberg Tokyo

Printed on acid-free paper

Library of Congress Cataloging-in-Publication Data
Atlas of exocrine pancreatic tumors: morphology, biology, and diagnosis, with an international guide for tumor classification/P.M. Pour . . . [et al.] (eds.). p. cm. Includes bibliographical references and index. ISBN 4-431-70129-X.—ISBN 3-540-70129-X. —ISBN 0-387-70129-X. 1. Pancreas—Tumors—Classification—Atlases—Congresses. I. Pour, P.M. (Parviz M.), 1933- . [DNLM: 1. Pancreatic Neoplasms—atlases. 2. Pancreatic Neoplasms—classification—congresses. WI 17 A87945 1994] RC280.P25A87 1994, 616.99′437—dc20, DNLM/DLC, for Library of Congress

Typesetting, printing, and binding: Best-set Typesetter Ltd., Hong Kong

Background

The classification of tumors is important for understanding tumor histogenesis, for predicting prognosis, for differential diagnosis, and for recommending appropriate therapy. Since 1836, when pancreatic cancer was first described, progress has been made in pancreatic cancer morphology, and a number of classifications have been proposed. All of these classifications are mainly based on morphological characteristics. Some are too detailed to be of practical use while others are more pragmatic. Some of the inherent problems in the previous classifications included difficulties in obtaining an adequate number of pancreatic tumors for examination and insufficient clinical data and follow-up. With the increasing incidence of pancreatic cancer in many parts of the world during the past six decades, and with the availability of more tumors to pathologists, advances have been made in pancreatic tumor studies. Classifications by Cubilla and Fitzgerald and by Klöppel, which are generally similar, mostly considered prominent morphological features and their histogenesis. These pathology-oriented classifications, although complete, were not practical from the standpoint of clinicians concerned with the prognosis of individual tumors. The recent development of sophisticated diagnostic instruments, awareness of the increasing incidence of the disease by clinicians, increased governmental funding of pancreatic cancer studies, improved follow-up procedures, development of various tumor markers, discovery of growth factors and their receptors, and the use of flow cytometry, DNA analysis, and molecular biological techniques have all contributed to a significant advancement in understanding the biology and morphogenesis of pancreatic neoplasms. The need for a revised pancreatic cancer classification arose, in part, from greater collaboration between pathologists, surgeons, clinicians, and basic researchers. The worldwide use of a single classification system would standardize data bases and facilitate international comparisons of incidences and results of treatment.

In August 1990, members of the International Pancreatic Cancer Study Group (IPCSG), which was established in 1987 to provide an international forum for pancreatic cancer researchers, met in Nagasaki, Japan, to discuss the existing problems of pancreatic tumor classification and biological characteristics of pancreatic cancer cells, and to propose a practical and clinically useful classification system. Experts from different biomedical fields, including pathologists, clinicians, surgeons, immunologists, and basic researchers, including molecular biologists, attended this meeting in which clinical, histomorphological and biological data of pancreatic exocrine tumors, selected from different institutions in the United States, Europe, and Japan, were reviewed and discussed. The researchers agreed that some of the previously described lesions, which were thought to represent an entity, are in reality a different phenotypical expression of a more common neoplasm. For example, the "pleomorphic or giant cell type" in the classification of several authors is a variant of ductal adenocarcinoma and has no prognostic significance. Another example is the mixed duct-islet, duct-islet-acinar, and acinar-islet tumors proposed by Cubilla and Fitzgerald and by Sommer and Meissner. Based on several recent studies, more than 80% of exocrine pancreatic carcinomas (ductal adenocarcinoma, mucinous cystic tumor, acinar cell carcinoma, and pancreatoblastoma) contain endocrine cells, some in a pattern consistent with the mixed exocrine-endocrine cell tumors and, therefore, their consideration as an entity is debatable. However, because more well-differentiated ductal adenocarcinomas contain endocrine cell elements than the poorly differentiated variety, the presence of endocrine cells within the cancers may have a prognostic value.

Accumulating observations have clarified the histogenesis of some tumors that previously were thought to be of acinar cell origin or whose histogenesis was unknown. Solid cystic tumors with favorable prognosis, thought by Klöppel to be of acinar cell origin, seem to originate from primitive primordial pancreatic cells, with the tendency for differentiation into ductal, insular, and acinar cells. The same is true for pancreaticoblastoma, which appears to present as a more immature form of an embryonic tumor with a rather poor prognosis. Microadenocarcinoma, listed as a variant of ductal type carcinoma by Cubilla and Fitzgerald, appears to be a variant of acinar cell cancer. Other tumors described by Cubilla and Fitzgerald, such as oncocytic carcinoma, oncocytic carcinoid, and ciliated cell carcinoma have not been observed by other investigators. A more recent detailed and extended classification by some Japanese pathologists, who differentiate cystic tumors on the basis of their connection to the pancreatic ductal system, was considered to be of value for establishing pathogenesis but unneeded for practical clinical classification and determination of prognosis.

Moreover, the clinical experience has revealed that intraductal tumors have a better prognosis than others. An example is the intraductal papillary tumor with excess mucin production. Many investigators have recognized the entity of these tumors although it is still unclear whether these tumors were missed or misdiagnosed in the past or whether their incidence has increased.

Much discussion surrounded intraductal lesions. It was recognized that the prognosis of some of these lesions cannot be determined from the histomorphological appearance, and, therefore, their designation as either an adenoma or carcinoma was improper. It was agreed that until more is known about these lesions, the designation of "tumors" should be given to them. This rather ambiguous designation indicates the unpredictable nature of such neoplasms. Additional morphologic phrases, such as "non-invasive" and "invasive", reflects their "observed" biological behavior. However, this distinction is subjective and relative. Costly serial sectioning and time-consuming histological examination may or may not distinguish a potentially malignant version (with invasion) from another prognostically more favorable "non-invasive" counterpart. Future studies are needed to reveal markers useful in predicting their biological behavior.

This subject highlighted another problem in establishing a unified classification system—the lack of guidelines for preparation and processing of specimen for histological diagnosis. Personal perception also confounds tumor diagnosis. Some consider small papillary projections occurring in some cystic tumors as papillary neoplasms, whereas others require a dominant papillary structure as a prerequisite for lesions to be termed papillary tumors.

The distinction between the benign and malignant tumors is still muddled. Although previous classifications considered cystic serous tumors (microcytic adenoma) as benign, recent observations point to their malignant potential inasmuch as a few adenocarcinomas with this histologic type have been reported. Genetic alteration of pancreatic cancer cells seems to offer a partial explanation, but the available biological and molecular biological data are not sufficient to form the basis of a clear-cut distinction between benign and potentially malignant tumors. For example, although the c-Ki-*ras* mutation can be used to distinguish normal from malignant cells, the pattern of mutation is not useful in differentiating invasive from non-invasive adenocarcinoma. As described in this atlas, the current results on tumor antigenicity, growth factors and their receptors, chromosomal aberrations, and gene mutations have not demonstrated a useful correlation that can be used to predict the prognosis of the diseases. Consequently, we still rely on histopathological findings in assessing the malignancy, grade of differentiation, and staging of pancreatic cancer. It was also recognized that the patterns of tumor invasion and metastases, and definition and characterization of preneoplastic lesions need careful study. These data could help to better understand the biology of pancreatic cancer.

The participants of the meeting considered the above problems and proposed a revised classification presented in this atlas and also recommended practical hints for tissue examination, fixation, and preparation for histological, immunological, and molecular biological studies with the hope that such standardization will facilitate common understanding.

These recommendations can guide pathologists, clinicians, and basic researchers in developing standardized techniques for tumor examination that will improve the understanding of the biology of pancreatic cancer. The classification represents a step in developing a clinically useful system with international acceptance. Further change and refinement of the classification on the basis of new data should be anticipated.

Other inherent problems that need collaborative efforts for resolution relate to the grading system of the tumors and their correlation with the prognosis. Because the method of surgical resection (partial, total, curative), availability of pancreatic and parapancreatic tissues for examination, and preoperative and postoperative patient treatment are all important factors in prognostic considerations and survival, current data do not provide a reliable base to determine which correlations exist and we await prospective studies.

The Editors

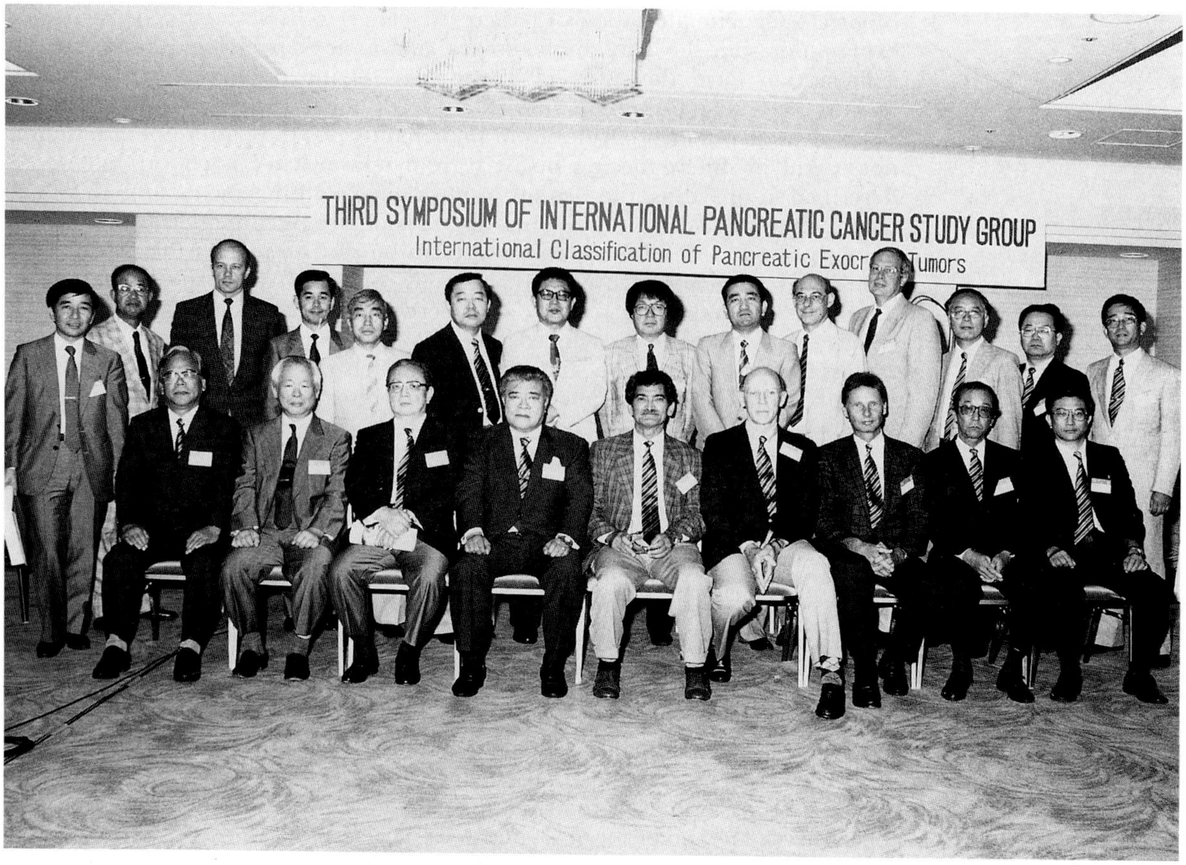

Members of the International Pancreatic Cancer Study Group participating in the classification of pancreatic cancer. *Rear row* (left to right): Akira Wada, Tetsuo Hayakawa, Reinhard Klapdor, Akinori Ishihara, Takahiko Funabiki, Yoshifumi Kawaharada, Akira Kuroda, Katsusuke Sataka, Tsukasa Tsunoda, Martin Sarner, Eugene DiMagno, Toshio Morohoshi, Shigetoshi Matsuo, Tsutoma Tomioka

Front row (left to right): Kohtaro Uchida, Hideo Harada, Hideo Ozaki, Ryoichi Tsuchiya, Parviz M. Pour, Daniel S. Longnecker, Günter Klöppel, Yoichi Konishi, Yo Kato

Histological Classification of Exocrine Pancreatic Tumors

Benign

Serous cystadenoma

Tumors with uncertain malignant potential

Intraductal (papillary-mucinous) tumors
  non-invasive (adenoma, severe dysplasia)
Mucinous cystic tumors
  non-invasive (adenoma, severe dysplasia)
Solid (papillary)-cystic tumors

Malignant

Serous cystadenocarcinoma
Intraductal (papillary-mucinous) carcinoma (invasive)
Ductal adenocarcinoma
Mucinous cystadenocarcinoma
Mucinous noncystic carcinoma
Adenosquamous carcinoma
Squamous cell carcinoma
Anaplastic (undifferentiated) carcinoma
Acinar cell carcinoma
Pancreatoblastoma
Small cell carcinoma

Contents

Contributors

Background . . . P.M. Pour*, Y. Konishi, G. Klöppel, D.S. Longnecker

Gross Anatomy of the Pancreas . . . A. Kuroda*, H. Nagai

Microanatomy and Fine Structure of the Pancreas . . . T. Morohoshi*, D.E. Bockman

Serous Cystadenoma. *Microcystic Type* . . . T. Funabiki*, K. Kamei. *Macrocystic Type* . . . K.B. Lewandrowski*

Intraductal Papillary Mucinous Tumors, Non-Invasive and Invasive. *Mucin Hypersecreting Tumors* . . . K. Yamao*, S. Nakazawa, M. Fujimoto, M. Yamada. *Papillary Tumors* . . . S. Milchgrub*, J. Albores-Saavedra

Mucinous Cystic Tumors, Non-Invasive and Invasive . . . Y. Wada*

Solid Cystic Tumors . . . K. Yamaguchi*, T. Morohoshi, G. Zamboni

Serous Cystadenocarcinoma . . . T. Funabiki*, K. Kamei

Ductal Adenocarcinoma . . . P.M. Pour*, T. Morohoshi

Mucinous (Noncystic) Adenocarcinoma, Including Signet-Ring Carcinoma . . . A. Yanagisawa*, Y. Kato, G. Klöppel

Adenosquamous Cell Carcinoma . . . S. Matsuya*, P.M. Pour

Squamous Cell Carcinoma . . . S. Matsuya*, P.M. Pour

Anaplastic (Undifferentiated) Carcinoma . . . M. Tsutsumi*, T. Morohoshi, Y. Konishi. *Pleomorphic Giant Cell Carcinoma* . . . K.B. Lewandrowski, W.H. Yong. *Mixed Pleomorphic, Osteoclastic Carcinoma* . . . B. Gatteschi*, V. Pugliese, P.M. Pour

Acinar Cell Carcinoma . . . A. Ishihara*

Pancreatoblastoma . . . T. Morohoshi*, G. Klöppel

Small Cell Carcinoma . . . G. Klöppel*

Preneoplastic Lesions of the Exocrine Pancreas . . . D.S. Longnecker*, G. Klöppel, P.M. Pour

Pathology of Metastatic Patterns of Pancreatic Cancer. *General Metastatic Patterns* . . . K. Kishi*, T. Uehara, T. Izumo, M. Kurosumi, S. Hirohashi, K. Mukai. *Lymphatic and Neural Invasion* . . . T. Nagakawa*, M. Kayahara

Tumor Spread and the Factors Influencing Prognosis in Patients with Resected Pancreatic Carcinoma . . . M. Yamamoto*, Y. Saitoh

---

* Asterisks indicate the principal authors; for their affiliations *see* back matter.

Staging for Carcinoma of the Pancreas: Japanese Stage Classification Compared to UICC Stage Classification . . . T. Tsunoda*, T. Eto, K. Ura, T. Matsumoto, R. Tsuchiya

Molecular Biology. *Growth Factors, Growth Factor Receptors, Tumor Suppressor Genes* . . . N.R. Lemoine*, P.A. Hall. *c-Ki-ras Mutation, Correlative Biological and Clinical Findings* . . . K. Motojima*, T. Urano, Y. Nagata, H. Shiku, T. Tsunoda, T. Kanematsu. *Geographical Patterns of c-Ki-ras and p53 Mutations and p53 Protein Accumulation* . . . A. Scarpa*, G. Zamboni, S. Hirohashi

Sampling Method for Pancreatic Tissue Examination. *General Method* . . . T. Tomioka*, M. Shimizu, K. Mukai. *Intraoperative Sampling* . . . O. Ishikawa*, H. Ohigashi, S. Imaoka

Color Plates

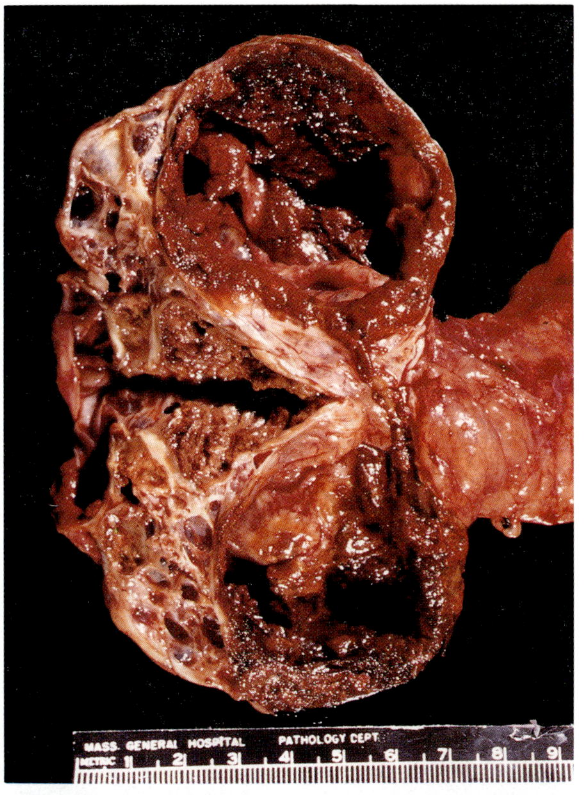

Fig. 5 (Chapter: Serous cystadenoma). Gross appearance of a macrocystic serous tumor with a dominant 8.0 cm macrocyst. This 66-year-old woman presented with a 2-year history of upper abdominal fullness. Physical examination revealed a palpable epigastric mass. CT showed a 10- to 15-cm multiseptic mass involving the head, body, and uncinate process of the pancreas. A subtotal pancreatectomy was performed (from [1] with permission) (*p. 34*)

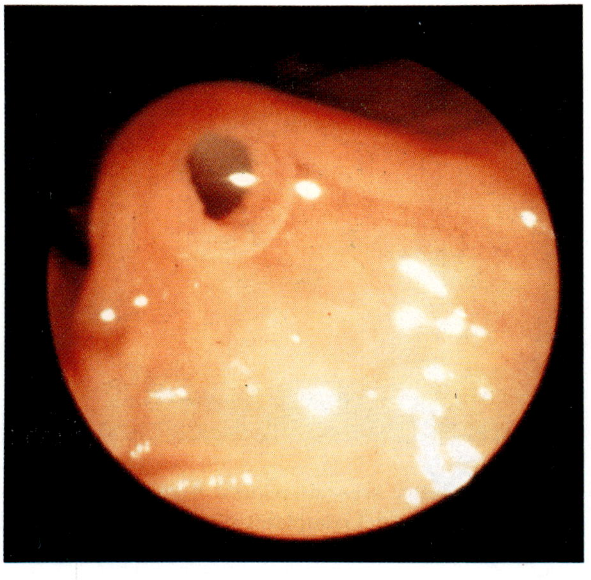

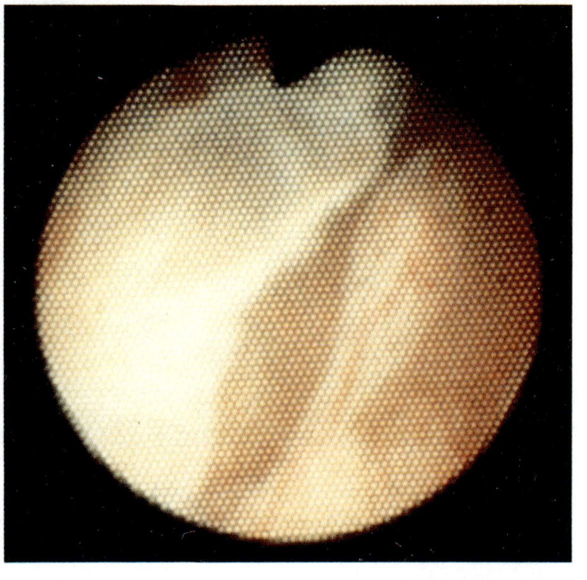

Fig. 6 (Figs. 6, 8 of Chapter: Intraductal Papillary Mucinous Tumors, Non-Invasive and Invasive). Intraductal papillary adenocarcinoma in a 61-year-old man with a complaint of epigastralgia. Duodenoscopy revealed characteristic features of this tumor: enlargement of the papilla, widely opened orifice of the papilla, and mucus excretion from the orifice (*p. 47*)

Fig. 8. Invasive type of intraductal tumor in a 70-year-old man with a complaint of jaundice. Peroral transpapillary pancreatoscopy showed papillary tumor (fish-egg-like appearance) in the main pancreatic duct (*p. 48*)

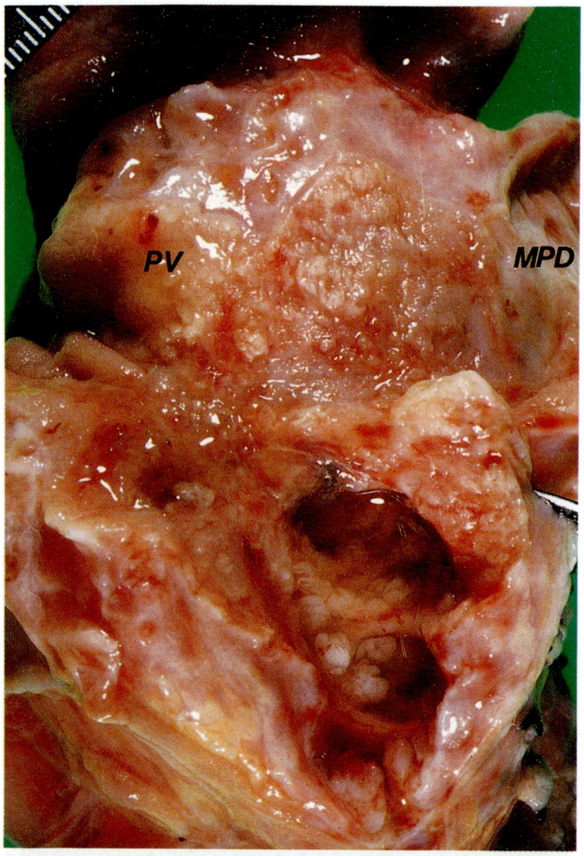

Figs. 15 (Figs. 15–18, 26 of Chapter: Intraductal Papillary Tumors, Non-Invasive and Invasive). Non-invasive intraductal tumor, branch duct type in a 74-year-old man with a complaint of diarrhea. Macroscopic examination revealed polyposis in the dilated inferior branch duct and a granular mucosa that extends from the branch to the dilated main pancreatic duct. *PV*, papilla of Vater; *MPD*, main pancreatic duct (*p. 51*)

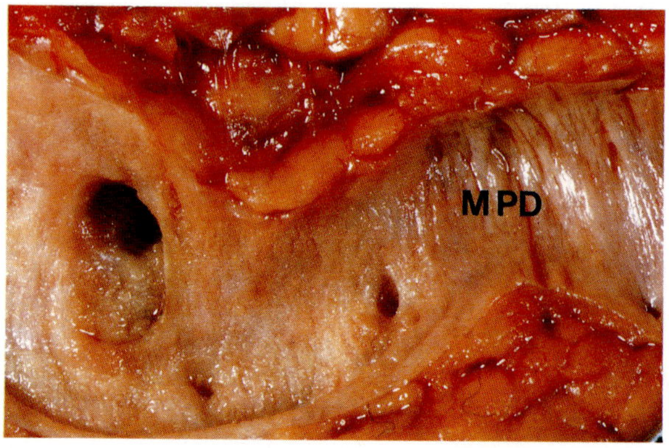

Fig. 16. Intraductal papillary tumor, main duct type in a 71-year-old man without symptoms. A granular mucosa extends from the dilated main duct to the branch ducts. Distended orifice of the branch ducts can be observed. *MPD*, main pancreatic duct (*p. 52*)

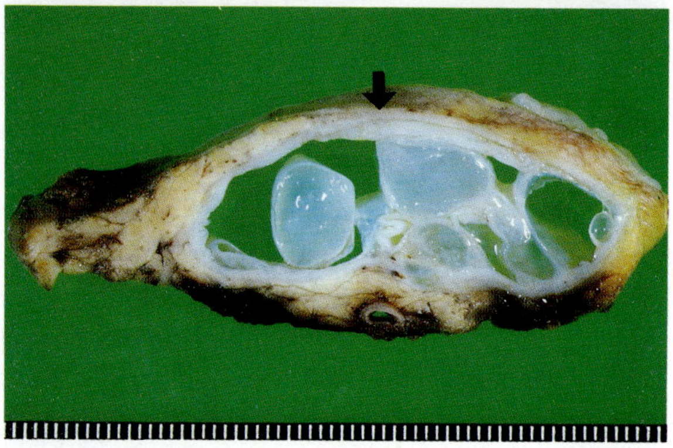

Fig. 17. Classical type of mucinous cystic tumor, non-invasive in a 37-year-old woman without symptoms. The cut surface of the tumor shows multilocular cyst. Thick fibrous capsule which surrounds the whole cyst is seen (*arrow*). (*p. 52*)

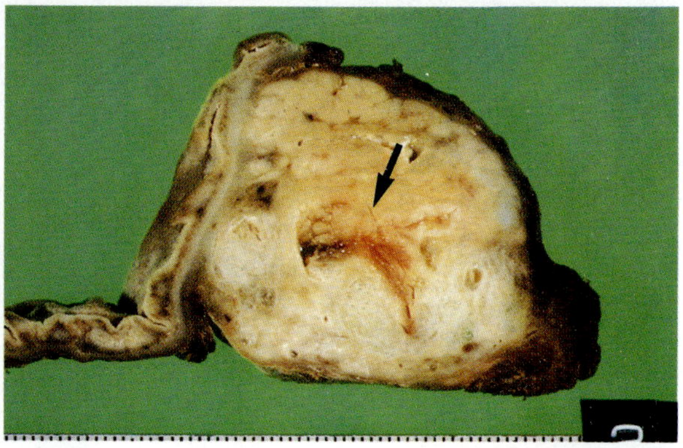

Fig. 18. Invasive type intraductal tumor in a 59-year-old man with a chief complaint of jaundice. He died of cancer recurrence within a year after operation. Lower half of the tumor shows a soft, medullary, yellow-white mass. Papillary tumor is present in the dilated main pancreatic duct and branch ducts (*arrow*) (*p. 53*)

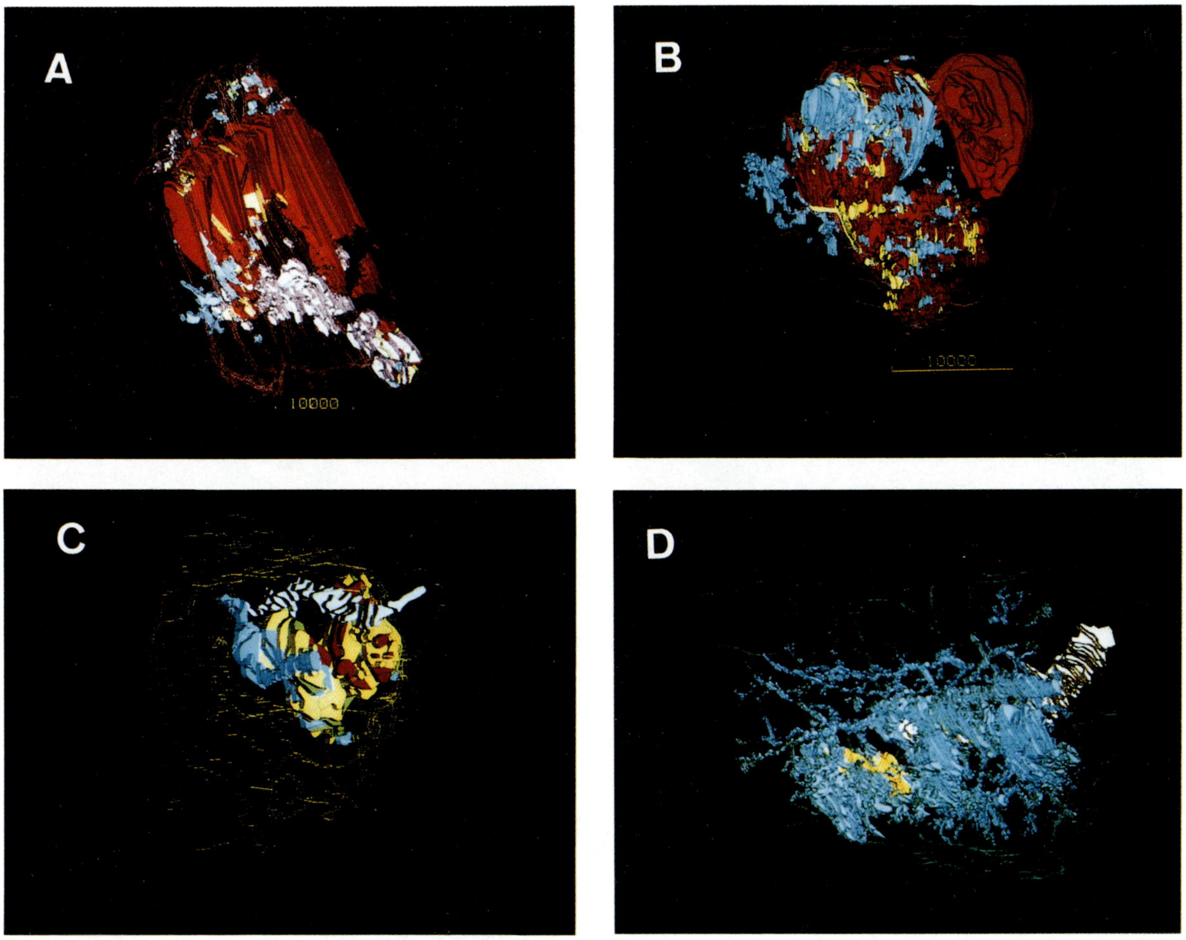

Fig. 26A–D. Computer assisted 3-D mapping of the mucus-hypersecreting tumor along the pancreatic duct. Epithelial changes are expressed with different colors: carcinoma in situ (*CIS*) in *red*, dysplasia in *yellow*, hyperplasia in *green*, ordinary epithelia in *blue*. ***A*** The main duct and subbranches, markedly dilated, are almost exclusively lined with CIS. Colored in pink are mucus lakes in periductal tissues. ***B*** The main duct is focally dilated corresponding to a major cyst, which is lined with CIS. Note the extension of CIS into several subbranches and nondilated part of the main duct. ***C*** A cystic sub-branch was found to have dysplasia of inner lining epithelium. Note the multicentric development of CIS in the area of dysplasia. ***D*** Two ductal subbranches are dilated, with the inner surfaces partially involved in dysplasia. No carcinoma was found. (From [32] with permission) (*pp. 57–58*)

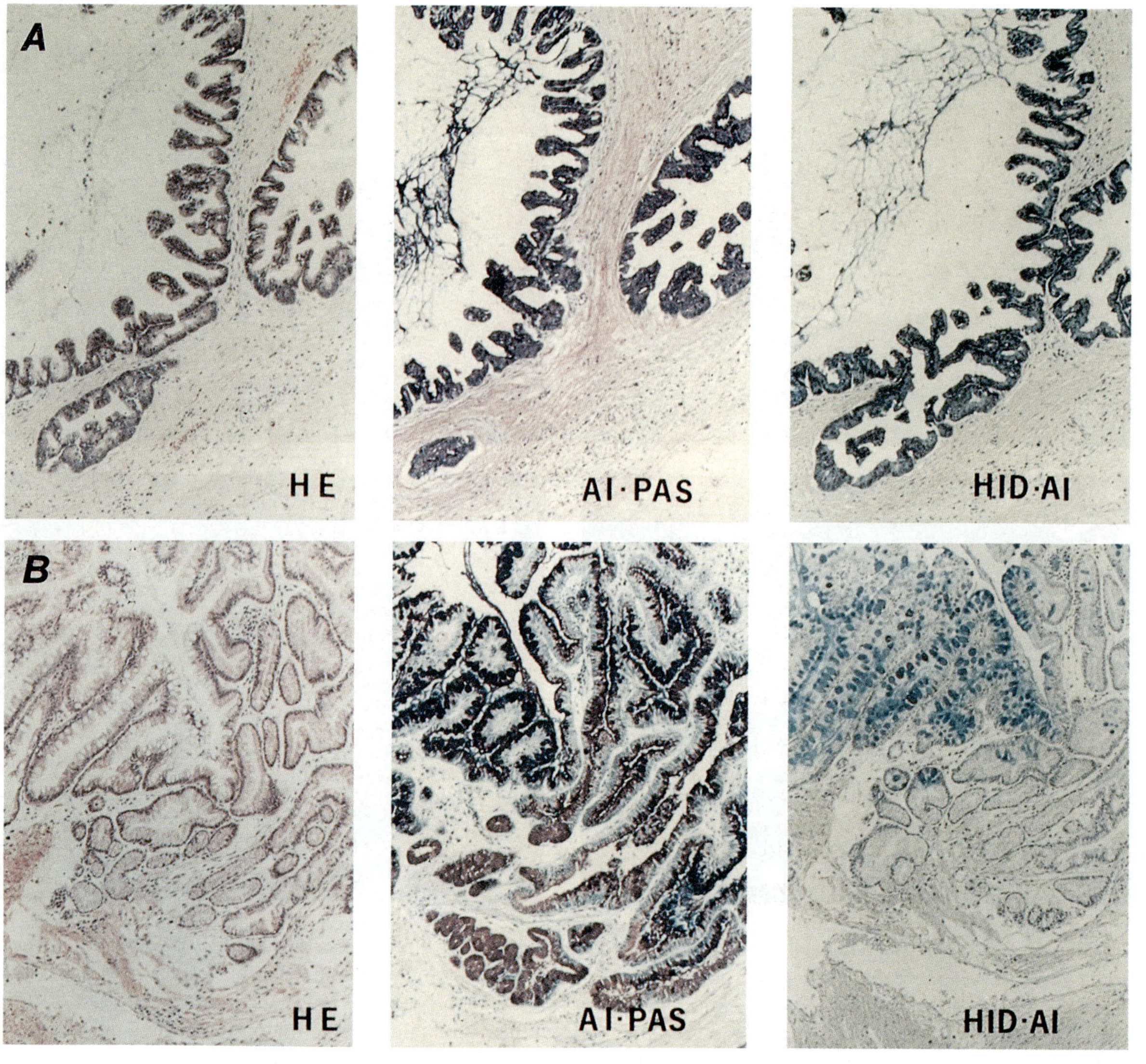

Fig. 32A,B (Chapter: Intraductal Papillary Tumors, Non-Invasive and Invasive). Double-staining with alcian blue (pH 2.5), periodic acid-Schiff (*PAS*) and with high-iron diamine (*HID*)-alcian blue (pH 2.5). ***A*** Invasive intraductal papillary tumor (IDT). Sialomucin can be observed in most of the tumor cells. ***B*** Noninvasive IDT. Neutral mucin is also observed in another portion of this tumor (*p. 63*)

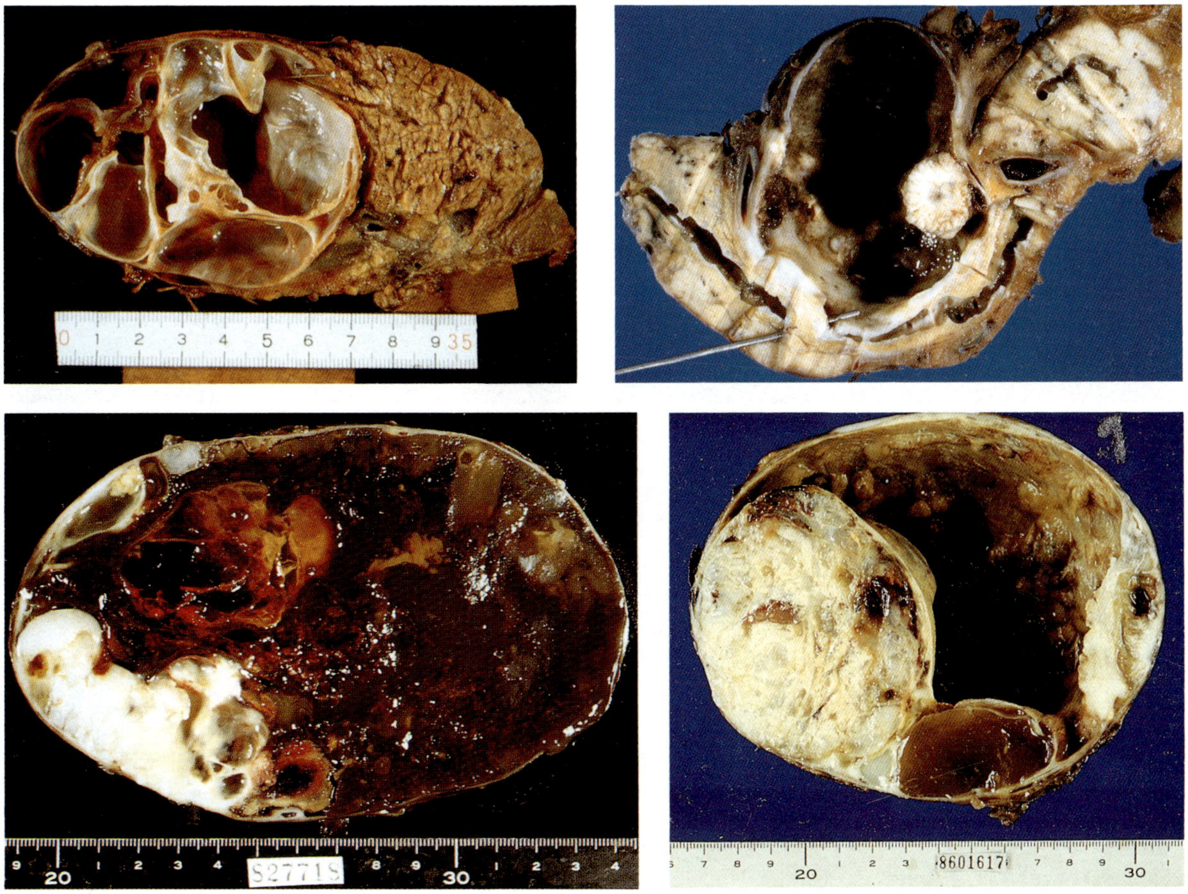

a b c d

Fig. 6a–d (Chapter: Mucinous Cystic Tumors, Non-Invasive and Invasive). Gross appearance of sectioned mucinous cystic tumor. ***a*** Mucinous cystadenoma (mucinous cystic tumor with benign appearance). A 38-year-old female who presented with epigastric discomfort for several months. Computed tomography (*CT*) scan demonstrated a cystic tumor in the tail of the pancreas which was resected by distal pancreatectomy. The cut surface of the surgical specimen reveals an encapsulated multilocular cyst composed of several large cystic spaces separated by thin fibrous septae. The cyst walls are smooth. Some cysts are filled with thick gelatinous mucin. The patient was alive and well 12 years after the operation. ***b*** Mucinous cystic tumor of borderline malignancy from the same patient as in Fig. 4. A unilocular cyst enclosed by a thick fibrous capsule is seen in the horizontally sectioned surgical specimen obtained by distal pancreatectomy. The tumor measures 4.5 cm in maximum diameter, and contains a polypoid papillary tumor projecting from the cyst wall. A bougie indicates a communication between the cyst lumen and the main pancreatic duct. There is a small pseudocyst just distal to the cystic tumor. The patient died 6 years after the surgery. ***c*** Mucinous cystadenocarcinoma from the same patient as in Figs. 2 and 3. The cut surface of the tumor resected by distal pancreatectomy shows a large cystic cavity filled with hemorrhagic and necrotic tissue. There are irregular excrescences from the cyst wall, which appear solid in some parts, but are actually composed of multiple small cysts containing mucoid material. This tumor demonstrated focal stromal invasion of the fibrous septae. The patient was alive 9 years after surgery with no evidence of tumor recurrence, in spite of preoperative rupture of the tumor suggested by the fistular tract extending into the thorax, associated with strong inflammatory adhesions of neighboring organs. ***d*** Mucinous cystadenocarcinoma from the same patient as in Figs. 1 and 5. The sectioned tumor reveals a multilocular cyst with solid-appearing large nodular excrescences protruding into the lumen of a major cyst. The external surface of the tumor is smooth. Some cysts demonstrate retention of thick gelatinous mucin. This tumor showed extensive stromal invasion of the fibrous septa and capsule with lymph node metastases. The patient died of carcinomatous peritonitis 3 months after radical operation (*p. 72, 73*)

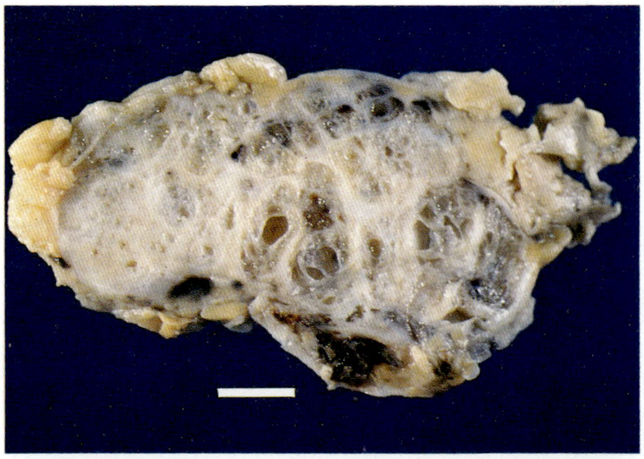

9a

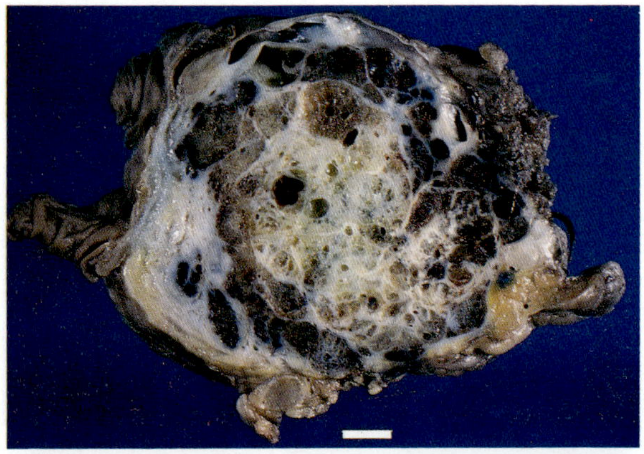

9b

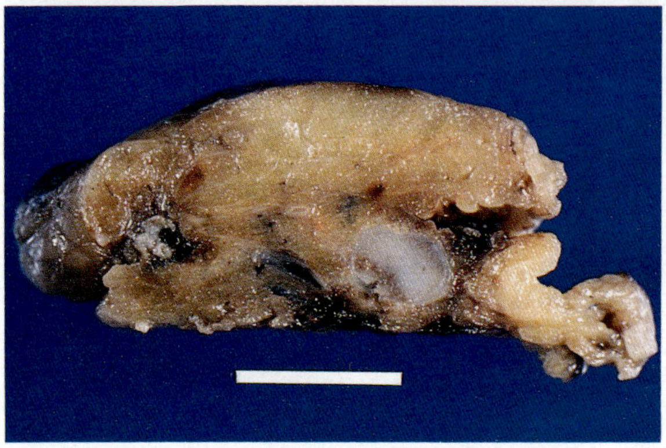

9c

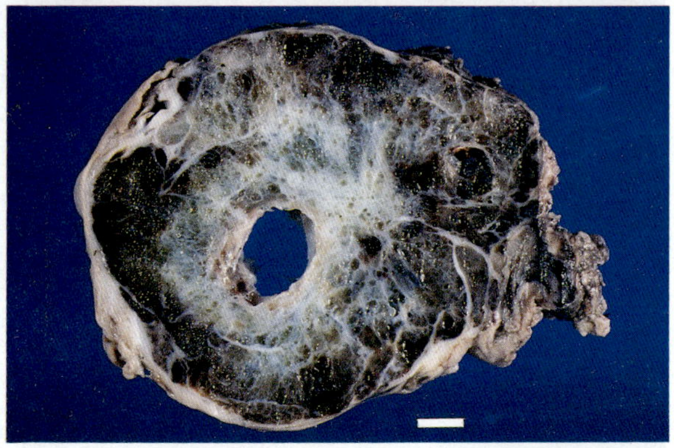

10

Fig. 9 (Figs. 9, 10, 12, 16–18 of Chapter: Serous Cystadenocarcinoma). **a** Multiple spongy cysts segmented by white fibrous tissue in a serous cystadenoma, and ***b*** in a serous cystadenocarcinoma in the pancreatic head. ***c*** The serous cystadenocarcinoma in the pancreatic body exhibits white and solid areas (*p. 106*)

Fig. 10. A serous cystadenocarcinoma of the pancreatic head. Necrotic appearance is evident (*p. 107*)

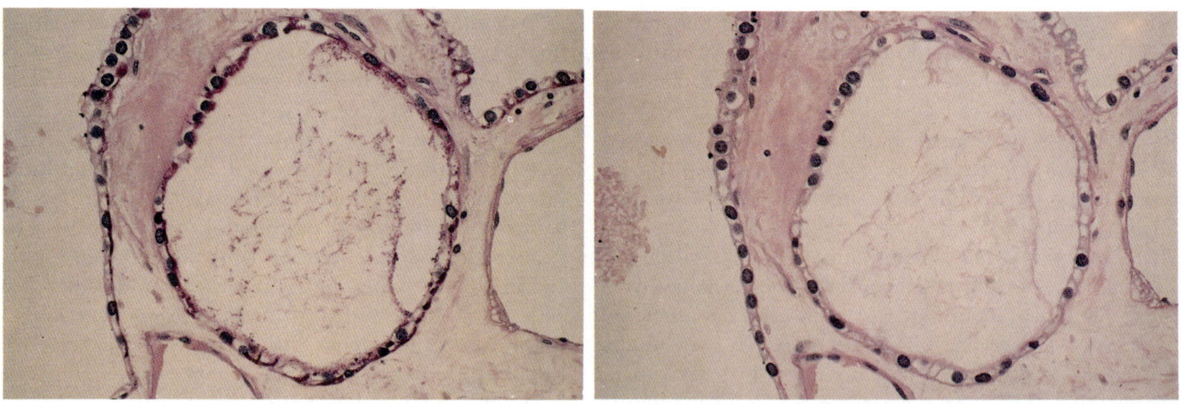

Fig. 12. Serous cystadenocarcinoma. Both fields stained with the periodic acid-Schiff reaction. The tissue on the right was predigested with diastase. ×100 (original magnification) (*p. 109*)

a 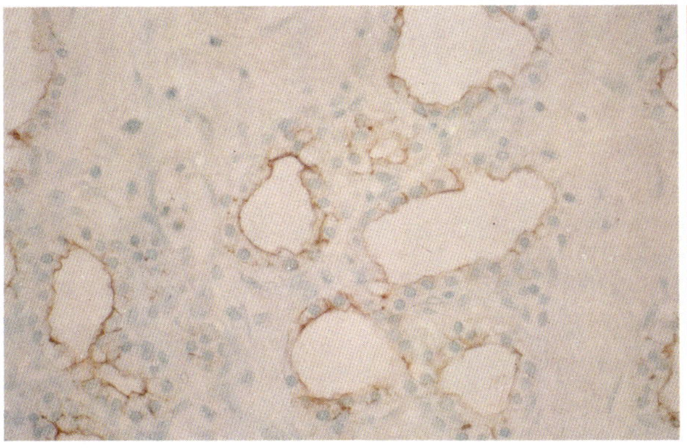 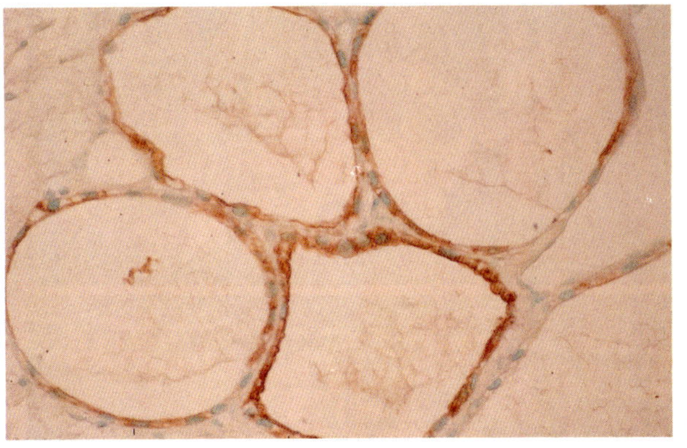 b

Fig. 16a,b. CA19-9 expression in a serous cystadenoma. ***a*** Tumor cells are stained only on the apical cell membrane (the same patient as in Fig. 9). ***b*** Tumor cells are stained diffusely in serous cystadenocarcinoma (tumor of the pancreatic head, the same patient as in Fig. 9). ×100 (original magnification). (*p. 112*)

a 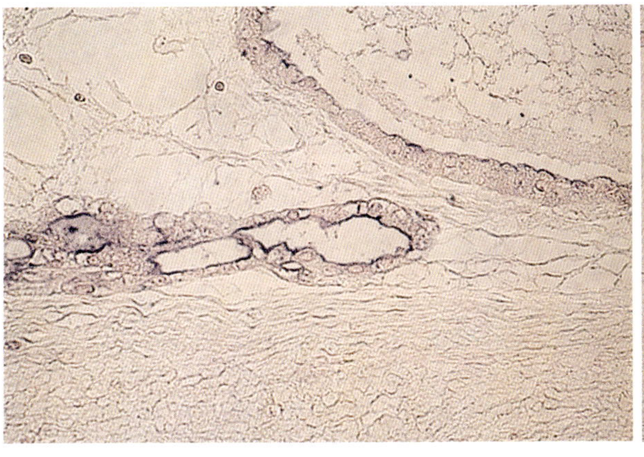 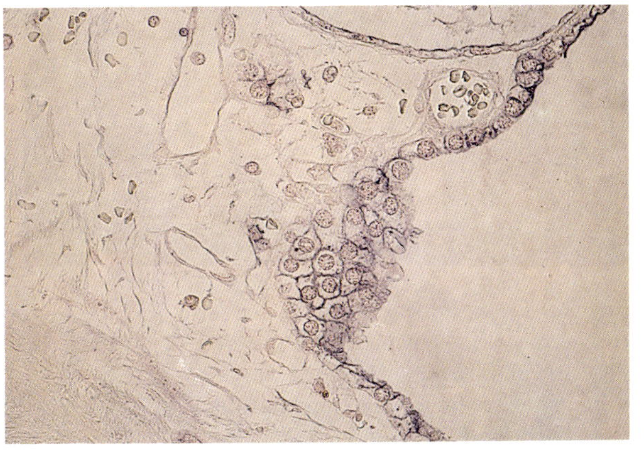 b

Fig. 17a,b. NCC-ST-439 expression in a serous cystadenoma (***a***) and in a serous cystadenocarcinoma (***b***) (the same patient as in Fig. 9). ×100 (original magnification). (*p. 113*)

a 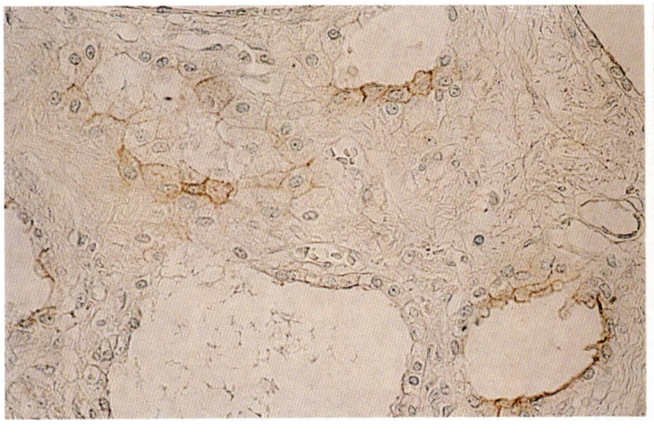 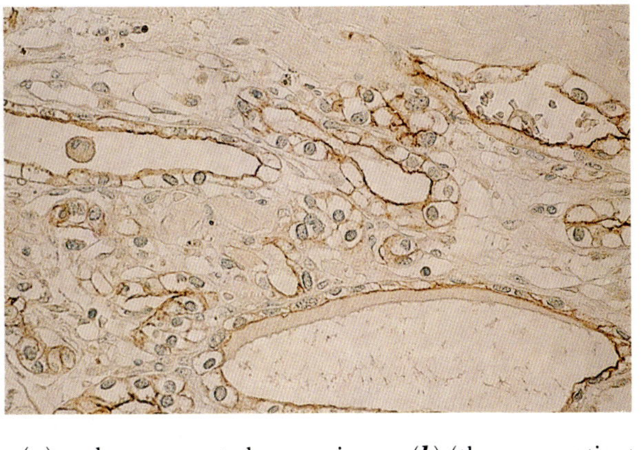 b

Fig. 18a,b. Anti c-*erb*B-2 expression in serous cystadenoma (***a***) and serous cystadenocarcinoma (***b***) (the same patient as in Fig. 9). ***a*** Only a few tumor cells are stained in serous cystadenoma, ***b*** but all tumor cells are stained in serous cystadenocarcinoma. ×100 (original magnification). (*p. 114*)

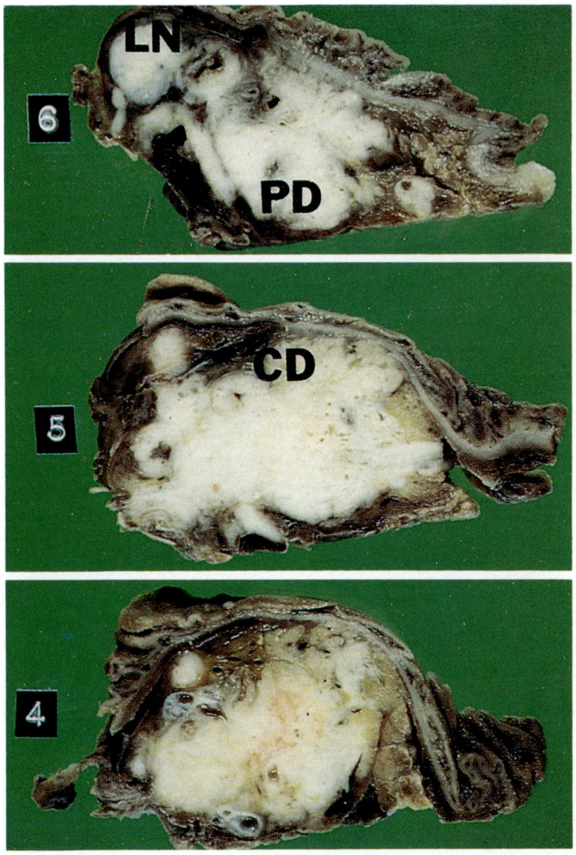

Fig. 2e. Gross appearance of pancreatic ductal adenocarcinoma (PDA), which had invaded the wall of the portal vein. The cut surface of the 3.5 × 3.0 × 5.5 cm tumor shows stenotic common bile duct (*CD*), pancreatic duct (*PD*), and lymph node metastasis (*LN*) (*p. 125*)

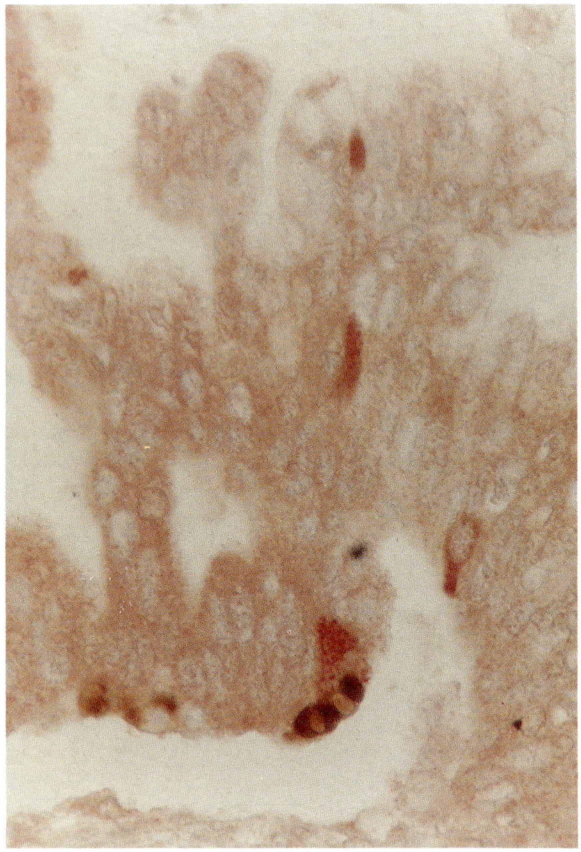

Fig. 13 (Figs. 2e, 13, 19, 22–24 of Chapter: Ductal Adenocarcinoma). Insulin (*brown*) and somatostatin (*red*) cells in a well-differentiated PDA. Note the presence of somatostatin cells in different heights of the malignant epithelium. ABC method, ×210 (*p. 135*)

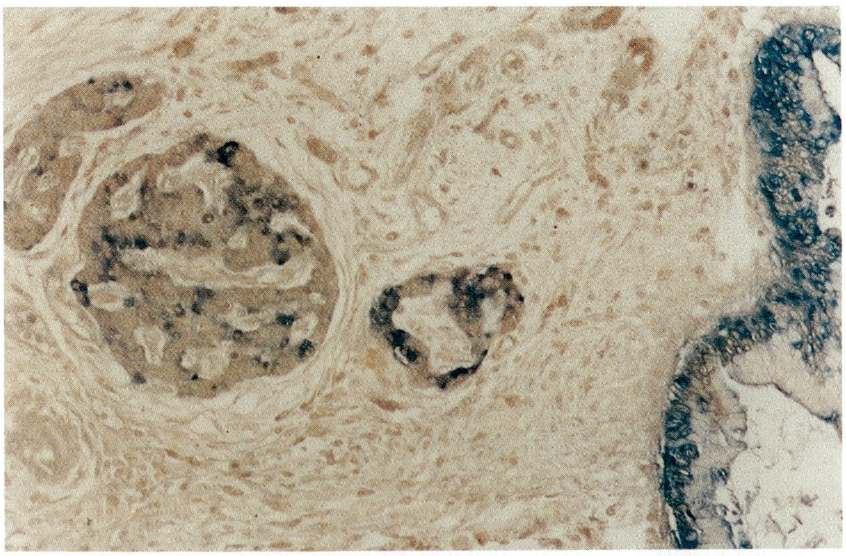

Fig. 19. Expression of CA19-9 antigen (*blue*) in the islets of a 64-year-old women with a well-to-moderately differentiated PDA. CO19-9, ABC, ×210 (*p. 139*)

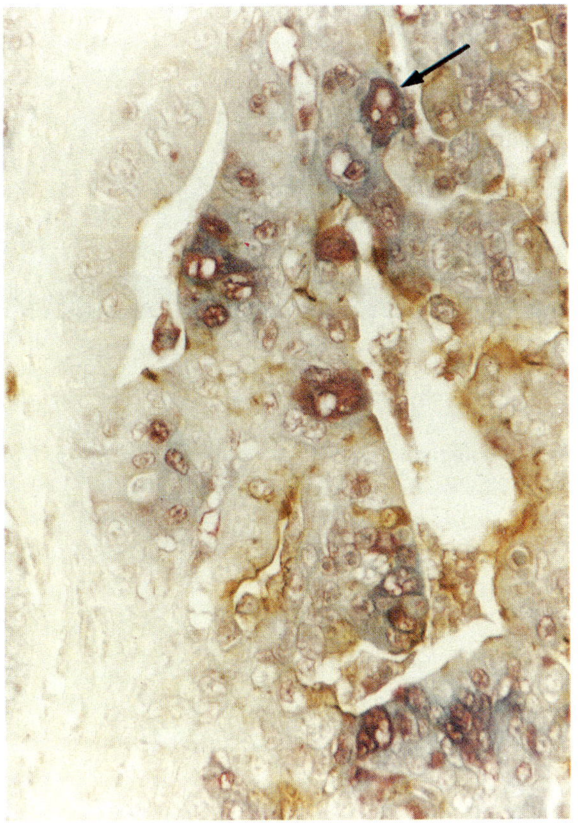

22

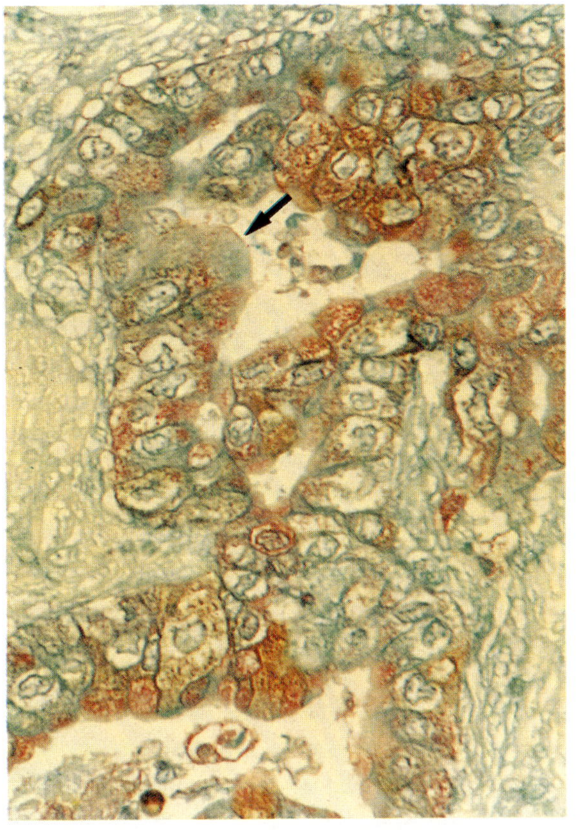

23

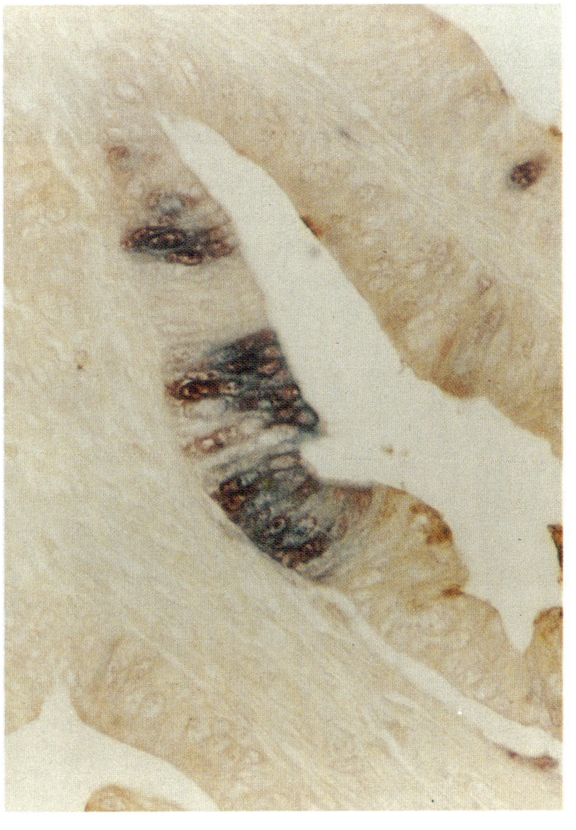

24

Fig. 22. Expression of CA19-9 (*blue*), DU-PAN-2 (*brown*) and TAG-72 antigens (*red*) in a poorly differentiated area of a PDA. Some cells (for example that shown by an *arrow*) express two antigens. ABC method, ×210 (*Figs. 22–24, p. 143*)

Fig. 23. A well-differentiated PDA, the cells of which express either CA19-9 (*green*), DU-PAN-2 (brown) and/or TAG-72 (*red*). Because of different cellular localization of each antigen, expression of two or three antigens can be found in some tumor cells. *Arrow* points to a cell expressing all of the three antigens. ABC method, ×210

Fig. 24. Heterogeneity of antigen expression in a well-differentiated PDA. Only a few cells express CA19-9 (*blue*), DU-PAN-2 (*brown*) or/and TAG-72 (*red*). ABC method, ×210

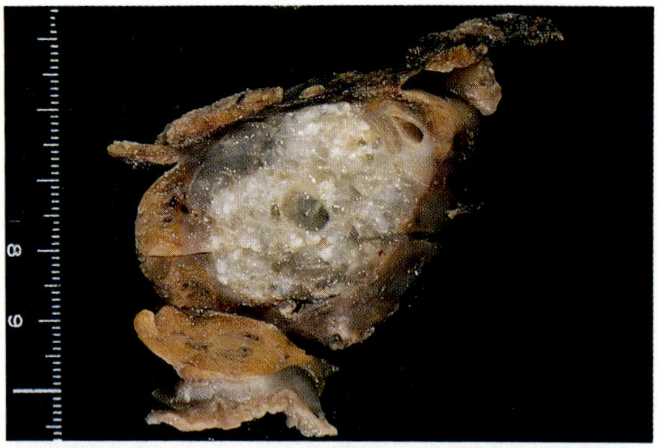

Fig. 1 (Chapter: Mucinous (Noncystic) Adenocarcinoma, Including Signet-Ring Carcinoma). Gross appearance of a mucinous (non-cystic) carcinoma. Pools of mucous are visible. The tumor occurred in the tail of the pancreas (*p. 156*)

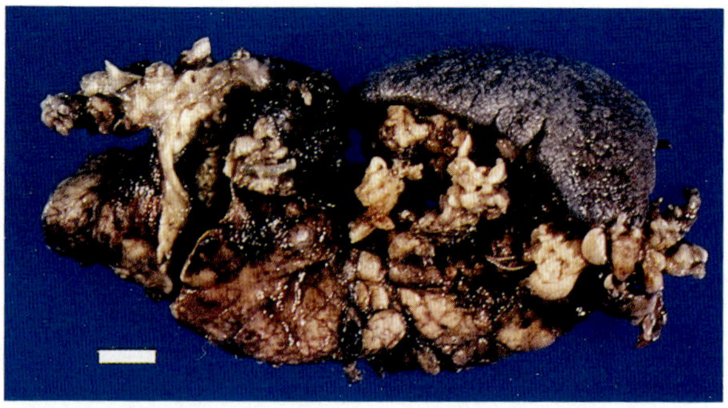

Fig. 3. The protruding tumor located in the pancreatic body was well-circumscribed with a fibrous capsule, measuring 3.2 × 2.8 × 3 cm, situated in the pancreas body and about 2.5 cm from the proximal stump (*p. 170*)

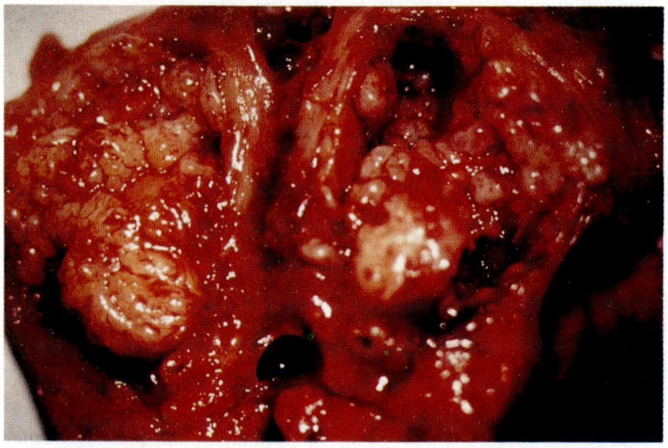

Fig. 2 (Figs. 2, 3, 9 of Chapter: Squamous Cell Carcinoma). The cut surface of a squamous cell carcinoma of the pancreas. The tumor was adherent to the surrounding tissues by dense connective tissue (*p. 170*)

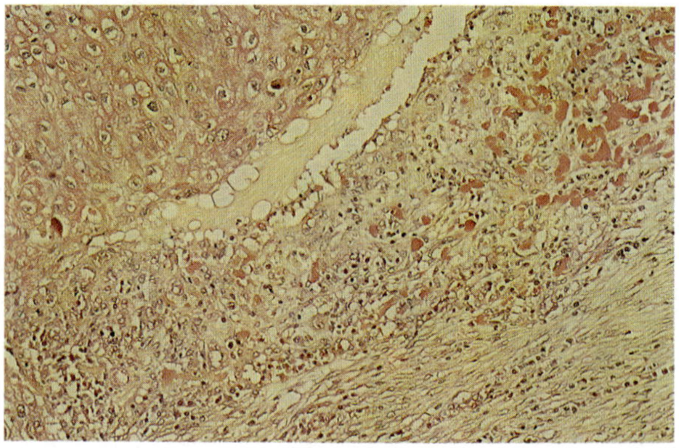

Fig. 9. Immunohistochemistry for cytokeratin revealed a positive reaction in squamous cell carcinoma cells, in the remaining keratinocytes, and in the breakdown products of keratohyalin in the surrounding granulation tissue. This may indicate that the granulation tissue developed secondary to the degeneration of squamous cell carcinoma. Immunohistochemistry with anticytokeratin antibody, ×120 (*p. 173*)

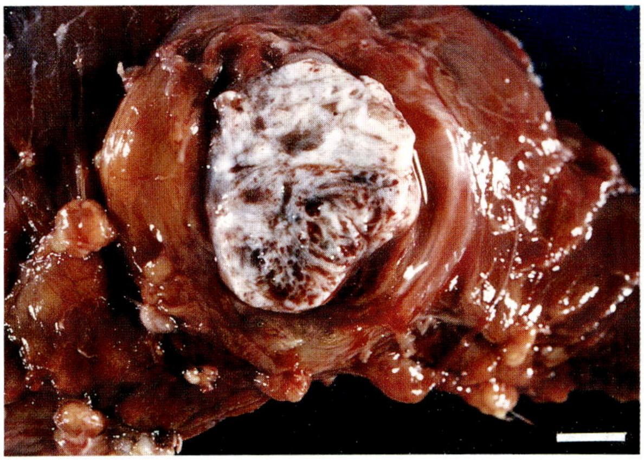

Fig. 3 (Figs. 3, 11 of Chapter: Acinar Cell Carcinoma). Gross of an acinar cell carcinoma of the pancreas. Specimen from a Whipple resection of the head of the pancreas in a 77-year-old female admitted to hospital with complaints of abdominal pain and vomiting. The patient was readmitted with multiple liver metastases 12 months after operation. The cut surface shows a well defined, white, firm neoplasm with hemorrhage, measuring 4.5 cm in its largest dimension. (*p. 190*)

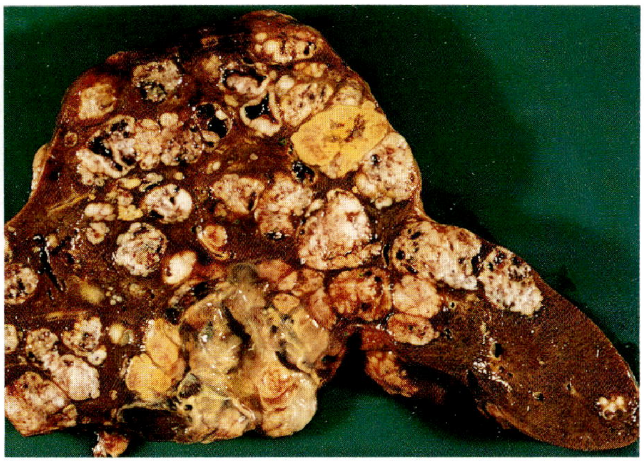

Fig. 11. Multiple liver metastases of pancreatic acinar cell carcinoma. The liver weighed 2380 g at autopsy, and contained numerous white-to-yellow metastatic nodules. The patient died of hepatic failure 18 months after Whipple operation. Serum elastase-1 level ranged from 3089 to 19 572 ng/dL, but serum amylase and lipase levels were in the normal range. Moderate elastase-1 activity was demonstrated in tissue homogenates of liver metastases (*p. 195*)

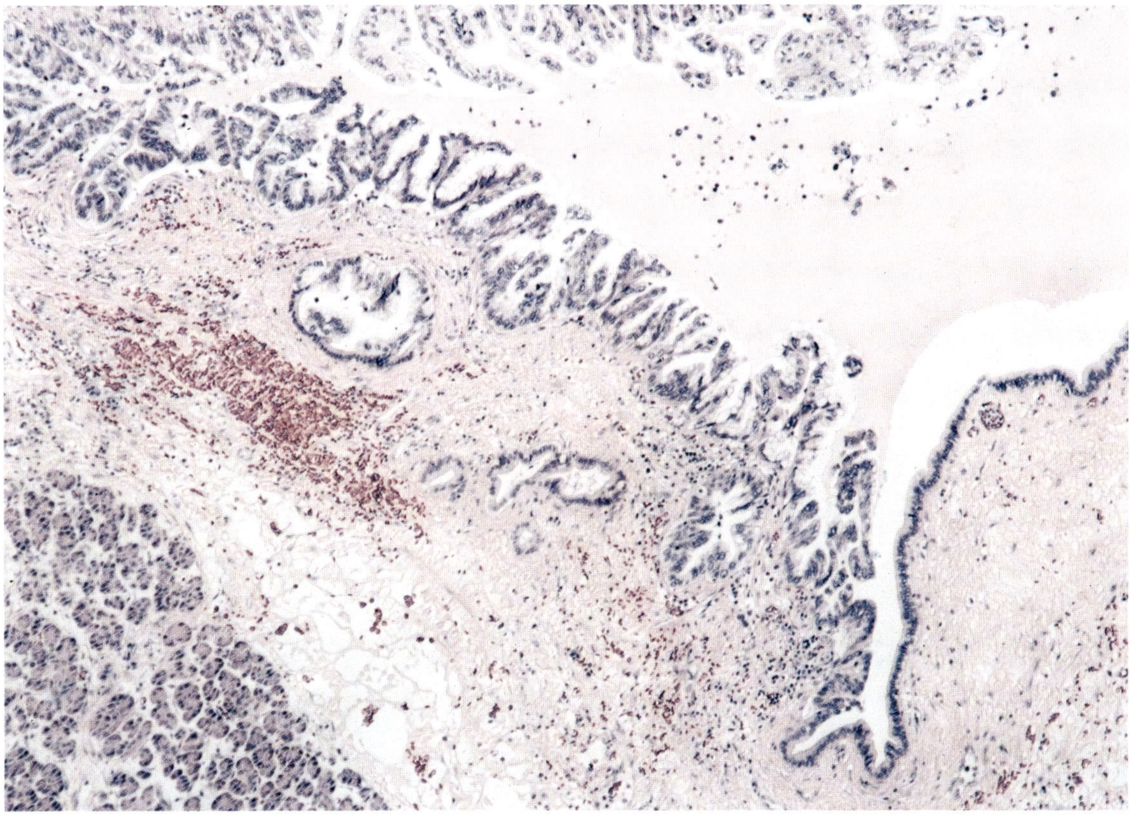

Fig. 11 (Chapter: Pathology of Metastatic Patterns of Pancreatic Cancer). Intraductal contiguous tumor spread into Wirsung's duct from a cancer of the head of the pancreas (*p. 234*)

Gross Anatomy of the Pancreas

Macroscopy and Topography

The pancreas is a soft, pale-yellow, coarsely lobulated organ 12–20 cm in length, 3–5 cm in width, and 1–3 cm in thickness, weighing 60–125 g in adults [1–3].

The topography of the pancreas is shown in Fig. 1. It lies relatively fixed in the retroperitoneum behind the peritoneal floor of the lesser sac, extending from the medial margin of the duodenum to the hilum of the spleen, in an oblique position, higher on the left at about the L1–L2 level.

Anatomically, the pancreas is divided into four portions: the head (the portion to the right of the superior mesenteric vein), the neck (the portion lying over the superior mesenteric vessels), the body, and tail (the portion to the left of these vessels). The border of the latter two portions is not clearly defined. According to the "General Rules for Describing Cancer of the Pancreas" proposed by the Japan Pancreas Society in 1986, the head of the gland is the portion to the right of the left border of the superior mesenteric and portal vein, and the remaining gland is bisected into the body (the right half) and the tail (the left half) [4].

The width and thickness of the pancreas are greatest at the head and tapers through the body to the tail. The anterior surface of the pancreas is covered by the peritoneum, but the posterior surface has no peritoneal covering except in the tail.

The head is intimately surrounded by the duodenal loop. The distal common bile duct usually passes through the parenchyma of the head, although in about 15% of subjects in the general population it remains externally in a groove on the posterior aspect before entering the second portion of the duodenum [2].

Anteriorly, the head is covered by the first portion of the duodenum, the pylorus, and the transverse colon. The posterior surface of the head is opposite the right renal vessels, the vena cava, and the aorta.

The uncinate process is an inferior projection of the head of the pancreas that extends behind the superior mesenteric vessels and the portal vein, and lies anterior to the vena cava and the aorta.

The neck is a narrow portion of the pancreas overlying the superior mesenteric, and portal veins. Its posterior surface is grooved by the portal vein which is formed by the confluence of the superior mesenteric and splenic veins. Anteriorly, the neck is covered by the pylorus and the duodenal bulb.

The body and tail extend to the left, anterior to the superior mesenteric artery, the aorta, the inferior mesenteric and splenic veins, the left adrenal gland, and the left kidney. Superiorly, the body and tail are related to the celiac axis and the splenic artery. Anteriorly, these portions are covered by the stomach, the gastrocolic ligament, and the transverse colon. Inferiorly, the body lies adjacent to the fourth portion of the duodenum and the ligament of Treitz. The tail may or may not reach the hilum of the spleen.

The transverse mesocolon attaches to the anterior surface of the head and the inferior aspect of the body and tail of the pancreas.

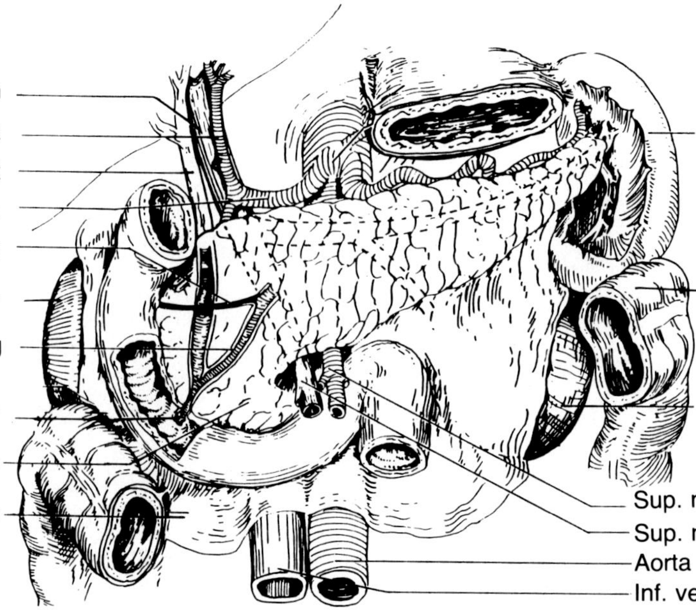

Fig. 1. Topography of the pancreas

Pancreatic Duct

Anatomy

The anatomy of the pancreas is shown in a pancreatic ductogram (Fig. 2). The pancreas develops from both ventral and dorsal pancreatic anlages which arise from the endodermal epithelium of the duodenum. Both anlages and their ducts usually fuse during the 7th embryonic week [5]. The ventral anlage becomes the dorsocaudal portion and uncinate process of the head of the pancreas, while the dorsal anlage becomes the ventrocephalic portion of the head and the body and tail of the gland.

The duct of the ventral anlage and of the dorsal anlage distal to the junction of both ducts serves as the main pancreatic duct (duct of Wirsung). The duct of the dorsal anlage proximal to the junction becomes the accessory pancreatic duct (duct of Santorini) [5].

The main pancreatic duct begins at the terminus of the tail of the gland, and runs closer to the posterior surface and midway between the superior and inferior margins through the body and neck into the head of the gland.

In the head, the main duct inclines caudally and dorsally, and passes to the left caudal side of the intrapancreatic portion of the common bile duct, with which it usually unites while running obliquely through the duodenal wall, and opens into the major duodenal papilla (the papilla of Vater), a prominence located on the posteromedial wall of the second portion of the duodenum (Fig. 3).

The main duct generally drains the dorsocaudal portion of the head, together with the body and tail of the pancreas. The accessory pancreatic duct usually begins near the neck of the gland at its junction with the main duct, and runs above the main duct, anterior to the common bile duct and opens into the minor duodenal papilla, about 2 cm superior and anterior to the major duodenal papilla [2]. The accessory duct drains the ventrocephalic portion of the head of the pancreas.

The main pancreatic duct has about 20–30 side branches which drain the superior and inferior portions of the gland.

Variations

Pancreatic Ducts

During the embryologic development of the main and accessory pancreatic ducts, several variations may result [1, 6].

The usual pattern of the pancreatic duct is that shown in Fig. 4a, in which the accessory duct is connected with the main duct, and opens into the duodenum. The accessory duct is smaller in caliber

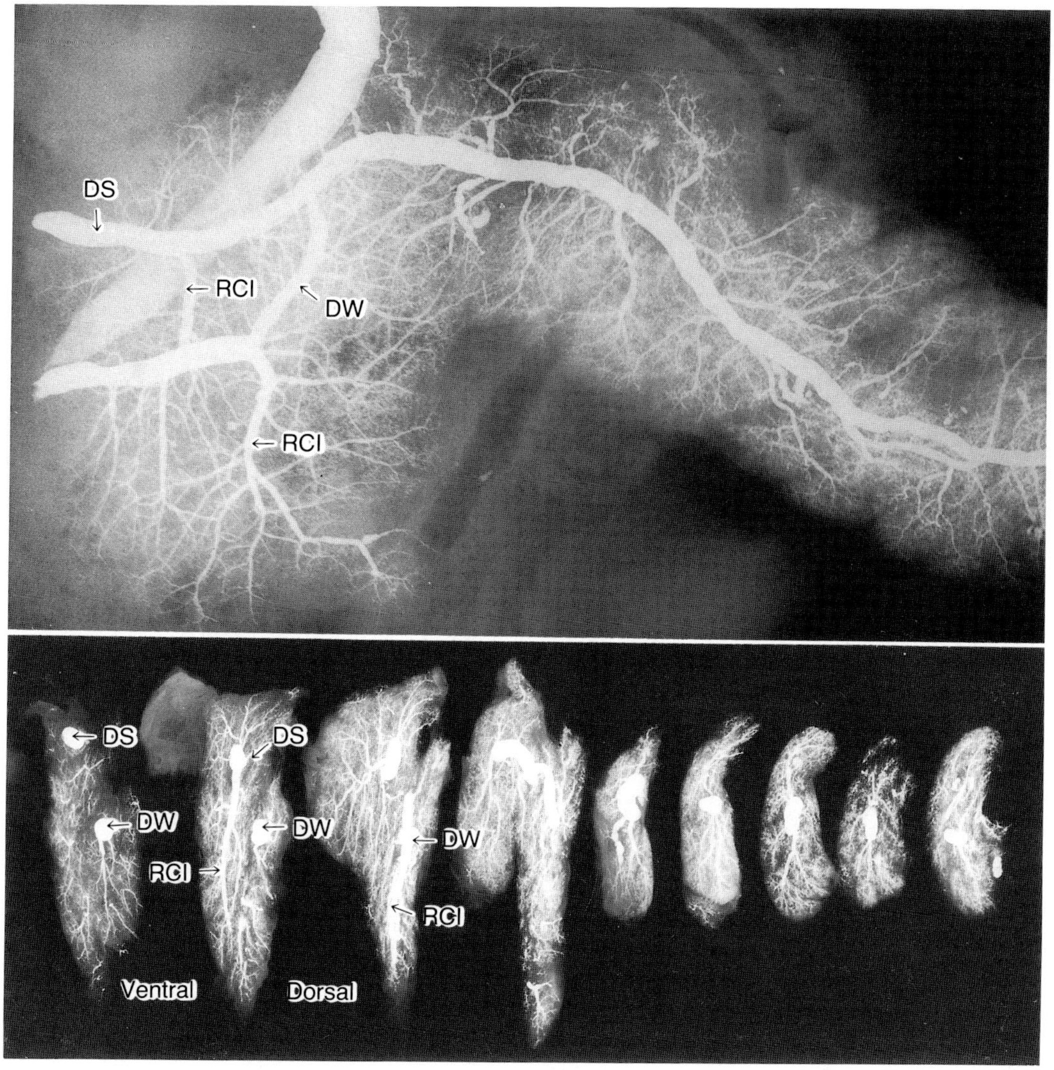

Fig. 2. Pancreatic ductogram of autopsy material. *DS*, duct of Santorini; *DW*, duct of Wirsung; *RCI*, ramus capitis inferior

than the main duct. Figure 4b,c show hypo- and aplastic variations of the accessory duct and Fig. 4d shows nonunion of both ducts. In these patterns, the main pancreatic duct carries most or all of the pancreatic secretion. Less common patterns in which the accessory pancreatic duct carries most or all of the secretion are shown in Fig. 4e,f. The variation shown in Fig. 4f is termed pancreas divisum.

The communication of the accessory and main ducts is present in 90% of patients and the patency of the accessory duct orifice is reported in 33%–60% of cases [6]. The frequency of the variations of the ducts is 60% in the usual configuration (Fig. 4a), 30% in the suppression of the accessory duct (Fig. 4b–d), and 10% in the suppression of the main duct (Fig. 4e,f) [7].

Termination of the Common Bile Duct and the Main Pancreatic Duct

The main pancreatic and common bile ducts unite in the duodenal wall in 85% of cases to form a common channel which has been termed the ampulla of Vater [6]. The common channel, 1–14 mm in length, opens on the major duodenal papilla with a single opening (Fig. 5a). Rare types in the termination of both ducts are shown in Fig. 5b,c. Both ducts open on the major duodenal papilla via sepa-

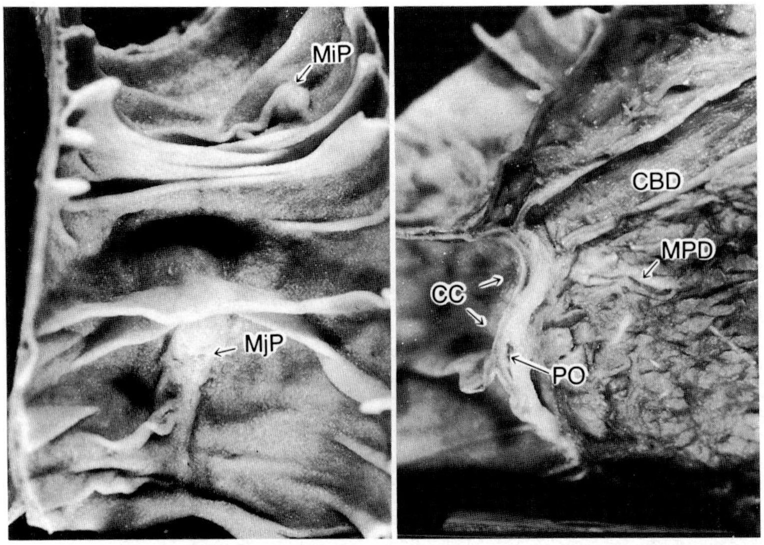

Fig. 3. The major and minor duodenal papilla viewed from the inside of the duodenum. Autopsy material. *CBD*, Common bile duct; *CC*, common channel; *MiP*, minor papilla; *MjP*, major papilla; *MPD*, main pancreatic duct; *PO*, papillary orifice

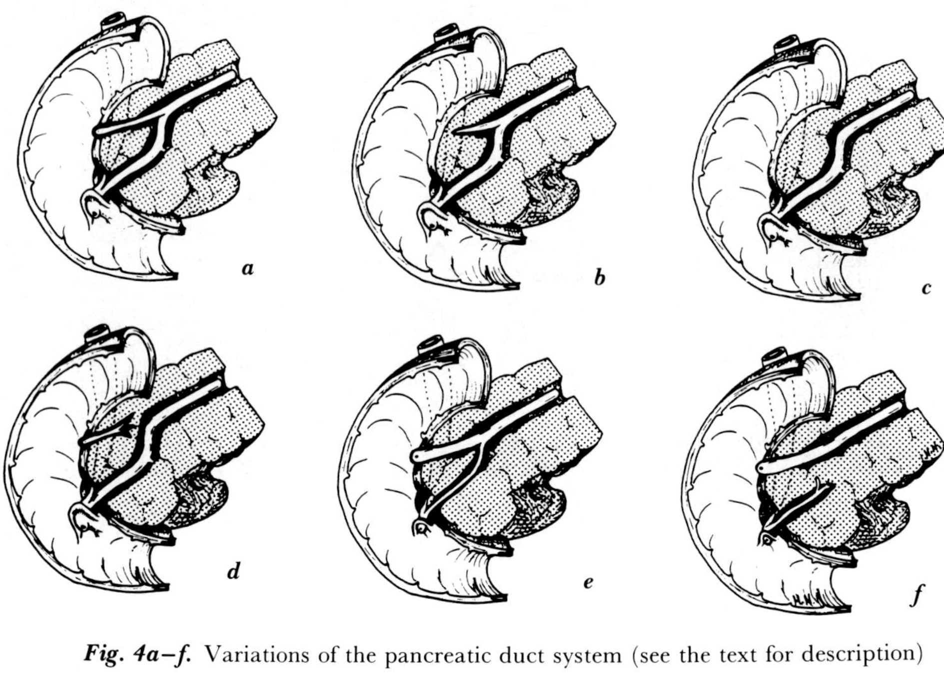

Fig. 4a–f. Variations of the pancreatic duct system (see the text for description)

rate orifices (Fig. 5b) or open into the duodenum at separate points (Fig. 5c).

Radiologically Normal Appearance

Endoscopic Retrograde Cholangiopancreatography

Endoscopic retrograde cholangiopancreatography (ERCP) is, at present, the only imaging technique which can demonstrate all the ducts of the pancreas.

The main pancreatic duct arches in an anterior direction and follows a variety of courses. The patterns of the course are described as ascending (49.6%), horizontal (35.8%), sigmoid (10.3%), and descending (4.3%) [3].

The main pancreatic duct is largest in the head of the gland with fusiform dilatation just before the duodenal entrance and tapers gradually to the tail.

Fig. 5a–c. Variations in termination of the common bile and main pancreatic ducts. *CBD*, Common bile duct; *MPD*, main pancreatic duct

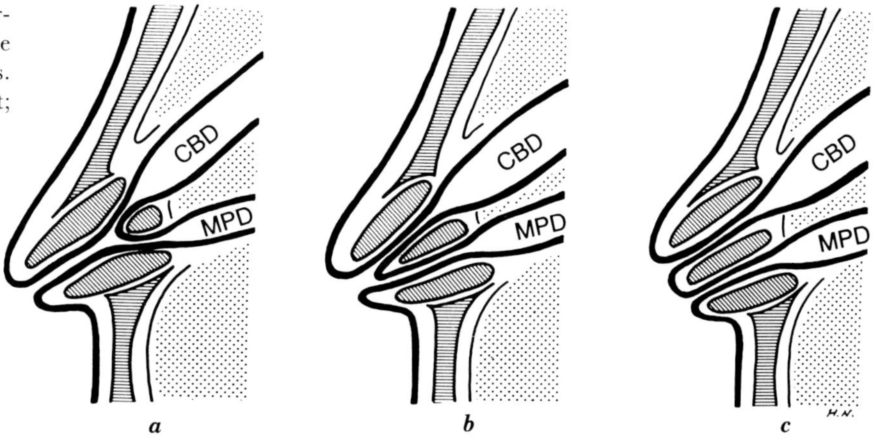

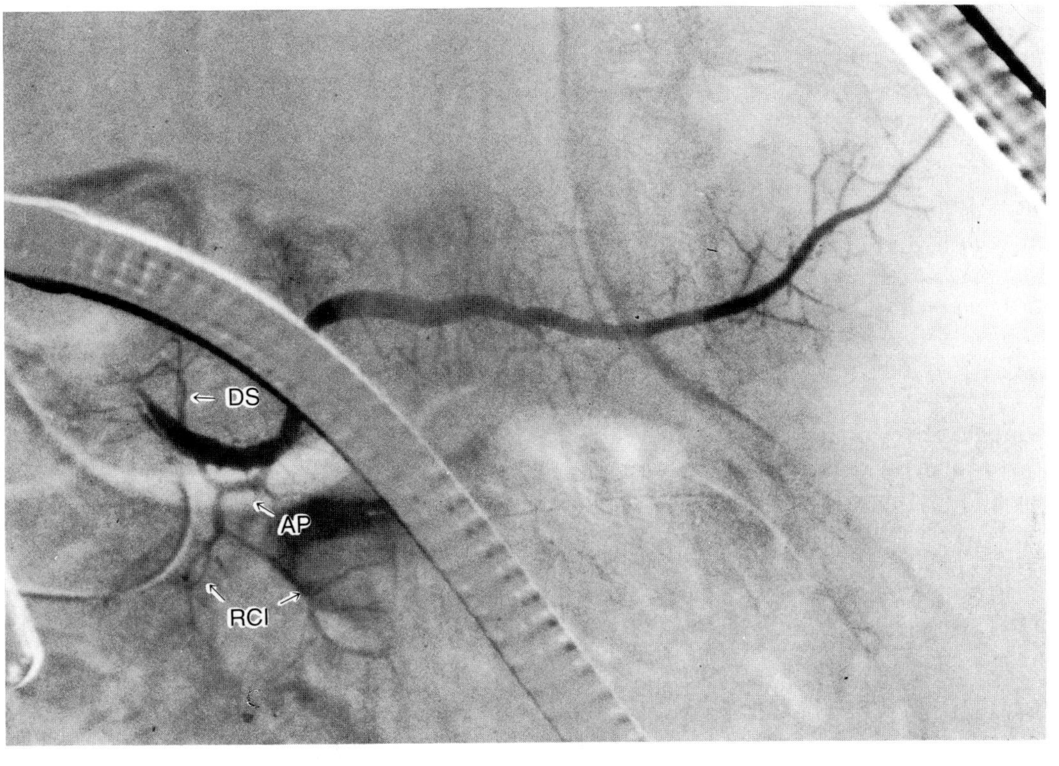

Fig. 6. Endoscopic retrograde cholangiopancreatogram (subtraction). *AP*, Ansa pancreatica; *DS*, duct of Santorini; *RCI*, ramus capitis inferior

The terminal portion of the main duct in the duodenal wall is narrowed like that of the common bile duct.

Published values of the mean diameter of the each portion of the main duct are shown in Table 1.

A short smooth segmental narrowing of the main duct may be seen normally in the neck of the gland where embryologic fusion of the ducts of Wirsung and Santorini occurs [3]. The terminus of the main pancreatic duct in the tail may be seen as a single tapering duct or as a confluence of two large ducts, the rami cauda superior and inferior [8].

The accessory pancreatic duct is usually smaller and in a more ventral and cephalad position than

Table 1. Main pancreatic duct caliber (mm) on ERCP.

Author	No. of cases	Head	Body	Tail
Classen et al. (1973) [18]	48	4.8	3.5	2.4
Kasugai et al. (1972) [19]	68	3.5	2.7	1.7
Ogoshi et al. (1973) [20]	25	3.4	2.9	2.0
Sivak and Sullivan (1976) [21]	35	3.2	2.4	1.2
Varley et al. (1976) [22]	102	3.1	2.0	0.9
Average	278	3.6	2.7	1.6

ERCP, Endoscopic retrograde cholangiopancreatography

the main duct. Rarely, the accessory duct may form an inferior loop which was termed "ansa pancreatica" by Dawson [9].

In the body and tail of the pancreas, approximately 15–20 short tributaries enter the main duct at almost right angles in a characteristic "herring-bone" pattern. In the head of the gland, the "herring-bone" pattern becomes less obvious and a larger side branch draining the uncinate process is usually seen. Occasionally, there is seen a similar large branch duct arising from the accessory pancreatic duct (Fig. 2). These large branch ducts were termed "ramus capitis inferior" by Anacker [8].

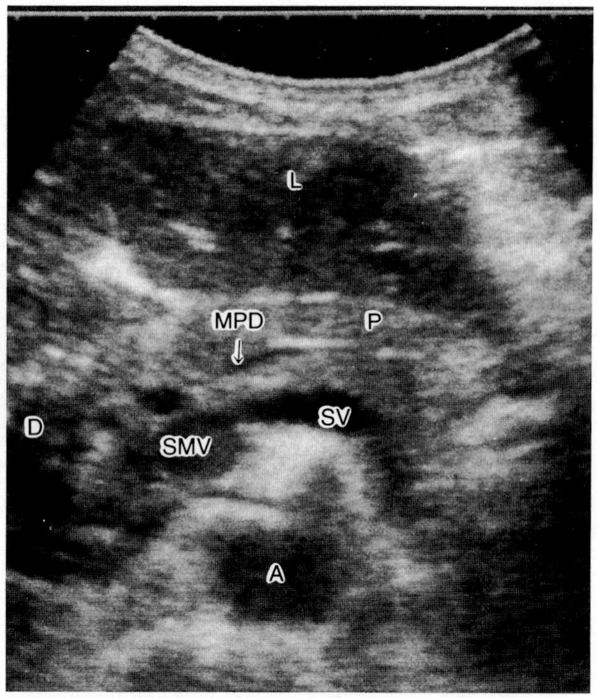

Fig. 7. Ultrasonogram of the pancreas. *A*, Aorta; *D*, duodenum; *L*, liver; *P*, pancreas; *MPD*, main pancreatic duct; *SMV*, superior mesenteric vein; *SV*, splenic vein

Ultrasonography

The main pancreatic duct can be seen normally on ultrasonography (Fig. 7) in about 80% of patients in the body and less frequently in the head and tail of the gland [3]. The main duct may be seen as a tubular structure when filled with fluid, and only as a linear structure when little fluid is present in the lumen.

The normal width of the main pancreatic duct on sonogram is 1–3 mm [5]. The normal accessory pancreatic duct and any side branches are not usually seen sonographically.

Computed Tomography

The normal main pancreatic duct is rarely visualized by routine computed tomography (CT) (Fig. 8) without contrast medium, and may be identified in about 50% of patients by optimum techniques using contrast medium [3, 5].

The normal main duct is identified as a thin linear area of low attenuation in only a short segment of the pancreas which runs in a horizontal fashion along the axis of the transverse X-ray beam of the CT scan. The normal accessory duct and side branches are not visualized by CT.

Arterial Anatomy

The pancreas receives its blood supply from branches of the celiac axis and the superior mesenteric artery (Fig. 9) [1, 2, 5].

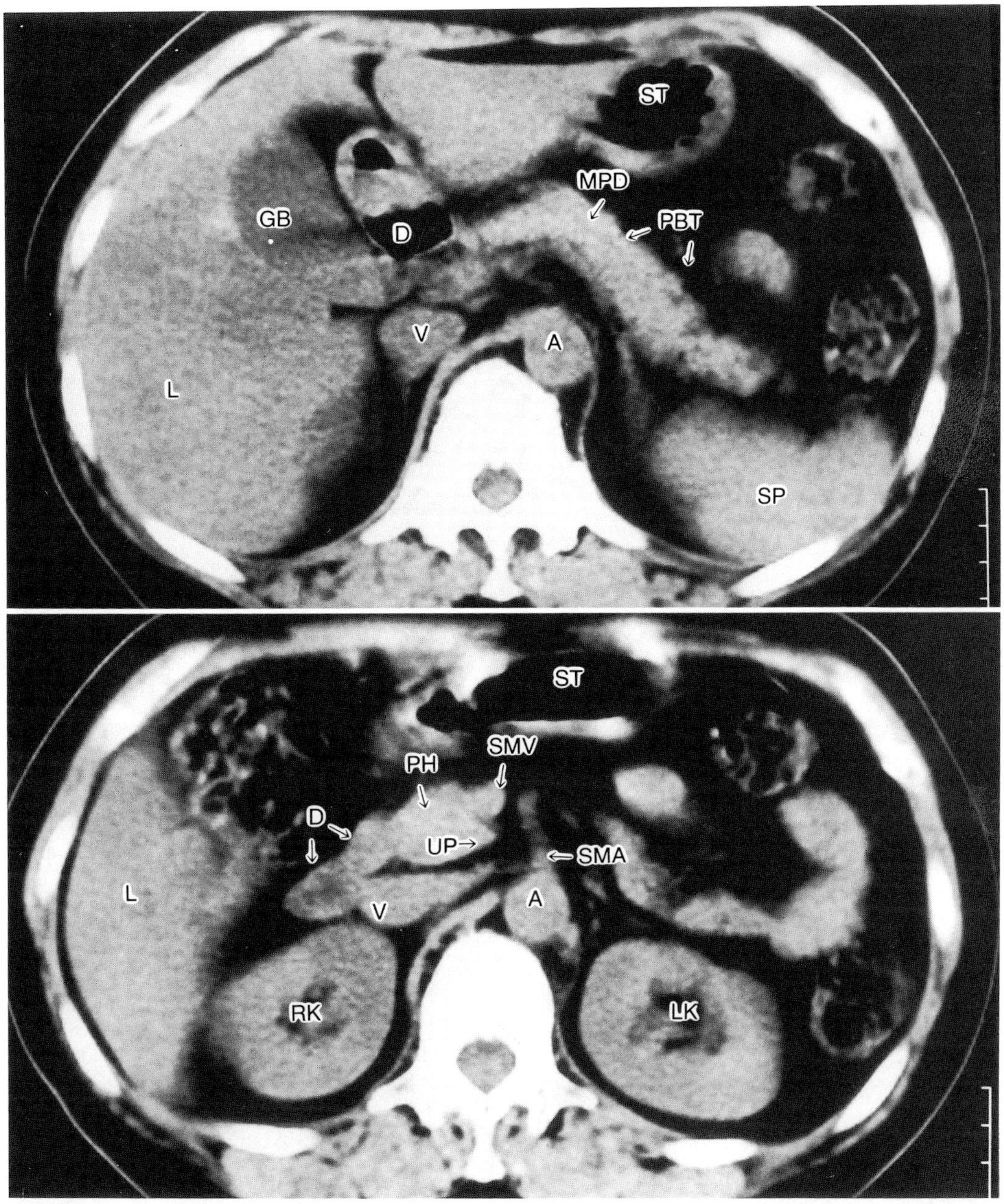

Fig. 8. Computed tomogram (*CT*) of the pancreas. *A*, Aorta; *D*, duodenum; *LK*, left kidney; *PBT*, pancreas body and tail; *PH*, pancreas head; *RK*, right kidney; *SMA*, superior mesenteric artery; *SMV*, superior mesenteric vein; *SP*, spleen; *ST*, stomach; *UP*, uncinate process; *V*, inferior vena cava

The Head

The gastroduodenal artery, which is typically the first major branch of the common hepatic artery arising from the celiac axis (Fig. 10), gives off a pair (posterior and anterior, in this order) of the superior pancreaticoduodenal arteries. The superior pancreaticoduodenal arteries descend on the posterior and anterior surfaces of the head of the pancreas to anastomose with a pair (posterior and anterior) of the inferior pancreaticoduodenal arteries, forming the posterior and anterior pan-

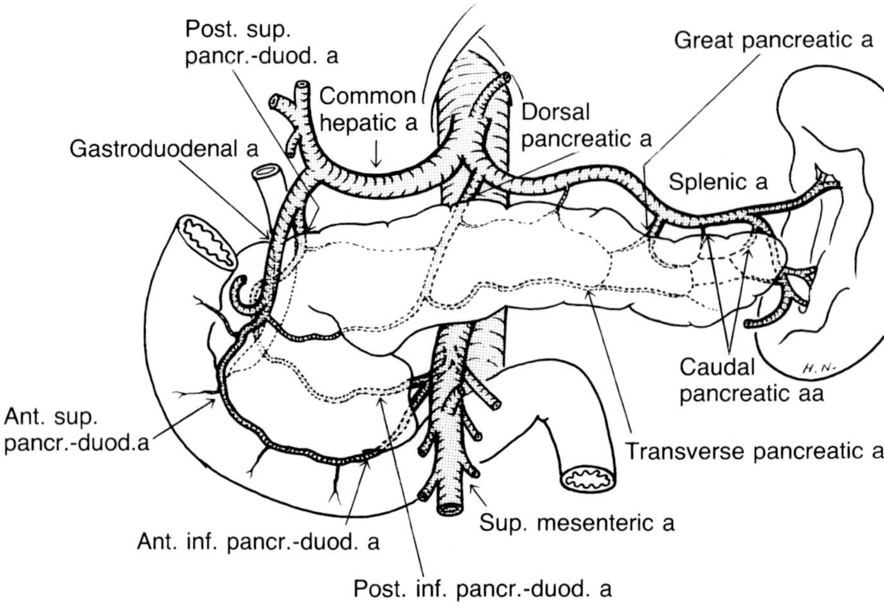

Fig. 9. Pancreatic arterial anatomy. *a*, Artery; *ant.*, anterior; *sup.*, superior; *post.*, posterior; *inf.*, inferior

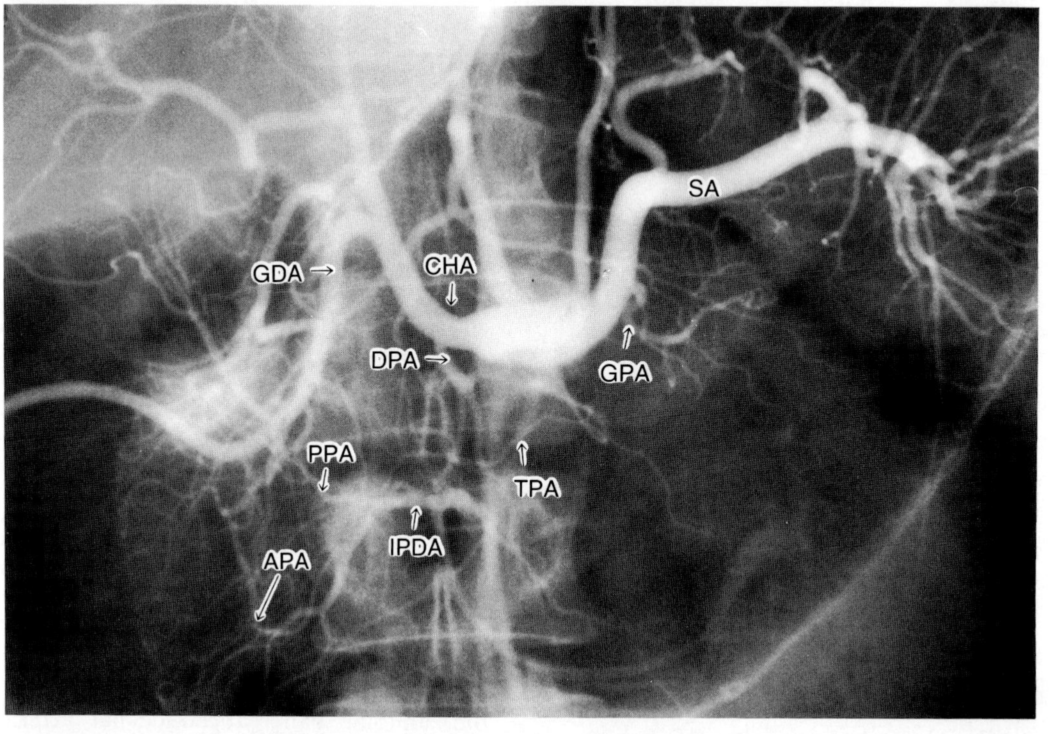

Fig. 10. Selective celiac arteriogram. *APA*, Anterior pancreatic arcade; *CHA*, common hepatic artery; *DPA*, dorsal pancreatic artery; *GDA*, gastroduodenal artery; *GPA*, great pancreatic artery; *IPDA*, inferior pancreaticoduodenal artery; *PPA*, posterior pancreatic arcade; *SA*, splenic artery; *TPA*, transverse pancreatic artery

creatic arcades. The anterior and posterior superior pancreaticoduodenal arteries are constant in origin, while the anterior and posterior inferior pancreaticoduodenal arteries arise separately or have a common trunk from the superior mesenteric artery. The posterior arcade passes behind the common bile duct, and is farther from the duodenum and in a more cephalad position than the anterior arcade. The head of the pancreas and duodenum are supplied with blood mainly from these arcades.

The Body and Tail

The dorsal pancreatic artery lies behind the neck of the gland, arising from the splenic (40%), the celiac, the common hepatic, or the superior mesenteric artery [5]. It runs downward to the lower border of the pancreas and divides into the left and right branches. To the left, it gives off the transverse (inferior) pancreatic artery and to the right, sends branches to the head and the uncinate process to anastomize with the superior pancreaticoduodenal or the gastroduodenal artery.

The dorsal pancreatic artery provides the main blood supply to the neck and body of the pancreas.

The transverse (inferior) pancreatic artery is the left branch of the dorsal pancreatic artery in 90% of cases, and may arise from the gastroduodenal, the right gastroepiploic, or the superior pancreaticoduodenal artery [5]. It runs along the inferior margin of the pancreas to anatomize with the great pancreatic and the caudal pancreatic arteries.

The great pancreatic (pancreatic magna) artery is the greatest artery among the two to ten branches of the splenic artery which courses along the superior margin of the body and tail of the gland. It usually arises around the border between the body and tail of the gland and divides into left and right branches to anastomize with the transverse pancreatic, the dorsal pancreatic, and the caudal pancreatic arteries.

The caudal pancreatic arteries are small branches of the splenic or the left gastroepiploic artery. The transverse pancreatic, the great pancreatic and the caudal pancreatic arteries supply blood to the body and tail of the pancreas.

Venous Anatomy

The venous blood of the pancreas (Figs. 11, 12) drains into the portal system around the gland: The splenic, the superior mesenteric, the inferior mesenteric, and the portal veins [2, 5, 6].

The splenic vein running inferior to the splenic artery along the posterior aspect of the pancreas joins the superior mesenteric vein which passes anterior to the inferomedial aspect of the uncinate process to form the portal vein behind the neck of the pancreas. The inferior mesenteric vein drains into the splenic (60%) or the superior mesenteric vein [5].

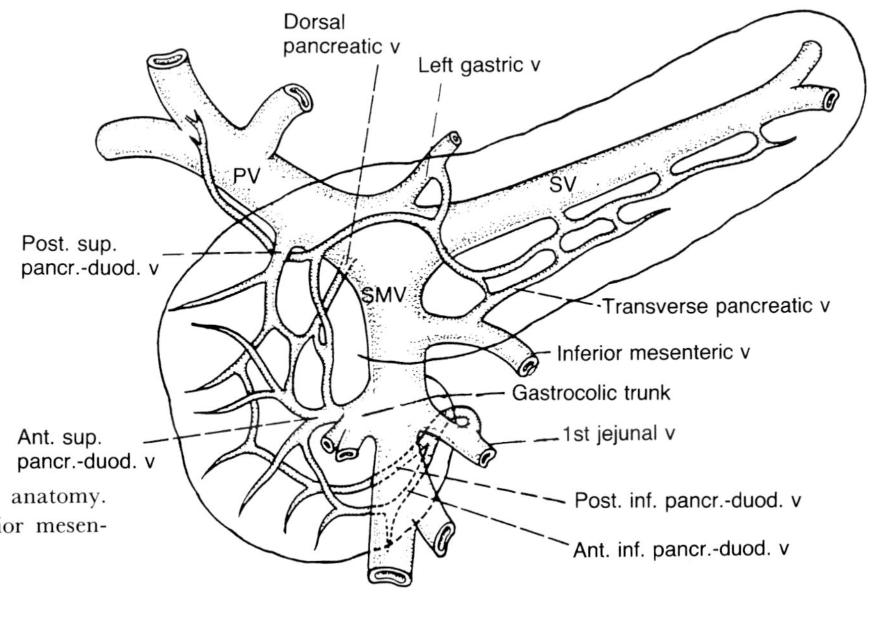

Fig. 11. Pancreatic venous anatomy. *PV*, Portal vein; *SMV*, superior mesenteric vein; *SV*, splenic vein

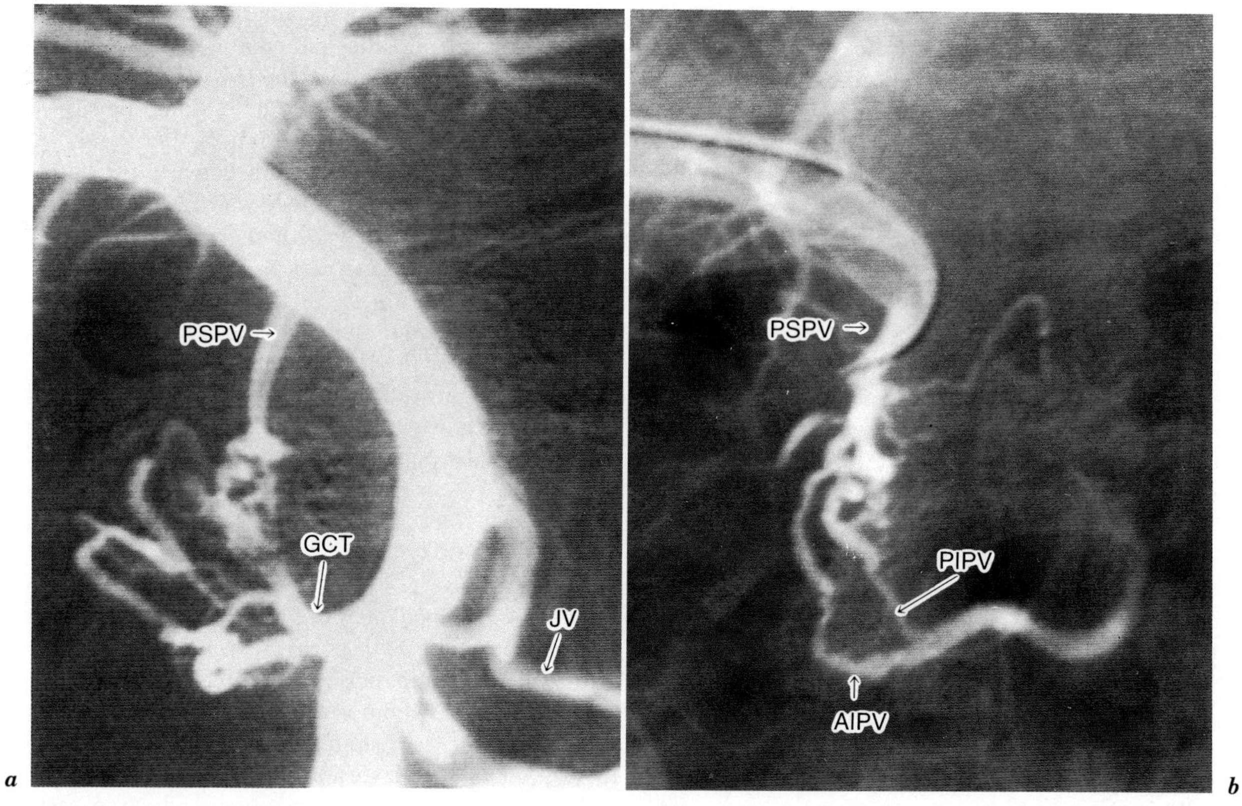

Fig. 12a,b. Percutaneous transhepatic portogram. ***a*** Transhepatic portogram. ***b*** Transhepatic portogram (selective injection of the posterior superior pancraticoduodenal vein). *AIPV*, Anterior inferior pancreaticoduodenal vein; *GCT*, gastrocolic trunk; *JV*, first jejunal vein; *PIPV*, posterior inferior pancreaticoduodenal vein; *PSPV*, posterior superior pancreaticoduodenal vein

In general, the pancreatic veins parallel the arteries and lie superficial to them.

The Head of the Pancreas is Drained by the Anterior and Posterior, Superior, and Inferior Pancreaticoduodenal Veins

The posterior superior pancreaticoduodenal vein terminates in the right posterior wall of the portal vein and the posterior inferior pancreaticoduodenal vein enters the first jejunal branch of the superior mesenteric vein.

The anterior superior pancreaticoduodenal vein terminates in the superior mesenteric vein via the gastrocolic trunk, a vessel formed by the confluence of the right gastroepiploic and the right colic veins. The anterior inferior pancreaticoduodenal vein drains into the first jejunal vein, frequently to form a common trunk with the posterior inferior pancreaticoduodenal vein.

The Body and Tail of the Pancreas are Drained by the Splenic Vein Above and the Transverse Pancreatic Vein Below

The splenic vein receives 3–13 short pancreatic venous branches. The transverse pancreatic vein terminates in the superior mesenteric vein, the inferior mesenteric vein, or occasionally, the splenic vein or the gastrocolic trunk.

Lymphatic Anatomy

The intralobular tissue of the pancreas is devoid of lymphatics, and lymph capillaries of the gland arise in the interlobular tissue. Lymph capillaries are collected by anastomosing networks to form large lymph ducts which reach the surface of the pancreas, usually along blood vessels.

The lymphatics from the pancreas empty into the regional lymph nodes. Various classifications

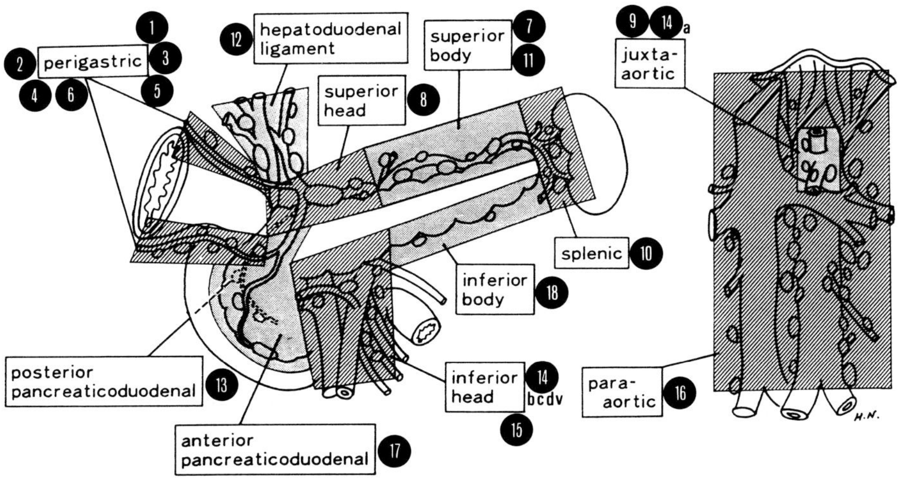

Fig. 13. The authors' classification of the regional lymph nodes of the pancreas. The numbers indicate the numerical grouping of the regional lymph nodes of the pancreas classified in the "General rules for describing cancer of the pancreas," proposed by the Japan Pancreas Society [4]

of the regional nodes of the pancreas have been proposed by several authors. We have divided the regional lymph nodes into 11 groups according to their sites, as shown in Fig. 13, and have studied lymphatic flow from the pancreas with autopsy material (Fig. 14) [10–12].

Lymph Drainage from the Head of the Pancreas

The main lymphatic flow from the head of the pancreas reaches the anterior and posterior pancreaticoduodenal nodes. Some lymphatics from the head of the pancreas skip the pancreaticoduodenal nodes to flow directly into the inferior head, juxta-aortic or para-aortic nodes.

The efferent lymphatics from the anterior pancreaticoduodenal nodes reach the inferior head lymph nodes or directly flow into the intestinal lymph trunks which terminate in the juxta-aortic and para-aortic lymph nodes. Most of the efferent lymphatics from the posterior pancreaticoduodenal nodes course down towards the juxta-aortic and para-aortic nodes.

The para-aortic lymph nodes receiving the direct or indirect lymphatic flow from the pancreas are mainly located on the bilateral and anterior aspects of the aorta ranging from the celiac axis to the origin of the inferior mesenteric artery. Some of the lymphatics from the pancreas directly flow into the following collecting lymphatic trunks: Lumbar lymphatic trunks, cisterna chyli, and thoracic duct [12].

Lymph Drainage from the Body and Tail of the Pancreas

The majority of lymphatics from the body and tail of the pancreas empty into the splenic and superior body lymph nodes. Some lymphatics flow into the inferior head, inferior body, juxta-aortic, or para-aortic nodes.

Efferent lymphatics from the splenic, superior body, inferior body, and inferior head nodes proceed to the juxta-aortic and para-aortic nodes.

Nervous Anatomy

Similar to other abdominal organs, the pancreas is innervated by sympathetic and parasympathetic nerves, as shown in Fig. 15.

The sympathetic nerves of the pancreas mainly originates from the greater and lesser splanchnic nerves. The greater splanchnic nerve is usually formed by branches from T4–T10 sympathetic ganglia, and the lesser splanchnic nerve consists of the nerve fibers from T9–L2 sympathetic ganglia. These splanchnic nerves pass through the diaphragmatic crura to enter the celiac plexus and ganglia, and make synaptic connections with neurons in the ganglia.

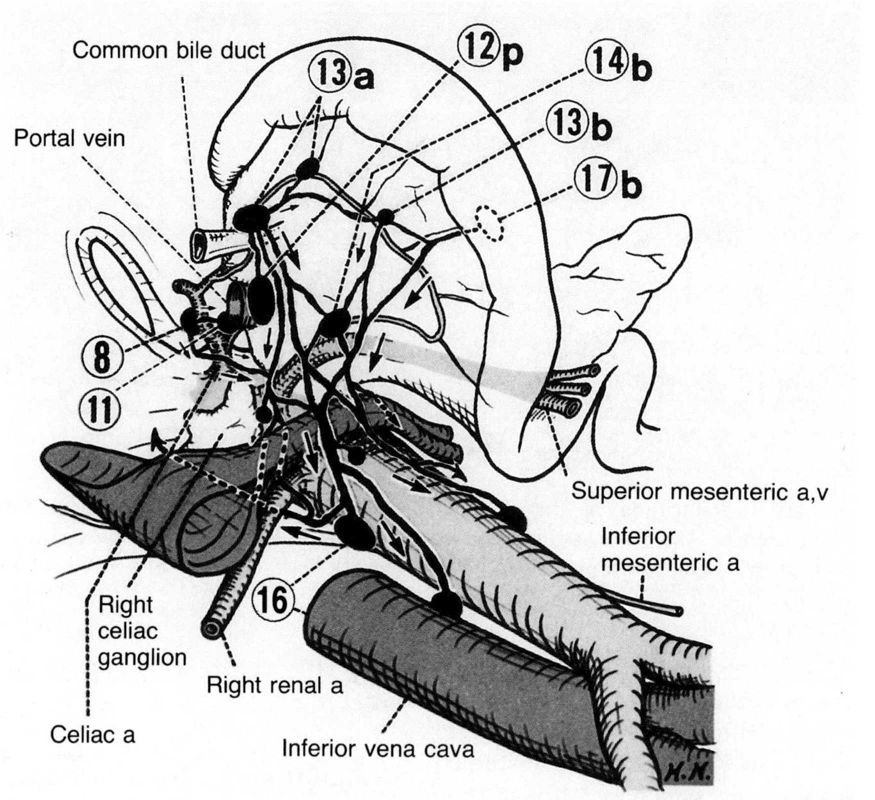
Common bile duct
13a
12p
14b
13b
17b
Portal vein
8
11
Superior mesenteric a,v
Inferior
mesenteric a
16
Right
celiac
ganglion
Right renal a
Celiac a
Inferior vena cava
H.N.

a

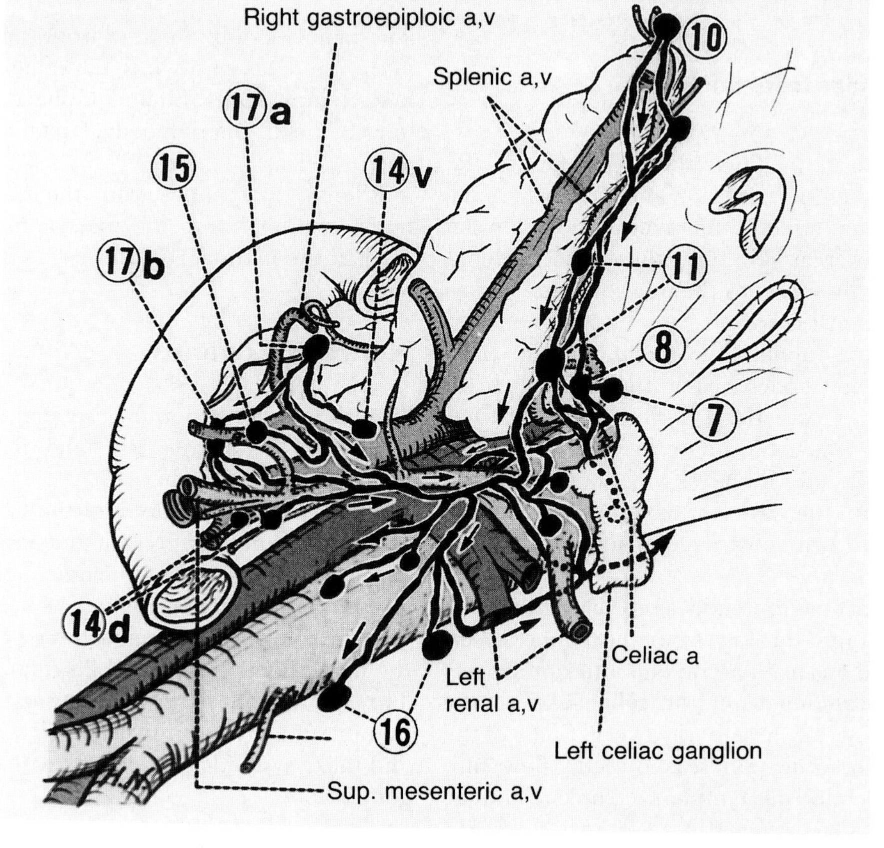
Right gastroepiploic a,v
10
Splenic a,v
17a
15
14v
17b
11
8
7
14d
Celiac a
Left
renal a,v
16
Left celiac ganglion
Sup. mesenteric a,v

b

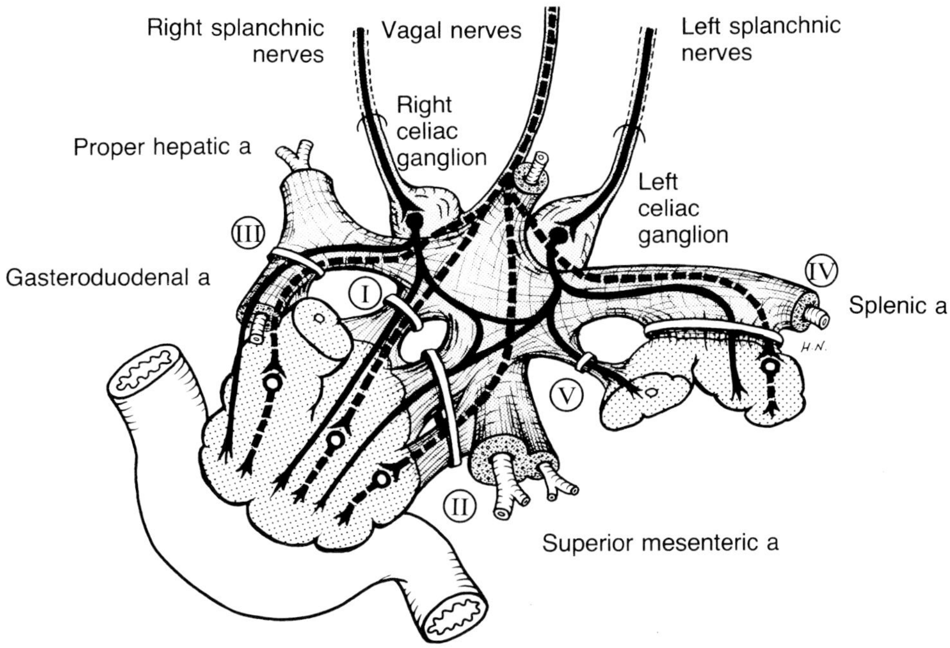

Fig. 15. The nervous anatomy of the pancreas. Only efferent fibers are shown. *I*, Plexus pancreaticus capitalis I; *II*, plexus pancreaticus capitalis II; *III*, plexus along the gastroduodenal artery; *IV*, plexus from around the splenic artery; *V*, plexus from the left celiac ganglion and the celiac plexus

The parasympathetic innervation of the pancreas originates from the vagus nerve. Although most of the vagus nerve fibers related to the pancreas pass through the celiac ganglia without synapsing, some reach the pancreas directly via the hepatic and gastric rami of the vagus nerve.

The main routes of both the sympathetic and parasympathetic nerves from the celiac plexus and ganglia to the pancreas are as follows:

1. The direct route from the celiac ganglion to the posterior surface of the head of the pancreas ("plexus pancreaticus capitalis I") [13],
2. The route from the bilateral celiac ganglion to the left margin of the uncinate process via the plexus around the superior mesenteric artery ("plexus pancreaticus capitalis II") [13],
3. The route from the plexus around the common hepatic artery to the anterior region of the

Fig. 14a,b. Lymphatic pathways from the pancreas. ***a*** Pathways from the posterior aspect of the head of the pancreas. ***b*** Pathways from the anterior aspect of the head and from the body and tail. The numbers in Figs. 13 and 14 indicate the numerical grouping of the regional lymph nodes (*LN*) proposed by the Japan Pancreas Society [4]. *1*, LN of the right cardiac region; *2*, LN of the left cardiac region; *3*, LN along the lesser curvature of the stomach; *4*, LN along the greater curvature of the stomach; *5*, LN of the supraphyloric region; *6*, LN of the infrapyloric region; *7*, LN along the left gastric artery; *8*, LN along the common hepatic artery; *9*, LN of the celiac axis; *10*, LN at the hilum of the spleen; *11*, LN along the splenic artery; *12*, LN of the hepatoduodenal ligament; *12p*, LN along the portal vein; *13*, LN of the posterior region of the pancreatic head; *13a*, LN of the superior part of 13; *13b*, LN of the inferior part of 13 (13a and 13b are divided at the level of the papilla of Vater); *14*, LN at the radix mesenterii; *14b*, LN at the origin of the inferior pancreaticoduodenal artery; *14c*, LN at the origin of the middle colic artery; *14d*, LN at the origin of the jejunal arteries; *14v*, LN along the superior mesenteric vein; *15*, LN along the middle colic artery; *16*, LN along the abdominal aorta; *17*, LN of the anterior region of the pancreatic head; *17a*, LN of the superior part of 17; *17b*, LN of the inferior part of 17 (17a and 17b are divided at the level of the papilla of Vater)

head of the pancreas coursing along the gastroduodenal artery and its tributaries,
4. The route from the left celiac ganglia to the body and tail of the pancreas via the plexus around the splenic artery and its tributaries, and
5. The direct route from the left celiac ganglion and the celiac plexus to the posterior region of the pancreatic body.

Via these routes, numerous extrinsic nerve fibers enter the gland through the capsule, often following the course of the vascular supply.

The postganglionic sympathetic fibers innervate directly blood vessels and islets, while the parasympathetic fibers terminate in intrapancreatic ganglia and the postganglionic fibers are distributed to acini and ducts. In addition, the pancreas are richly innervated by intrinsic peptidergic nerves [14].

The nerve plexuses of the pancreas, especially the plexus pancreaticus capitalis I and II, serve as the main routes of perineural extrapancreatic spread of cancer of the head [10–12].

Accessory Pancreas

Pancreatic tissue may develop in various sites remote from the pancreas. This has been referred to as ectopic, aberrant, or accessory pancreas.

Most accessory pancreata have been found in the wall of the stomach or the duodenum close to the opening of the major and minor duodenal papillae. Less frequent sites are the esophagus, small bowel, Meckel's diverticulum, colon, spleen, biliary tract, liver, and mesentery [2, 5].

The clinical incidence of accessory pancreas in several large series ranges from 1% to 13% [15–17]. Because the majority of accessory pancreata are asymptomatic, they are probably more common than their clinical incidence would suggest.

Accessory pancreatic nodules in the gastrointestinal tract are usually submucosal, well-circumscribed, smooth masses. The nodules vary in diameter from a few millimeters to several centimeters, and their summits often have a central umbilication representing the orifice of a ductal structure.

Since they contain normal exocrine tissue in all and islet-cell tissue in one-third of subjects, they may be subject to the same diseases, such as pancreatitis and pancreatic neoplasm, including islet-cell tumors.

References

1. Cubilla LA, Fitzgerald PJ Tumors of the exocrine pancreas. (1984) Gross anatomy. In: Hartmann WH, Sobin LH (eds) Atlas of tumor pathology, 2nd series, Fascicle 19. AFIP, Washington
2. Quinlan RM (1991) Anatomy and embryology of the pancreas. In: Zuidema GD (ed) Shackelford's surgery of the alimentary tract, 3rd edn, vol III. W B Saunders, Philadelphia, pp 3–18
3. Friedman AC, Birns MT (1987) Section III. The pancreas. Embryology, anatomy, histology, and physiology. In: Friedman AC (ed) Radiology of the liver, biliary tract, pancreas, and spleen. Williams and Wilkins, Baltimore, pp 619–642
4. The Japan Pancreas Society (1986) The general rules for describing cancer of the pancreas (in Japanese). Kanehara, Tokyo
5. Freeny PC, Lawson TL (1982) Radiology of the pancreas. Springer, Berlin Heidelberg New York
6. Skandalakis JE, Gray SW, Skandalakis LJ (1987) Surgical anatomy of the pancreas. In: Howard JM, Jordan JR, Reber HA (eds) Surgical diseases of the pancreas. Lea and Febiger, Philadelphia, pp 11–36
7. Gray W, Skandalakis JE, Skandalakis LJ (1987) Embryology and congenital anomalies of the pancreas. In: Howard JM, Jordan JR, Reber HA (eds) Surgical disease of the pancreas. Lea and Febiger, Philadelphia, pp 37–45
8. Anacker H (1975) Radiological anatomy of the pancreas. In: Anacker H (ed) Efficiency and limits of radiological examination of the pancreas. Georg Thieme, Stuttgart, pp 29–42
9. Dawson W, Langman J (1961) An anatomical-radiological study on the pancreatic duct pattern in man. Anat Rec 139:59–68
10. Nagai H, Kuroda A, Morioka Y (1986) Lymphatic and local spread of T1 and T2 pancreatic cancer. A study of autopsy material. Ann Surg 204:65–71
11. Nagai H, Kuroda A, Morioka Y (1983) An appraisal of radical operation for pancreatic cancer in view of modes of cancer spread (in Japanese). J Bili Tract Panc (Tan to Sui) 4:1091–1104
12. Nagai H (1987) An anatomical and pathological study of autopsy material on metastasis of pancreatic cancer to para-aortic lymph nodes (in Japanese). J Jpn Surg Soc (Nihon Geka Gakkai Zasshi) 88: 308–317
13. Yoshioka H, Wakabayashi T (1958) The pancreatic neurotomy on the head of the pancreas for relief of pain due to chronic pancreatitis. A new technical procedure and its results. Arch Surg 76:546–554

14. Holst JJ Neural regulation of pancreatic exocrine function. (1986) In: Go VLW, Gardner JD, Brooks FP, Lebenthal E, DiMagno EP, Scheele GA (eds) The exocrine pancreas. Biology, pathology and diseases. Raven, New York, pp 287–300
15. Dolan RV, Remine WH, Dockerty MB (1974) The fate of heterotopic pancreatic tissue. A study of 212 cases. Arch Surg 109:762–765
16. Feldman M, Weiberg T (1952) Aberrant pancreas: A cause of duodenal syndrome. JAMA 148:893–898
17. Barbosa J de C, Dockerty MB, Waugh JM (1946) Pancreatic heterotopia: Review of the literature and report of 41 authenticated surgical cases, of which 25 were clinically significant. Surg Gynecol Obstet 82:527–542
18. Classen M, Hellwing H, Rosch W (1973) Anatomy of the pancreatic duct. A duodenoscopic-radiological study. Endoscopy 5:14–17
19. Kasugai T, Kuno N, Kobayashi S, Hattori K (1972) Endoscopic pancreatocholangiogram. Gastroenterology 63:217–226
20. Ogoshi K, Niwa M, Hara Y, Nebel OT (1973) Endoscopic pancreatocholangiography in the evaluation of pancreatic and biliary disease. Gastroenterology 64:210–216
21. Sivak MV, Sullivan BH Jr (1976) Endoscopic retrograde pancreatography. Analysis of the normal pancreatogram. Am J Dig Dis 21:263–269
22. Varley PF, Rohrmann CA Jr, Silvis SE, Vennes JA (1976) The normal endoscopic pancreatogram. Radiology 118:295–300

Microanatomy and Fine Structure of the Pancreas

Introduction

The pancreas is the second largest gland in the digestive system and is exceeded only by the liver. It lies retroperitoneally in the upper abdominal cavity, with its head enclosed by the curve of the duodenum and its tail reaching to the spleen. Its anterior surface is covered by the peritoneum. The pancreatic parenchyma is lobulated. Each lobule is surrounded by connective tissue and is served by blood vessels and nerves. The pancreas is both an exocrine and an endocrine gland. This chapter will focus on the features of the exocrine pancreas, although the endocrine pancreas and nonparenchymal elements will be included to some extent.

Acinar Units

The dominant histological elements in the normal human pancreas are the exocrine components, which comprise more than 90% of the pancreatic volume. The pancreas has been shown to be capable, under certain conditions, of secreting more than 25 ml/kg body weight of pancreatic juice per day, including more than 25 g of secretory proteins, which are mainly digestive enzymes [1]. The exocrine pancreas is classified as a compound tubuloalveolar gland. It consists of areas of acinar cells, which synthesize and secrete the digestive enzymes, and a system of ducts. Pancreatic acinar cells are arranged both as tubules and as alveoli, as the classification of the gland suggests. The tubuloalveolar units, usually referred to as alveoli or acini, branch and sometimes anastomize with each other [2]. Each pancreatic lobule contains many of these units.

Each acinar unit consists of a group of acinar cells arranged in a single layer around a central lumen (Fig. 1). Centroacinar cells, containing no secretory granules, frequently comprise part of the acinar unit (Fig. 1). At the boundary of the cells with the surrounding connective tissue, there is a basal lamina. The lumen of the acinar unit is variable in size. After stimulation of secretion, for example after a meal, pancreatic enyzmes are secreted into the lumen that becomes larger than during rest. No myoepithelial cells (basket cells) are present in the pancreas, although they are a regular component of salivary and mammary glands.

Acinar cells are pyramidal-shaped cells with their base on the basal lamina and their apex bordering the lumen. Their large nuclei are located in the basal area. The nuclei are generally round, with one or two nucleoli. It is not unusual to find two nuclei in one cell. Abundant rough endoplasmic reticulum is concentrated in the infra-and paranuclear region of the abundant cytoplasm, an area sometimes referred to as the ergastoplasm or Nebenkern. The apical cytoplasm of acinar cells contains zymogen granules and is acidophilic, or eosinophilic.

Immunocytochemically, acinar cells show a positive reaction with antisera against various pancreatic enzymes, including alpha-amylase, alpha-1-antitrypsin, alpha-1-antichymotrypsin, trypsin, and chymotrypsin. They are negative for tumor markers, including carcinoembronic antigen (CEA) and CA19-9, for alpha-fetoprotein, and for endocrine markers including neuron-specific

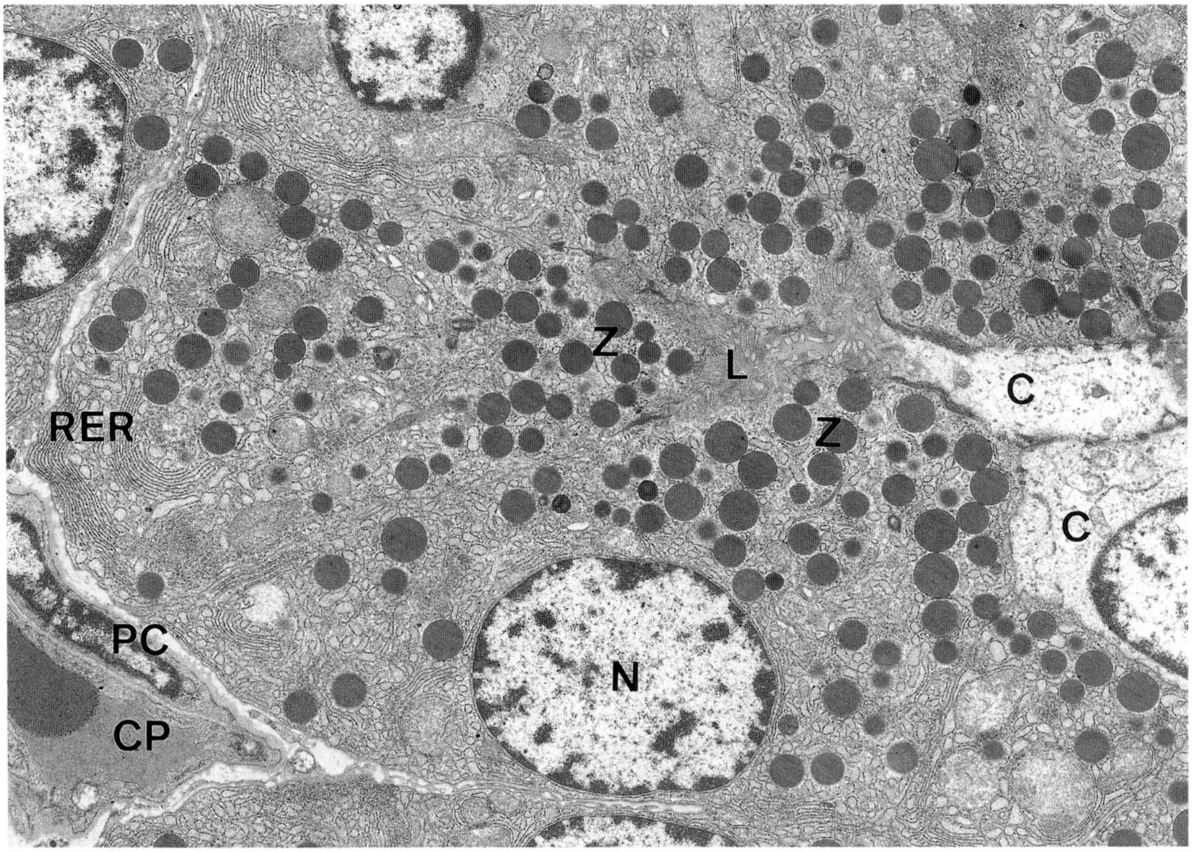

Fig. 1. Fine structure of human pancreatic acinus. Zymogen granules (*Z*) are numerous in the apical region (*close to the lumen*) of the acinar cells, but may be seen also in the more basal regions. Rough endoplasmic reticulum (*RER*) is prominent in the infranuclear region. *N*, Nucleus of acinar cell; *C*, centroacinar cell; *L*, acinar lumen; *CP*, capillary; *PC*, pericyte. (×5600)

enolase and other islet hormones such a insulin, glucagon, somatostatin, and pancreatic polypeptide [3]. Well-differentiated acinar tumor cells, including those of acinar cell carcinoma or pancreatoblastoma, are positive with the above antisera, including alpha-fetoprotein [4] (see Chapters "Acinar Cell Carcinoma" and "Pancreatoblastoma" in this volume).

Adjacent acinar cells are connected by junctional complexes apically, completely separating the lumen from the intercellular space below. The junctional complexes consist of a tight junction (zonula occuludens) closest to the lumen, an intermediate junction (zonula adherens), and desmosomes (maculae adherens). The plasma membranes of adjacent acinar cells adhere completely to each other at the tight junctions, so that a belt-like arrangement completely surrounds each cell [5, 6]. Electron microscopic examination reveals that in many places, adjacent acinar cells are connected by a gap junction (nexus). At each of these junctions, the plasma membranes of adjacent cells approach within 2 nm of each other. Freeze fracture replicas of the membranes have shown packed arrays of intramembranous particles [6–8]. Gap junctions provide sites for communication between adjacent cells.

The zonula adherens surrounds each acinar cell in belt-like fashion [5, 6]. The plasma membrane in this region is not well defined. Tonofilaments in the cytoplasm insert on the membrane. At the desmosomes, the intercellular gap is wider (30–50 nm). A desomsomal plaque serves as a site for attachment of tonofilaments. The desmosomes are in a rivet-like arrangement along the lateral plasma membrane.

Short microvilli, approximately 0.5 μm in length and 0.1 μm in diameter, protrude into the lumen from the apical surface of acinar cells. Here, the covering plasma membrane is coated with a thin

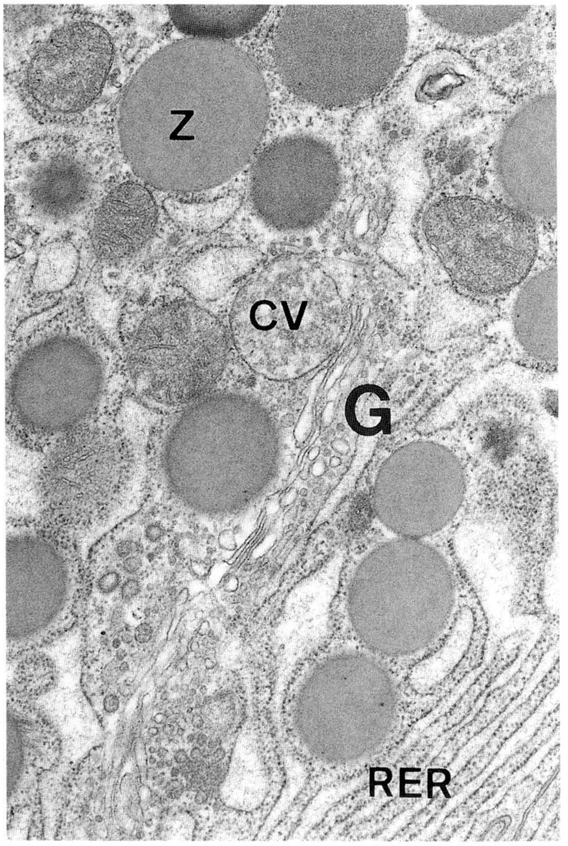

Fig. 2. Golgi complex (*G*) in an acinar cell. *Z*, Zymogen granules; *CV*, condensing vacuole; *RER*, rough endoplasmic reticulum. (×20 000)

mucoprotein layer. Bundles of microfilaments from the core of the microvilli. They are actin filaments, as demonstrated immunocytochemically [9]. These filaments join with the terminal web in the apical cytoplasm.

The rough (or granular) endoplasmic reticulum, concentrated in the infra- and para-nuclear region, is characterized by stratified or laminated cisterns circumscribed by a single membrane. Ribosomes, frequently arranged as polysomes, adhere to the outer surface of this membrane. The majority of the cellular RNA is located in this area, which is considered the site of protein synthesis [1, 5, 6, 10]. As the pancreatic enzymes are synthesized, they are first accumulated in the cisternae of the rough endoplasmic reticulum. The cisternae sometimes are dilated, forming vesicle-like structures with intracisternal granules. This may be an indication of accelerated protein synthesis.

Golgi complexes (Fig. 2) are located in the supranuclear region of acinar cells. They frequently are composed of three to five layers of cisternae. Each Golgi cisterna is surrounded by a membrane. Numerous vesicles, the majority of which are devoid of ribosomes, are present. Some vesicles, usually located at the periphery of the complex, are covered with a fuzzy material and are, therefore, referred to as coated vesicles. Rough endoplasmic reticulum in the region also produces vesicles, some of which lack ribosomes. This arrangement is regarded as evidence that secretory proteins are segregated from the rough endoplasmic reticulum, migrating to join the Golgi complex [6, 10]. The convex surface of the Golgi complex is referred to as the forming face, while the concave surface is called the maturing face. Some larger vacuoles, with varying electron densities, separate from the maturing face, and are regarded as the initial stage of formation of zymogen granules [1, 6, 10]. These are referred to as presecretory or prezymogen granules. Secretory proteins mature and are concentrated within these granules.

Mature zymogen granules characteristically are stored in the apical part of the cytoplasm of acinar cells (Figs. 1–5). These granules are spherical and, therefore, appear round in thin sections. They are approximately 1 μm in diameter and are circumscribed by a limiting membrane. Pancreatic enzymes are secreted into the acinar lumen by the process of exocytosis. The zymogen granules approach the apical plasma membrane. The membranes of the granules and the cell apex touch and then fuse. The contents of the granules are then discharged into the acinar lumen (Fig. 3a,b). Secreted material frequently appears as filamentous (Fig. 4a) or flocculent material in the lumen. With heightened stimulation of secretion, zymogen granules beneath the surface may fuse with those at the surface, forming a chain of granules releasing their product into the lumen [6].

Primary lysosomes are a normal component in the region of the Golgi complex. A segregation process in the complex separates the lysosomal enzymes from the zymogens that are packaged in the zymogen granules. The formation of lysosomes may be considered, therefore, an important part of the maturation process of zymogen granules [5, 6].

Other cellular organelles are characteristic of acinar cells. Large mitochondria are numerous, frequently interposed between adjacent strands of rough endoplasmic reticulum. A pair of centrioles (diplosome), composed of nine triplets, is present in the perinuclear region. Multivesicular bodies are

a b

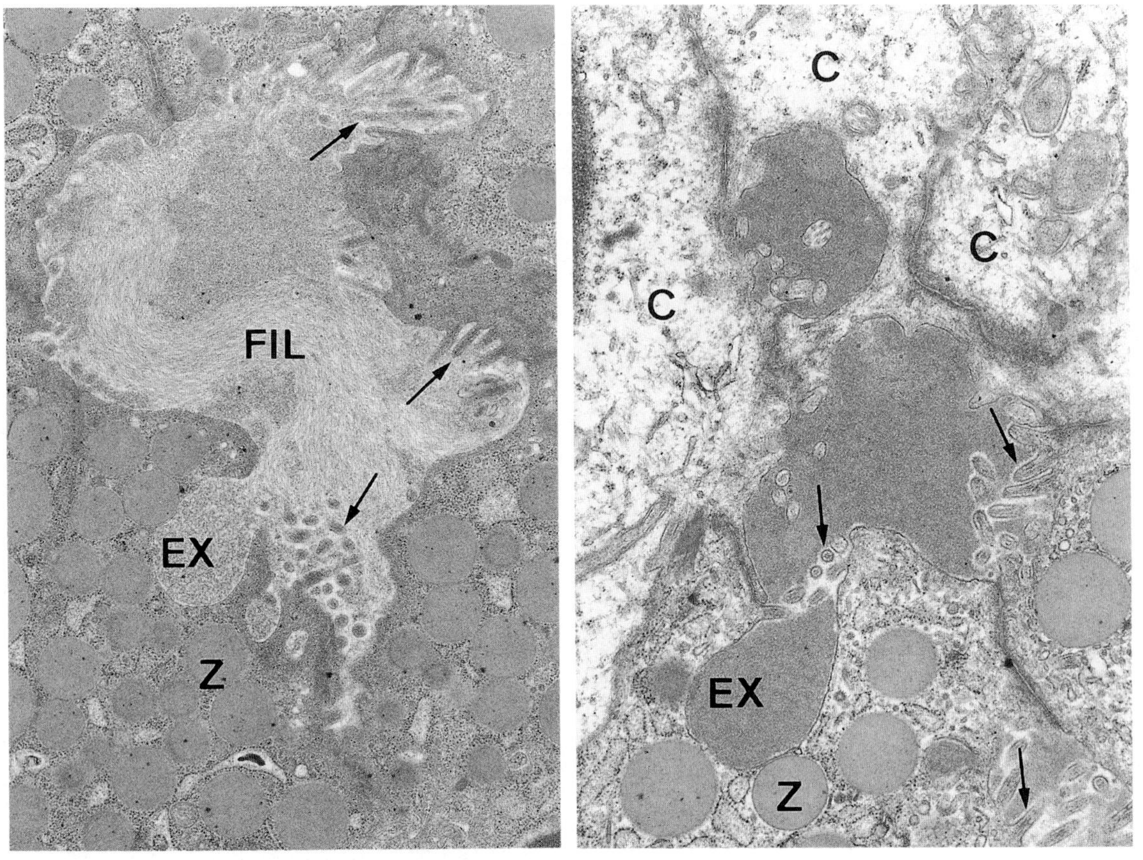

Fig. 3a,b. Two views of the acinar lumen, which is surrounded by acinar and centroacinar (*C*) cells, and is filled with secretion products, some of which appear filamentous (*FIL*). Numerous zymogen granules (*Z*) are present in the acinar cells. Exocytosis of zymogen granule contents into the lumen is obvious (*EX*). *Arrows* point to microvilli. (×14 000)

found frequently. Tonofilaments and microtubules are scattered in the cytoplasm. A few lipid droplets are present in normal acinar cells. Lipid droplets may be greatly increased in patients with diabetes mellitus, obesity, or alcohol abuse [11]. Annulate lamellae, which are normal components of ova and Sertoli cells, are not found in normal acinar cells. However, they may be found in tumor cells showing acinar differentiation (such as acinar cell carcinoma and pancreatoblastoma) [12].

Pancreatic Ductal System

Two large ducts drain pancreatic juice into the duodenum. These are the main and accessory pancreatic ducts (ducts of Wirsung and Santorini, respectively). The ductal system begins at the acinar unit, where intercalated ducts (ductules) are continuous with centroacinar cells. The juice passes, in turn, through intralobular ducts and interlobular ducts before entering the main and accessory ducts. Ductal cells are the site of secretion of bicarbonate ion and fluid into the pancreatic juice [13, 14]. The ducts often are involved in the initiation of pancreatitis and cancer.

Centroacinar cells are recognized in the electron microscope as relatively clear cells that make up part of the acinar unit. They are joined to adjacent acinar cells by junctional complexes, and their lateral membranes form interdigitations (Fig. 5). Their basal membrane rests on a basal lamina that is continuous with that underlying the adjacent acinar cells. They have rounded nuclei like acinar cells, but they do not contain zymogen granules (Fig. 4). Their cytoplasm appears clear because it

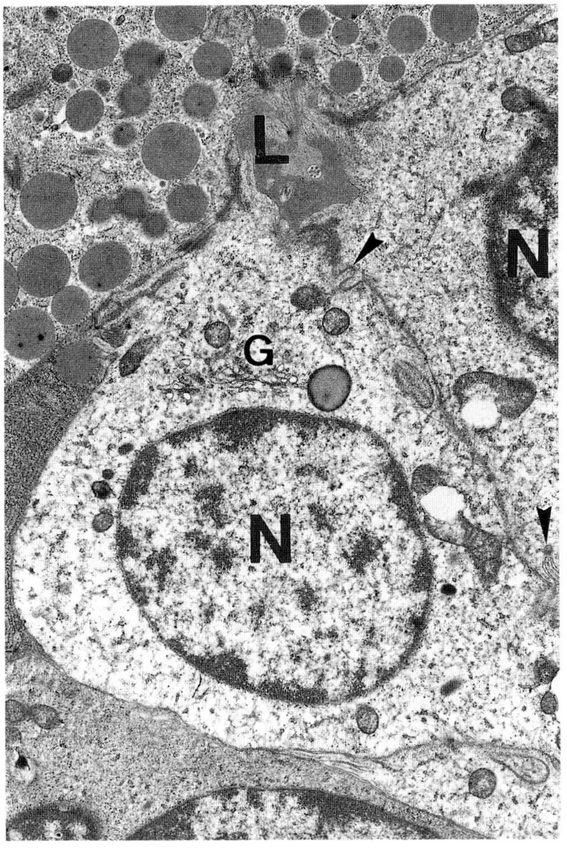

Fig. 4. Fine structure of centroacinar cells, which contain a large nucleus (*N*) and a few organelles. A supranuclear Golgi complex (*G*) is present. The *arrowhead* points to interdigitation of adjacent cells. *L*, Acinar lumen. (×10 000)

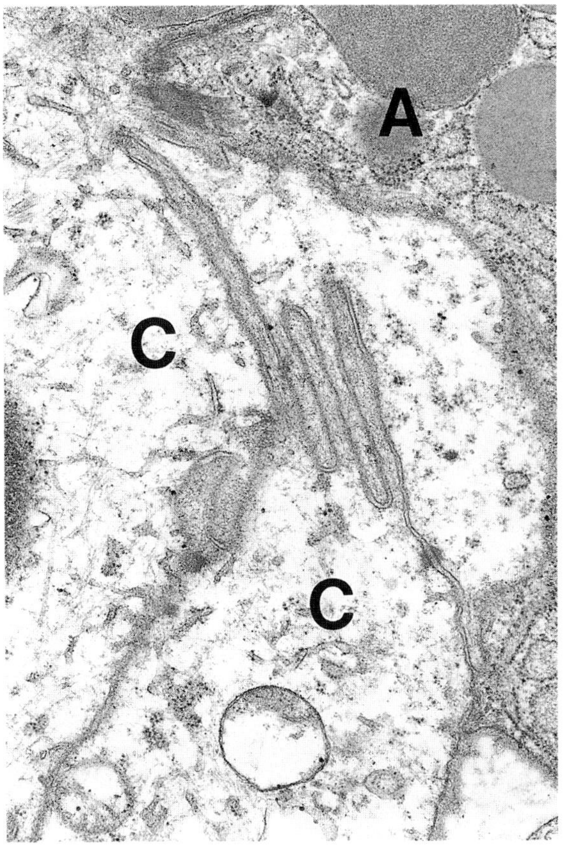

Fig. 5. Interdigitation of adjacent centroacinar cells (*C*). The edge of an acinar cell (*A*) is seen. (×21 000)

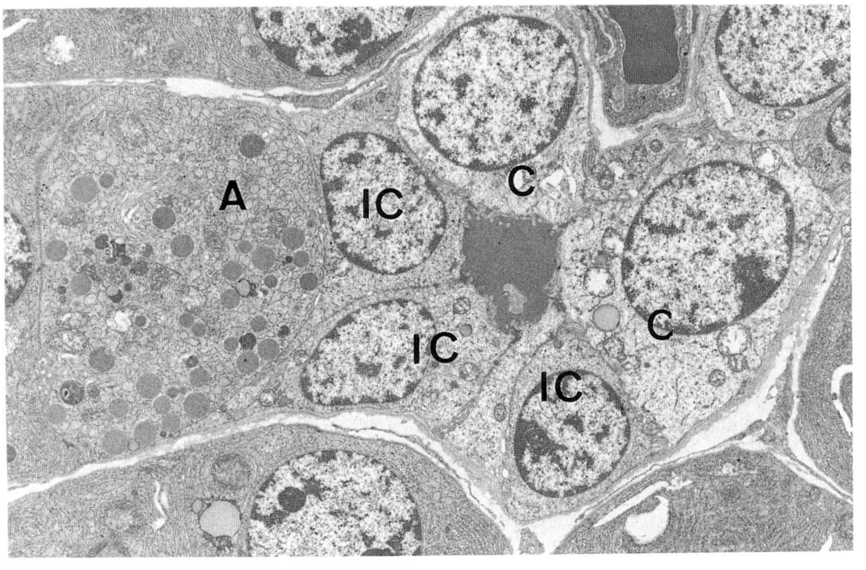

Fig. 6. Fine structure of the initial part of intercalated ductules. Two of the epithelial cells that comprise the ductule are labeled (*IC*). *A*, Acinar cell; *C*, centroacinar cell. (×3800)

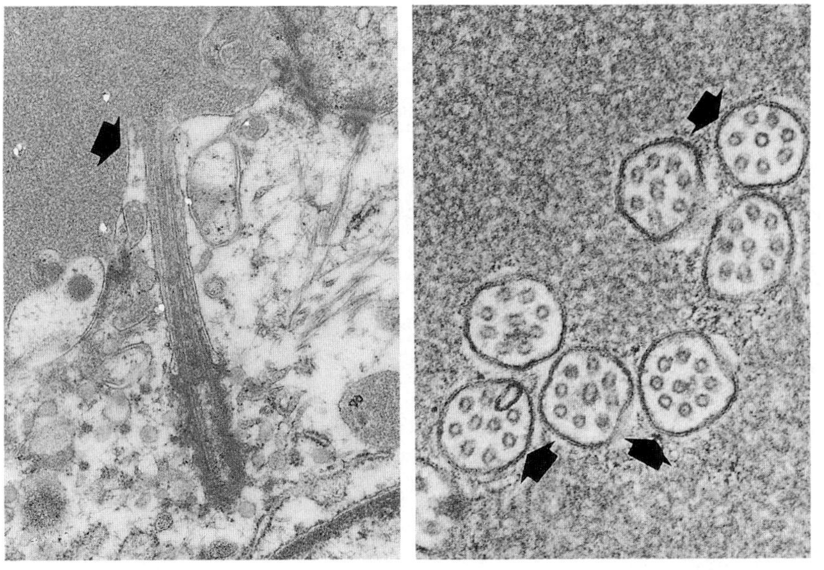

Fig. 7a,b. ***a*** Longitudinal and ***b*** cross sections of modified ciliae (*arrows*) in pancreatic ductular system. Note that none of the cross sections have the characteristic "9 plus 2" arrangement of microtubules expected for motile kinocilia. ***a***, ×18 000; ***b***, ×69 000

contains little rough endoplasmic reticulum and fewer ribosomes than acinar cells. The luminal surface is smooth, with a few microvilli (Fig. 4).

Intercalated ductules are formed by single flat to low cuboidal epithelial cells that have a clear cytoplasm (Fig. 6). They are quite similar morphologically to centroacinar cells. Their cytoplasm contains a few organelles. Mitochondria are present but they are not very numerous. One or two modified ciliae project into the ductular lumen from intercalated cells (Figs. 3b 7a,b). The ciliae are approximately 5–10 μm long and 0.2–0.3 μm in diameter [6]. They project along the same direction in which the pancreatic juice flows. It has been suggested that they are kinociliae which mix the pancreatic juice and help move it along the ductal system [6, 15]. However, because they usually do not display the characteristic microtubular arrangement (nine peripheral and two central) of kinociliae, it is thought that they resemble more the modified ciliae of the olfactory epithelium, and may act in a sensory capacity for contents of the pancreatic juice [16].

Although it has been proposed that ductular cells contain carbonic anhydrase [17, 18], and are the main site of transportation of bicarbonate ion and fluid into the pancreatic juice, the fine structure is not what is expected for such a function [6, 15]. Whereas the kidney tubules, where ion and fluid transport takes place, have elaborately infolded basal membranes associated with numerous mitochondria, the ductular cells lack these features and contain only a few smooth-surfaced vesicles near the apical and lateral plasma membrane.

Intralobular ducts continue from intercalated ductules. The content of the epithelial cells changes little from that described for intercalated ductules. The cells lining intralobular ducts usually are cuboidal, and a small amount of connective tissue adds to the thickness of the wall. One occasionally finds acidophilic epithelial cells in these ducts, which, by electron microscopy, are found to have a cytoplasm that is packed with mitochondria. Although these cells have been called oncocytes (Fig. 8), indicating that they are foci for oncocytic metaplasia, this interpretation is doubtful [15].

Interlobular ducts are lined with a single layer of cuboidal or low columnar cells lying on a basement membrane. The epithelial cells have round or oval nuclei, some rough endoplasmic reticulum, mainly basal mitochondria, and a well-developed Golgi apparatus. The cells are connected with each other by junctional complexes and elaborate interdigitations. These epithelial cells are similar to those in the intralobular ducts. Numerous microvilli project into the lumen. The membrane in this area is covered by a fuzzy surface coat that stains with the periodic acid-Schiff reaction and with Alcian blue. This proteoglycan coat is regarded as a protective barrier [6, 15]. According to Nagata and Monno [15], some goblet cells and Paneth cells are scattered in the epithelium of the interlobular ducts of nor-

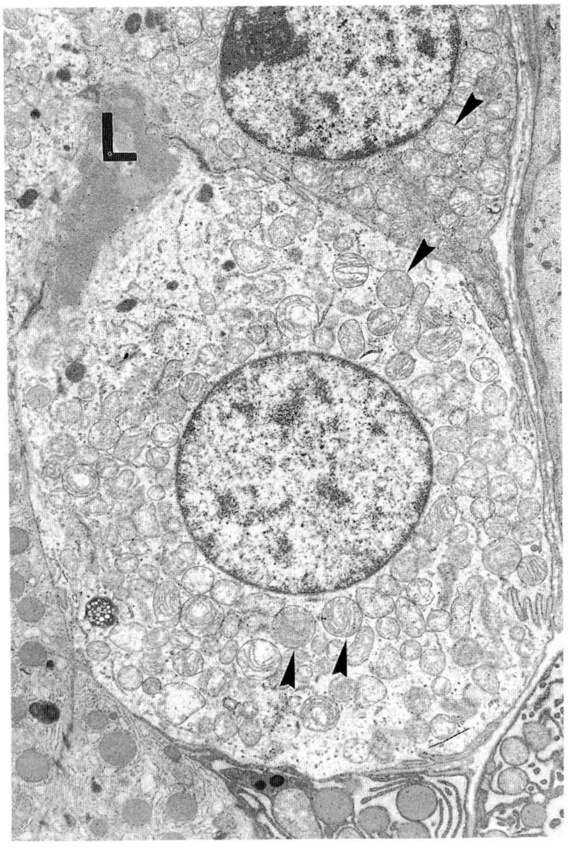

Fig. 8. Oncocytes containing numerous mitochondriae (*arrowheads*) throughout the cytoplasm surround the ductular lumen (*L*). (×5600)

mal pancreas. The mucin-secreting cells have secretory granules in the apical cytoplasm. The granules are discharged by exocytosis.

The main pancreatic duct is lined by a single layer of tall columnar cells with oval nuclei in the basal region (Fig. 9). The epithelium expands basally to provide mucous glands in some areas (Fig. 10). The epithelial cells of the main pancreatic duct have a greater proportion of mucus-secreting cells, which have an abundance of mucin granules in the apical region (Fig. 11). Surface epithelial cells, complete with nuclei and cellular organelles, may be seen to exfoliate, and are thought to be replaced by cells in the basal area [6]. Scattered endocrine cells may also be found in the basal region of the epithelium [15]. These are cuboidal, and react positively with Glimerius' stain. Characteristic dark granules are observed in the cytoplasm by electron microscopy (Fig. 12). Normal pancreatic duct epithelium and ductal carcinoma react positively with antisera to CA19-9, but normal duct epithelium is negative with antisera against CEA [3].

Endocrine Pancreas

Pancreatic endocrine components consist of several cell types producing different hormones. Four main types include A-cells secreting glucagon, B-cells secreting insulin, D-cells secreting somatostatin, and PP-cells secreting pancreatic polypeptide. They are inserted into the lobules among the acinar units forming spheroidal islets (of Langerhans) which appear round or oval in sections. They are 85–210 μm in diameter [19]. The total number of islets in the whole pancreas has been estimated to be about 30 000, and the total weight to be less than 1 g [19].

A few solitary endocrine cells are scattered between acini and in the epithelium of the ductal system. A larger number are found in the larger pancreatic ducts, especially the main pancreatic duct in the head portion.

Non-epithelial Elements of the Pancreas

The normal pancreas includes several tissue elements in addition to the epithelial cells that form the acini and ductal system. They include, as in other organs, blood and lymph vessels, nerves, adipocytes, fibroblasts, and extracellular matrix.

Blood and Lymphatic Vessels

The pancreas is supplied mainly by three arterial streams. The first supply is branches of the gastroduodenal artery, including the superior pancreaticoduodenal artery. The second is branches of the inferior pancreaticoduodenal artery, which is derived from the superior mesenteric artery. The third is branches from the splenic artery; these supply mainly the body and tail of the pancreas from the posterior-superior surface. The pancreaticoduodenal arteries primarily supply the head, forming arcade-like shunts there [1].

The arterial supply merges into arterioles which course first in the interlobular connective tissue,

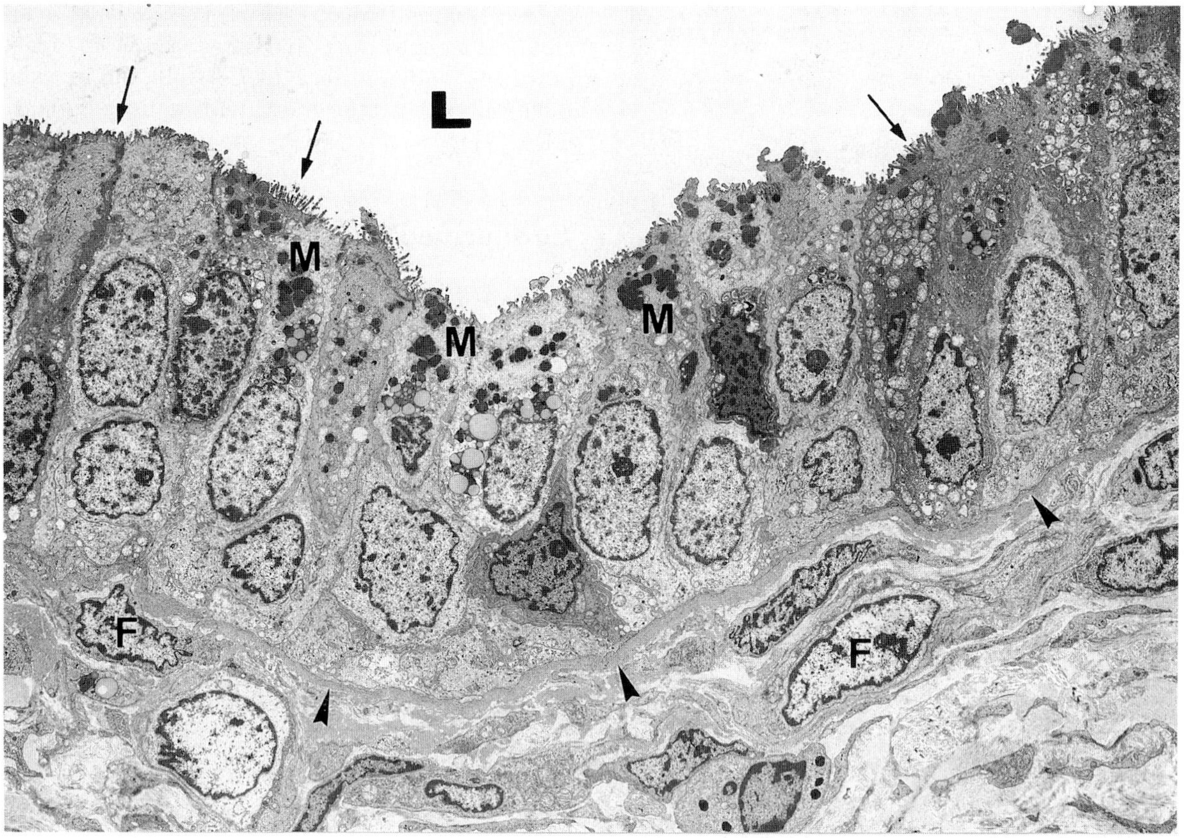

Fig. 9. Fine structure of the main pancreatic duct. Tall columnar epithelial cells rest on a basement membrane (*arrowheads*). Mucin granules (*M*) are present in the apical cytoplasm and microvilli (*arrows*) and project into the lumen (*L*). Fibroblasts (*F*) and extracellular matrix are distributed around the duct. (×2400)

then penetrate into the lobule. Much of the blood supply to the lobule goes first to the islets through afferent arterioles, forms a glomerulus-like arrangement of capillaries there, then passes on through efferent capillaries to supply the capillary plexus around the acinar units. Some of the blood supply to the acinar units goes directly to the periacinar plexus. (For reviews of pancreatic microcirculation, see Heitz [1] and Bockman [20]). The capillaries are thin, fenestrated endothelial cells surrounded by a basal lamina. The capillaries lie in the interacinar space, and pericytes often are observed immediately surrounding the endothelial cells (Figs. 1, 13).

Drainage of blood is initially through intralobular and interlobular venules, then through veins draining into the pancreaticoduodenal and pancreatic veins, and eventually into the hepatic portal system. Lymphatic capillaries form networks in the lobules, then join to form larger vessels draining to the surface, where primary lymph nodes receive the lymph. Further lymph drainage is through preaortic nodes at the base of the celiac and superior mesenteric arteries, and eventually into the thoracic duct.

Nerves

The pancreas has an abundant nerve supply that includes sensory nerves as well as those of the sympathetic and parasympathetic divisions of the autonomic nervous system. The pancreatic nerves are mainly unmyelinated, although some myelinated fibers are present (Fig. 14). Each major nerve branch has mixed nerve fibers that are separated from the surrounding connective tissue by a perineurium, providing for a specialized microenvironment within which the nerve fibers func-

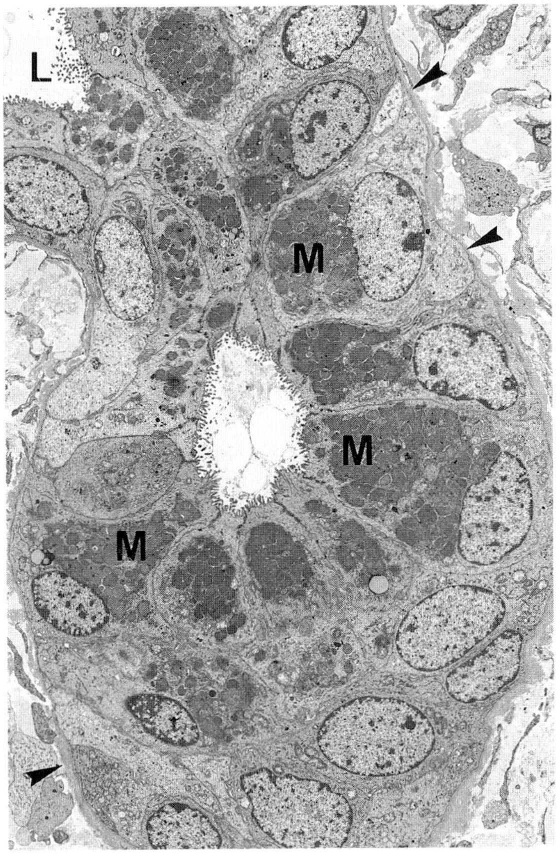

Fig. 10. Mucin-secreting cells of the main pancreatic duct. Mucin granules (*M*) fill the apical region of most cells. *Arrowheads* indicate the basement membrane. *L*, Lumen. (×1800)

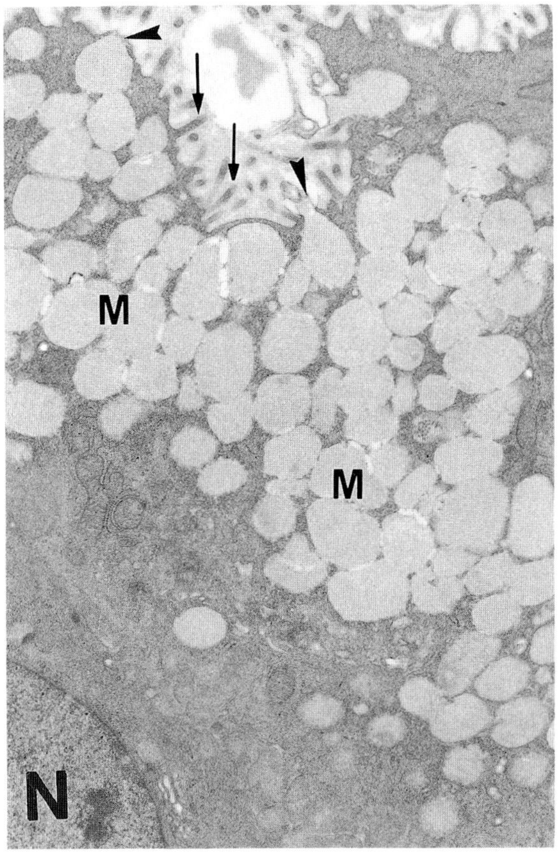

Fig. 11. Exocytotic discharge (*arrowheads*) of mucin granules (*M*) in a mucin-secreting cell of the main pancreatic duct. *Arrows* point to microvilli. *N*, Nucleus. (×8500)

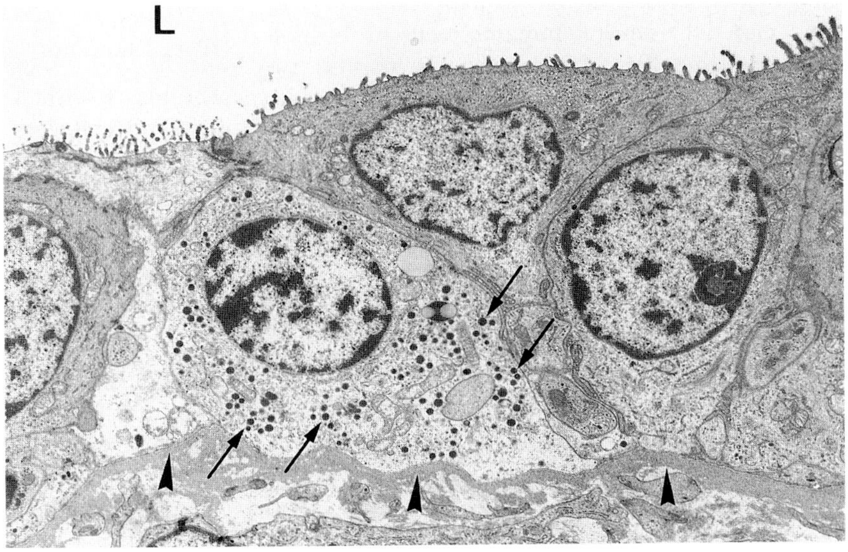

Fig. 12. Endocrine cell in duct epithelium. It borders on the basement membrane (*arrowheads*), endocrine granules (*arrows*), but does not reach the lumen (*L*). (×6000)

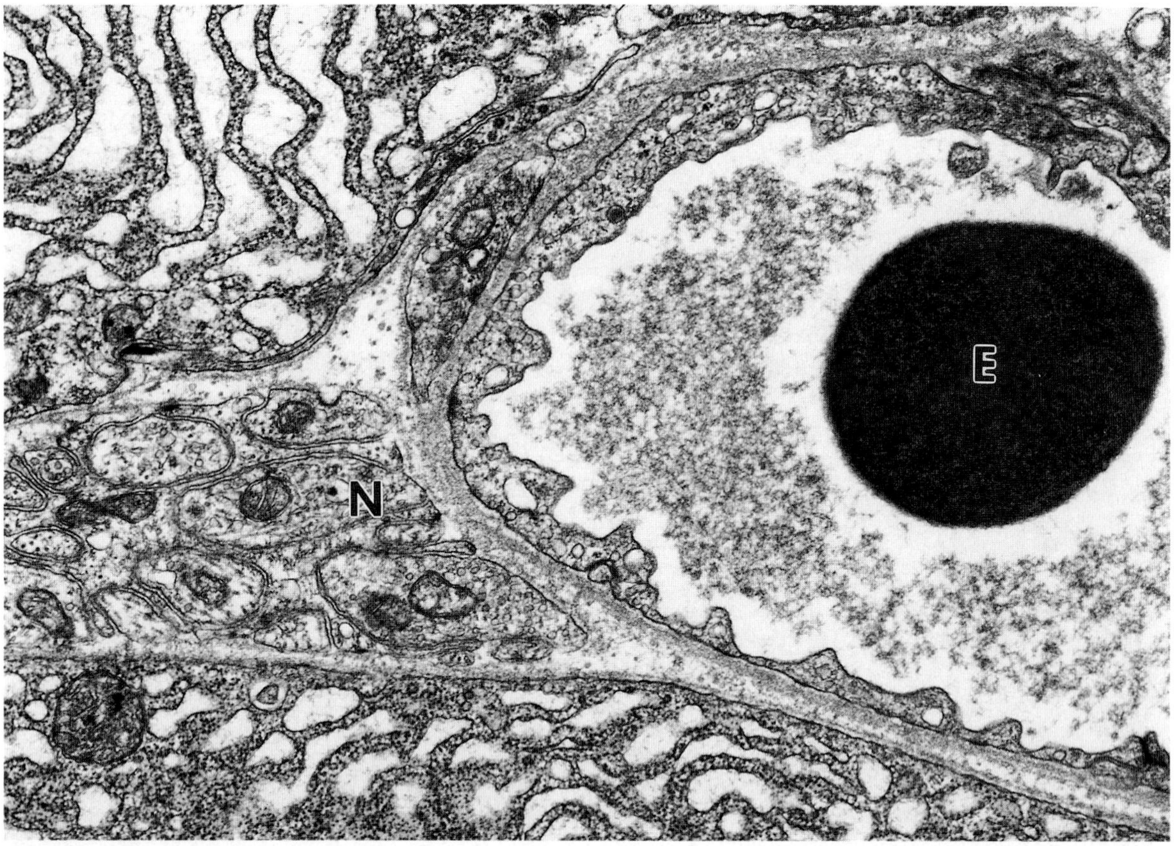

Fig. 13. A capillary in the interacinar space. The thin endothelial cell is surrounded by a basal lamina. Nerve fibers (*N*) are adjacent to the blood vessel. *E*, Erythrocyte. (×17 200)

tion. In some conditions, the protective barrier provided by the perineurium is breached, making the nerve fibers vulnerable to biologically active substances, such as activated pancreatic enzymes and material from inflammatory cells in the connective tissue [21]. In chronic pancreatitis, the inflammatory cells are mostly lymphocytes, with smaller numbers of macrophages and neutrophils (Fig. 15).

Pancreatic adenocarcinoma usually invades nerves (Fig. 16). This process breaches the protective perineurium and makes it possible for the adenocarcinoma cells to affect the nerves directly. It is believed that these processes are involved in the generation of pain in patients with pancreatic cancer.

Small branches of nerves, both extrinsic and intrinsic (from nerve cell bodies located in parasympathetic ganglia within the pancreas) extend throughout the pancreas (Fig. 17). They affect secretion of the exocrine and endocrine pancreas, and blood flow. Sensory fibers are transmitted to the central nervous system through the splanchnic and vagus nerves.

Other Elements

Fibroblasts with associated extracellular matrix, including collagen fibers, are more abundant in the interlobular space than within the lobules. In pathological conditions, especially chronic pancreatitis, these elements increase greatly and are recognized as fibrosis.

Fat storage cells (Ito's cells) are sometimes found in the extracellular matrix of normal animal pancreas [22] and in human pancreas [23]. These cells characteristically have multiple fatty vacuole in the cytoplasm. It is thought that this type of cell is fibrogenic under a variety of conditions, including alcohol abuse, because it usually is closely associated with collagen fibers (Fig. 18). Adipocytes, rare in the normal young pancreas, increase in

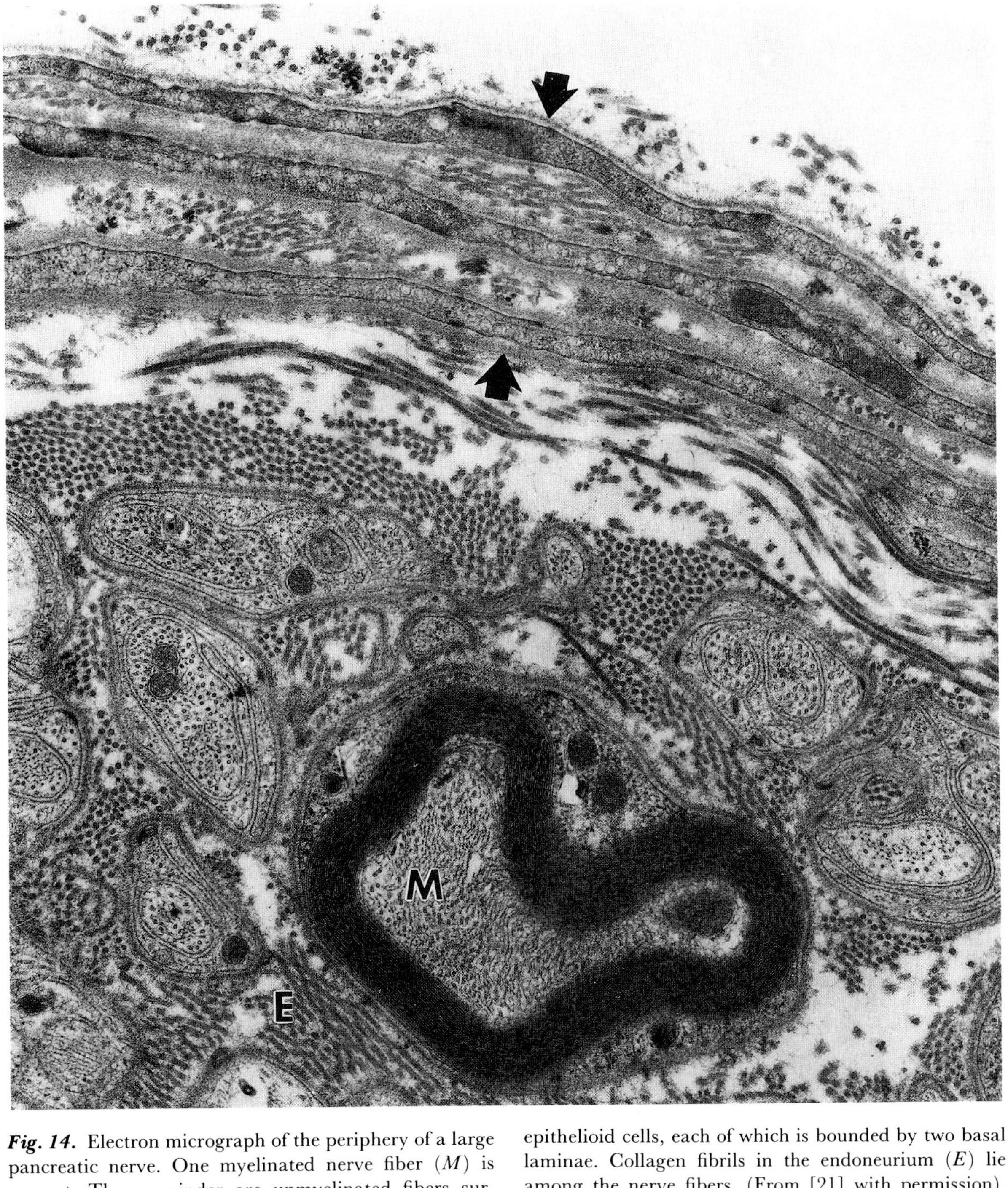

Fig. 14. Electron micrograph of the periphery of a large pancreatic nerve. One myelinated nerve fiber (*M*) is present. The remainder are unmyelinated fibers surrounded by extensions of Schwann cells. The perineurium (between *arrows*) consists of three layers of thin epithelioid cells, each of which is bounded by two basal laminae. Collagen fibrils in the endoneurium (*E*) lie among the nerve fibers. (From [21] with permission). (×20 880)

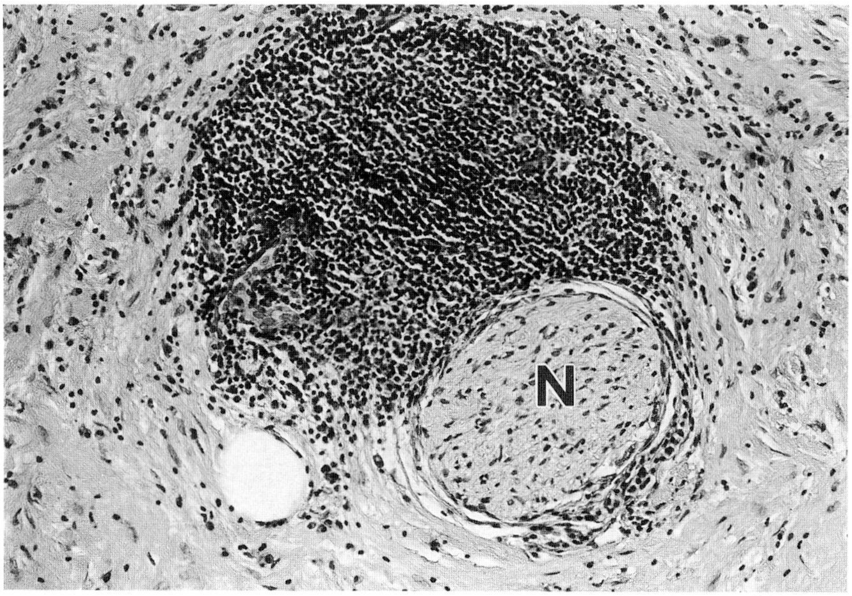

Fig. 15. Nerve (N) from a patient with chronic pancreatitis. A focus of chronic inflammatory cells lies adjacent to the nerve, and some of the cells have penetrated the perineurium. (×400)

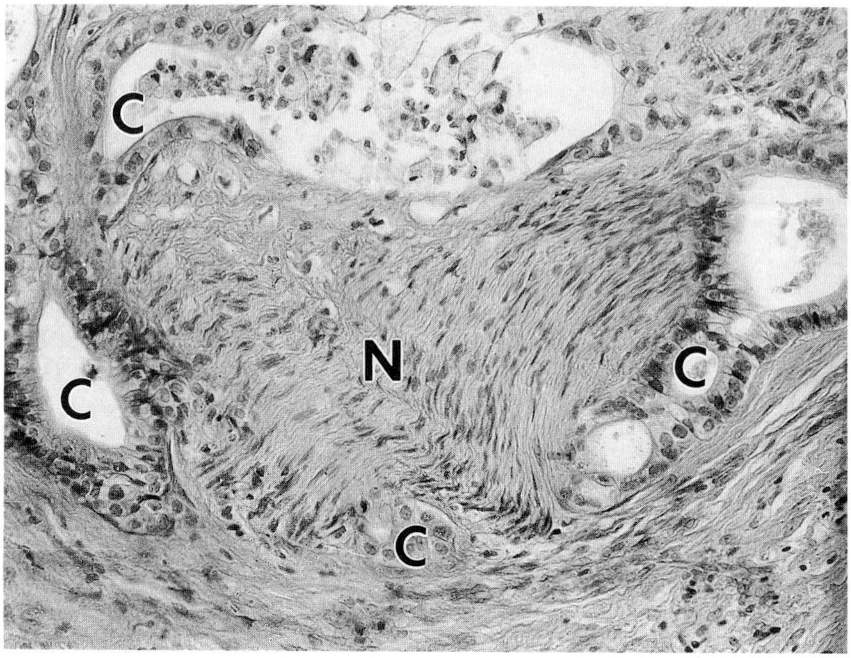

Fig. 16. Nerve from patient with pancreatic cancer. The nerve (N) has been penetrated by the cells of the adenocarcinoma (C). The perineurium has been breached by the invasion. (From [24] with permission). (×240)

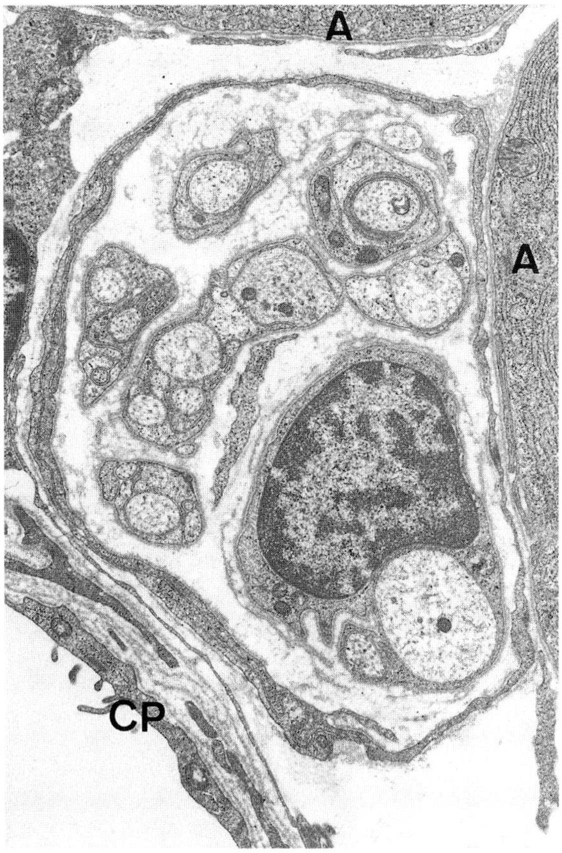

Fig. 17. Nerve fibers in the periacinar space. *A*, Acinar cells; *CP*, capillary. (×9000)

frequency with age. They are quite numerous in some individuals, especially those who are obese and have hepato-choledocho-choledocystic diseases. Necrosis of the adipose tissue is a serious part of acute necrotizing pancreatitis.

References

1. Heitz PU, Beglinger C, Gyr K (1984) Anatomy and physiology of the exocrine pancreas. In: Klöppel G, Heitz PU (eds) Pancreatic pathology. Churchill Livingstone, London, pp 3–21
2. Akao S, Bockman DE, Lechene de la Porte S, Sarles H (1986) Three-dimensional pattern of ductuloacinar associations in normal and pathological human pancreas. Gastroenterology 90:661–668
3. Morohoshi T, Kanda M, Horie A, Chott A, Dreyer T, Klöppel G, Heitz UP (1987) Immunocytochemical markers of uncommon pancreatic tumors. Acinar cell carcinoma, pancreatoblastoma, and solid cystic (papillary-cystic) tumor. Cancer 59:739–747
4. Morohoshi T, Sagawa F, Mitsuya T (1990) Pancreatoblastoma with marked elevation of serum alpha-fetoprotein. An autopsy case report with immunocytochemical study. Virchows Arch [A] 416: 265–270
5. Fujita H (1981) II. The cell, and III. The tissue. In: Fujita H, Fujita T (eds) Textbook of histology (in Japanese), Part I. Igaku-Shoin, Tokyo, pp 85–264
6. Kern HF (1986) Fine structure of the human exocrine pancreas. In: Go VLW, Gardener JD, Brooks FP, Lebenthal E, Di Magno E, Scheele GA (eds) The exocrine pancreas. Raven, New York, pp 9–19

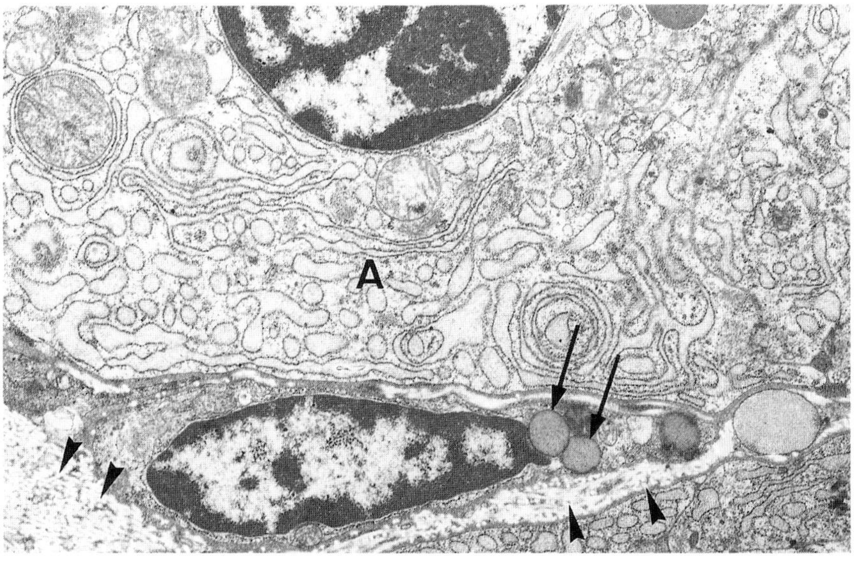

Fig. 18. Fat-storage cell (of Ito) adjacent to an acinar cell (*A*). Fatty vacuoles are indicated by the *arrows*, fine collagen fibrils by the *arrowheads*. (×9000)

7. Adler G, Bieger W, Kern HF (1978) Amino acid transport in the exocrine pancreas. Effect of maximal and supramaximal hormonal stimulation in vivo. Cell Tissue Res 194:447–462
8. Gorelick FS, Jamieson JD (1981) Structure-function relationship of the pancreas. In: Johnson LR (ed) Physiology of the gastrointestinal tract. Raven, New York, pp 773–794
9. Drenckhahn D, Mannherz HG (1983) Distribution of actin and the actin-associated proteins myosin, tropomyosin, alpha-actinin, vinculin, and villin in rat and bovine exocrine glands. Eur J Cell Biol 30:167–176
10. Watanabe Y (1977) Fine structure of pancreatic acinar cell (in Japanese). Igakuno Ayumi 103: 261–270
11. Bordalo O, Baptista A, Dreiling D, Noronha M (1984) Early pathomorphological pancreatic changes in chronic alcoholism. In: Gyr KE, Singer MV, Sarles H (eds) Pancreatitis—concepts and classification. Elsevier, Amsterdam, pp 57–60
12. Horie A, Morohoshi T, Klöppel G (1987) Ultrastructural comparison of pancreatoblastoma, solid-cystic tumor, and acinar cell carcinoma. J Clin Electron Microscopy 20:353–362
13. Schulz I (1981) Electrolyte and fluid secretion in the exocrine pancreas. In: Johnson LR (ed) Physiology of the gastrointestinal tract. Raven, New York, pp 795–819
14. Case RM, Argent BE (1986) Bicarbonate secretion by pancreatic duct: Mechanisms and control. In: Go VLW, Gardner JD, Brooks RP, Lebenthal E, DiMagno E, Scheele GA (eds) The exocrine pancreas. Raven, New York, pp 213–243
15. Nagata A, Monno S (1984) Ultrastructure of pancreatic duct and pancreatic ductal cells (in Japanese). The Cell 16:397–402
16. Bockman DE, Büchler M, Beger HG (1986) Structure and function of specialized cilia in the exocrine pancreas. Int J Pancreatol 1:21–28
17. Churg A, Richter WR (1972) Histochemical distribution of carbonic anhydrase after ligation of the pancreatic duct. Am J Pathol 68:23–30
18. Spicer SS, Sens MA, Tashian RE (1982) Immunocytochemical demonstration of carbonic anhydrase in human epithelial cells. J Histochem Cytochem 30:864–873
19. Klöppel G (1984) Anatomy and physiology of the endocrine pancreas. In: Klöppel G, Heitz PU (eds) Pancreatic pathology. Churchill Livingstone, London, pp 133–153
20. Bockman DE (1992) Microvasculature of the pancreas: Relation to pancreatitis. Int J Pancreatol 12:11–21
21. Bockman DE, Büchler M, Malfertheiner P, Beger HG (1988) Analysis of nerves in chronic pancreatitis. Gastroenterology 94:1459–1469
22. Watari N (1984) Ultrastructural studies on the connective tissues in the pancreas (in Japanese). The Cell 16:402–408
23. Morohoshi T, Kanda M (1985) Periacinar fibroblastoid cell—its action on early stage of alcoholic pancreatitis (in Japanese). Tann to Sui 6:1205–1211
24. Bockman DE (1993) Surgical anatomy of the pancreas and adjacent structures. In: Beger HG, Büchler M, Malfertheiner P (eds) Standards in pancreatic surgery. Springer, Berlin Heidelberg New York (in press)

Serous Cystadenoma

Synonyms

Microcystic adenoma; glycogen-rich cystadenoma; nonmucous-secreting adenoma

Definition

Serous cystadenoma is a benign pancreatic tumor that is usually composed of small (micro) cystic spaces containing serous material. Therefore, the term microcystic serous adenoma is applied to this lesion. However, recent observations show that this tumor may occur in a macrocystic form [1, 2]. Consequently, serous cystadenoma appears to be a more appropriate term. The macrocystic or lymphangiomatoid variant [2], is radiologically and gross morphologically different from the more common microcystic form [1], and should be recognized as a variant of serous cystadenoma. Macrocystic tumors are not uncommon compared to other cystic pancreatic neoplasms. Of 80 cystic tumors treated at Massachusetts General Hospital over the past 15 years, 5 (6.3%) were macrocystic serous cystadenomas [1].

Incidence

Serous cystadenoma is rare. However, with improvements in computed tomography (CT) and ultrasonography (US), these tumors are being recognized with increasing frequency. The pathological concept of pancreatic serous cystadenoma was first established by Compagno and Oertel [3]. Numerous case reports and small series of this tumor have been reported since then. This neoplasm is usually regarded as a benign unifocal lesion. However, recently six cases have been reported [4–9] as malignant (serous cystadenocarcinoma) or multifocal (see Chapter "Serous Cystadenocarcinoma" in this volume).

Sex

Serous cystadenoma occurs more frequently in women than in men. Compagno and Oertel [3] reported that 21 of their 34 patients (62%) with this tumor were women. In our study [10], there were four women and one man. The reported female to male ratio ranges up to 6:1 [3, 11]. The macrocystic form occurred in three women and two men [1].

Age

Most cases occur in patients above 60 years of age (range: 34–88 years, with a mean of 68 years). The age of the 5 patients with macrocystic serous cystadenoma was between 46 and 67 [1].

Etiology and Pathogenesis

The etiology of serous cystadenoma is unknown. This tumor is sometimes associated with diabetes mellitus, von Hippel-Lindau syndrome, and extrapancreatic neoplasms. Diabetes mellitus is found in about 20% of the patients. Extrapancreatic neoplasms including carcinoma of the colon, larynx, lung, thyroid, kidney, cervix, breast, as well as leukemia and lymphoma are found in some patients with serous cystadenoma, but it is difficult to prove that these conditions are significantly associated factors.

Serous cystadenoma possibly derives from the centroacinar or proximal ductal cells. However, the coexistence of serous cystadenoma and ductal adenocarcinoma [12] suggests a common precursor cell in these two tumors. The cells of serous cystadenoma are similar to centroacinar cells or ductal cells based on immunohistochemical findings with anti-CA19-9, anti-epithelial membrane antigen (EMA), anti-cytokeratin and other antibodies [13, 14]. Serous cystadenoma cells (of both microcystic and macrocystic forms) contain characteristic cytoplasmic deposits of glycogen, as do other tubular or centroacinar cells of the human fetal pancreas [1, 3, 15].

Clinical Presentation

Serous cystadenoma is characterized by slow growth and by the absence of early symptoms. The most common symptoms are abdominal pain or discomfort and back pain. Other symptoms include weight loss, fatigue, nausea, vomiting, melena, recurrent pancreatitis and hematoperitoneum [16]. Some patients present with obstructive jaundice and abodominal masses. Sometimes the tumor is found incidentally during an operation for other reasons. The duration of symptoms ranges from a few days to 5 years [3, 14], although most patients have histories of several months' duration. Plain radiographs often show an upper abdominal soft tissue mass and sometimes calcifications within the tumor. Gastrointestinal barium series occasionally demonstrate a widening of the duodenal loop or external displacement of the stomach or colon.

Ultrasonographic Findings

Most microcystic forms of serous cystadenomas show solid masses without cystic components on ultrasonography (US). Reticular septum-like structures and calcifications were reported in 7% and 17%, respectively [17]. High-echo patterns may be observed in 47% and low-echo patterns in 42%. For example, the tumor in Fig. 1 showed

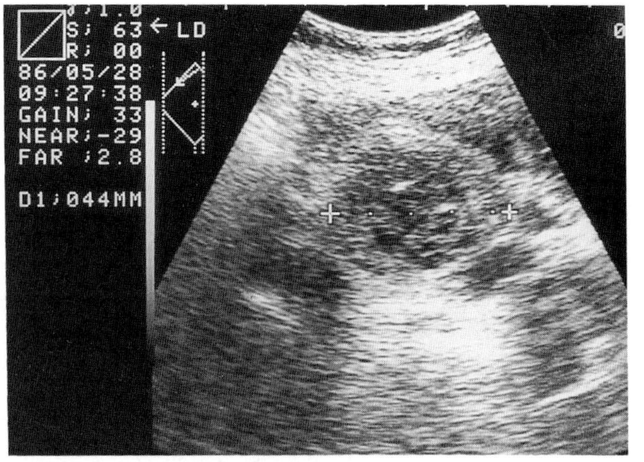

Fig. 1. Ultrasonographic finding of serous cystadenoma in a 71-year-old woman. The tumor showed a low-echoic mass with clear margins

a low-echoic mass with clear margins and a high-echoic area resembling a map inside the tumor [18].

Computed Tomography Findings

The microcystic form of serous cystadenoma has the appearance of a round, homogeneous, low-density mass with clear margins on a precontrast scan. A central stellate scar with a starburst pattern

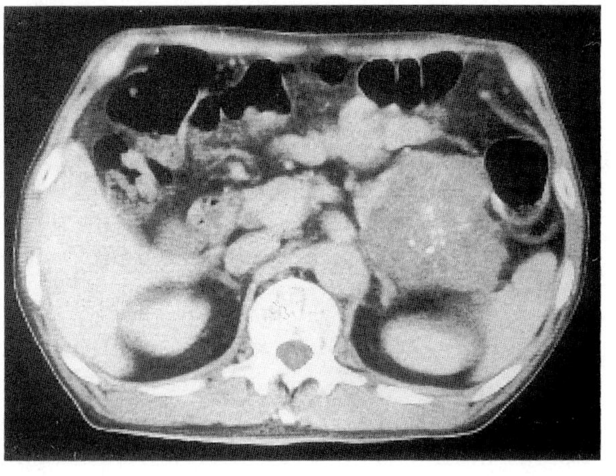

Fig. 2. Computed tomography (CT) findings of a serous cystadenoma in a 71-year-old man. The tumor revealed a low-density mass with a clear margin, and central stellate calcifications. Following the intravenous administration of contrast material, the low-density mass was enhanced and assumed a honeycomb structure

of fine calcifications can be demonstrated in about 20% of the cases. Following the intravenous administration of contrast material, the low-density mass is enhanced and assumes a honeycomb structure (Fig. 2). The macrocystic variant may show a unilocular cyst [1, 2] and may be interpreted as a solitary cyst of other pathology. In a 60-year-old Japanese woman, multiple macrocystic lesions were present in the head of the pancreas with dilatation of the distal common bile duct. Endoscopic retrograde cholangiopancreatography (ERCP), revealed an irregular stricture of the main pancreatic duct and a filling defect in the common bile duct due to the compression of the common bile duct by one of the large cysts [2]. Magnetic resonance imaging is of no additional diagnostic value [16].

Angiographic Findings

Abundant "neoplastic" vessels can be observed in approximately 40% of cases. The feeding arteries are dilated (Fig. 3a) and the surrounding arteries deviate with expansive tumor growth, but encasement of the artery is not found. In the venous phase, the drainage vein is dilated and winds along the surface of the tumor along with prominent tumor staining (Fig. 3b). A macrocystic variant was hypovascular and showed a stricture of the portal vein with no staining [2].

Macroscopic Findings

The microcystic form of serous cystadenomas is usually unifocal with the greatest diameter from 0.5 to 25 cm, with a mean of about 10 cm. The tumor is located more frequently in the body and

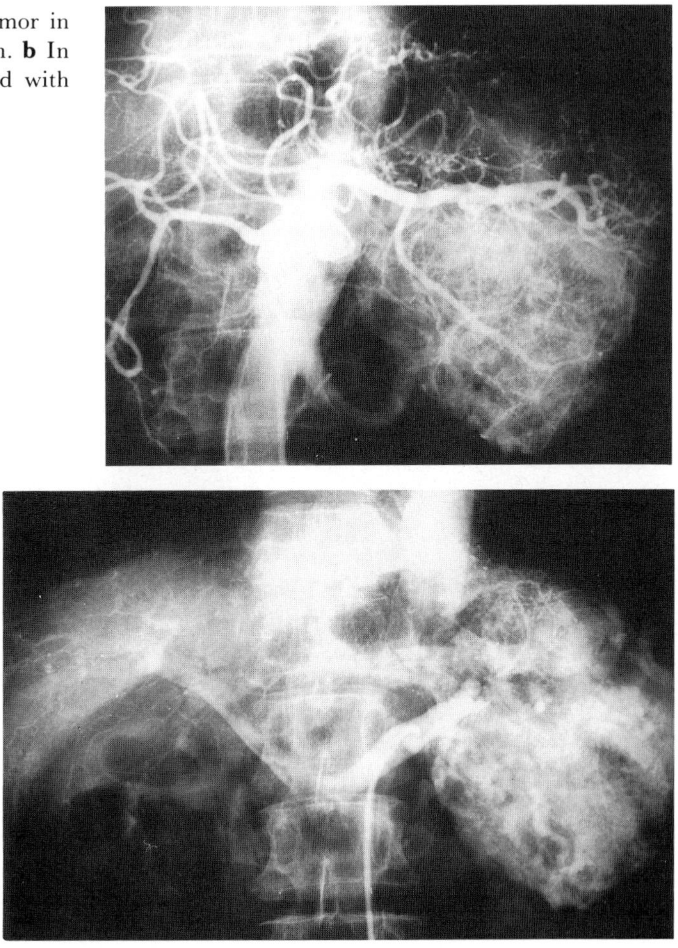

a

b

Fig. 3a,b. Angiographic pattern of the same tumor in Fig. 2. **a** Abundant "neoplastic" vessels are seen. **b** In the venous phase, the drainage vein was dilated with prominent pooling stain tail than in the head of the pancreas. In a series of 40 patients, 17 were located in the head, 5 in the uncinate process, 3 in the neck, 16 in the body, and 6 in the tail; seven of these patients had multiple tumor sites [16]. The location of macrocystic serous cystadenomas was head, body and the uncinate process; head; body and tail; and body [1]. The size of the macrocystic variant ranges between 2.5 to 8 cm, and can compress the common bile duct and cause chronic pancreatitis [2]. The microcystic form is usually a global or ovoid rubbery firm nodule with an irregular nodular external surface. The tumor is brown, grayish-white or grayish-pink. There is a well-defined margin between the tumor and pancreatic parenchymal tissue, with no capsule although a zone of thin fibrous tissue may surround the tumor. In contrast, 4 out of 5 macrocystic variants showed fibrous capsules of 0.2 to 0.5 cm thickness [1]. The microcystic tumor usually consists of multiple spongy cysts, varying from less than 1 mm to several centimeters in diameter. The cysts are separated from one another by connective tissue and usually contain nonviscous clear fluid (Fig. 4). The cysts are often larger peripherally than centrally. Focal hemorrhage or calcification may be observed but usually no necrosis is found.

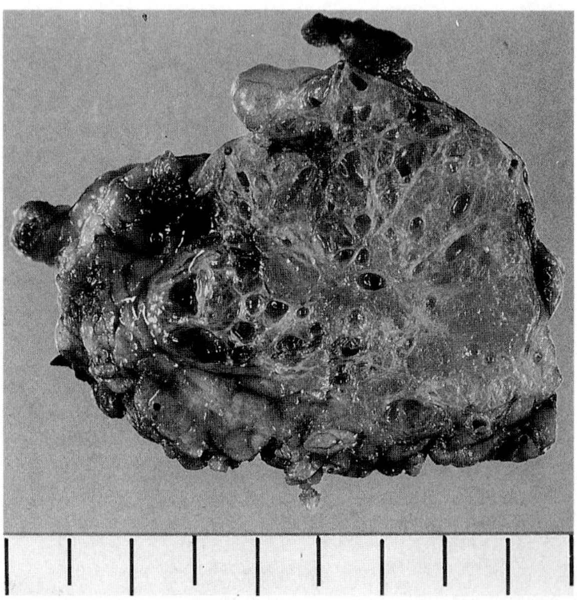

Fig. 4. Gross appearance of a serous cystadenoma in a 81-year-old woman. Sponge-like multilocular cysts separated by radiating fibrous trabeculae are seen on a cut surface

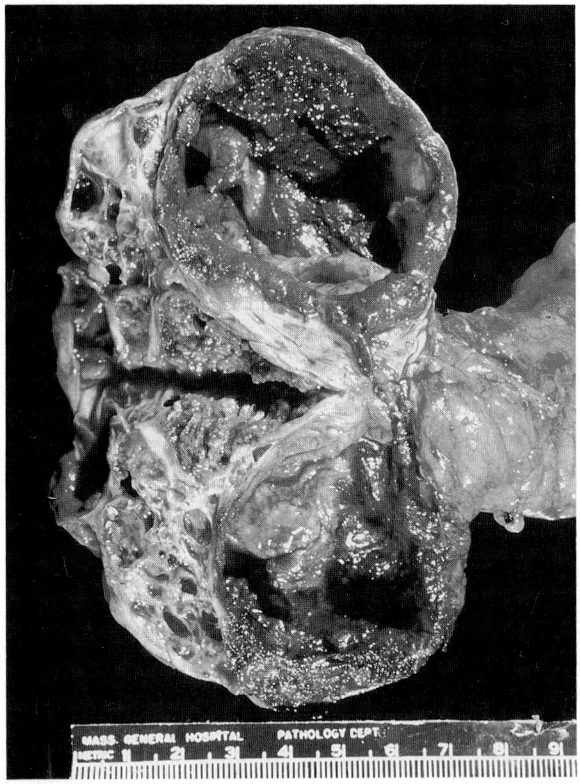

Fig. 5. Gross appearance of a macrocystic serous tumor with a dominant 8.0 cm macrocyst. This 66-year-old woman presented with a 2-year history of upper abdominal fullness. Physical examination revealed a palpable epigastric mass. CT showed a 10- to 15-cm multiseptic mass involving the head, body, and uncinate process of the pancreas. A subtotal pancreatectomy was performed (from [1] with permission). (*For color reproduction see color insert in the frontmatter*)

The macrocystic variant is composed of cystic spaces, ranging from 0.3 to 8.0 cm, often with one large dominant cyst (Fig. 5) filled with turgid, brown watery fluid and semisolid debris. A central stellate scar may not be present and no connection to pancreatic ducts is seen.

Microscopic Findings

The microcystic tumor consists of innumerable small cysts (Fig. 6). Each cyst is lined by a single layer of flat or cuboidal epithelial cells. Papillary tufts (without fibrovascular cores) or true papillae (with fibrovascular cores) are present in some microcystic forms. The macrocystic variant usually contains a large cyst and a few smaller cysts (Fig.

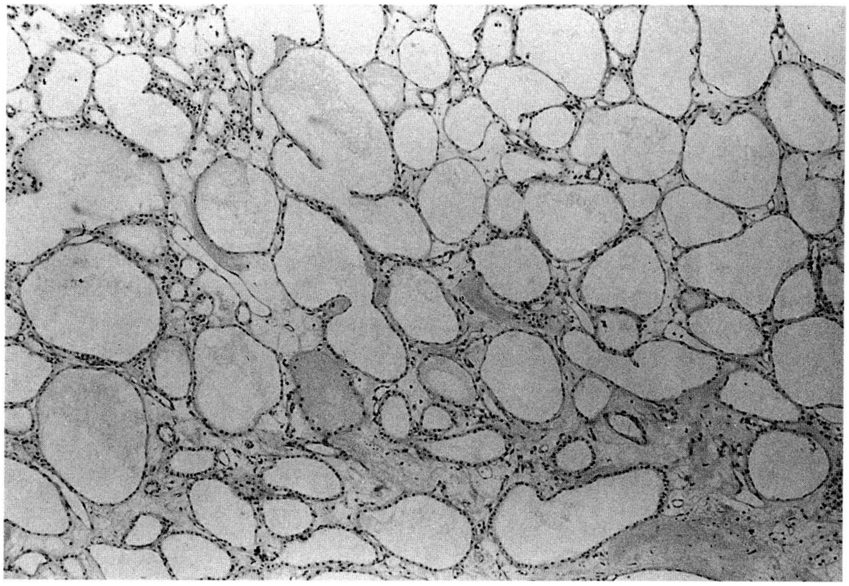

Fig. 6. Microscopic view of the same tumor in Fig. 4. The tumor consists of various sized cysts (×10)

7a) that are not apparent on gross examination. Characteristically, the epithelial linings of the large cysts are denuded (Fig. 7b,c). In one case, 98% denudation of the epithelium was found [1]. Desquamated epithelium and iron-laden macrophages may be found in the lumen of some cysts (Fig. 7c). When an epithelial lining is present, the cells are identical to those seen in the microcystic form.

Serous cystadenoma cells of both forms have clear cytoplasm with centrally located nuclei (Fig. 8). Mitotic figures are absent and there is no cytologic atypia. The nucleoli are indistinct and the chromoplasm is finely granular. The epithelial cells of both tumors possess abundant cytoplasmic periodic acid schiff (PAS)-positive granules that can be completely digested by diastase (Fig. 9). No mucin is demonstrated by special stains. The cysts are separated by collagenous tissue with a capillary network. This stromal component is extremely scant in some areas, while it is abundant and markedly hyalinized in others. The stroma often contains calcification, hemosiderin granules, and cholesterol clefts. Two cases of serous cystadenoma coexistent with ductal adenocarcinoma have been reported so far [12].

Electron Microscopy

The epithelial cells of serous cystadenoma are mostly cuboidal. Nuclei with prominent clumps of chromatin are generally ovoid and the nuclear membrane is smooth. The nucleolus is visible. The cytoplasm contains many glycogen granules and a few mitochondria, lysosomes, and lipid vacuoles. Secretory granules are rarely found (Fig. 10). Desmosomal junctions are present between these cells and microvilli can be seen occasionally. The epithelial cells are separated by a well-developed basal lamina from the underlying stroma. Capillaries and a collagen framework are found in the stroma. Nyongo and Huntrakoon [19] observed myoepithelial cells at the periphery of cuboidal cells, although Shorten et al. [14] could not confirm this finding.

Immunohistochemistry

Only a few immunohistochemical studies have been reported. Shorten et al. [14] reported that monoclonal anticytokeratin, with a broad range of molecular weights (AE1 and AE3) is reactive with the cytoplasm of many epithelial cells lining the cysts. No immunoreactivity was found with anti-carcinoembryonic antigen (CEA), factor VIII-, Uro-2-, Uro3-, or Uro-4-related antigens. Alpert et al. [13] observed a positive staining of the tumor cells for EMA, cytokeratin of lower molecular weight (PKK1), AE1/AE3 and neuron-specific enolase (NSE), but negative reactivity with CEA, chromogranin, insulin, glucagon, somatostatin, vasoactive intestinal peptide (VIP), pancreatic polypeptide (PP), and gastrin [10, 20]. Tumor cells

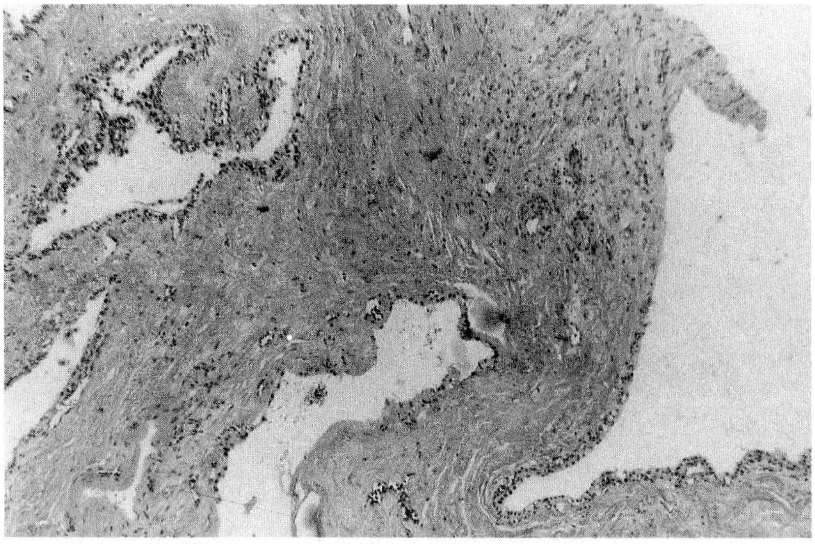

a

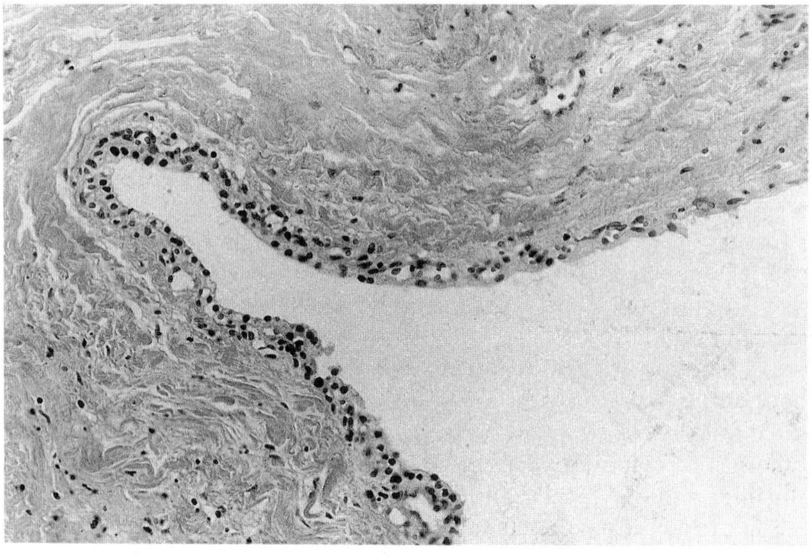

b

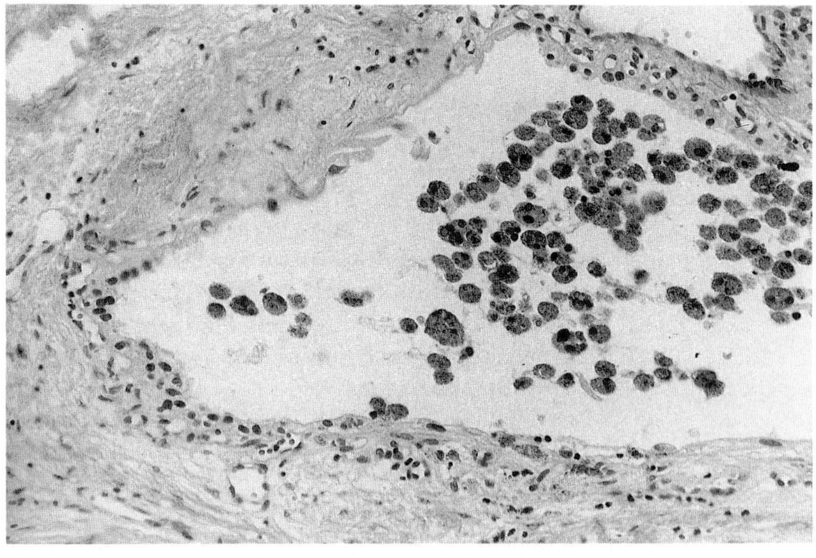

c

Fig. 7a–c. Histological appearance of the tumor shown in Fig. 5. **a** The large cyst (*right*) and the smaller cysts (*left* and *center*) show focal desquamation of the epithelium. The small cysts were macroscopically invisible. Note the abundance of collagen between the cysts. (H&E, ×32). **b** High-power view of the large cyst depicted in **a**. Partial denudation of the epithelium, which is composed of uniform cells with dark nuclei. (H&E, ×210). **c** A small cyst filled with desquamated epithelium and hemosiderin-laden macrophages. Most of the cyst wall is denuded. (H&E, ×210)

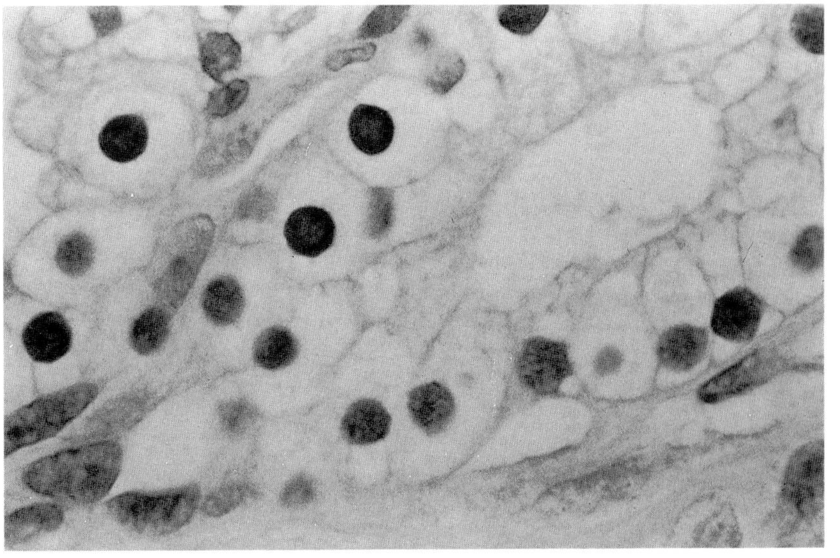

Fig. 8. Cuboidal, polygonal, or occasionally flat epithelial cells of a microcystic form of a serous cystadenoma have clear cytoplasm and round or oval dense nuclei in the center (×400)

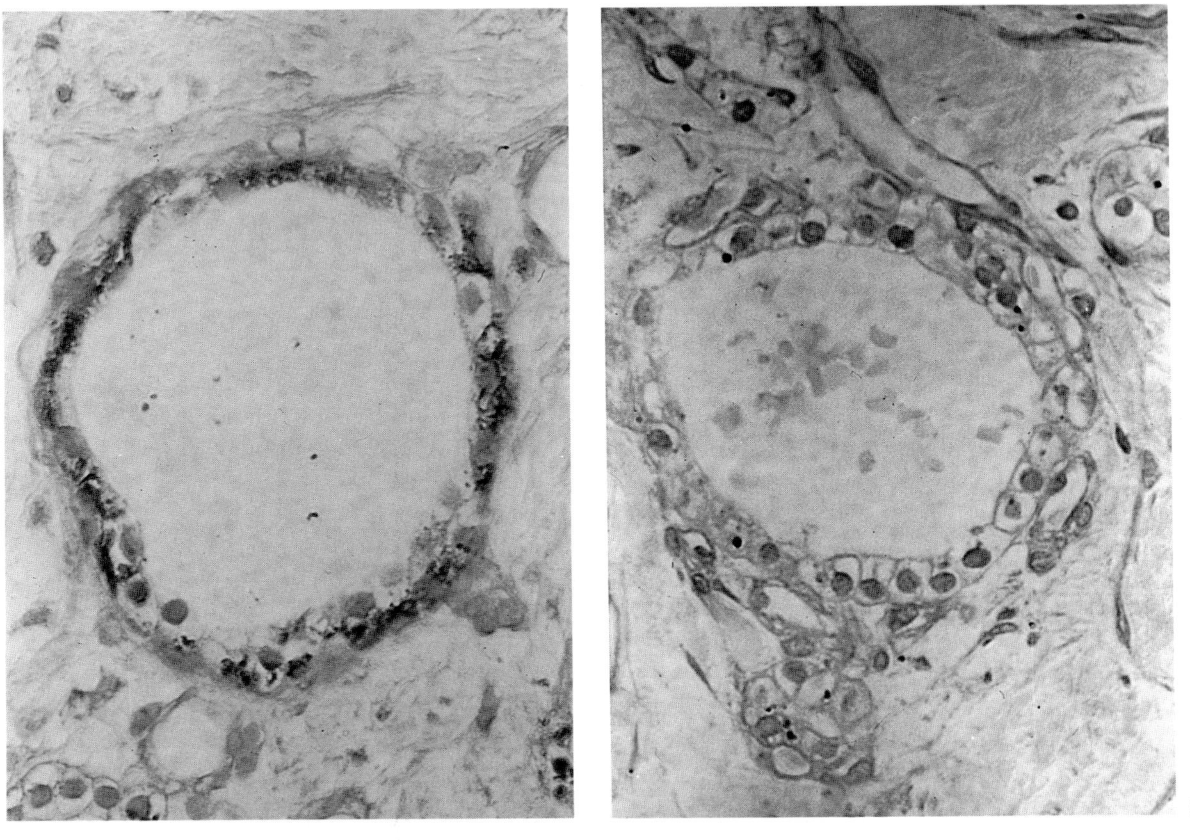

a *b*

Fig. 9.a,b. The same tumor as in Figs. 2 and 3, **a** showing abundant cytoplasmic periodic acid Schiff (PAS)-positive granules, **b** which were completely digested by diastase

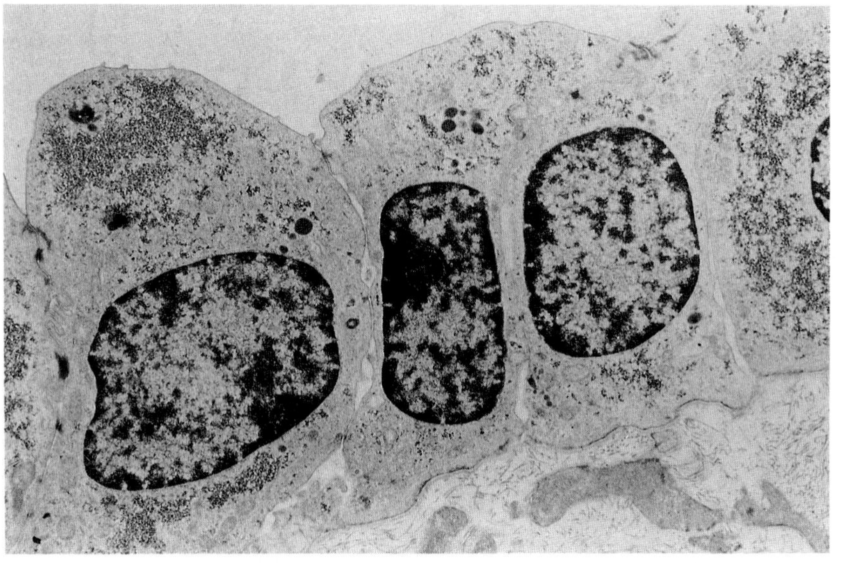

Fig. 10. Electron micrograph of the tumor in Fig. 2. The epithelial cells contain intracytoplasmic glycogen granules (×5000)

stain with anti-CA125, anti-CA19-9 (Fig. 11a), anti-NCC-ST-439 (Fig. 11b) and anti-c-*erb*B-2 antibodies (Fig. 11c). Serous cystadenoma cells stain only on the apical membrane with anti-CA125, anti-CA19-9, and anti-NCC-ST-439 antibodies. A few tumor cells stain with anti-c-*erb*B-2 antibodies (Table 1). Also, in the macrocystic variant, positive staining has been shown for cytokeratin and EMA but not for factor VIII antigen [1].

Table 1. Immunohistochemical findings.

Cases	CEA	CA19-9	NCC-ST-439	C-*erb*B-2
1	—	A	A	—
2	—	A	A	M
3	—	A	A	—
4	—	A	A	—

A, apical side; M, membrane; —, negative.

Nuclear DNA Analysis

Only a limited analysis of the DNA content of the microcystic form of serous cystadenoma has been reported [10, 21]. Unger et al. [21] studied seven serous cystadenomas by flow cytometry. Five cases showed diploid nuclear DNA, and 2 cases had aneuploid nuclear DNA with a DNA index under 1.3. The ratio of S-phase (proliferative activity) ranged from 0.1% to 3.1% in all seven cases. In our four serous cystadenomas [10], tumor cells exhibited diploidy with a DNA index of 1.0. Proliferative indices varied from 4.9% to 20.9%, with a mean of 14.4% (Table 2).

Ag-NOR Expression

We have conducted the only study on argyrophilic nuclear organizer region (Ag-NOR) number [18]

Table 2. Findings of nuclear DNA analysis.

Cases	CV	FPCN	Ploidy pattern	DNA index	Proliferation index
1	8.0	36	Diploidy	1.0	16.9
2	8.0	33	Diploidy	1.0	4.9
3	9.3	34	Diploidy	1.0	20.9
4	9.7	27	Diploidy	1.0	14.9

CV, coefficient of variation; FPCN, first peak channel number.

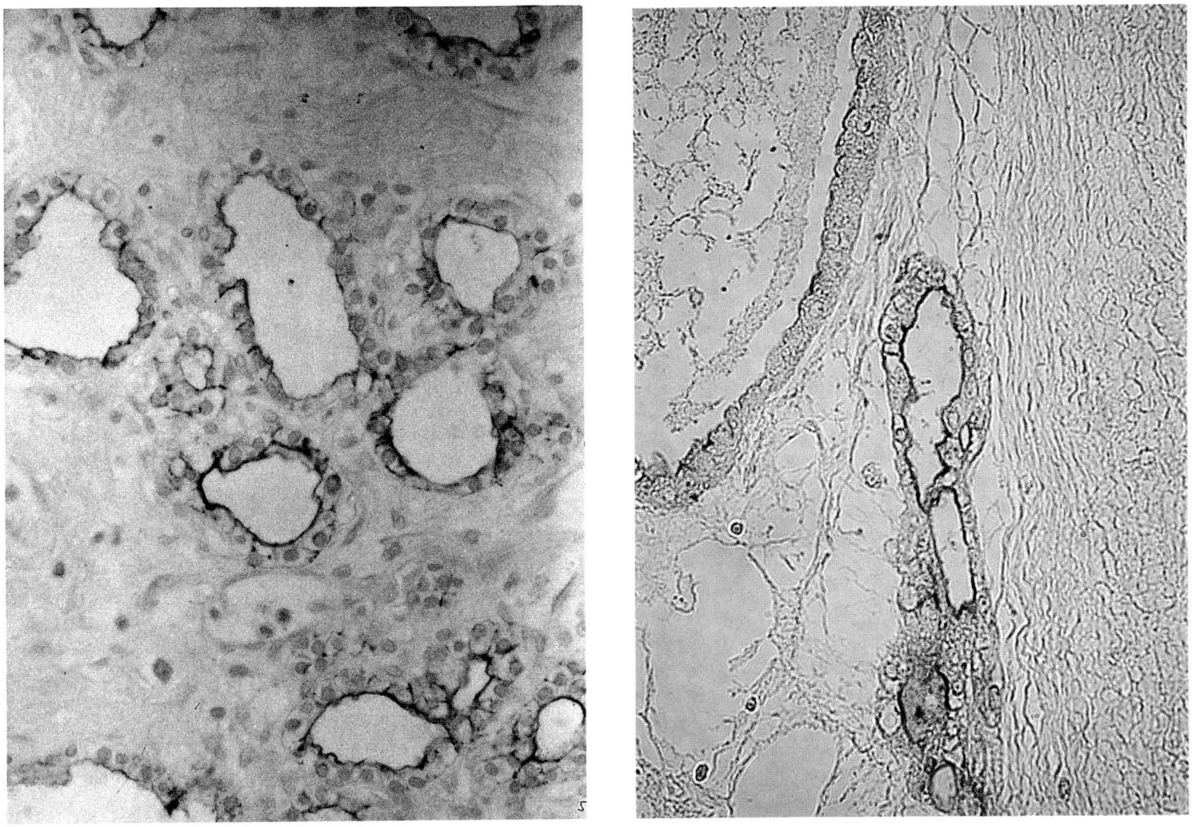

a *b*

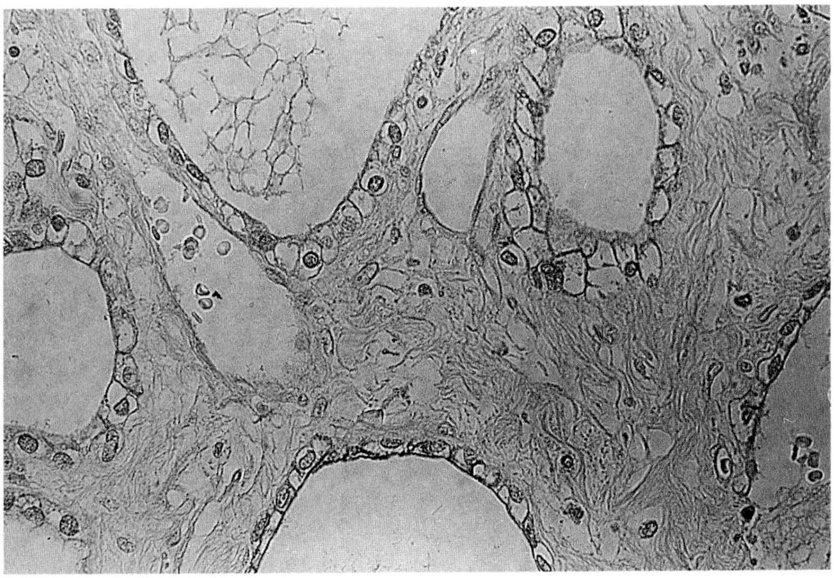

c

Fig. 11.a-c A serous cystadenoma in a 81-year-old woman **a** showing staining with anti-CA19-9 and **b** anti-NCC-ST-439. The tumor cells are stained only on the apical membrane. **c** Anti-c-*erb*B-2 staining shows staining of only a few tumor cells

in the microcystic form of serous cystadenoma (Fig. 12). In four serous cystadenomas, the Ag-NOR number was from 1.75 to 1.93, with an average of 1.85 (Table 3). The average Ag-NOR number was 1.39 in normal pancreatic ductal cells and 3.00 in pancreatic ductal carcinoma cells. The Ag-NOR number of serous cystadenoma cells is significantly higher than that of pancreatic normal ductal epithelium, but lower than that of pancreatic ductal carcinoma cells.

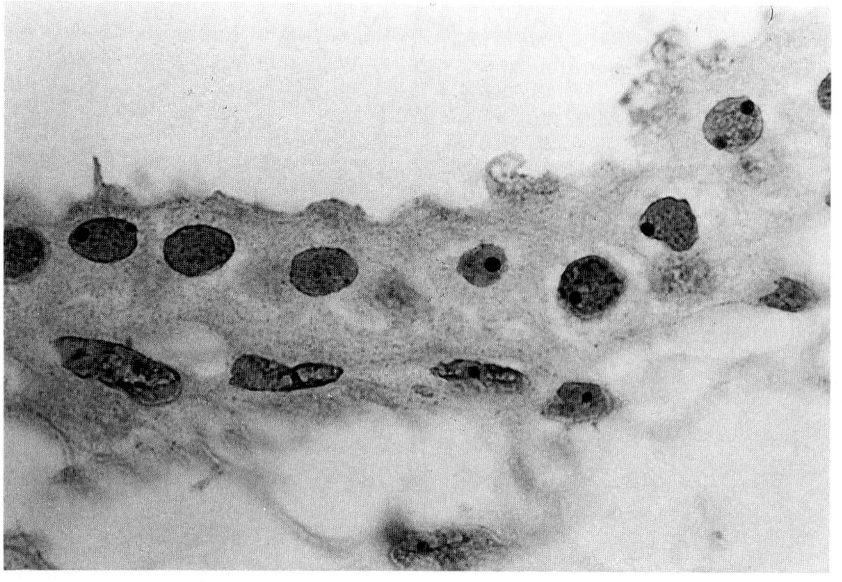

Fig. 12. Demonstration of argyrophilic nuclear organizer regions (Ag-NOR) in the tumor in Fig. 8. The Ag-NOR number was defined as the mean count of black granules in a nuclei of 100 cells

Table 3. Ag-NOR number.

Cases	Number	Standard Deviation	Dispersion
1	1.93	0.70	0.49
2	1.85	0.74	0.55
3	1.87	0.73	0.54
4	1.75	0.74	0.55

Ag-NOR, argyrophilic nuclear organizer regions.

Prognosis

The prognosis of serous cystadenomas is generally favorable. Compagno and Oertel [3] reported on 34 patients with this tumor, including 10 incidental findings at autopsy. Thirteen patients survived 2 months to 25 years. Four of these patients underwent tumor biopsy only, eight partial pancreatectomy, and one pancreatoduodenectomy. Twenty-one of the 34 patients died. Thirteen died of unrelated causes and four had operative deaths (including three of the pancreatoduodenectomy cases). Four died as a result of pancreatic tumors. In the report of Shorten et al. [14], six of eight patients had a long survival, and three were alive postoperatively at 2, 3, and 5 years. Three, in whom only a diagnostic biopsy was made, were alive at 2 years. Yearly CT scans in one biopsy case indicated no change in the tumor. Two patients died, one from chemically induced peritonitis 6 days after local excision of a 2-cm tumor and the other 6 months postoperatively from complications of Hodgkin's disease.

Diagnosis and Differential Diagnosis

The clinical and radiologic features of serous cystadenoma are unreliable in distinguishing this tumor from other types of pancreatic cysts. In a study by Warshaw et al. [22], fully 33% of serous tumors referred to Massachussetts General Hospital had been misdiagnosed as pseudocysts. However, the morphological findings of serous cystadenoma are straightforward. Careful sampling of tissues is required to exclude focal malignancy or the coexisting ductal carcinoma [12]. Differentiation of serous cystadenoma from other cystic lesions, including true congenital cysts (usually small and mostly associated with polycystic disease of other organs), acquired parasitic cysts, enterogenous cysts, dermoid cysts, retention cysts presents no difficulty. The macrocystic form should be distinguished from pseudocysts and the potentially malignant mucinous cystadenoma. The presence of multiloculation on CT is generally reliable for distinguishing serous cystadenoma from pseudocysts because the latter is unilocular. However, a macrocystic variant with a unilocular cyst may mimic the appearance of a pseudocyst. The lack of a central stellate scar or a delicate fibrous septa in macrocystic tumors is similar to mucinous cystic tumors and pseudocysts. The histopathological findings may mimic a pseudocyst when the epithelial lining of the macrocystic form is extensively denuded. This is especially true in frozen sections. In such cases, extensive sampling may be necessary. The presence of glycogen, the lack of mucin and the presence of numerous cysts are the hallmarks of serous cystadenoma. Serous cystadenoma should be distinguished from its malignant counterpart, serous cystadenocarcinoma (see chapter "Serous Cystadenocarcinoma", this volume).

References

1. Lewandrowski K, Warshaw AL, Compton C (1992) Macrocystic serous cystadenoma of the pancreas: A morphologic variant differing from microcystic adenoma. Hum Path 23:871–875
2. Nan Y, Kurimoto K, Nakamura T, Kuno N, Kobayashi S (1993) A case of serous cystadenoma of the pancreas protruding into the common bile duct. J Jpn Pancreas Soc 8:201–206
3. Compagno J, Oertel JE (1978) Microcystic adenomas of the pancreas. A clinicopathologic study of 34 cases. A J C P 69:289–298
4. Kim YI, Seo JW, Suh JS, Lee KU, Choe KJ (1990) Microcystic adenomas of the pancreas. Report of three cases with two of multicentric origin. Am J Clin Pathol 94:150–156
5. Friedman HE (1990) Nonmucinous, glycogen-poor cystadenocarcinoma of the pancreas. Arch Pathol Lab Med 114:888–891
6. George DH, Murphy F, Michalski R, Ulmer BG (1989) Serous cystadenocarcinoma of the pancreas. A new entity. Am J Surg Pathol 13:61–66
7. Kamei K, Funabiki T, Ochiai M, Amano H, Kasahara M, Sakamoto T (1991) Multifocal pancreatic serous cystadenoma with atypical cells and focal perineural invasion. Int J Pancreatol 10:161–172
8. Okada T, Nonami T, Miwa T, Yamada F, Ando K, Tatematsu A, Sugie S, Kondo T (1991) Hepatic metastases of serous cystadenocarcinoma resected 4 years after operation of primary tumors (in Japanese). Jpn J Gastroenterol 88:2719–2723
9. Yoshimi N, Sugie S, Tanaka T, Aijin W, Bunai Y, Tatematsu A, Okada T, Mori H (1992) A rare case of serous cystadenocarcinoma of the pancreas. Cancer 69:2449–2453
10. Kamei K, Funabiki T, Ochiai M, Amano H, Maragami Y, Kasahara M, Sakamoto T (1992) Some considerations on the biology of pancreatic serous cystadenoma. Int J Pancreatol 11:97–104
11. Bogomoletz W, Adent J, Widgren S, Staroll M, McLaughlin J (1980) Cystadenoma of the pancreas: A histological, histochemical, and ultrastructural study of seven cases. Histopathology 4:309–320
12. Montag AG, Fossati N, Michelassi F (1990) Pancreatic microcystic adenoma coexistent with pancreatic ductal carcinoma. A report of two cases. Am J Surg Pathol 14:353–355
13. Alpert LC, Truong LD, Bossart MI, Spjut HJ (1988) Microcystic adenoma (serous cystadenoma) of the pancreas. Am J Surg Pathol 12:251–263
14. Shorten SD, Hart WR, Petras RE (1986) Microcystic adenomas (Serous cystadenoma) of pancreas. Am J Surg Pathol 10:365–372
15. Lo JW, Fung CHK, Yonan TN, Martinez N (1977) Cystadenoma of the pancreas: An ultrastructural study. Cancer 39:2470–2474
16. Pyke CM, VanHeerden JA, Colby TV, Sarr MG, Weaver AL (1992) The spectrum of serous cystadenoma of the pancreas. Ann Surg 215:132–139
17. Naganuma S, Ishida H, Igarashi K, Ohyama Y, Morikawa P, Naganuma T, Hoshino T, Ishioka T, Masamune O (1990) Two cases of serous cystadenoma of the pancreas. Jpn J Med Ultrasonics 17:444–450
18. Funabiki T, Kamei K, Fukui H, Ochiai H, Marugami Y, Suganuma M, Imazu H, Matsubara T, Futawatari H, Hasegawa S (1993) Diagnostic imaging and histopathological findings of the pancreatic serous cystadenoma (in Japanese). Diagnostic Imaging of the Abdomen 13:388–396
19. Nyongo A, Huntrakoon M (1985) Microcystic adenoma of the pancreas with myoepithelial cells. Am J Clin Pathol 84:114–120
20. Kamei K, Horibe Y, Kuroda M, Tashiro K, Kasahara M, Funabiki T, Occhiai M, Amano H, Hosoda Y, Shiina E (1988) Two cases of pancreatic serous cystadenoma (in Japanese). J Jpn Panc Soc 3:569–576
21. Unger PD, Danque PO, Fuchs A, Kaneko M (1991) DNA flow cytometric evaluation of serous and mucinous cystic neoplasms of the pancreas. Arch Pathol Lab Med 115:563–565
22. Warshaw A, Compton C, Lewandrowski K, Cardenosa G, Mueller P (1990) Cystic tumors of the pancreas. Ann Surg 212:432–445

Intraductal Papillary Mucinous Tumors Non-Invasive and Invasive

Intraductal Tumor: Noninvasive and Invasive

Initial studies on premalignant lesions of pancreatic cancer showed that hyperplastic and metaplastic ductal proliferations, including papillary hyperplasia, are often found in association with pancreatic carcinoma [1, 2]. Although subsequent reports have confirmed these observations, it has been established that most of these lesions do not serve as cancer precursors [3–5]. In fact, papillary hyperplasia is now considered to be a nonspecific response of the ductal epithelium to various stimuli, especially ductal obstruction [6]. Only one case of papillary hyperplasia of the pancreas unassociated with preexisting chronic pancreatitis or pancreatic cancer has been reported [7]. Histologically, papillary hyperplasia may involve the intralobular, interlobar, and main ducts. Tall columnar mucin-secreting cells with regular basal nuclei line the papillary projections. Cytologic atypia and mitotic figures are not seen and, therefore, this lesion does not represent a diagnostic problem and should not be confused with intraductal papillary tumor.

Recent efforts to detect early pancreatic carcinoma by endoscopic retrograde cholangiopancreatography (ERCP), computed tomography (CT), and ultrasound (US), or by careful examination of the pancreas at autopsy have resulted in the characterization of papillary intraductal carcinoma.

Definition

Intraductal tumor corresponds well to a tumor of type III cancer of the pancreatographic classification proposed by Ohashi and Takagi [8] in 1980 (Fig. 1). Because they established clinical criteria for this cancer, much information concerning this type of cancer has accumulated and the definition of the tumor has been revised. Currently, the definition of this type of cancer is approached from two points of view: consideration from a clinical standpoint (narrow view) and from a pathological or clinicopathological context (broad view). The narrow view of this cancer was advocated by Ohashi et al. [9]. This definition is based on clinical concepts and, more specifically, on the characteristic features of the papilla of Vater (excretion of mucin through the patulous orifice and accumulation of mucin in the dilated pancreatic duct). The broad view of this cancer is defined pathologically by Kato and Yanagisawa [10] as a "pancreatic cancer with a large volume of extracellular mucin production or retention" or clinicopathologically by Yamao et al. [11] as a "pancreatic cancer in which the mucin produced by the tumor can be clinically or macroscopically recognized." Intraductal mucin hypersecreting tumor is the clinical term (narrow view). The cancer that is defined by the clinicopathological concept (broad view) consists of intraductal papillary cancer of a mucin-producing type, mucinous cystadenocarcinoma, and mucinous adenocarcinoma.

By histology, immunohistochemistry, and intraductal growth pattern, two types of intraductal tumors can be distinguished: intraductal mucin hypersecreting and intraductal papillary neoplasms [12]. These two tumor types may be found together in a single tumor with varying degrees of each [13]. The criterion for a common classification of these tumors is their intraductal growth pattern. There-

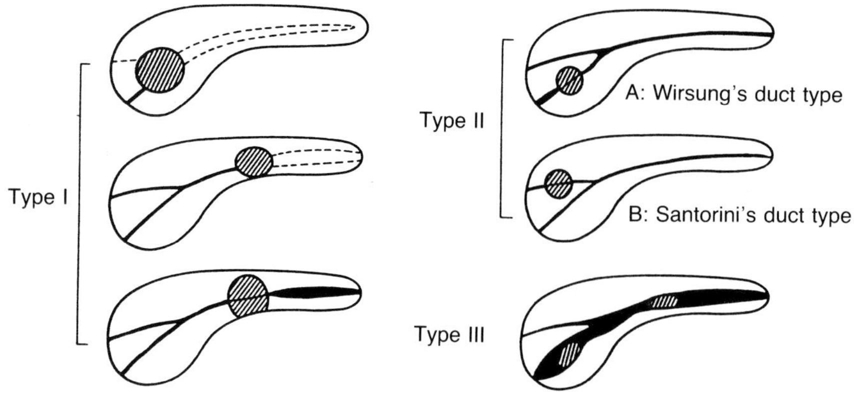

Fig. 1. New classification of endoscopic retrograde cholangio pancreatography findings of pancreatic cancer proposed by Ohashi and Takagi. (From [8], with permission)

fore, the intraductal mucin hypersecreting tumors, intraductal papillary neoplasms, and duct-ectatic type of pancreatic carcinoma [14] represent variants of intraductal tumors and not separate entities. However, most of the intraductal papillary neoplasms that were clinically diagnosed are mucin hypersecreting. Only a few cases with non-duct-ectatic type intraductal papillary tumors were reported [15].

To avoid confusion, the term "intraductal tumor" should be applied to both of these neoplasms and the presence of excess mucin or the predominance of papillary structures should be indicated as an additional characteristic (i.e., intraductal "papillary" and/or "mucin-hypersecreting" tumor). Because even benign-appearing tumors show focal atypia or malignant changes and because the unpredictable biological behavior of this tumor and the presence of c-Ki-*ras* mutation (even in benign-looking epithelia) [16, 17], the term "adenoma" should be reserved for only those intraductal lesions which do not show any cytomorphological and molecular biological evidence for malignancy.

Synonyms and Related Terms

Mucous-secreting cancer [9]; mucin-producing cystic adenocarcinoma [18]; duct-ectatic mucinous cystadenocarcinoma [10]; and mucin-hypersecreting cancer [19] are terms used to describe similar findings, and this has led to a certain amount of confusion.

The spectrum of tumors that show characteristic features of the papilla of Vater and pancreatogram include: mucin-producing tumor [20, 21]; intraductal mucin-hypersecreting neoplasms [13]; intraductal papilloma [12]; villous adenoma of the main pancreatic duct [22]; intraductal cystadenoma [23]; diffuse intraductal papillary adenocarcinoma [24]; diffuse villous carcinoma of the duct of Wirsung [25]; diffuse villous adenoma of the pancreatic duct [26]; and mucinous pancreatic duct ectasia [27].

Incidence

Intraductal tumor (IDT) accounts for 0.5% of pancreatic tumors found at autopsy, 7.5% of clinically diagnosed tumors, and 16.3% of tumors in resected cases [14]. With regard to only resected ductal cancers, IDT comprises from 5.8% [28] to 9.5% [29]. Until the first proposal on a detailed definition of this cancer was presented in 1982, only a few cases were reported in Japan and other countries; however, the number of documented cases has increased remarkably in recent years, especially in Japan. The reason for this increase is unknown, but it might be related to a better understanding of the characteristic clinical features of this tumor and improvement of diagnostic methods such as US, CT, and endoscopic retrograde cholangiopancreatography (ERCP).

Age and Sex

IDT is usually found in the 60–70 year age group. The tumors are most frequently found in the head of the pancreas in men [28, 29], while mucinous cystic neoplasms often occur in the body or tail of the pancreas in middle-aged women. Yamao et al. [29, 30] studied 34 cases with this tumor. The age of the 13 patients with this invasive type (9 men and 4 women) ranged from 50 to 87 years (mean age: 69 years); of 14 patients with noninvasive type (10 men and 4 women), the ages ranged from 47 to 74 years (mean age: 64 years); and of 7 patients with ductal hyperplasia (6 men and 1 woman), the ages ranged from 53 to 71 years (mean age: 63 years). Benign lesions preceded malignant lesions by several years.

Etiology and Pathogenesis

In an analogy to the adenoma-cancer sequence found in mucinous cystic neoplasms [31], the sequence between hyperplasia, adenomatous changes of the pancreatic duct epithelium, and cancerous lesions has been suggested for IDT [29, 32]. However, many authors feel that the benign-appearing epithelium of the mucinous cystic neoplasm is potentially malignant because such "benign" epithelium can be seen in metastatic deposits.

A diversity of opinions exists as to the similarities and differences between IDT and mucinous cystic neoplasm. Table 1 summarizes the similarities and differences between them [33]. Although certain pathological findings are common, differences exist in the location, sex ratio, and macroscopic findings. Because of the predilection of the head of the pancreas in men for IDT and of the morphological differences between IDT and mucinous cystic neoplasm, some authors believe that a clear distinction should be made between the two [34, 35]. Others claim that morphological differences between the two depend mainly on the location of the tumor (Fig. 2) and on the amount of mucus flow into the main pancreatic duct [33, 36]. Thus, if the tumor arises from the main duct (main duct type) or from a branch duct (branch duct type), it develops into IDT; whereas if it originates from a peripheral branch duct (peripheral type), it develops into a mucinous cystic neoplasm. Higa et al. [37] postulated the same situation in appendiceal "mucocele". The hypothesis is supported by: (1) pathological similarities between IDT and mucinous cystic tumors, (2) some morphologically transitional forms between the two (Fig. 3), and (3) the presence of a comparatively high percentage of the communication between cysts and the pancreatic duct in mucinous cystic neoplasm when examined by preoperative and postoperative pancreatogram [29]. Cystic spaces found in IDT are all in the ductal system, usually in the main duct and the subbranches. These spaces still form a continuous tree-like system [32]. Neoplastic or hyperplastic epithelia line the inner surface of these dilated ducts, a finding which suggests that ductal ectasia is attributed to the growth of the lining of cells, which advances in such a way as to extend the ductal surface [32]; however, elevated intraductal pressure from impaction of overproduced mucus may contribute as well. Nevertheless, three-dimensional reconstruction revealed no mechanical obstruction of pancreatic ducts that could cause dilatation [32].

Table 1. Similarity and difference between IDT and mucinous cystic neoplasm (from [33], with permission).

Similar findings
1. Tumors originating from pancreatic duct epithelium
2. High columnar tumor cells with a large amount of mucin production
3. A large amount of mucin macroscopically recognized
4. Tumor consisting of mixture of carcinoma, adenoma and hyperplasia
5. Similar invasive pattern in the form of muconodular carcinoma or tubular adenocarcinoma
6. The existence of precancerous lesions, adenoma-carcinoma sequence
7. Almost the same findings in immunohistochemical and mucous histochemical analysis

Different findings
1. Sex, age, location
2. Macroscopic and pancreatographic appearance

Clinical Presentation

IDT is markedly different from the common type of pancreatic cancer with regard to the patient's symptoms and the clinical course. While the major symptoms include abdominal pain, jaundice, fever, diabetes mellitus, and weight loss, a few patients with IDT are asymptomatic. A history of acute or chronic pancreatitis has been noted in about one-fourth of the patients [38, 39]. In the studies of Yamao et al., [29, 30], jaundice was the most frequent clinical symptom in 9 of 13 cases (70%) with the invasive type, while abdominal pain was a complaint in 4 of 6 cases (67%) with the non-invasive (carcinoma in situ) type. Icterus was closely related to the invasive type with parenchymal invasion when it was located in the head of the pancreas or when the tumor extended into the common bile duct or ampulla of Vater. Episodes of jaundice may also result from detachment of the papillary structures with subsequent biliary obstruction [35]. In the noninvasive type, two-thirds of the patients were asymptomatic, and most of the

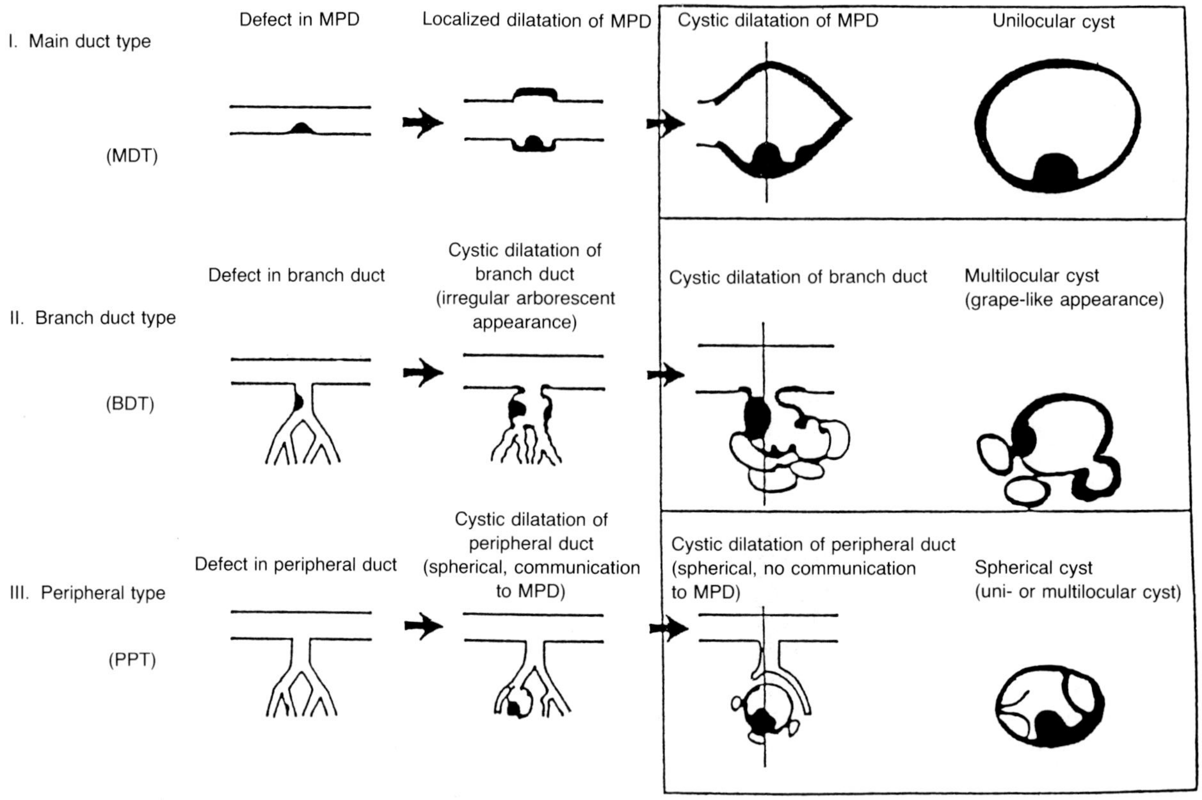

Fig. 2. Pancreatographic findings in the case of intraductal mucin-hypersecreting pancreatic tumor. The change seems to depend upon the site of the tumor growth and the stage of the tumor

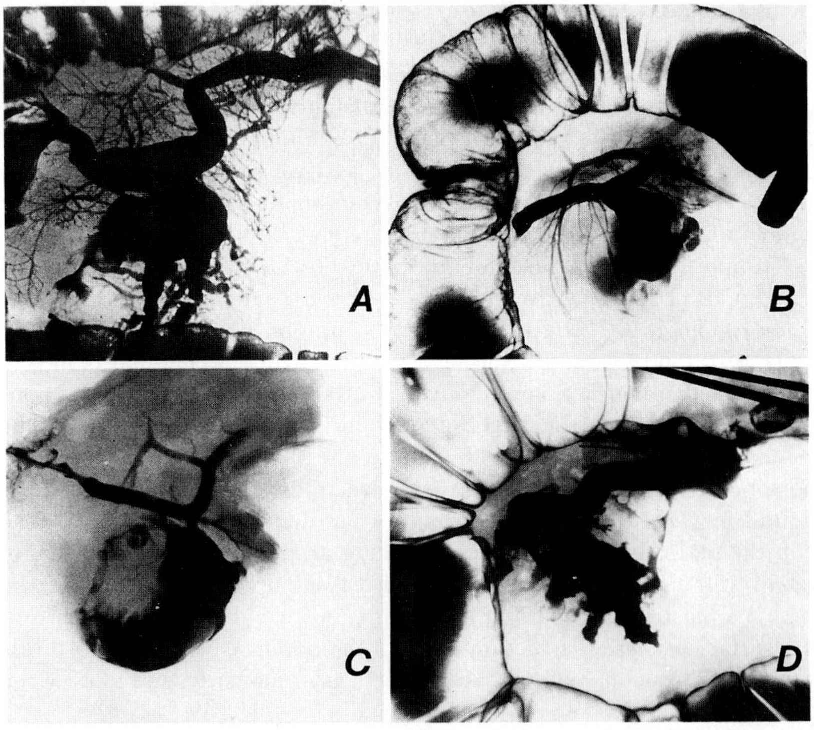

Fig. 3A–D. A Intraductal papillary tumor (duct-ectatic mucinous cystadenoma). ***B*** Mucinous cystadenoma, grape-like appearance. Intermediate type on pancreatogram between ***A*** and ***C***. ***C*** Mucinous cystadenoma, spherical cyst. ***D*** Intraductal tumor (duct-ectatic mucinous cystadenocarcinoma)

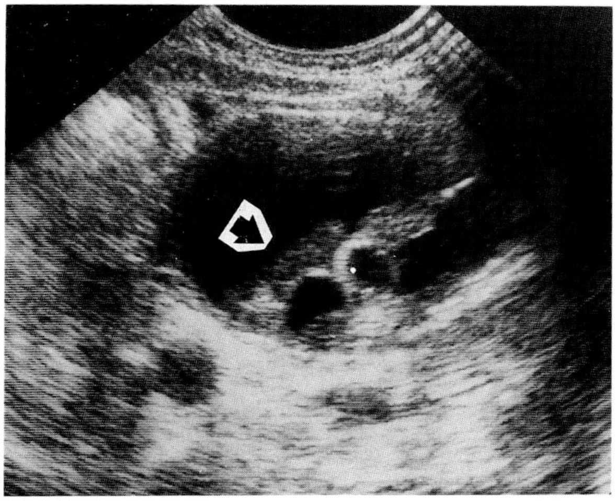

Fig. 4. Invasive intraductal papillary tumor with liver metastasis in a 41-year-old woman with a complaint of anorexia. Ultrasonography showed a multilobular cyst with mural nodule (*arrow*)

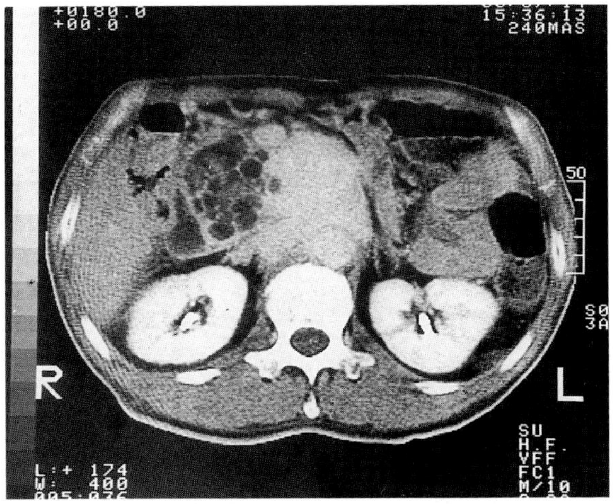

Fig. 5. Invasive intraductal tumor in a 60-year-old man with a complaint of body weight loss. Computed tomography showed multilobular cysts with wall thickenings in the head of the pancreas. Solid part of this tumor adjacent to the cystic area, invaded to the retroperitoneum and abdominal aorta

tumors were found by a routine checkup or at autopsy.

Diagnosis

Generally, there are no specific laboratory findings. Some studies have demonstrated elevated levels of serum amylase or elastase 1, which may contribute to the early detection of this tumor [28, 29].

Plasma CA19-9 showed a positivity of 29% in the noninvasive type of IDT and of 44% in the invasive type [40]. The respective rates for the positivity of carcinoembryonic antigen (CEA) were 12% and 50%.

The imaging modalities useful for the diagnosis of this tumor include abdominal echography (44%), and computed tomography (22%) [41]. Abdominal echography has contributed much to its detection and ERCP is effective for the definitive diagnosis of this tumor [41]. Characteristic findings obtained by US or endoscopic ultrasonography (EUS) are: (1) dilatation of the main pancreatic duct, (2) a multilobular cyst, (3) a solid tumor, mural nodule, or localized wall thickening, and (4) a mucus echo. US or EUS show irregularity of the wall of the pancreatic duct or a thickened septum-like structure. The most important findings for differential diagnosis between the noninvasive and the invasive type of this tumor are the presence or absence of a solid mass (low or mixed echo pattern) or a mural nodule (hyperechoic mass) in the dilated duct or cyst (Fig. 4).

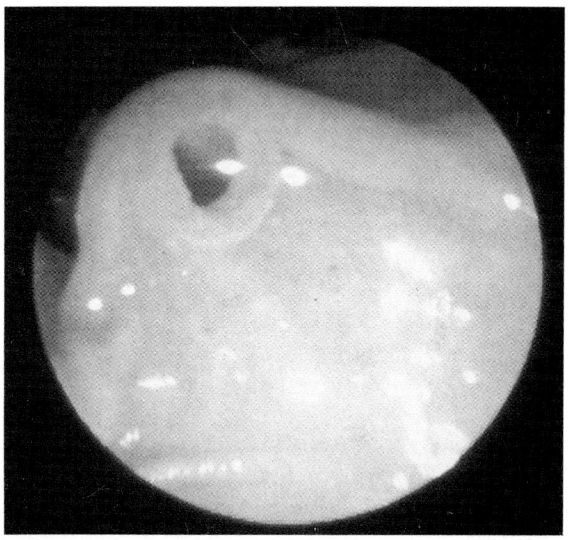

Fig. 6. Intraductal papillary adenocarcinoma in a 61-year-old man with a complaint of epigastralgia. Duodenoscopy revealed characteristic features of this tumor: enlargement of the papilla, widely opened orifice of the papilla, and mucus excretion from the orifice. (*For color reproduction see color insert in the frontmatter*)

CT shows almost the same features as those obtained by US. Enhanced CT scans, especially dynamic scans, are useful for the diagnosis of

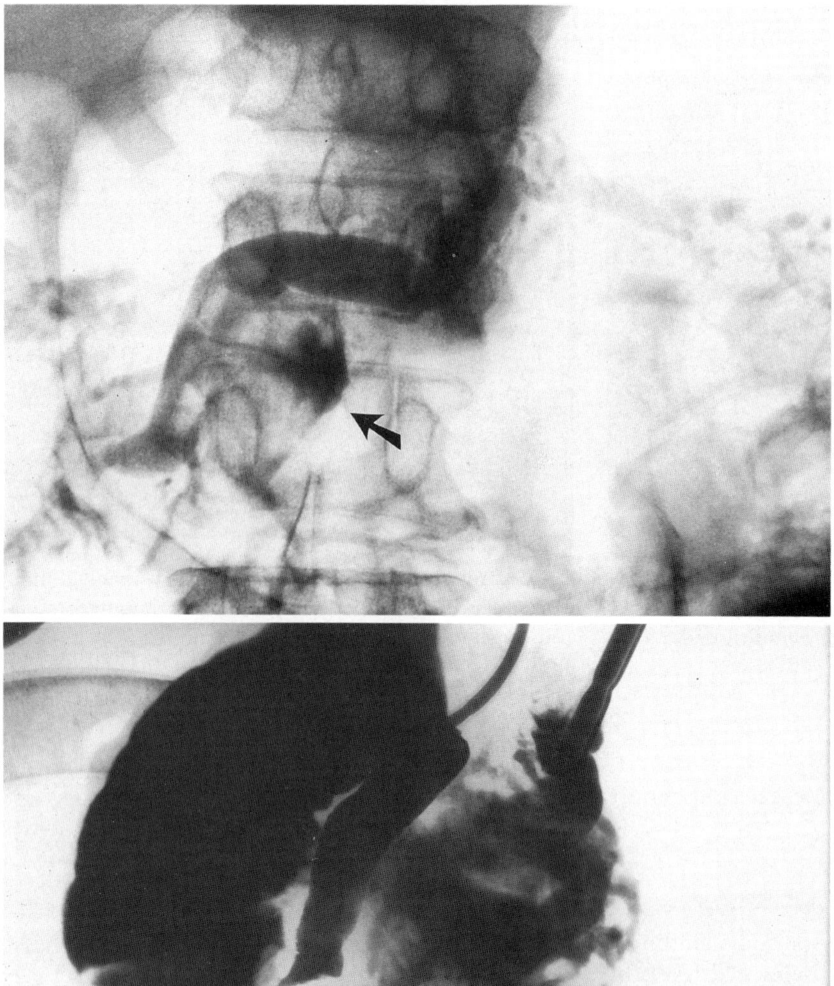

A

B

Fig. 7A,B. Intraductal tumor (*IDT*) in a 70-year-old man with a complaint of abdominal pain and backache. ***A*** Endoscopic retrograde cholangiopancreatography demonstrated remarkably dilated main pancreatic duct and inferior branch duct (*arrow*) with filling defect. ***B*** A typical pancreatogram of the IDT

the extrapancreatic tumor extension and for the determination of operability (Fig. 5).

ERCP findings are the most characteristic and conclusive. In the mucin-producing type, duodenoscopy at the time of ERCP shows characteristic enlargement of the papilla, the widely opened orifice of the papilla, and mucin excretion from the orifice (Fig. 6). Characteristic features are sometimes seen at the site of the accessory papilla.

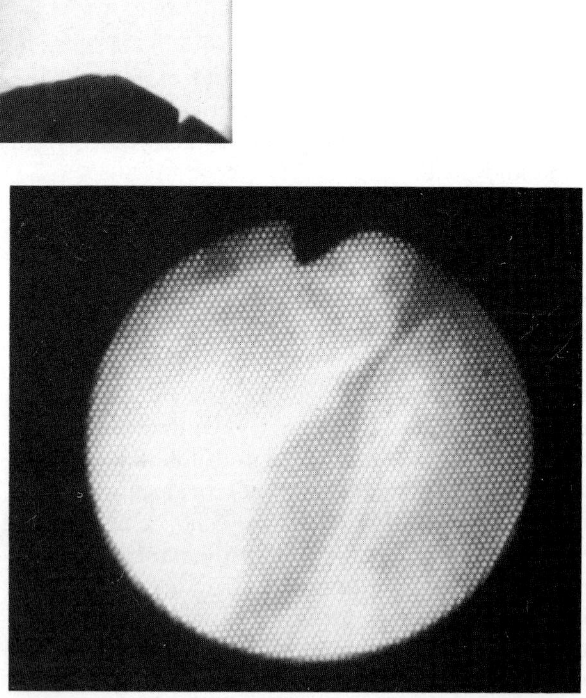

Fig. 8. Invasive type of intraductal tumor in a 70-year-old man with a complaint of jaundice. Peroral transpapillary pancreatoscopy showed papillary tumor (fish-egg-like appearance) in the main pancreatic duct. (*For color reproduction see color insert in the frontmatter*)

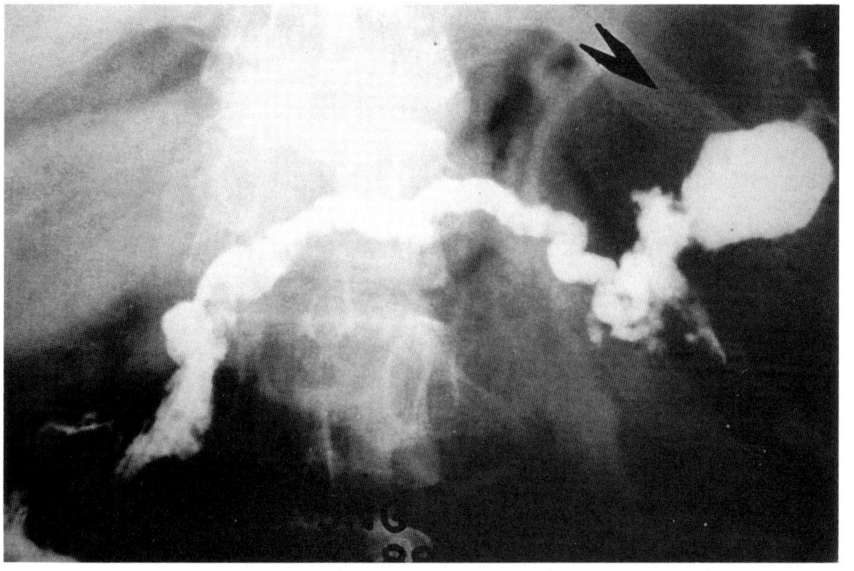

Fig. 9. Retrograde cholangiopancreatography showing uniform dilatation of the main pancreatic duct with a cystic dilatation in the tail (*arrow*). A lesser concentration media is seen in the cephalic portion of the duct. (From [35], with permission)

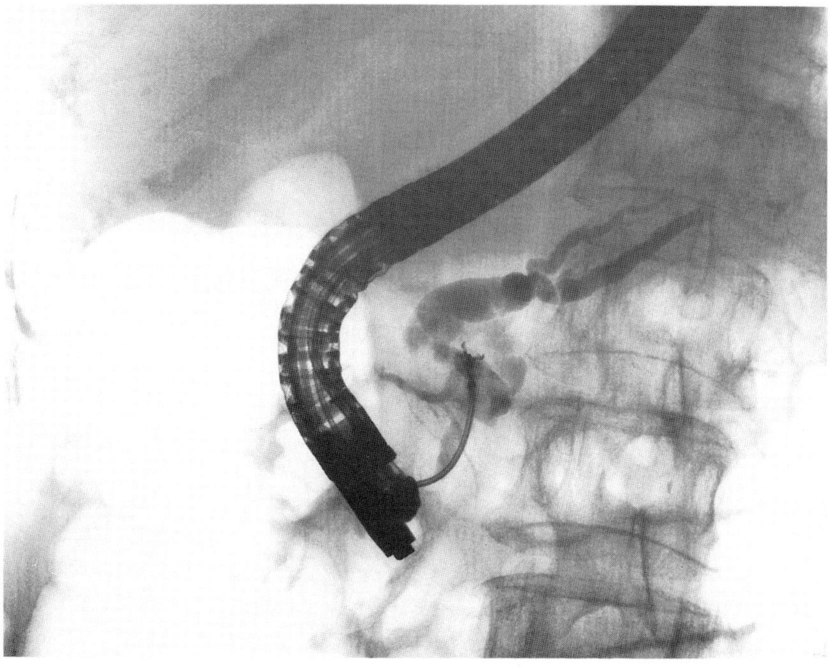

Fig. 10. Endoscopic transpapillary pancreatic duct biopsy. Biopsy forceps are introduced to the target point in the dilated branch duct under fluoroscopic guidance after endoscopic retrograde cholangiopancreatography

Pancreatograms reveal dilatation of the main pancreatic duct (main duct type) and cystic dilatation of its branches (branch duct type). A filling defect caused by mucus or a tumor can be seen in the dilated main duct or in its branches (Fig. 7). In the predominantly papillary type, the main pancreatic duct is found uniformly dilated (Fig. 9).

In the main duct type, peroral transpapillary pancreatoscopy (POPS) shows a papillary tumor with a "fish egg" appearance (Fig. 8), granular mucosa, polyp, or rough mucosa. In the branch duct type, the existence of mucin can be seen, but no tumor in the main duct can be observed. POPS can make a differential diagnosis between tumors and chronic pancreatitis and reveal intrapancreatic growth of the tumor [23, 30].

Percutaneous biopsy under ultrasonic guidance or the laparoscopic method for pancreatic biopsy is hazardous, because the leakage of the mucin from the puncture site may cause pseudomyxoma peritonei. Transpapillary biopsy (Fig. 10) and cytology are somewhat effective with the main duct

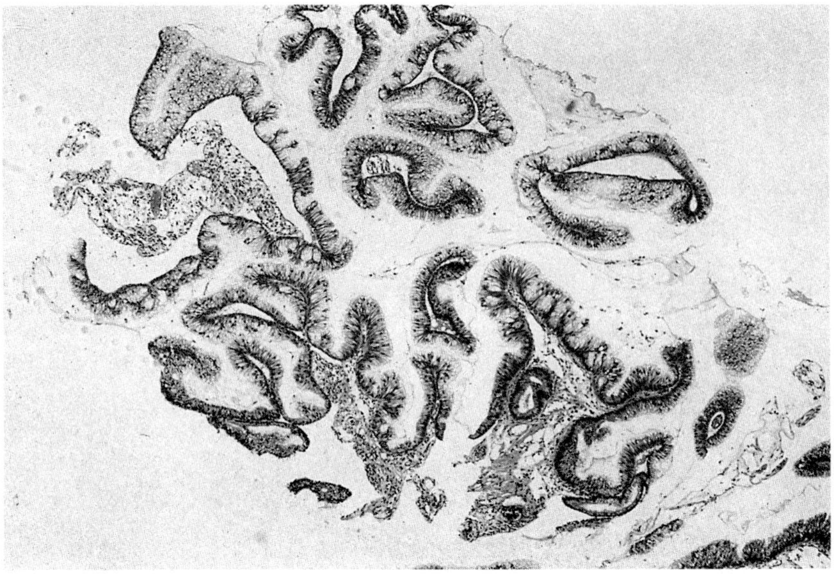

Fig. 11. Invasive form of intraductal tumor. Transpapillary pancreatic biopsy shows papillary projections of tall columnar epithelium with various kinds of cellular atypism. (H&E ×40)

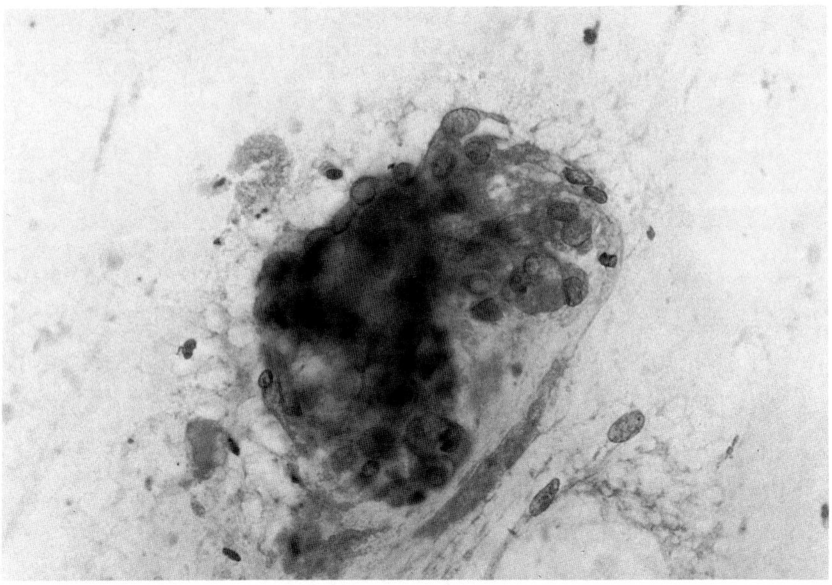

Fig. 12. Transpapillary brushing cytology reveals papillary clump of atypical columnar cells. The nuclear polymorphism is also seen (Papanicolou stain, ×200)

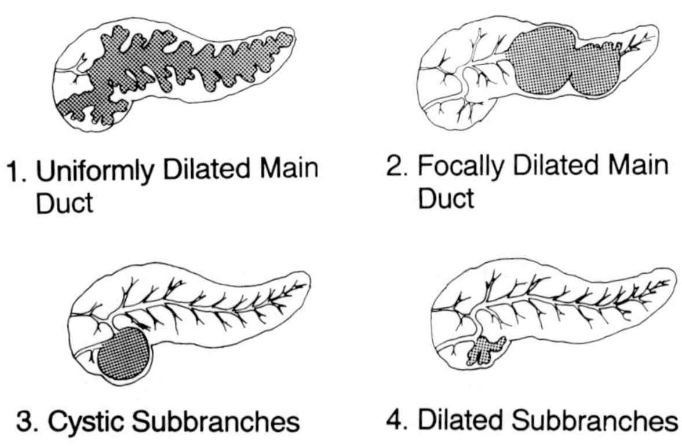

Fig. 13. Classification of intraductal tumor of mucus-hypersecreting type based on gross features. (From [32], with permission)

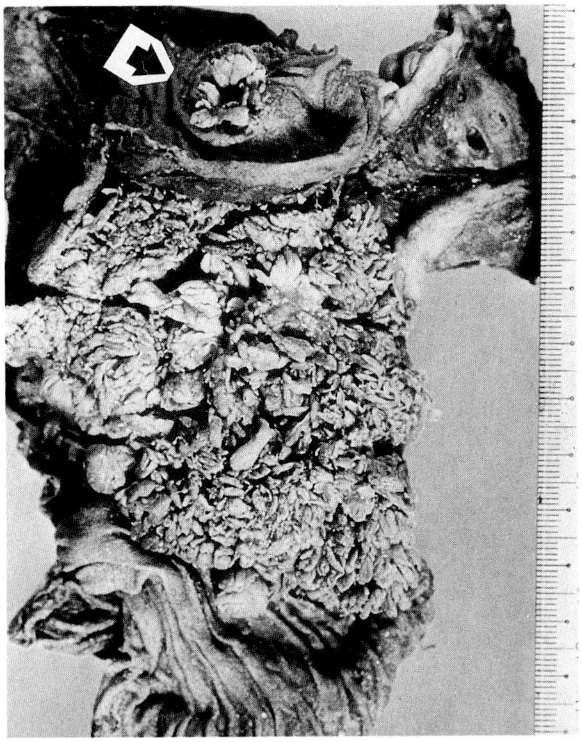

Fig. 14. Invasive type of intraductal tumor, main duct type in a 72-year-old man with a complaint of peripheral edema. Villous tumor filled the dilated main duct and inferior branch duct in the pancreatic head. Papillary growth of tumor perforated into the duodenal lumen from the dilated pancreatic duct (*arrow*)

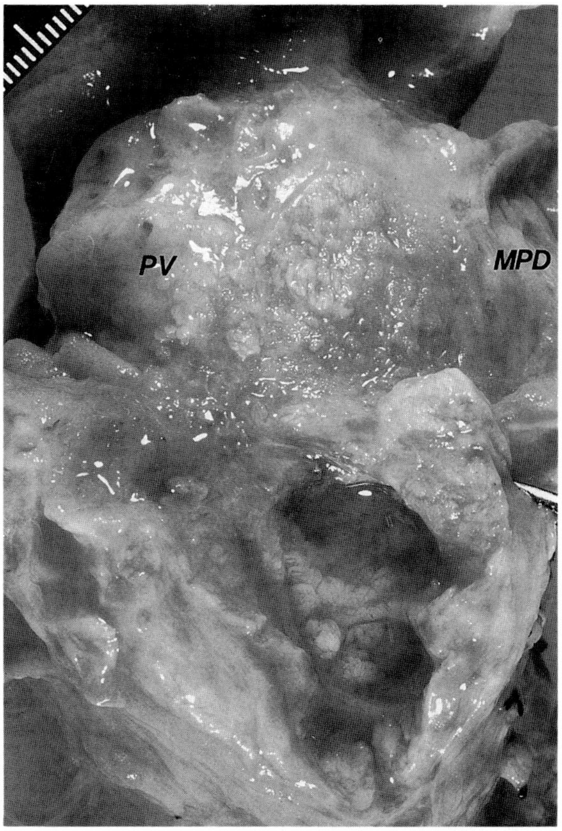

Fig. 15. Non-invasive intraductal tumor, branch duct type in a 74-year-old man with a complaint of diarrhea. Macroscopic examination revealed polyposis in the dilated inferior branch duct and a granular mucosa that extends from the branch to the dilated main pancreatic duct. *PV*, papilla of Vater; *MPD*, main pancreatic duct. (*For color reproduction see color insert in the frontmatter*)

type and the branch duct type in which the tumor has spread into the main pancreatic duct (Figs. 11 and 12). The positive rate of malignancy detection with these techniques is only 50% or below [40]. The reasons are: (1) highly differentiated cellular patterns, and (2) intratumor heterogeneity from mild to severe atypia within the same tumor.

Angiography rarely shows abnormal images when a tumor (or cyst) is small in size and localized only within the pancreatic duct epithelium. As the tumor (cyst) grows, abnormal findings such as stretching and displacement of intrapancreatic or peripancreatic vessels may be observed. Once the tumor invades into the pancreatic parenchyma, encasement of the intrapancreatic arteries, as seen in the common type of ductal cancer, is found.

Gross Findings

It is rather difficult to differentiate between noninvasive and invasive types of IDT if there are no massive invasions.

Noninvasive Type of Intraductal Tumor. The cut surface of the main duct type in the noninvasive type (adenoma, carcinoma in situ) reveals an extremely dilated main pancreatic duct. In the predominantly papillary type, the pancreatic duct is partially or completely filled with a papillary or granular gray-white mass, which may spread into the common bile duct and ampulla of Vater. The distal portion of the main pancreatic duct is often dilated, tortuous, and sometimes even cystic [35]. In the mucin-hypersecreting type, grape-like clusters of cystic branch ducts filled with mucin are observed in the branch duct type [11, 29; Fig. 3B]. Tumors with remarkably dilated main ducts are often misdiagnosed as mucinous cystic tumors connected to the pancreatic duct because there are almost no pathological differences between a large cyst and

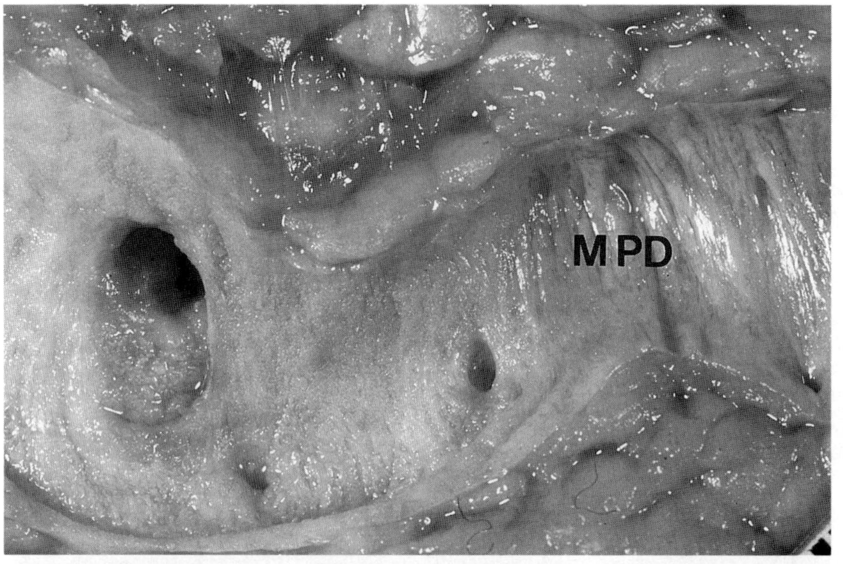

Fig. 16. Intraductal tumor, main duct type in a 71-year-old man without symptoms. A granular mucosa extends from the dilated main duct to the branch ducts. Distended orifice of the branch ducts can be observed. *MPD*, main pancreatic duct. (*For color reproduction see color insert in the frontmatter*)

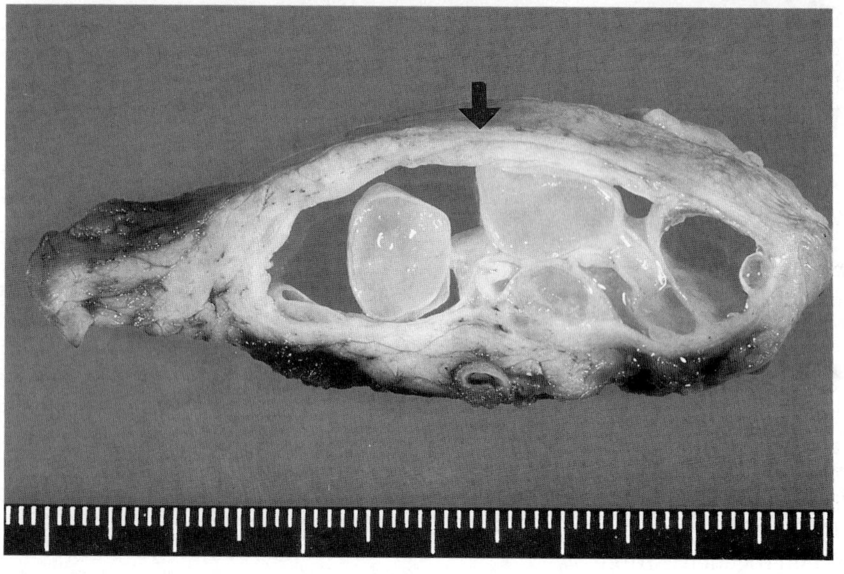

Fig. 17. Classical type of mucinous cystic tumor, non-invasive in a 37-year-old woman without symptoms. The cut surface of the tumor shows multilocular cyst. Thick fibrous capsule which surrounds the whole cyst is seen (*arrow*). (*For color reproduction see color insert in the frontmatter*)

the dilated main duct. In this situation, a pancreatogram is useful for making the correct diagnosis. Three-dimensional reconstruction of 12 IDTs [31] disclosed the following 4 types: type 1, uniformly dilated main duct; type 2, focally (or segmentally) dilated main duct; type 3, cystic subbranches; and type 4, dilated subbranches (Fig. 13).

The inner surface of the dilated pancreatic duct may display papillary excrescences: villous tumor (Fig. 14), polypoid tumor, granulous mucosa (Fig. 15), localized mucosal thickenings, or rough mucosa (Fig. 16). The more visible the papillary projections, the greater the possibility of malignancy.

A thick fibrous capsule surrounding the whole cyst can be seen in mucinous cystic neoplasms [10] (Fig. 17), whereas such a capsule is missing in the branch duct type of IDT.

Invasive Type of Intraductal Tumor. Macroscopically, an IDT with minimal invasion (intraductal "papillary" and/or "mucinous" carcinoma) presents findings similar to the noninvasive type. On the other hand, the cut surface of some areas of the invasive type is poorly demarcated and may show a soft, medullary, yellowish-white mass (Fig. 18), different from the appearance of a common type of cancer which presents a hard, scirrhous, white

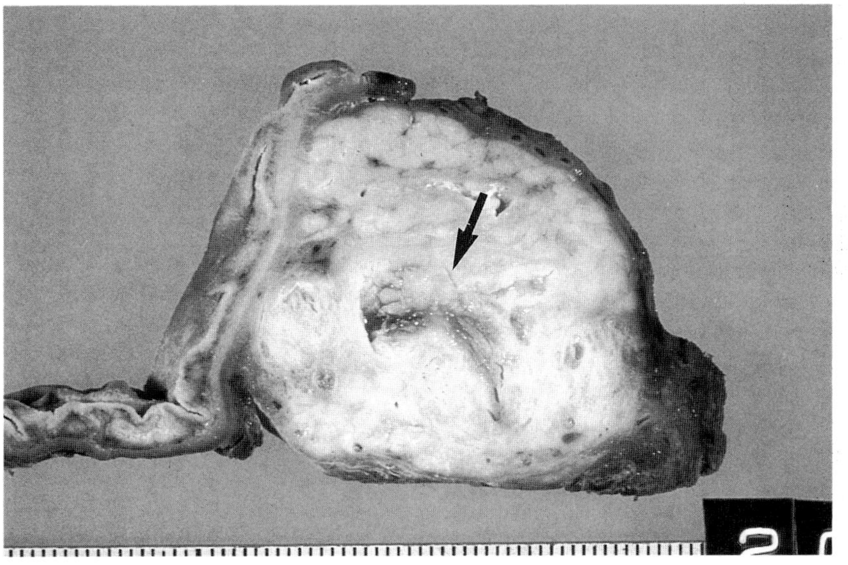

Fig. 18. Invasive type intraductal tumor in a 59-year-old man with a chief complaint of jaundice. He died of cancer recurrence within a year after operation. Lower half of the tumor shows a soft, medullary, yellow-white mass. Papillary tumor is present in the dilated main pancreatic duct and branch ducts (*arrow*). (*For color reproduction see color insert in the frontmatter*)

mass [29, 30]. Papillary configuration is also seen in the invasive type.

Both invasive IDT and the mucinous cystic neoplasm [18, 43], when located in the head of the pancreas, can cause a fistula into the bile duct (Fig. 19), duodenum, and stomach at a rate of about 10%. No benign cases with perforation into these three tissues have been reported. Lymph node metastases may occur, but are less frequent in IDT than in the common type of pancreatic ductal adenocarcinoma.

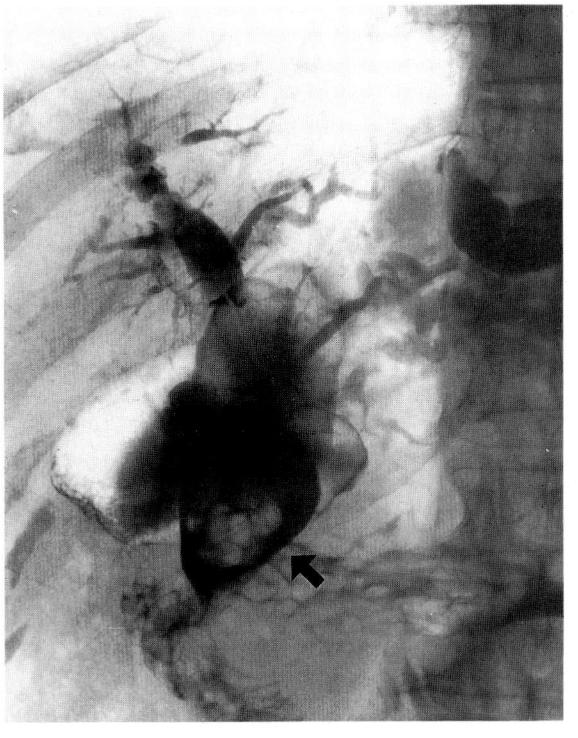

Fig. 19. Invasive form of intraductal tumor in an 80-year-old woman with a complaint of jaundice. Cholangiography revealed a large amount of mucus (*arrow*), which flowed into in the common bile duct through a fistula from the pancreatic duct

Microscopic Features

Noninvasive Type of Intraductal Tumor. In the noninvasive type of IDT, the tumor is confined within the duct, and tumor cells either appear normal (adenoma) or malignant (carcinoma). Because IDT may be multifocal and may show different histopathological features ranging from benign to dysplastic, atypical, and malignant changes in different foci, the term intraductal adenoma should be employed only after extensive sampling. The term "intraductal (papillary) carcinoma," or "carcinoma in situ" may be applied to the malignant changes confined to the lining of the epithelium.

In the predominantly papillary type, numerous papillary projections obstruct the lumen of the main pancreatic duct or its branches (Fig. 20). Focal intraluminal bridging results in a cribriform pattern reminiscent of breast carcinoma (Fig. 21).

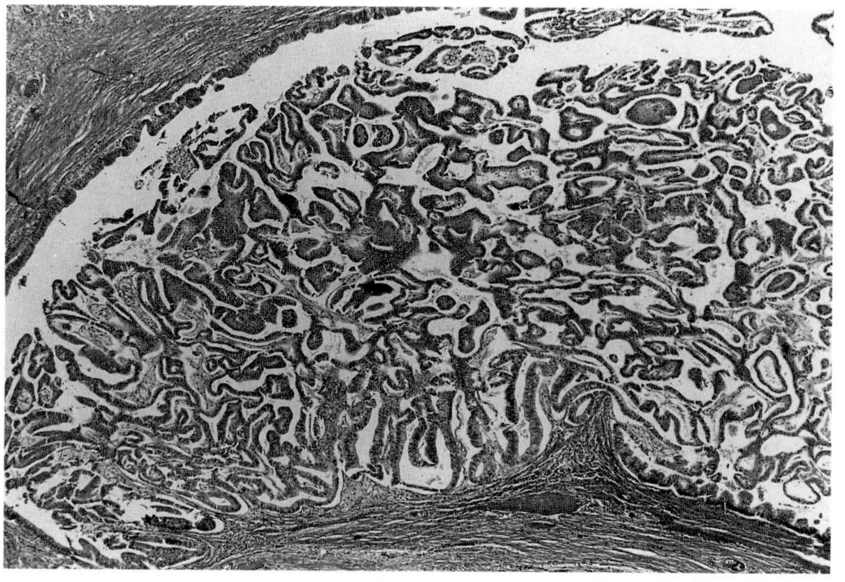

Fig. 20. Main pancreatic duct distended and filled with intraductal papillary structure. Flat epithelium is seen in the *left upper* portion of the photograph. (From [35] with permission)

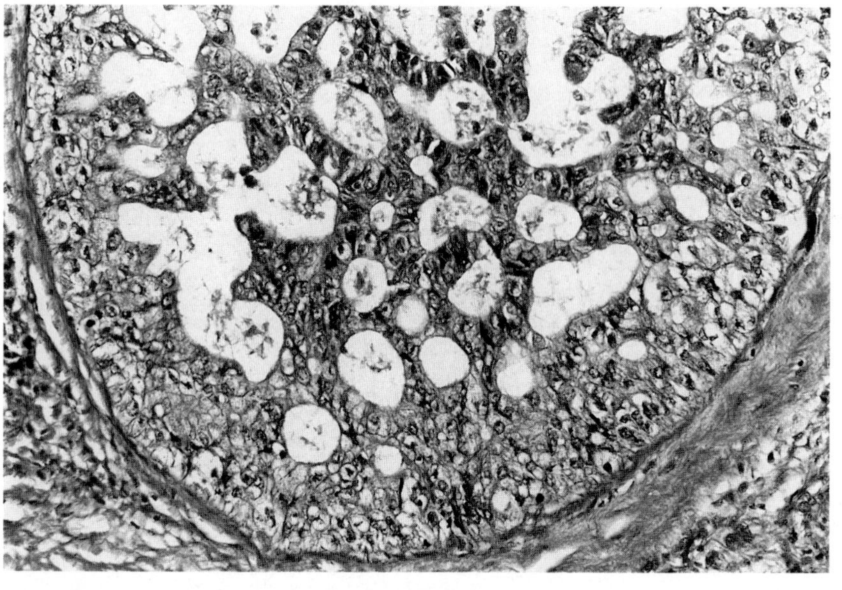

Fig. 21. Prominent epithelial bridging resulting in a cribriform pattern reminiscent of breast carcinoma (H&E ×400). (From [35], with permission)

Central necrosis rarely gives rise to a comedo carcinoma pattern (Fig. 22). These three growth patterns usually coincide in different areas of the same tumor. Often, there is a sharp transition between normal or hyperplastic to neoplastic ductal epithelium (Fig. 23). Most neoplastic cells are cuboidal or columnar and contain hyperchromatic or vesicular nuclei and a variable amount of mucin. Columnar cells, with elongated pseudostratified nuclei and without cytoplasmic mucin resembling those of colonic adenocarcinomas, predominate in some tumors. Goblet and Paneth cells have also been described [35]. The appearance of tumor cells ranges from atypical to clearly malignant (Fig. 24). Mitotic figures are not common. Tumors showing minimal cytologic atypia and few mitosis have been interpreted in the past as papilloma or papillomatosis [43]. Areas of carcinoma in situ in smaller ducts can be demonstrated and most likely present multifocality (Fig. 25).

In the mucin-hypersecreting type, dilated main pancreatic duct and branch ducts contain a large amount of sticky mucin. As in benign cases, most cells in malignant cases have a benign appearance,

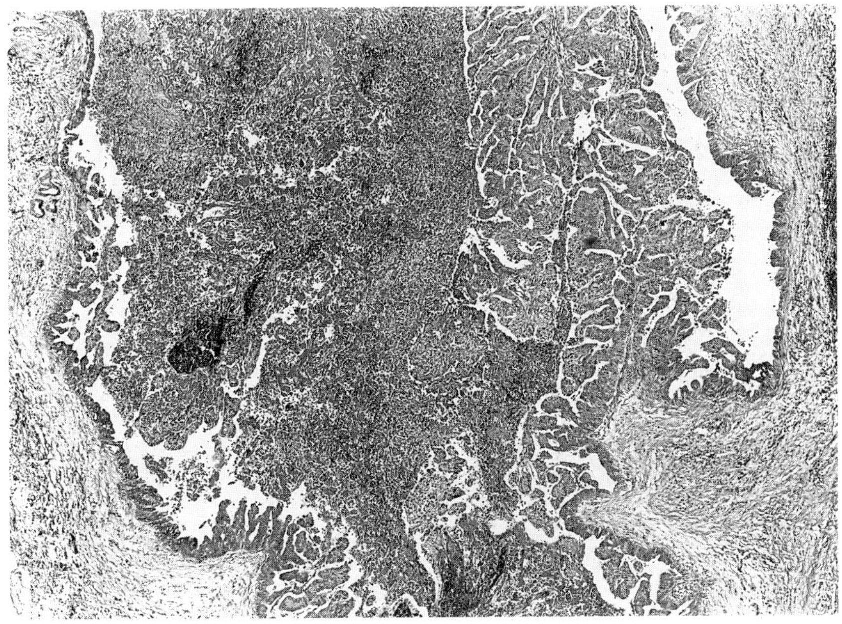

Fig. 22. Low power view of an intraductal papillary tumor with extensive necrosis (H&E ×100). (From [35], with permission)

and a continuous extension of the tumor cells can be seen in the duct system [32, 44].

Also, most of the mucin-hypersecreting type consist of papillary and atypical hyperplasia, with only a small area showing malignant changes. A considerable sampling variation is found within the same tumor, with some areas showing mild dysplasia and the others being unquestionably malignant [45]. Therefore, this type of tumor (as well as mucinous cystic neoplasm), should be extensively sampled. Multiple sections every 5 mm should be sufficient for diagnosis. In some cases, it is rather difficult or even impossible to distinguish between the atypical form of hyperplasia and carcinoma in situ [35]. In such instances, morphological criteria such as the degree of cellular atypia, as defined by Kozuka et al. [4], may be adopted to differentiate between hyperplasia, atypical hyperplasia, and carcinoma in situ.

A three-dimensional analysis of type 1 lesion (Figs. 13 and 26A) showed in 4 out of 12 cases diffuse dilatation of the main duct involving also some subbranches to a lesser degree, creating an impression of multiple cysts on the cut surfaces. The entire area of the dilated main duct and subbranches were lined primarily with malignant cells. Areas of dysplasia were found adjacent to those of carcinoma in situ [32].

Type 2 presented large and small cysts, all filled with mucin. The major cyst (Figs. 13 and 26B) corresponded to the main duct and a subbranch

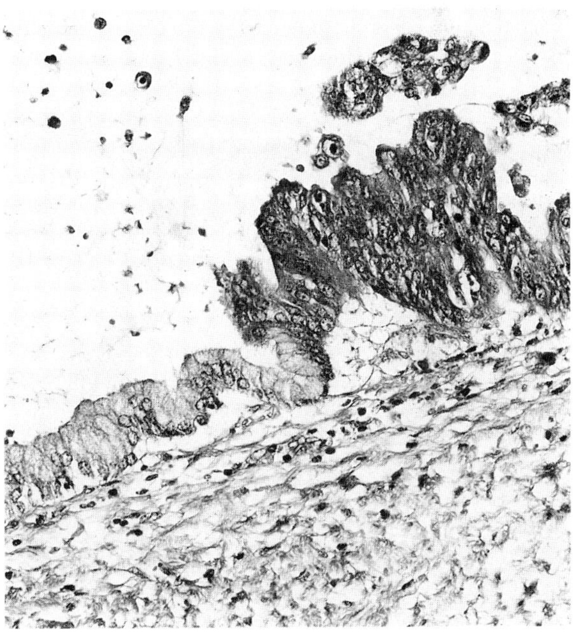

Fig. 23. Sharp transition between benign hyperplastic and neoplastic epithelium of a main pancreatic duct. (H&E ×400)

A 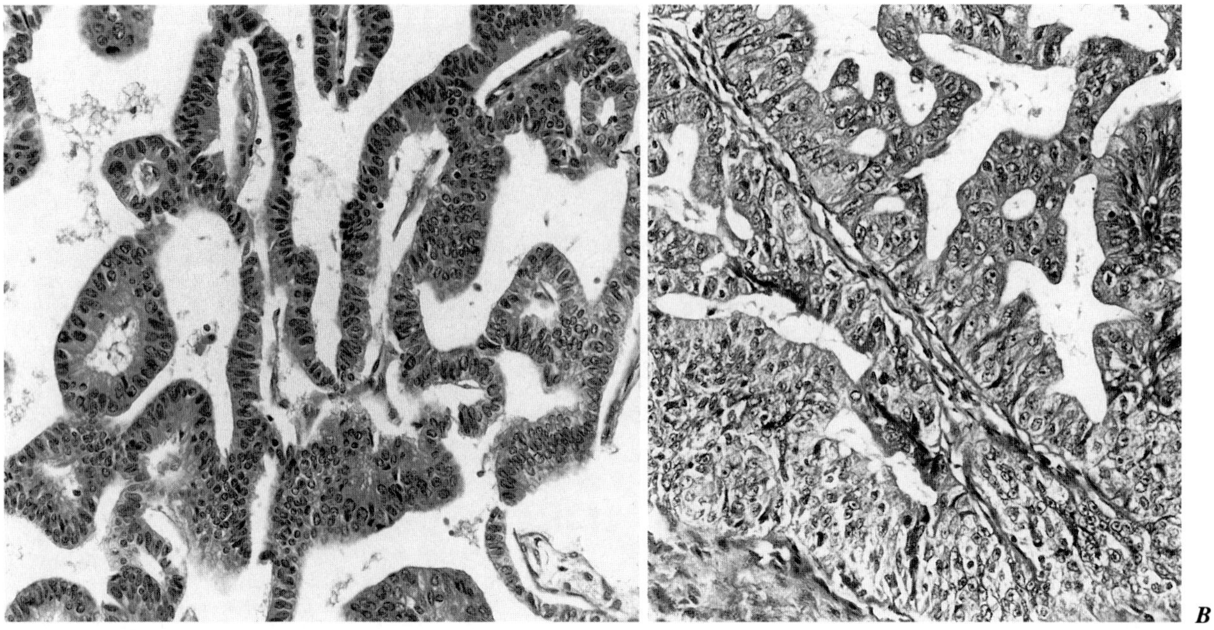 B

Fig. 24A,B. Papillary intraductal tumor ***A*** with minimal variation in size and shape of the nuclei and moderate hyperchromatism. However, nucleoli and mitoses are absent. ***B*** In contrast, a higher degree of nuclear pleomorphism and mitotic activity can be seen. (H&E ×300)

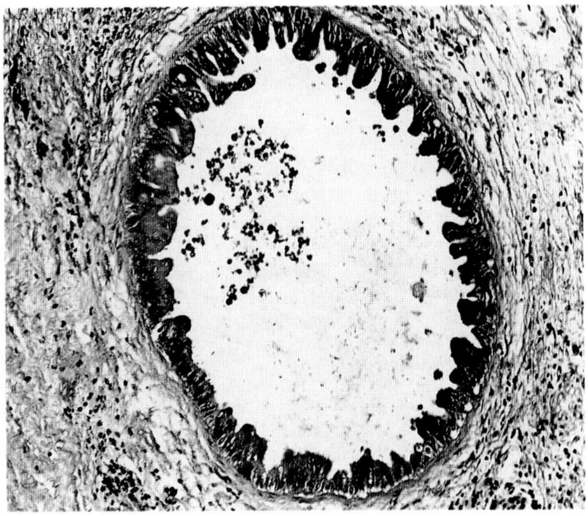

Fig. 25. Carcinoma in situ in a small pancreatic duct away from an intraductal papillary carcinoma that arose in the main pancreatic duct. (H&E ×200)

with a surface epithelium of carcinoma in situ alternating with patches of dysplasia. It was found that the carcinomatous epithelium can spread into a duct without causing ectasia [32]. Two of 12 specimens were type 2. Type 3 lesions (Figs. 13 and 26C) presented a cystic subbranch and were lined entirely with dysplastic cells with foci of carcinoma in situ between them. Two of the 12 specimens belonged to type 3 [32].

Type 4 presented involvement of at least two subbranches and several ductules (Figs. 13 and 26D) and spared the main duct. The major part of the ectatic ducts had hyperplastic epithelia and ordinary cells, but in its central part there was an area of dysplasia. No carcinoma was seen. Four of 12 tumors were classified as type 4 [32].

Some cases with characteristic findings of papilla of Vater and pancreatogram are diagnosed as hyperplasia or even as an inflammatory disease such as a chronic pancreatitis. In such cases, careful tissue samplings for histological diagnosis is essential.

Invasive Type of Intraductal Tumor. It is easy to make a diagnosis of invasive cancer when the tumor shows a massive invasion into the pancreatic parenchyma or pancreatic capsule, but it is rather

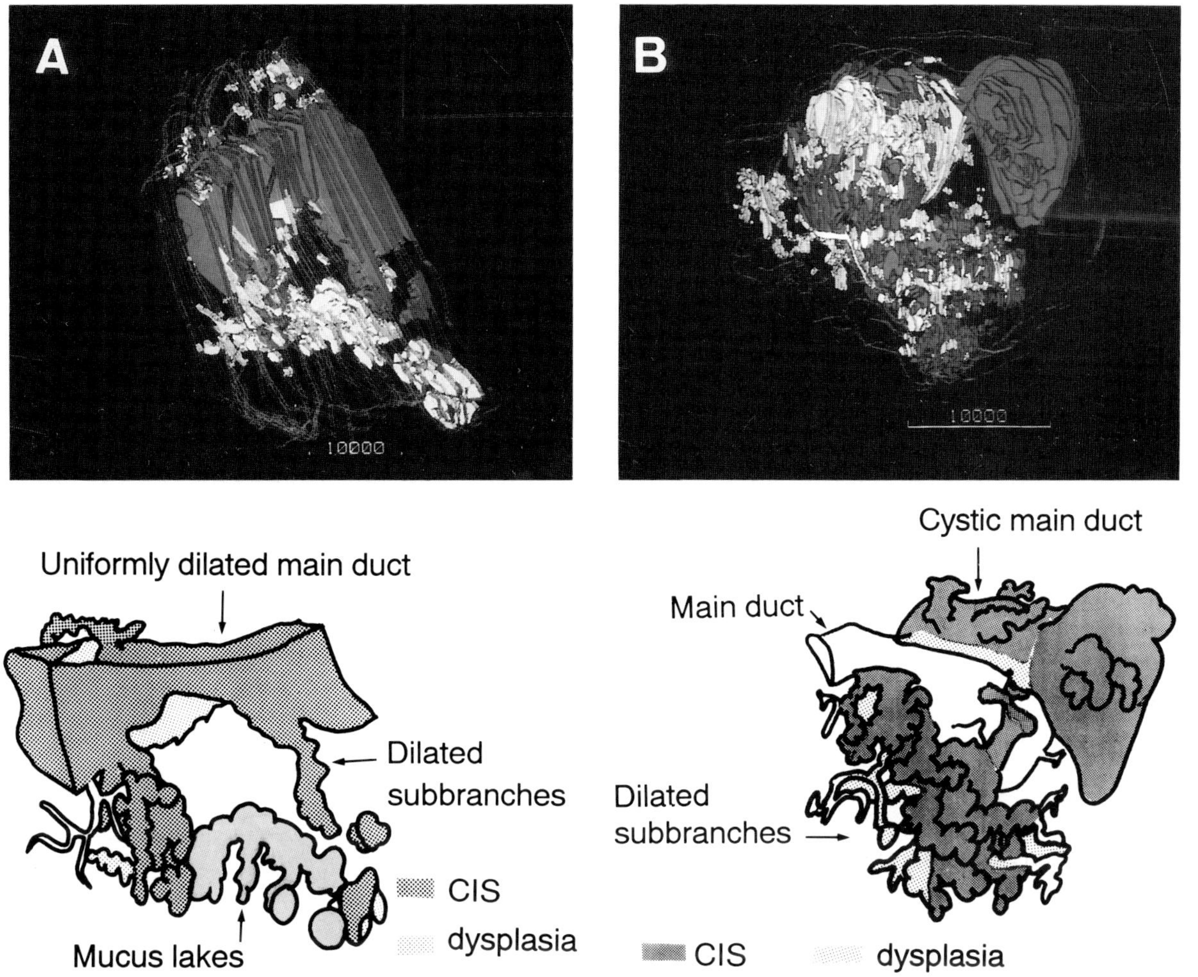

Fig. 26A–D. Computer assisted 3-D mapping of the mucus-hypersecreting tumor along the pancreatic duct. Epithelial changes are expressed with different colors: carcinoma in situ (*CIS*) in *red*, dysplasia in *yellow*, hyperplasia in *green*, ordinary epithelia in *blue*. ***A*** The main duct and subbranches, markedly dilated, are almost exclusively lined with CIS. Colored in pink are mucus lakes in periductal tissues. ***B*** The main duct is focally dilated corresponding to a major cyst, which is lined with CIS. Note the extension of CIS into several subbranches and nondilated part of the main duct. (*For color reproduction see color insert in the frontmatter*; *continued on p. 58*)

difficult to make a correct diagnosis of invasive cancer with minimal invasion. Specimens obtained from suspected malignant cases should be examined meticulously for infiltration into the pancreatic parenchyma. Three-dimensional analysis [32] has shown that focal invasion can be found in some areas of epithelium of carcinoma in situ type.

In the predominantly papillary type, the invasive component is nonpapillary and indistinguishable from conventional ductal carcinoma (Figs. 27 and 28). In the mucin-producing variety, muconodular infiltration (Fig. 29) also may be seen [44]. An IDT with muconodular infiltration shows a papillary tumor in the main pancreatic duct and branch duct with mucus lakes spread over a wide range of pancreatic parenchyma. The muconodular infiltrating pattern is claimed to be the principle infiltration pattern in mucin-producing tumors, while the principle pattern in mucinous cystic neoplasm is tubular infiltration [44]. The pancreatic parenchyma distal to the IDT usually shows variable degrees of atrophy of the acinar tissue accompanied by fibrosis and chronic inflammation. These histologic changes result from ductal obstruction.

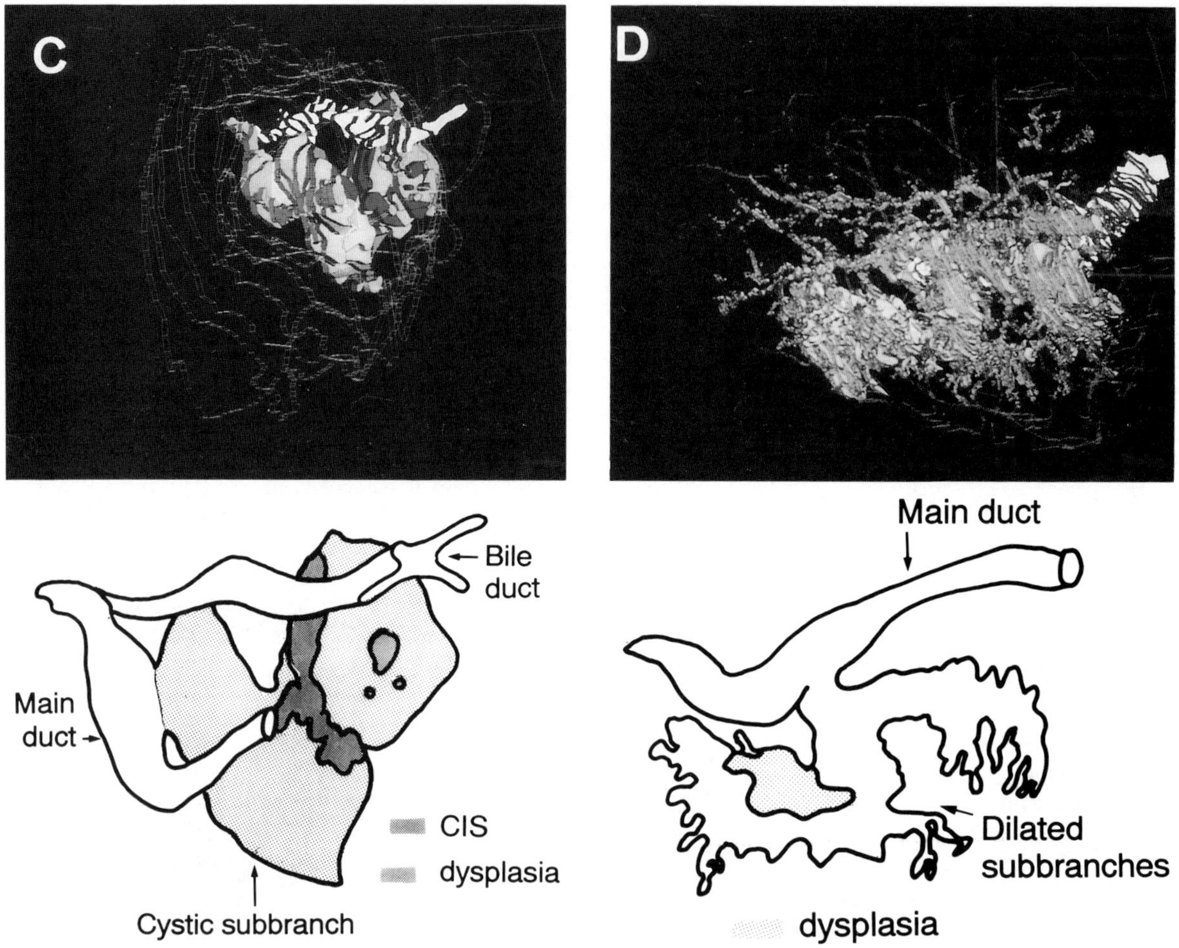

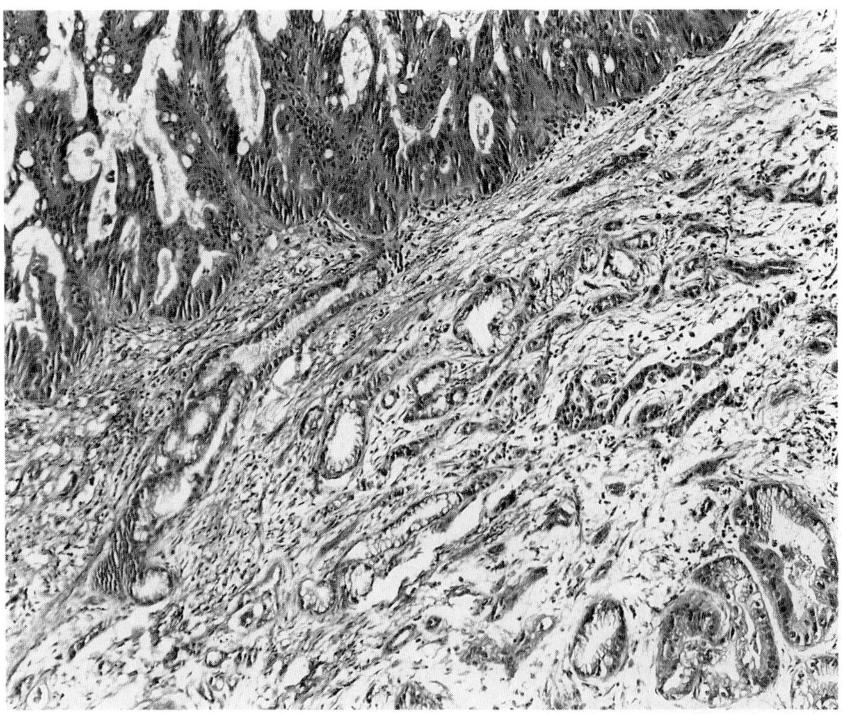

Fig. 27. Intraductal papillary carcinoma with stromal infiltration. The invasive component is similar to conventional ductal carcinoma. (H&E ×300)

Fig. 26C. A cystic sub-branch was found to have dysplasia of inner lining epithelium. Note the multicentric development of CIS in the area of dysplasia. ***D*** Two ductal subbranches are dilated, with the inner surfaces partially involved in dysplasia. No carcinoma was found (*For color reproduction see color insert in front matter*). (From [32] with permission)

Electron Microscopy

There are no specific ultrastructural features for IDT. The few tumors that have been examined with the electron microscope have shown tall columnar epithelial cells resting on a basal lamina [12]. Microvilli emerged from the apical cytoplasm, a number of mitochondria, and a well-developed rough endoplasmic reticulum and Golgi apparatus are seen. Mucin droplets of variable size and electron density are present. The nuclei are indented and may show cytoplasmic inclusions. Electron microscopic study of the mucin-hypersecreting type [46] revealed that tumor cells are filled with mucus granules in the apical cell portion, resembling Goblet cells. They exhibit many intracellular organelles, mature microvilli, and junctional complexes (Fig. 30). However, tumor cells resembling Goblet cells have also been seen in some cases of conventional pancreatic ductal carcinoma and are not specific for mucin-hypersecreting IDT.

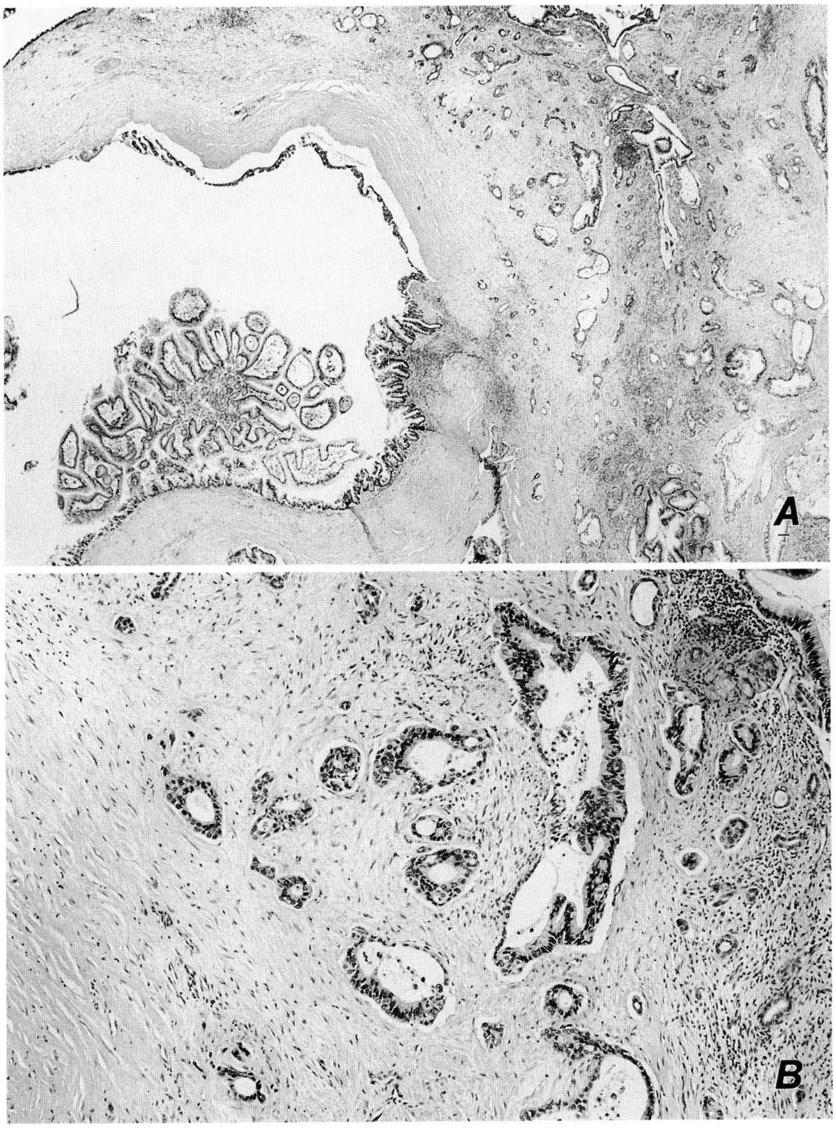

Fig. 28A,B. Invasive intraductal tumor. ***A*** Most of this tumor consists of well-differentiated tubular adenocarcinoma (*right*), whereas intraductal papillary tumor can be seen in the dilated main pancreatic duct (*left*) (H&E ×100). ***B*** A high power view of ***A*** tubular infiltration pattern is observed in the pancreatic parenchyma. (H&E ×200)

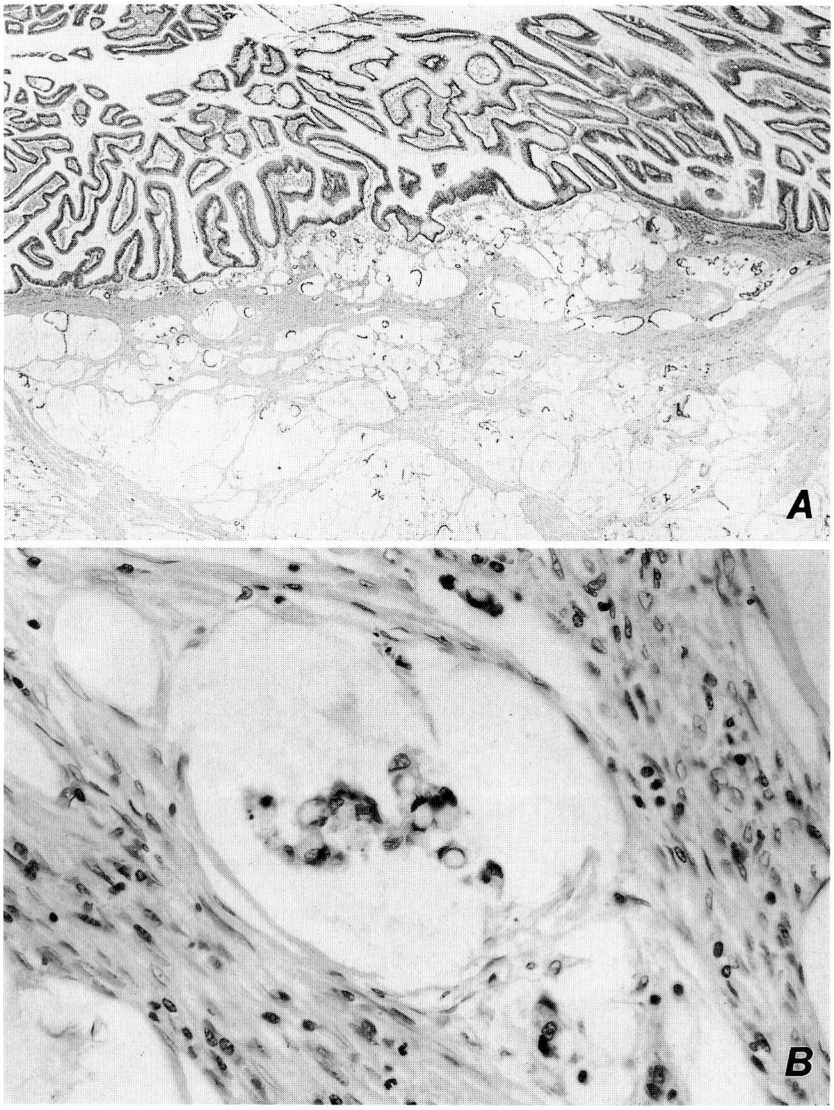

Fig. 29A,B. Invasive type intraductal tumor. The same case as in Fig. 18. ***A*** Low power magnification showing papillary tumor in the main duct (*upper*) and muconodular infiltration in the pancreatic parenchyma (*lower*). (H&E ×200). ***B*** Floating tumor cells including signet-ring cells lie within lakes of mucin. (H&E ×400)

Immunohistochemistry

Immunohistochemical staining for CEA and CA19-9 is positive in some cases [12, 47]. The degree of the staining is usually weaker in IDT than in the common type of cancer. A difference in the immunohistochemical staining was found between benign and malignant lesions: In malignant lesions, CA19-9 staining appears diffuse in the cytoplasm and stroma (Fig. 31), whereas in benign lesions, the staining is limited to the apical or supranuclear cell cytoplasm [47]. Immunohistochemical staining for DU-PAN-2 is negative or weakly positive at the apical pole of the tumor cells both in malignant and benign lesions [47]. Somatostatin cells [48] or serotonin-positive cells [35, 49, 50] may be found in some cases.

A mucous histochemical study has shown that mucus produced by malignant cells contains mainly sialomucin, whereas in benign tumors it is usually neutral mucin, and in the normal pancreatic ducts it is sulfated mucin (Fig. 32) [44]. During malignant development, mucus produced by hyperplastic cells changes from sulfated mucin and neutral mucin to sialomucin. This gradual change is more obvious in mucin-hypersecreting IDT than in the common type of ductal cancer [51].

Molecular Biology

The incidence of the point mutation of the c-Ki-*ras* oncogene in IDT is reported as zero [13], 60% [17] or higher both in the carcinoma area and in the

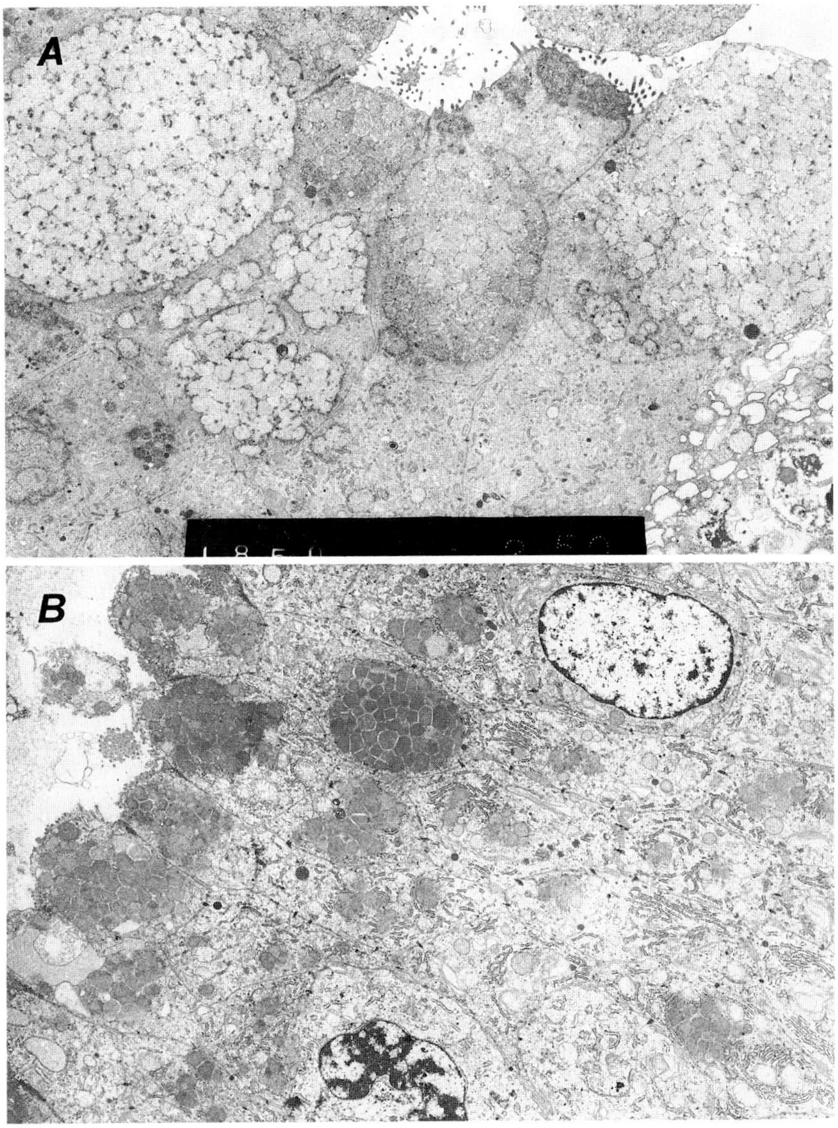

Fig. 30A,B. Electron microscopic findings. ***A*** Invasive form of intraductal tumor (*IDT*). Apical portion of the tumor cells is packed by mucus granules of low electron density. Microvilli are observed in the duct lumen (×2500). ***B*** IDT with minimal invasion. Apical portion of the tumor cells is filled with mucus granules of high density. Oval-shaped nucleus is located at the base. (×2500)

benign-appearing component [52]. The zero or moderate incidence may reflect the favorable prognosis of this tumor [13]. The high incidence may indicate the possible existence of an adenoma-carcinoma sequence in the evolution of this type of neoplasm.

No correlation has been found between the severity of the cytologic atypia and the c-Ki-*ras* mutation, but a direct relationship has been noticed between the size of the tumor and the mutation [17]: The smaller tumors lacked mutations. Therefore, it seems that the mutation is not the first genetic abnormality, but rather an expression of the progression of the disease [17]. However, additional studies are needed to confirm these observations.

Diagnosis and Differential Diagnosis

Mass survey by US can detect the dilated pancreatic duct and cystic lesions even in asymptomatic patients. EUS gives more precise information than conventional US. CT shows almost the same findings as US. CT complements US in that it can cover the blind points of US such as the periampullary region and the tail of the pancreas, but CT itself is not a reliable screening method for detection of IDT. ERCP is very effective in making the final diagnosis, because it demonstrates characteristic findings of major or minor papilla and the pancreatogram in almost all patients with this type of tumor. Angiography and enhanced CT are helpful in determining extrapancreatic growth and oper-

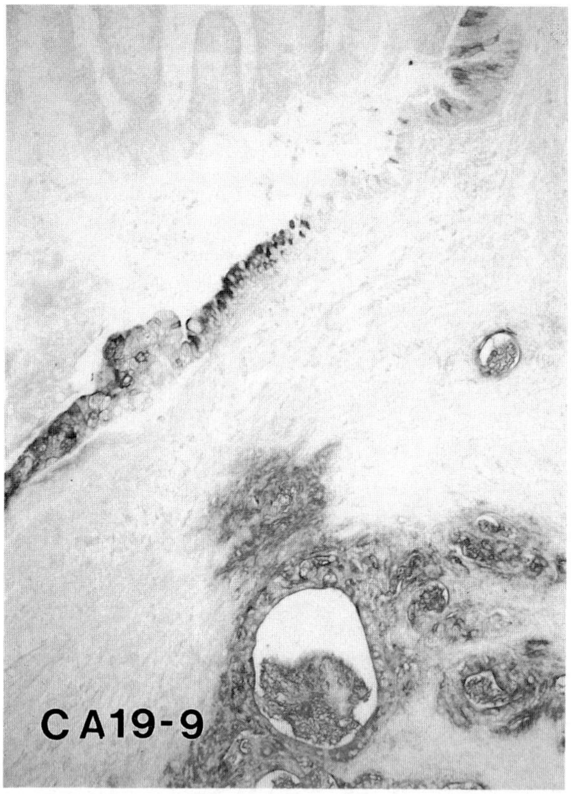

Fig. 31. Intraductal tumor with tubular infiltration. The same case as Fig. 27. Immunohistochemical staining for CA19-9 was negative in intraductal papillary tumor (*upper left*). Immunoactivity with CA19-9 is localized in the cytoplasm as well as on the apical and basolateral surfaces of the neoplastic cells lining the duct (*center*), whereas it is diffusely distributed in the cells and surrounding stroma adjacent to the malignant cells which infiltrate the pancreatic parenchyma (*lower portion*). (×200)

Table 2. Abnormal findings suspicious for malignancy in case of intraductal tumor.

1. Fistula formation to the common bile duct (obstructive jaundice, dilatation of the bile duct)
2. Fistula formation to the duodenum or the stomach
3. All three characteristic findings of the Papilla of Vater
4. Remarkably dilated main pancreatic duct more than 10 mm in diameter
5. Mural nodule in the cyst or dilated pancreatic duct described by US or CT
6. Encasement of the vessels by angiography
7. High degree of cellular atypia shown by biopsy or cytology

US, ultrasonography; CT, computed tomography

ability of the tumor. POPS, transpapillary biopsy, and cytology are additional aids in diagnosis. Thus, it is comparatively easy to separate this type of tumor from chronic pancreatitis and the common type of ductal cancer, when attention is paid to the characteristic features obtained by these imaging modalities. Because intraductal carcinomas may show focal intestinal differentiation and the dilated duct may be interpreted as a cyst, IDTs can be confused with mucinous cystic neoplasms. However, these cystic tumors are usually multilocular and more commonly located in the tail of the pancreas of middle-aged females [31, 53]. The epithelium of the cyst often shows the ductal-type of pancreatic differentiation as well as intestinal and gastric cell phenotypes [53]. A population of endocrine cells including enterochromaffin cells, somatostatin-producing cells, gastrin-producing cells, pancreatic polypeptide-secreting cells, and vasoactive intestinal peptide cells has been demonstrated in 70% of mucinous cystic tumors [49, 54]. In addition, the wall of the cyst shows a cellular mesenchymal stroma that is not present in the intraductal carcinoma.

However, clinically it is rather difficult to make a differential diagnosis between invasive or non-invasive types of IDT. Table 2 lists the abnormal findings suggesting malignancy and includes: (1) fistula formation to the duodenum and stomach detected by endoscopy, (2) the common bile duct demonstrated by cholangiography, (3) hypoechoic mass in the pancreatic parenchyma demonstrated by US, and (4) encasement of the peripancreatic vessels by angiography. When the diagnosis of IDT is made, resection would appear to be the treatment of choice, taking into account the patient's age, general condition, symptoms, the location of the tumor, the degree of difficulty of surgery, the degree of the malignancy of the tumor, and the pathological characteristics of the tumor (malignant potential, growth kinetics). When patients demonstrate abnormal findings as shown in Table 1, they should absolutely be operated upon because of the high possibility of malignancy.

Prognosis

Patients with intraductal tumors confined to the ducts or with limited stromal infiltration (micro-invasion) are cured by total pancreatectomy [15, 24, 55, 56]. However, intraductal tumors with

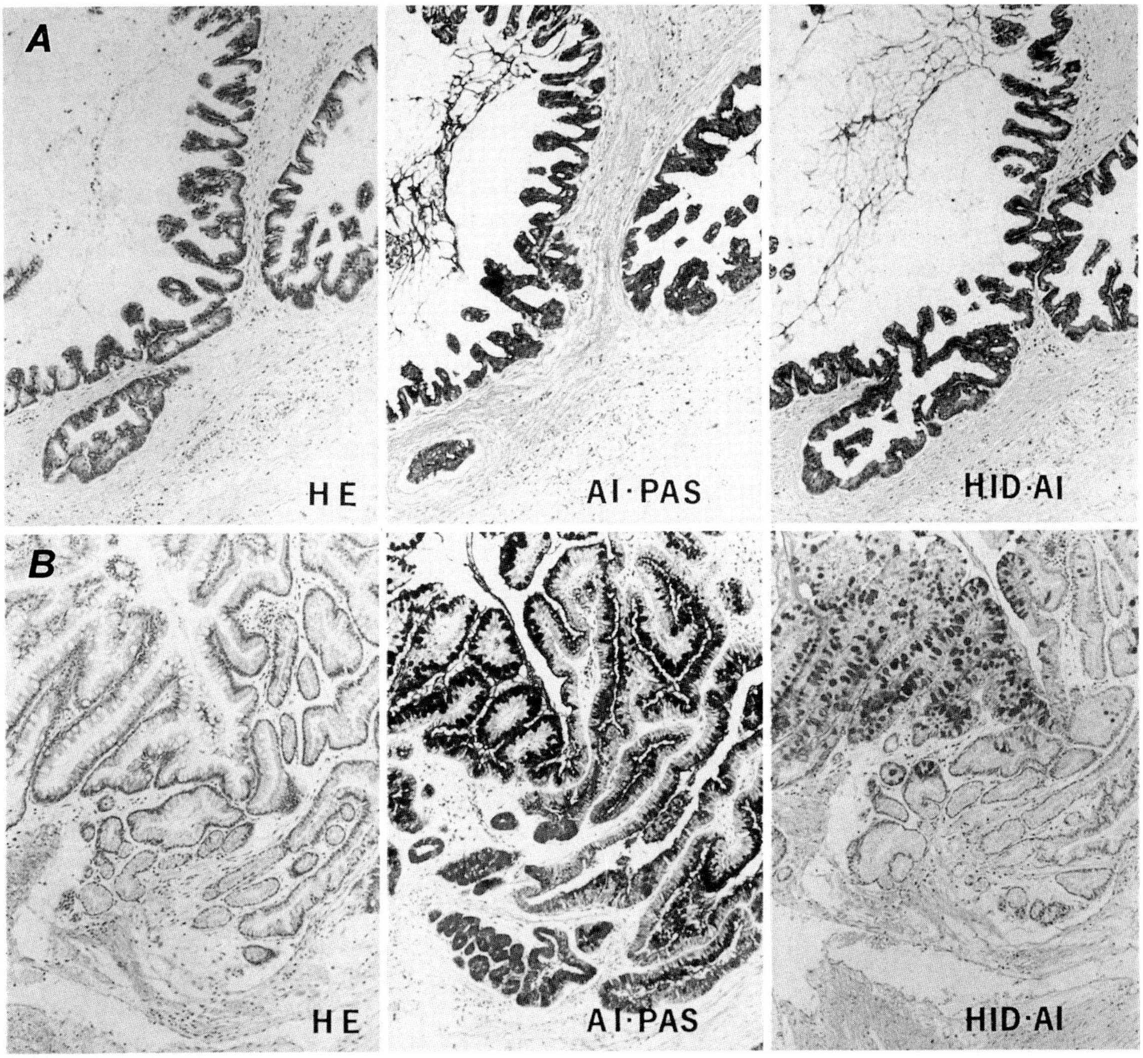

Fig. 32A,B. Double-staining with alcian blue (pH 2.5), periodic acid-Schiff (*PAS*) and with high-iron diamine (*HID*)-alcian blue (pH 2.5). ***A*** Invasive intraductal papillary tumor (IDT). Sialomucin can be observed in most of the tumor cells. ***B*** Noninvasive IDT. Neutral mucin is also observed in another portion of this tumor. (*For color reproduction see color insert in the frontmatter*)

extensive stromal infiltration behave aggressively as conventional ductal carcinomas. Most patients die soon after diagnosis [35]. In malignant cases, the postoperative cumulative 5-year survival rate was 60.7%, while the 3-year survival rate of patients with the common type of ductal cancer is 12% [57]. In the series of patients reported by Yamao et al. [29, 30], the 5-year survival rate of cases with the noninvasive type was 84.7% and of invasive cases was 68.8%. Six out of 13 invasive cases died of cancer recurrence after operation (Yamao, unpublished). A few cases had metastases to other organs, such as the liver, lung, pleura, and bones. The biological behavior of this cancer relates directly to the absence or presence of stromal invasion. Cases with carcinoma in situ or with minimal stromal invasion of cancer cells have a good prognosis after operation. The available results suggest that the extent of invasion is crucial to the prognosis [49]. It must be noted that macroscopically, the extent of tumors cannot be determined during surgery. According to Furukawa et al. [32], malignant epithelium can extend into ductal segments without remarkable dilation of the duct. That there can be such a discrepancy between the dilated ductal segments and the actual presence of tumor cells appears to be of great clinical significance. When CT or other diagnostic images are used to choose the area for resection, it should be remembered that the tumor previously may have extended over the boundaries of the cystic spaces into the surrounding undilated ducts. The reconstruction study by Furukawa et al. [32] showed that, in the lesions classified as the diffuse type, the tumor seemed to involve an unexpectedly wide ductal area (Fig. 26). This pattern of spread may justify a total pancreatectomy [24]. In the other three types, neoplastic cells also were found extending into segments where dilatation was not as remarkable [32]. Accordingly, it may not be sufficient in such patients to excise only the dilated segments. Removal of a pancreas with IDT should be done by excising not only the ectatic ducts but also some portion of the parenchymal zone that contains such ducts.

Acknowledgments. We would like to thank Prof. Sadao Kozuka (deceased) and Prof. Malcolm Moore for their guidance and suggestions. The authors are indebted to Dr. S. Akao, Department of Surgery, Kochigaya Hospital, Dokkyou Medical College, for providing electron microscopic pictures, and to Drs. N. Horibe and Imaeda, Department of Pathology, Second Teaching Hospital, Fujita Health University School of Medicine, for providing the pictures of biopsy and cytological specimens.

References

1. Sommers SC, Murphy SA, Warren S (1954) Pancreatic duct hyperplasia and cancer. Gastroenterology 27:629–640
2. Pour MP, Sayed S, Seyed G (1982) Hyperplastic, preneoplastic and neoplastic lesions found in 83 human pancreases. Am J Clin Pathol 77:137–152
3. Cubilla AL, Fitzgerald PJ (1976) Morphological lesions associated with human primary invasive nonendocrine pancreas cancer. Cancer Res 36:2690–2698
4. Kozuka S, Sassa R, Taki T, Masamoto K, Nagasawa S, Saga S, Hasegawa K, Takeuchi M (1979) Relation of pancreatic duct hyperplasia to carcinoma. Cancer 43:1418–1428
5. Fitzgerald PJ, Cubilla AL (1986) Pancreas. In: Henson DE, Albores-Saavedra J (eds) The pathology of incipient neoplasia. WB Saunders, Philadelphia, pp 217–231
6. Klöppel G, Bommer G, Ruckert K, Seifert G (1980) Intraductal proliferation in the pancreas and its relationship to human and experimental carcinogenesis. Virchows Arch [A] 387:221–233
7. Shimizu M, Itoh H, Okumara S, Hashimoto K, Hanoika K, Ohyanagi H, Yamamoto M, Kurada Y, Tanaka T, Saitoh Y (1989) Papillary hyperplasia of the pancreas. Hum Pathol 20:806–807
8. Ohashi K, Takagi K (1980) ERCP and imaging diagnosis of pancreatic cancer (in Japanese). Gastroenterol Endosc 77:1493–1495
9. Ohashi K, Murakami Y, Maruyama M, Takekoshi T, Ohta H, Ohashi I, Takagi K, Kato Y (1982) Four cases of mucus-secreting pancreatic cancer (in Japanese). Prog Dig Endosc 20:348–351
10. Kato Y, Yanagisawa A (1986) Mucus producing carcinoma of the pancreas. Its concept and classification (in Japanese). Biliary Tract and Pancreas 7:731–737
11. Yamao K, Nakazawa S, Naito Y, Kimoto E, Morita K, Inui K, Ohnuma T, Funakawa T, Hayashi Y (1986) Clinicopathological study of the mucus-producing pancreatic tumors. Jpn J Gastroenterol 83:2588–2597
12. Morohoshi T, Kanda M, Asanuma K, Klöppel G (1989) Intraductal papillary neoplasms of the pancreas. A clinicopathological study of six patients. Cancer 64:1329–1335
13. Rickert F, Cremer M, Deviere J, Tavarea L, Lamnilliotte JP, Schroder S, Wurbs D, Klöppel G (1991) Intraductal mucin-hypersecreting neoplasms of the pancreas: A clinico-pathological study of eight patients. Gastroenterology 101:512–519
14. Furuta K, Watanabe H, Ikeda S (1992) Differences between solid and ductal ectatic types of pancreatic ductal carcinomas. Cancer 69:1327–1333
15. Mizumoto K, Inagaki T, Koizumi M, Uemura M, Ogawa M, Kitazawa S, Tsutsumi M, Toyokawa M, Konishi Y (1988) Early pancreatic adenocarcinoma. Hum Pathol 19:242–244
16. Ohhashi K, Murakami Y, Yamada M, Ninomiya E, Takano K, Hori M, Seki M, Yanagisawa A, Kato Y, Takagi K (1992) Diagnostic progress of cystic lesion in the pancreas (in Japanese). Progress of Digestive Endoscopy 40:11–16
17. Tada M, Omata M, Ohto M (1991) Ras gene mutations in intraductal papillary neoplasms of the pancreas. Analysis in five cases. Cancer 67:634–637
18. Ito Y, Blackstone MO, Frank PH, Skinner DB (1977) Mucinous biliary obstruction associated with a cystic adenocarcinoma of the pancreas. Gastroenterology 73:1410–1412
19. Itai Y, Kokubo T, Atomi Y, Kuroda A, Haraguchi Y, Terano A (1987) Mucin-hypersecreting carcinoma of the pancreas. Radiology 165:51–55
20. Yamao K, Kajikawa M (1983) Reevaluation of the ERCP (in Japanese). Gann no Rinsho 29:1097

21. Takayama T, Kato K, Sano H, Katada N, Honda Y, Sugimoto Y, Koyama Y, Uemura M, Fukushima A, Takeichi M, Nimura Y, Maeda S, Kamiya J, Isogaya M (1984) Two cases of mucus-secreting pancreatic tumor (in Japanese). Biliary Tract and Pancreas 5:229–234
22. Payan MJ, Xerri L, Moncada K, Bastid C, Agostini S, Sastre B, Sahel J, Chouz R (1990) Vilous adenoma of the main pancreatic duct: A potentially malignant tumor? Am J Gastroenterol 85:459–463
23. Kohler B, Kohler G, Riemann JF (1990) Pancreoscopic diagnosis of intraductal cystadenoma of the pancreas. Dig Dis Sci 35:382–384
24. Conley CR, Scheithauer BW, Weiland LH, van Heerden JA (1987) Diffuse intraductal papillary adenocarcinoma of the pancreas. Ann Surg 205: 246–249
25. Hivet M, Maisel A, Horiot A (1975) Carcinome villeux diffus du Wirsurg: Pancréatectomie totale. Med Chir Dig 4: 159–162
26. Rogers PN, Seywright MM, Murray WR (1987) Diffuse villous adenoma of pancreatic duct. Pancreas 2:727–730
27. Agostini S, Choux R, Payan MJ, Sahel J, Clement JP (1989) Mucinous pancreatic duct ectasia in the body of the pancreas. Radiology 170:815–816
28. Takagi K, Takekoshi T, Ohashi K, Kasumi F, Maruyama M, Murakami Y, Gondo M, Hiraiwa T, Kato Y, Yanagisawa A (1982) Diagnostic ability and limitation of ERCP for pancreatic cancer (in Japanese). Stomach and Intestine 17:1065–1080
29. Yamao K, Nakazawa S, Naito Y, Kimoto E, Morita K, Inui K, Ohnuma T, Funakawa T, Hayashi Y, Fukui A (1986) Diagnosis of pancreatic cystic diseases by ERCP (in Japanese). I to chou (Stomach and Intestine) 21:745–753
30. Yamao K, Nakazawa S, Naito Y, Kimoto E, Inui K, Hayashi Y, Kano J, Yamada M, Mitake M, Ichikawa K, Onuma T (1988) The efficacy of peroral transpapillary pancreatoscopy (POPS) for the diagnosis of mucus-producing pancreatic tumors (in Japanese). Gastroenterol Endosc 30:563–569
31. Compagno J, Oertel JE (1978) Mucinous cystic neoplasms of the pancreas with overt and latent malignancy (cystadenocarcinoma and cystadenoma). A clinicopathological study of 41 cases. Am J Clin Pathol 69:573–580
32. Furukawa T, Takahashi T, Kobari M, Matsuno S (1992) The mucus-hypersecreting tumor of the pancreas. Development and extension visualized by three-dimensional computerized mapping. Cancer 70:1505–1513
33. Nakazawa S, Yamao K, Yamada M, Naito Y, Kimoto E, Inui K, Hayashi Y, Kano J, Mitake M, Kozuka S (1988) Study of the classification of mucin-producing cystic tumor of the pancreas (in Japanese). Jpn J Gastroenterol 85:924–932
34. Warshaw AL (1991) Mucinous cystic tumors and mucinous ductal ectasia of the pancreas. Gastrointest Endosc 37:199–201
35. Milchgrub S, Campuzano M, Casillas J, Albores-Saavedra JA (1992) Intraductal carcinoma of the pancreas. Cancer 69:651–656
36. Tian F, Myles J, John JM (1992) Mucinous pancreatic ductal ectasia of latent malignancy: An emerging clinicopathologic entity. Surgery 111: 109–113
37. Higa E, Rosai J, Pizzimbono CA, Wise L (1973) Mucosal hyperplasia, mucinous cystadenoma, and mucinous cystadenocarcinoma of the appendix. A re-evaluation of appendiceal "mucocele". Cancer 32:1525–1541
38. Ohashi K (1989) Clinical features of mucus-producing pancreatic tumor (in Japanese). In: Naito Y, Yamoa K (eds) Mucus-producing pancreatic tumor. Igakutosho, Tokyo, p 35
39. Obara T, Maguchi H, Saitoh Y, Ura H, Koike Y, Kitazawa S, Namiki M (1991) Mucin-producing tumor of the pancreas: A unique clinical entity. Am J Gastroenterol 86:1619–1625
40. Kuroda A, Motoyoshi M, Atomi H, Morioka K (1991) Problems of mucin-producing pancreatic tumor (in Japanese). Surgery 53:1441–1448
41. Nakazawa S, Yamao K (1991) Mucin-producing tumor of the pancreas. The proposal of the new clinical entity and its revision. Dig Endosc 3:144–156
42. Yamaguchi K, Tanaka M (1991) Mucin-hypersecreting tumor of the pancreas with mucin extrusion through an enlarged papilla. Am J Gastroenterol 86:835–839
43. Caroli J, Hadchouel P, Mercadier M, Lageron A (1975) Papillome bénin du canal de Wirsung. Diagnostic par cathéterisme rétrograde. Med Chir Dig 4:163–166
44. Yamada M, Kozuka S, Yamao K, Nakazawa S, Naitoh Y, Tsukamoto Y (1991) Mucin-producing tumor of the pancreas. Cancer 68:159–168
45. Nicholas NJ, Lawson JM, Cotton PB (1991) Mucinous pancreatic tumors: ERCP findings. Gastrointest Endosc 38:133–138
46. Akao S, Sasaki K, Horikawa S, Terada H, Kimura W, Fujita M, Nakamura T, Yoshida M, Iwami N, Hayashida K, Akiyama H, Takahashi S, Ishikawa H (1990) Electron microscopy study of two cases of mucin-producing pancreatic carcinoma (in Japanese). Pancreas 5:85–92
47. Yamao K, Nakazawa S, Yamada M, et al. (1987) Immunohistochemical study for CA19-9, CEA, and DUPAN-2 in case of mucin-producing cystic tumor of the pancreas (in Japanese). Dig Org Immunol 19:142–146
48. Mogaki M (1991) Lectin-histochemical and immunohistochemical studies on mucin-producing

tumor of pancreas (in Japanese). Pancreas 6:498–511
49. Albores-Saavedra J, Madji M, Henson DE, Angeles-Angeles A (1988) Enteroendocrine cell differentiation in carcinoma of the pancreas. Pathol Res Pract 183:169–175
50. Motojima K, Tomioka T, Kanamatu T (1992) Immunohistochemical study of pancreatic cystadenocarcinoma. Am J Gastroenterol 87:43–47
51. Chen J, Baithun SI, Ramsay MA (1985) Histogenesis of pancreatic carcinomas: A study based on 248 cases. J Pathol 146:65–76
52. Yanagisawa A, Kato Y, Ohtake K, Kitagawa T, Ohashi K, Hori M, Takagi K, Sugano H (1991) c-Ki-*ras* point mutation in ductectatic-type mucinous cystic neoplasms of the pancreas. Jpn J Cancer Res 82:1057–1060
53. Albores-Saavedra J, Gould EW, Angeles-Angeles A (1990) Cystic tumors of the pancreas. Pathol Annu, Second Part, 19–50
54. Albores-Saavedra J, Angeles-Angeles A, Nadji M, Henson DE (1987) Mucinous cystadenocarcinoma of the pancreas. Morphologic and immunocytochemical observation. Am J Surg Pathol 11:19–25
55. Place S, Louvel A, Farhi JP, Chapuis S (1985) Adénocarcinoma papillaire du canal de Wursurg. Gastroenterol Clin Biol 9:361–364
56. Smith RC, Kneale K, Goulston K (1986) In situ carcinoma of the pancreas. NZ J Surg 56:369–373
57. Abe Y, Okuyama K, Onoda S, Kozu T, Ryou M, Isono K (1988) A case of mucin-producing pancreatic cancer originating in Santorini's duct (in Japanese). Geka Shinryou 30:1586–1589
58. Kuroda A (1986) Problems of mucus-producing carcinoma of the pancreas (in Japanese). Biliary Tract and Pancreas 7:717–721

Mucinous Cystic Tumors Non-Invasive and Invasive

Synonyms and Terminology

Of the cystic neoplasms of the pancreas, tumors composed of mucus-secreting columnar epithelium had until recently been termed cystadenoma or cystadenocarcinoma [1–3], whereas prior to this they were called by various names, including macrocystic adenoma [4], multilocular cystoma [5], and papillary cystadenocarcinoma [6].

However, in 1978 Compagno and Oertel [7], and Hodgkinson et al. [8] clearly differentiated the mucinous tumors from the serous (microcystic) cystadenoma, a cystic neoplasm belonging to a separate category recognized as mostly benign. In addition, cases of non-mucinous variants of cystadenocarcinoma, although very rare, have been reported in recent years as acinar cell cystadenocarcinoma or serous cystadenocarcinoma [9–11].

Therefore, the mucinous tumors described here are now usually classified as mucinous cystadenoma or mucinous cystadenocarcinoma [12, 13]. However, it has been suggested to collectively refer to all these tumors by the term mucinous cystic tumor [7, 14, 15], because the distinction between benign and malignant is difficult in some instances, not only macroscopically but also microscopically, and even mucinous cystadenomas with benign histological appearance probably have a high potential for malignant transformation.

Intraductal mucin hypersecreting and papillary tumors of the pancreas [16, 17] or pancreatic mucinous ductal ectasia [18] are also mucinous neoplasms of pancreatic ducts showing cystic dilatation. Although these lesions may be intrinsically the same as mucinous cystic tumors and at times referred to as mucinous cystadenoma or cystadenocarcinoma of "ductectatic type" [19, 20], this tumor will be discussed in another section.

Incidence

Mucinous cystic tumors account for the large majority of neoplastic cysts of the pancreas [21, 22], about 10% of all cystic lesions [23, 24], and 1% to 2% of primary pancreatic exocrine malignancies [12, 14, 25]. A review of the literature by Segesser and Rohner [26] reported more than 300 cases of cystadenoma and over 100 cases of cystadenocarcinoma, and ReMine et al. [27] later stated that almost 500 neoplastic cysts of the pancreas had been reported.

A review of the Japanese literature revealed 138 cases of cystadenoma and 161 cases of cystadenocarcinoma [28], most of which corresponded to the mucinous cystic tumor. Out of 3821 malignant pancreatic tumors registered at the Japan Pancreas Society over the last 10 years (1981–1990), the frequency of cystadenocarcinoma was 3.2%. In my series at the Surgical Department of Tokyo University over a 25-year period (1965–1990), I have experienced ten patients with mucinous cystic tumor including two with benign appearance, three borderline, and five malignant varieties, together with nine cases of mucinous ductal ectasia.

Age and Sex

The mucinous cystic tumor, in particular non-invasive (benign) cystadenoma, occurs predominantly in middle-aged women. The clearly malignant cases, i.e., cystadenocarcinomas, in comparison to cystadenomas, tend to be found at a slightly older age with a less marked female predominance. In the cases reported in Japan, the mean age of patients with cystadenoma was 47 years (range: 13–78 years) and with cystadenocarcinoma was 56 years (range: 9–80 years). The male to female ratio was 1:3.4 for cystadenoma, and 1:1.8 for cystadenocarcinoma. This sex and age distribution is consistent with that described in the English literature [3, 7, 29].

Etiology

The pathogenesis of these tumors is unknown. However, it is of interest that similar lesions can be induced by parenteral administration of nitrosamine derivatives in Syrian hamsters [30]. The female predominance of the tumor suggests that genetic factors [14] or sex hormones may be related to the tumorigenesis.

Phenotypically, the cells of mucinous cystic tumors closely resemble pancreatic duct epithelium. Albores-Saavedra [13] postulated that they originate from an "endodermal stem cell" that differentiates into cells with intestinal phenotypes, on the basis of his ultrastructural and immunohistochemical observations.

Clinical Presentation

The clinical features depend largely on the size of the tumor. Small tumors are usually asymptomatic and are detected as an incidental finding at autopsy or during laparotomy for a concomitant disease. Even a large tumor may show no clinical manifestations if it does not significantly involve the duct of Wirsung, the common bile duct, or the gastrointestinal tract. Thus, the tumor location in the pancreas is one determinant of symptomatology. According to the literature, approximately 80% of tumors were situated in the body and/or tail of the pancreas, and in most cases they seemed to have developed from branch ducts rather than from major ducts of the pancreas.

The most frequent symptom is pain or discomfort of the upper abdomen, which at times radiates to the back. The pain is often vague in nature but occasionally is very severe like that of acute pancreatitis. Some patients have a history of pancreatitis with abdominal pain and transient hyperamylasemia, probably due to associated inflammation of the pancreas caused by the tumor. The other major symptoms include anorexia, weight loss, and steatorrhea, as well as diabetes, all of which are mainly present in patients with a large tumor of the pancreatic head. Jaundice is uncommon but can occur in some malignant cases as the result of biliary obstruction.

Regarding the clinical signs, a palpable, frequently enlarging mass in the upper abdomen is noted in at least one half of patients. The mass is usually round, firm, and nontender. In some instances, an asymptomatic abdominal mass that has been present for years is the only complaint of the patient.

Diagnosis

The clinical diagnosis of mucinous cystic tumors is mostly based on the findings of diagnostic imaging procedures, which correspond well with the macroscopic features of the tumor.

Barium meal study (Fig. 1) and occasionally bowel gas pattern on plain films (Fig. 2) demonstrate compression or displacement of the stomach, duodenum, or colon, highly suggestive of the presence of a pancreatic mass protruding from the retroperitoneum. Plain radiographs of the abdomen may demonstrate rough, nodular calcification localized in the capsule or septa of the tumor. Although calcification was reported in only 16% of patients by plain radiography [31], its detection will be increased by the use of various other diagnostic methods.

Ultrasonography (US) and computed tomography (CT) most precisely reveal the characteristics of tumors (Fig. 3), and are excellent tools for the detection and differential diagnosis. A considerable number of asymptomatic tumors have been detected by either US or CT performed for medical screening. In general, US and CT both demonstrate well-defined encapsulated hypoechoic or low density masses containing one or more large cysts. Particularly in malignant cases, irregular thickening of the cyst wall and/or papillary excrescences projecting into the cystic cavity are demonstrated. These complicated structures are more clearly defined by enhanced CT scan. Magnetic resonance (MR) imaging is considered equal or slightly superior to CT [32], even though it is still a developing modality.

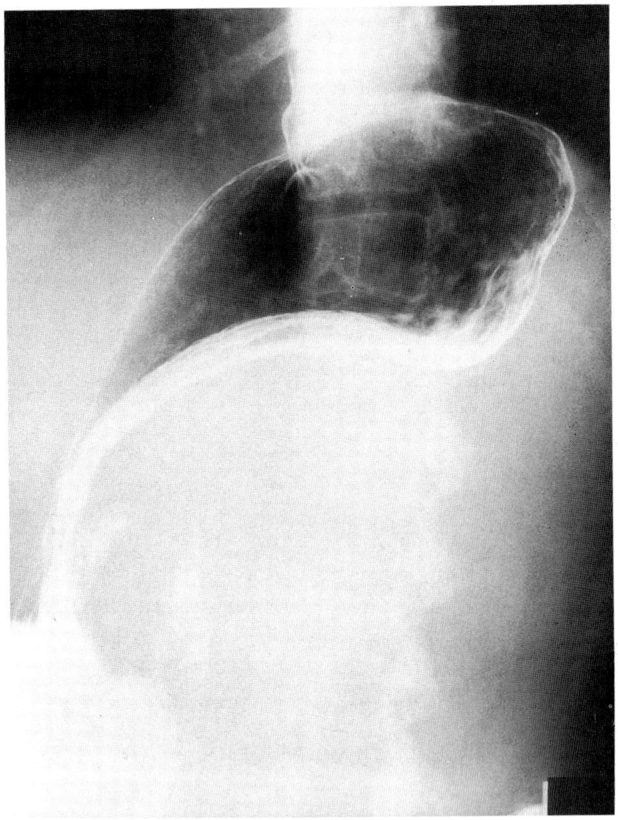

Fig. 1. Barium meal study. A 36-year-old female, who presented with an asymptomatic abdominal mass. The greater curvature of the stomach is markedly compressed by a large extragastric mass. The tumor was a mucinous cystadenocarcinoma (shown in Fig. 6d)

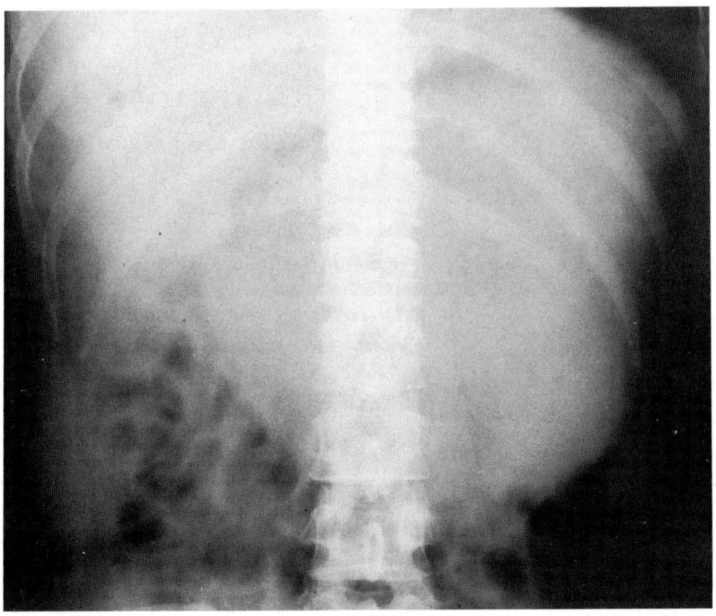

Fig. 2. Plain X-ray film of the abdomen. A 37-year-old female, who was admitted with sudden epigastric pain, high fever, and dyspnea. The gas pattern reveals superior displacement of the stomach and inferior displacement of the transverse colon, highly suggestive of the presence of a large retroperitoneal mass. Later, the diagnosis of mucinous cystadenocarcinoma (shown in Fig. 6c) with probable rupture into the pleural cavity was made

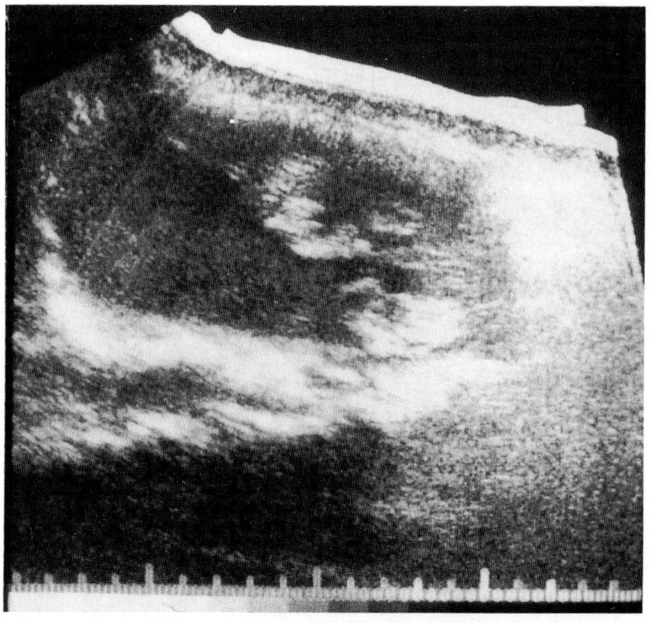

a

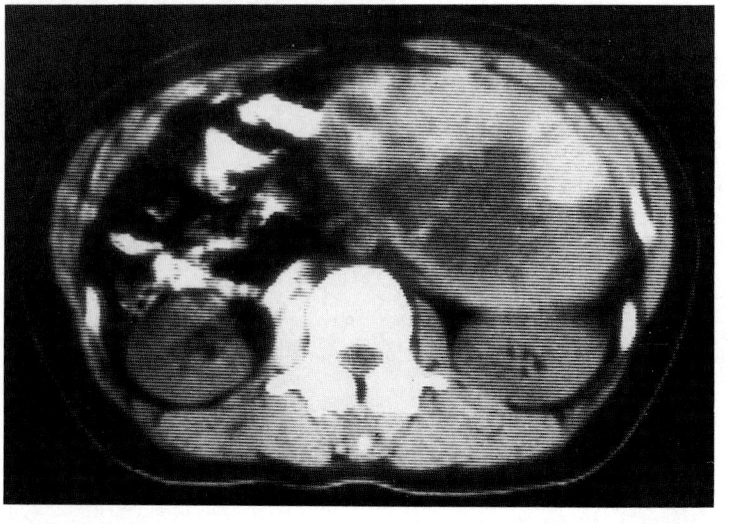

b

Fig. 3a,b. Ultrasonography (*US*) and computed tomography (*CT*). The same patient as in Fig. 2. US ***a*** and CT ***b*** both demonstrate a well-defined large cystic mass in the body of the pancreas. There are irregular intraluminal excrescences protruding from the wall of the cyst. The protrusions consisted of smaller cysts which appeared solid in some parts

The most common feature on endoscopic retrograde cholangiopancreatography (ERCP) is displacement of the main pancreatic duct with or without narrowing, due to compression by a large expanding pancreatic mass (Figs. 4, 5). The cystic space of the tumor is rarely opacified by contrast medium. Hence, in most cases of mucinous cystic tumor, clinically there is no communication between the cyst cavity and the ductal system. In contrast, a communication is usually present in the cystic lesion of mucinous ductal ectasia, which includes the lesions corresponding to ductectatic (intraductal) tumors [20].

On angiography, these tumors are generally hypovascular or avascular, with a few exceptions in malignant cases. Major vessels are displaced and sometimes encased. Vascular encasement or obstruction can occur in non-invasive as well as in invasive tumors, secondary to associated inflammation of the cyst wall or compression by the tumor.

Serum biochemistry is generally not useful in the diagnosis of this disease. Carcinoembryonic antigen (CEA) and carbohydrate antigen (CA19-9) are often elevated in patients with malignant tumor [33, 34], but are not specific findings. High levels

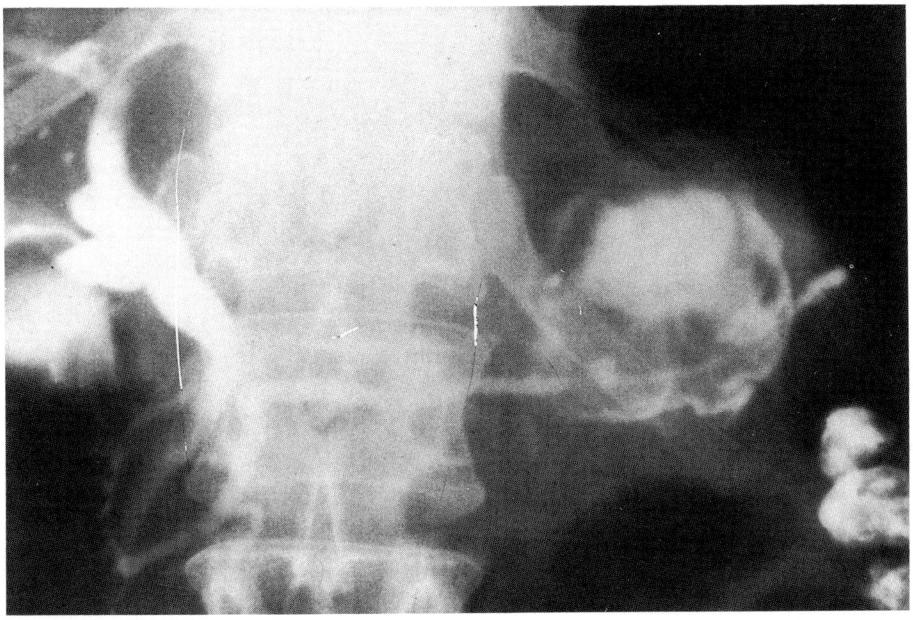

Fig. 4. Endoscopic retrograde cholangiopancreatography (*ERCP*). A 54-year-old female, with a repeated history of pancreatitis with severe abdominal pain and transient hyperamylasemia. The main pancreatic duct shows slight anterior displacement with narrowing, and a cystic cavity is opacified by contrast medium. Such a communication between the cyst cavity and the ductal system is a rare clinical finding in mucinous cystic tumors. The cystic lesion was identified as a non-invasive mucinous cystic tumor of borderline malignancy (shown in Fig. 6b)

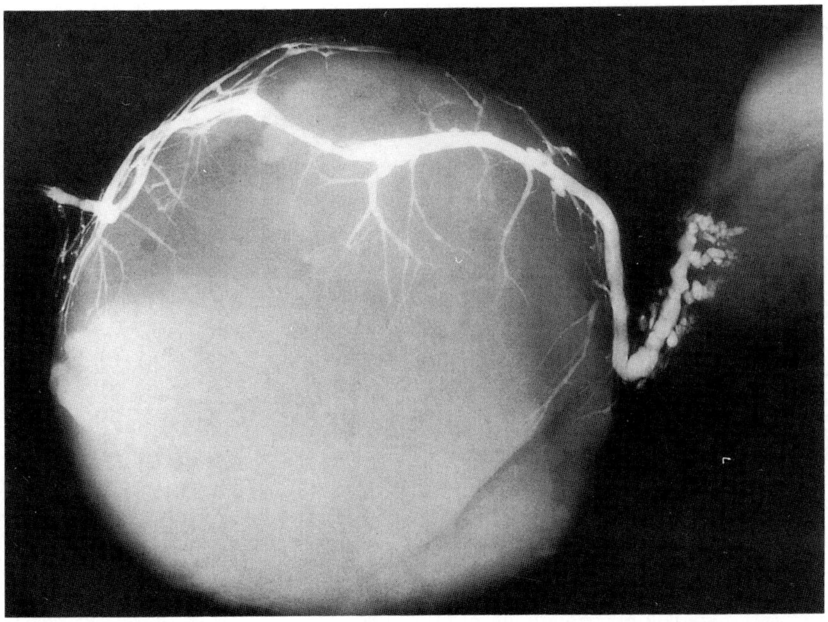

Fig. 5. Pancreatography of the surgical specimen. The same patient as in Fig. 1. The resected distal half of the pancreas clearly demonstrates stretching and displacement of the main pancreatic duct by an expanding tumor. The duct shows stenosis near the tumor and secondary dilatation distally. The cystic cavity of the tumor did not communicate with the duct

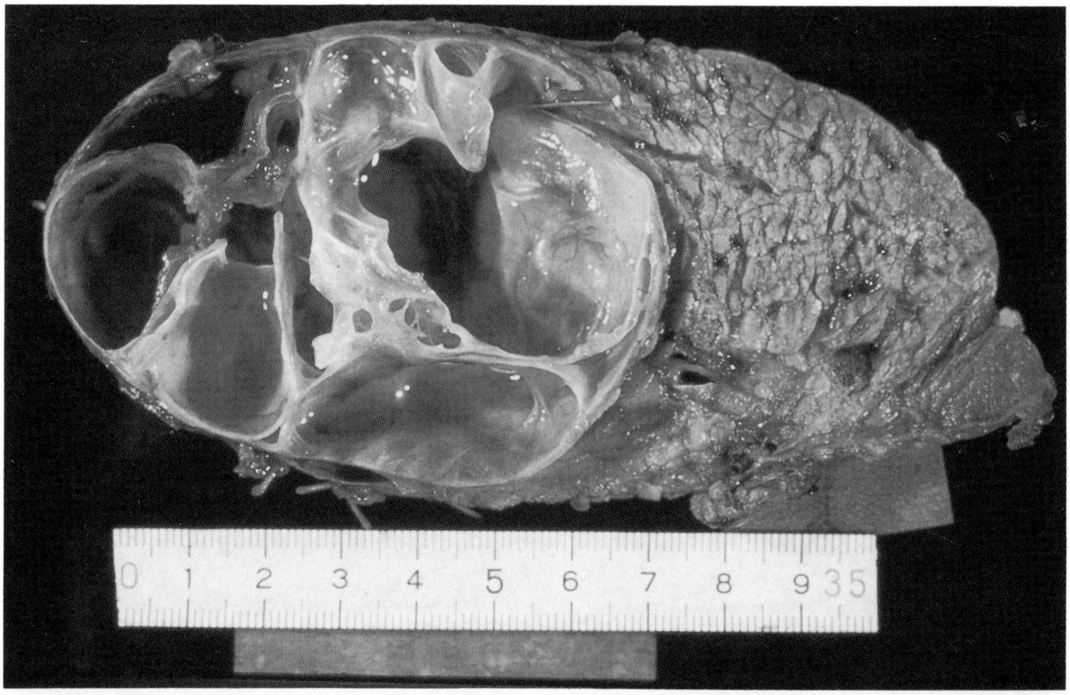

a

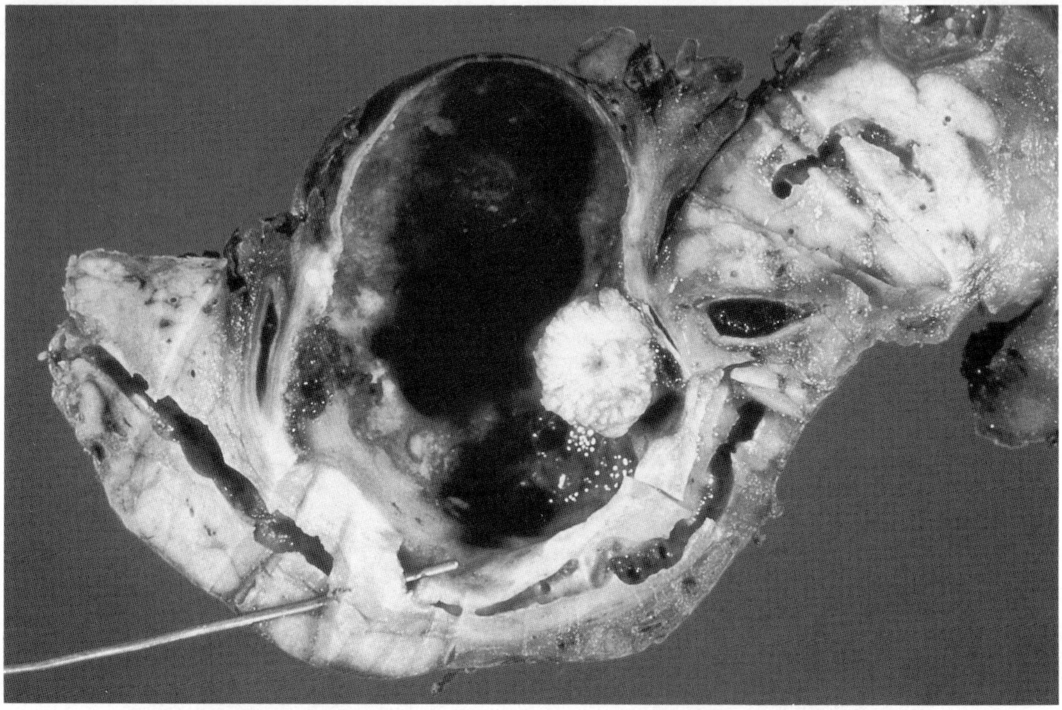

b

Fig. 6a–d. Gross appearance of sectioned mucinous cystic tumor. ***a*** Mucinous cystadenoma (mucinous cystic tumor with benign appearance). A 38-year-old female who presented with epigastric discomfort for several months. Computed tomography (*CT*) scan demonstrated a cystic tumor in the tail of the pancreas which was resected by distal pancreatectomy. The cut surface of the surgical specimen reveals an encapsulated multilocular cyst composed of several large cystic spaces separated by thin fibrous septa. The cyst walls are smooth. Some cysts are filled with thick gelatinous mucin. The patient was alive and well 12 years after the operation. ***b*** Mucinous cystic tumor of borderline malignancy from the same patient as in Fig. 4. A uni- ▷

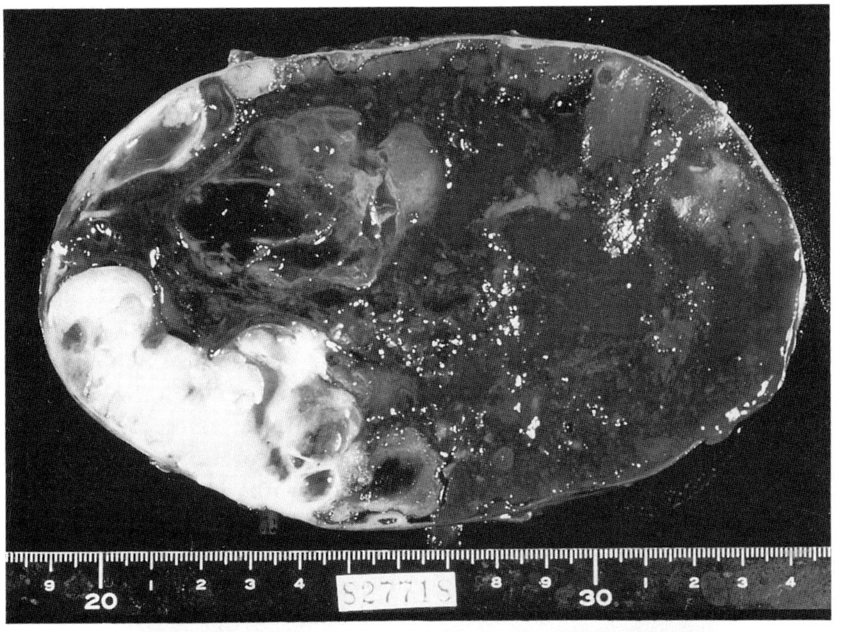

c

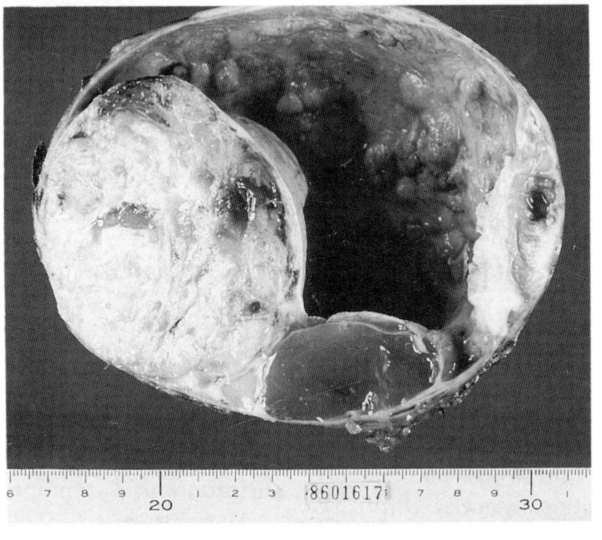

d

locular cyst enclosed by a thick fibrous capsule is seen in the horizontally sectioned surgical specimen obtained by distal pancreatectomy. The tumor measures 4.5 cm in maximum diameter, and contains a polypoid papillary tumor projecting from the cyst wall. A bougie indicates a communication between the cyst lumen and the main pancreatic duct. There is a small pseudocyst just distal to the cystic tumor. The patient died of a usual ductal cancer of the head of the pancreas 6 years after this surgery. ***c*** Mucinous cystadenocarcinoma from the same patient as in Figs. 2 and 3. The cut surface of the tumor resected by distal pancreatectomy shows a large cystic cavity filled with hemorrhagic and necrotic tissue. There are irregular excrescences from the cyst wall, which appear solid in some parts, but are actually composed of multiple small cysts containing mucoid material. This tumor demonstrated focal stromal invasion of the fibrous septa. The patient was alive 9 years after surgery with no evidence of tumor recurrence, in spite of preoperative rupture of the tumor suggested by the fistular tract extending into the thorax, associated with strong inflammatory adhesions of neighboring organs. ***d*** Mucinous cystadenocarcinoma from the same patient as in Figs. 1 and 5. The sectioned tumor reveals a multilocular cyst with solid-appearing large nodular excrescences protruding into the lumen of a major cyst. The external surface of the tumor is smooth. Some cysts demonstrate retention of thick gelatinous mucin. This tumor showed extensive stromal invasion of the fibrous septa and capsule with lymph node metastases. The patient died of carcinomatous peritonitis 3 months after radical operation. (*For color reproduction see color insert in the frontmatter*) of serum amylase or elastase 1 may be present, probably due to obstruction of the pancreatic duct by the tumor. Recently, percutaneous fine-needle aspiration of these tumors has been widely performed under ultrasonic guidance [34, 35, 36]. This technique has allowed pancreatic biopsy and also biochemical and cytological examination of the cyst fluid to be easily performed preoperatively. The aspirated fluid from malignant cysts frequently contains high levels of CEA, LDH, and CA19-9, and low levels of amylase and elastase 1. Pseudocyst of the pancreas usually shows the opposite results. However, there is considerable overlap of these values between benign and malignant cysts. Aspiration biopsy or cytology may lead to an accurate diagnosis of malignant tumor if a suitable sample is obtained; however, the data available at present are insufficient to evaluate the sensitivity and reliability of these parameters, and further studies are needed.

Gross Findings

The tumors consist of a bulky, round, lobulated mass, and have a thick fibrous capsule usually surrounded by normal pancreatic tissue. The external surface is generally smooth and glistening, but some tumors may have carcinomatous or inflammatory adhesions to the retroperitoneum and neighboring organs. The size of the tumor ranges from 1 to 30 cm in maximum diameter, with a mean of about 10 cm. The sectioned tumor reveals either a unilocular cyst or irregular multilocular cysts separated by thin fibrous septa. In either case, the cystic cavities are generally large, with smaller cysts sometimes observed within the fibrous capsule and septa. The cyst walls tend to be smooth in benign lesions (Fig. 6a), whereas the inner surface of malignant cysts often shows irregular protuberances or papillary excrescences projecting into the cyst lumen (Fig. 6b–d). These intraluminal protrusions may appear solid in some parts, but are actually composed of multiple small cysts containing mucoid material. Most cysts are filled with thick, gelatinous mucin, and at times with hemorrhagic or necrotic tissue.

Microscopic Findings

Microscopically, all these tumors consist of relatively well differentiated mucus-secreting epithelium. Low power view usually demonstrates cysts of varying size containing thick, mucoid material occasionally mixed with blood or debris (Fig. 7). The epithelial lining of these cysts is composed of high columnar mucinous cells, which are arranged in a single row in some cysts, but are often stratified and form small or large papillary projections (Figs. 8–10). The most notable feature is a wide range of variation in the lining, from histologically benign-appearing epithelium (Fig. 11), to atypical epithelium, to definite carcinoma in situ (Figs. 10–12). Marked variation of epithelium can be frequently observed even within the same cyst, with an abrupt transition from one type to another in some parts, whereas in other places the borderline is poorly defined with a gradual transition. Tumors with solely benign-appearing epithelium are known to exist, and have traditionally been called (mucinous) cystadenoma (Figs. 6a, 11). However, most tumors demonstrate atypical epithelia or foci of frank carcinoma if a sufficient number of histologic sections are examined. Atypical or carcinomatous epithelium is usually identified in the irregularly thickened cyst wall or intraluminal papillary excrescences. Cysts whose lining epithelium shows prominent intacystic papillary growth are mainly composed of definite carcinoma (Fig. 12).

Stromal invasion of adenocarcinoma is often found in malignant tumors (mucinous cystadenocarcinoma). The invasion generally shows well differentiated tubular adenocarcinoma limited to small areas of the fibrous capsule or septa (Fig. 13). However, in advanced cases, extracapsular invasion is not rare, and even if carcinoma is confined to within the capsule, diffuse and extensive infiltration of carcinoma with poor differentiation may be present in the fibrous stroma (Fig. 14a,b). Even in invasive tumors, it is also easy to find adenomatous areas with benign appearance. These microscopic findings suggest that cystadenocarcinomas probably arise by malignant transformation occurring in benign mucinous cystadenoma. The author and others [7, 12, 25], support the concept that all mucinous cystic tumors should be regarded as intrinsically malignant or as having a high potential for malignant transformation. Tumor spread is mainly limited to local invasion, and usually there is no evidence of lymphatic or vascular metastasis.

In association with these tumors, the cyst wall may become inflamed, and a small postinflammatory pseudocyst may develop in or adjacent

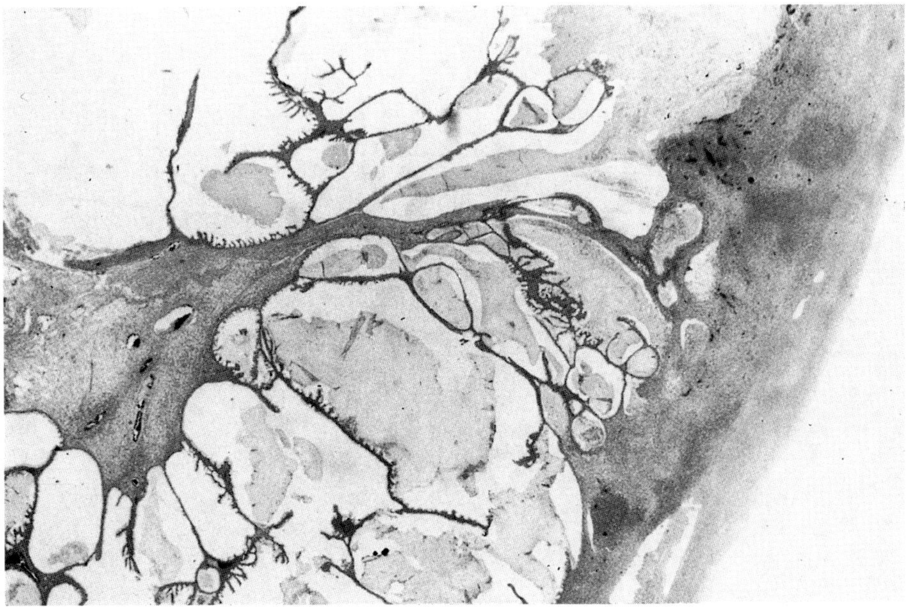

Fig. 7. Mucinous cystadenocarcinoma. Low power view of the solid-appearing part of the tumor shown in Fig. 6d, which is composed of varying sized cysts containing thick, mucoid material. The fibrous septa and capsule are thickened in places. (H&E ×40)

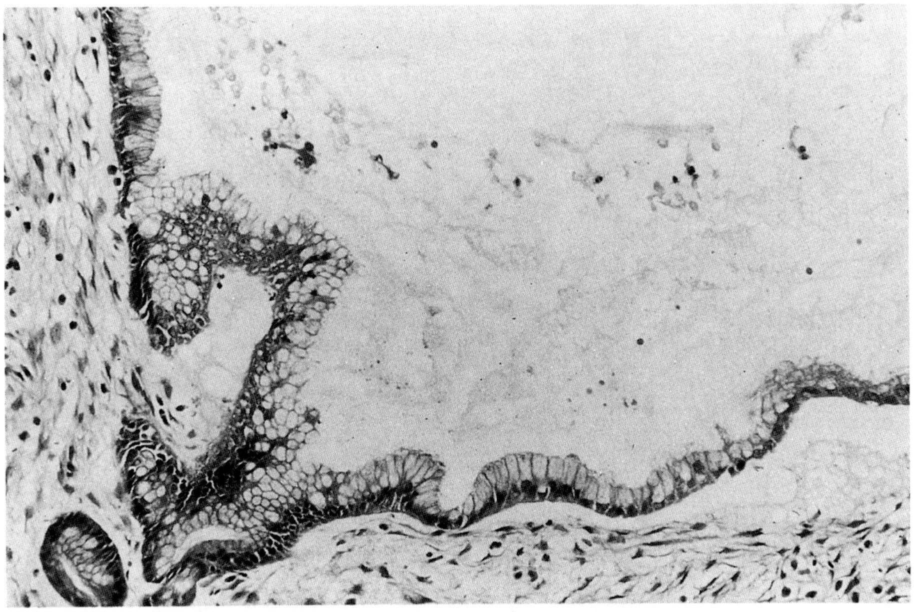

Fig. 8. Non-invasive mucinous cystic tumor of borderline malignancy. High columnar mucinous epithelium observed in the tumor of Fig. 6b. Well-differentiated epithelial cells are arranged in a single row or stratified. (H&E ×400)

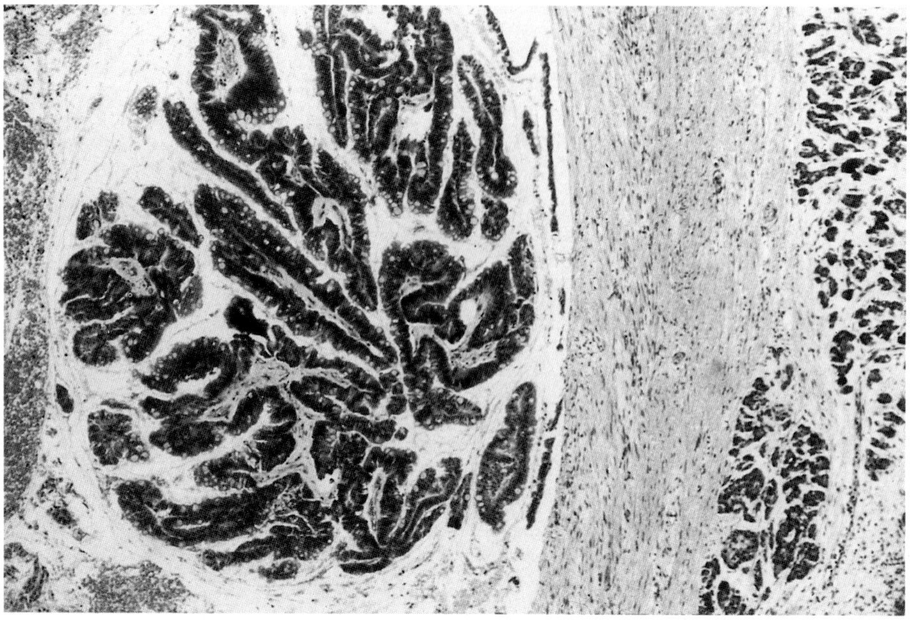

Fig. 9. Non-invasive mucinous cystic tumor of borderline malignancy. A polypoid papillary tumor projecting into the cyst lumen from the tumor of Fig. 6b, showing arborizing epithelial growth with thin fibrous stalks. The diagnosis of mucinous cystic tumor with moderate to severe atypia was made. Other parts of this cyst were also covered by atypical epithelium containing no foci of definite carcinoma. (H&E ×100)

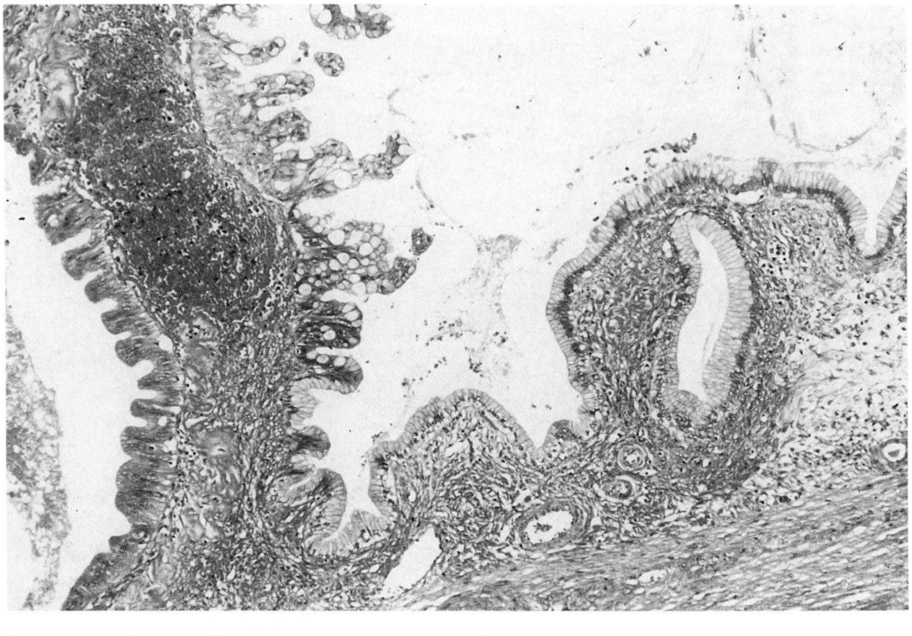

Fig. 10. Mucinous cystadenocarcinoma. Epithelial lining of the tumor shown in Fig. 6c. There is wide variation, from histologically benign, to atypical epithelium, to definite carcinoma in situ. (H&E ×200)

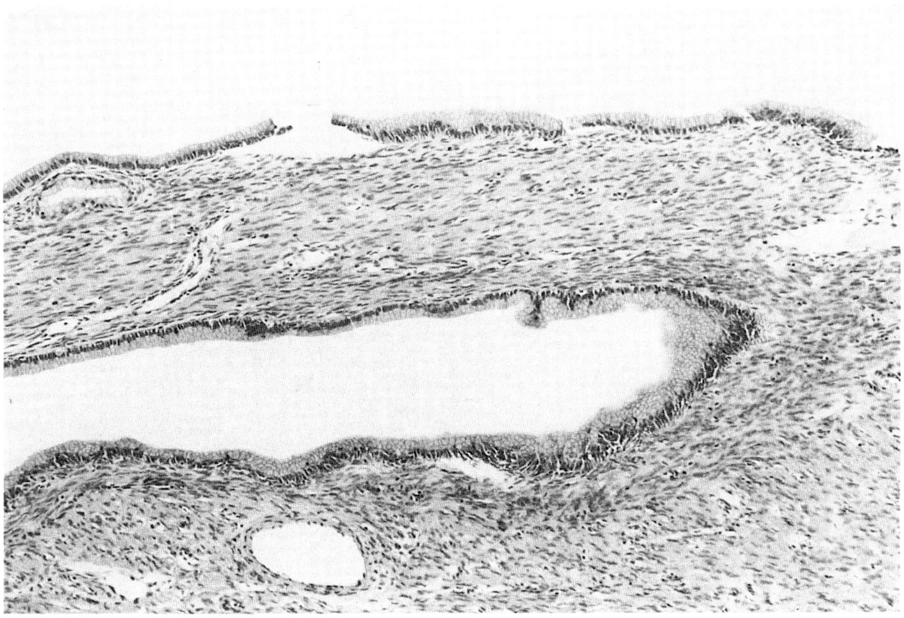

Fig. 11. Non-invasive mucinous cystadenoma (mucinous cystic tumor with benign appearance). Benign-appearing epithelium in the cysts of Fig. 6a. All the cysts were lined by this type of well-differentiated mucinous columnar epithelium. Papillary growth of the lining was rarely found, but such proliferative epithelia in small areas suggested the neoplastic nature of this lesion. (H&E ×200)

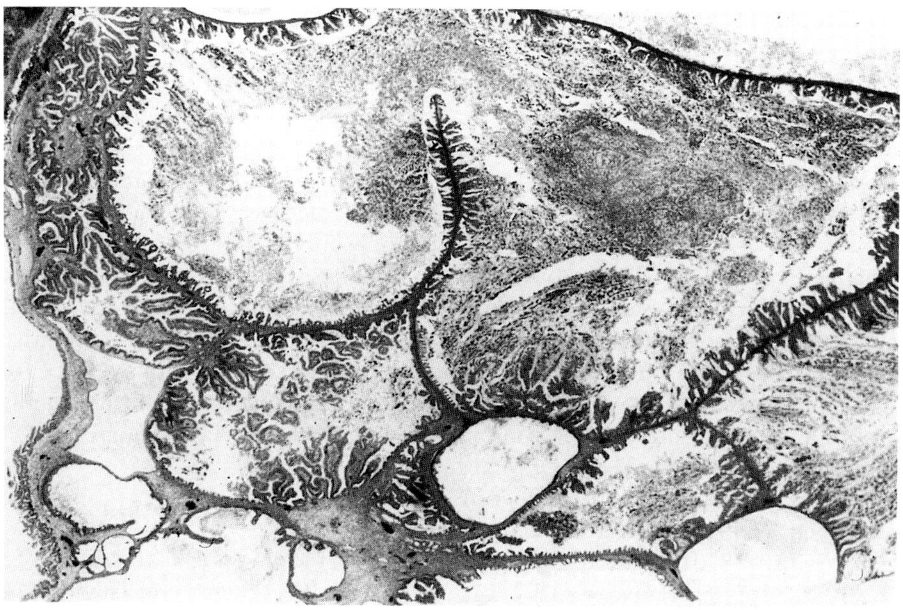

Fig. 12. Mucinous cystadenocarcinoma. Microscopic appearance of the irregular excrescences in the tumor shown in Fig. 6c. The lining epithelium shows marked intracystic papillary growth. Most of the epithelium can be identified as definite carcinoma in situ. (H&E ×100)

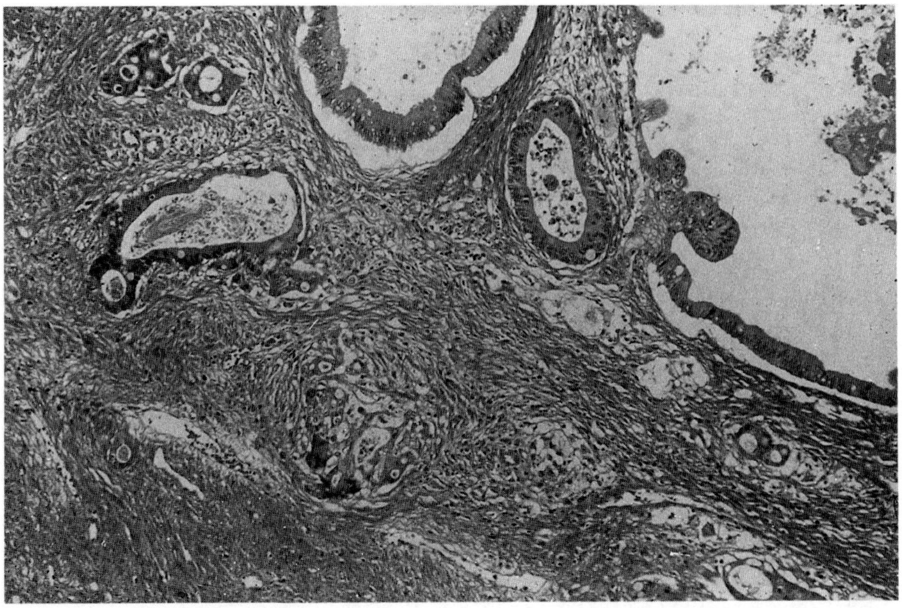

Fig. 13. Mucinous cystadenocarcinoma. Stromal invasion found in the tumor of Fig. 6c. Infiltrating tubular adenocarcinoma is seen in the fibrous stroma adjacent to a cystic space. In this tumor, a few small foci of stromal invasion were histologically confirmed in the fibrous septa. (H&E ×200)

to the tumor. The fibrous capsule of the tumor sometimes contains focal calcifications, granulomas, and atrophic pancreatic parenchyma including ducts and islets. The adjacent pancreatic tissue appears unremarkable unless it is markedly compressed by the tumor.

Histochemical and Ultrastructural Studies

Mucin histochemistry of tumor cells demonstrates a marked increase in neutral and sialomucins, which are absent or scanty in the epithelium of normal pancreatic ducts [37, 38]. These histochemical reactions are qualitatively identical with those of goblet cells. Some tumors contain cells with silver-positive intracytoplasmic granules [7], and immunohistochemically neuroendocrine elements have been confirmed in over half of mucinous cystic tumors [13, 21]. In addition, these tumors show an intense reactivity of CEA and CA19-9 in the epithelial cells and occasionally also in the stroma (Fig. 15a,b) [39, 40]. Yamaguchi and Enjoji [22] showed that the staining was stronger and more extensive in malignant tumors than in tumors of benign appearance or borderline malignancy. Based on the reactivity of tumor cells with anti-CEA antibody, Ohta et al. [41] concluded that severe atypical epithelial hyperplasia, composed primarily of mucus-poor columnar epithelium, represented a precursor to mucinous cystadenocarcinoma, and suggested that mucus-poor atypical epithelia may undergo malignant transformation. Ultrastructural study of tumor cells by Albores-Saavedra et al. [13] revealed mucin vacuoles and some colonic markers including microvilli with long rootlets of actin filaments and dense bodies located along the apical portion of the cytoplasm.

All these findings may provide evidence of intestinal differentiation of tumor cells. However, it should be noted that the characteristics described here are not specific to this type of tumor and may also be demonstrated in the common duct cell adenocarcinoma of the pancreas.

Differential Diagnosis

Because the imaging features of US and CT accurately reflect the macrocystic nature of mucinous cystic tumors, it is easy to differentiate this tumor from serous cystadenoma which shows coalescence of multiple small cysts of generally microscopic size (see Chapter "Serous Cystadenoma" in this volume). The clinical diagnosis may present some problems in the differentiation from pseudocyst, retention cyst, congenital cyst, and solid and cystic (papillary-cystic) tumor of the pancreas. Usually

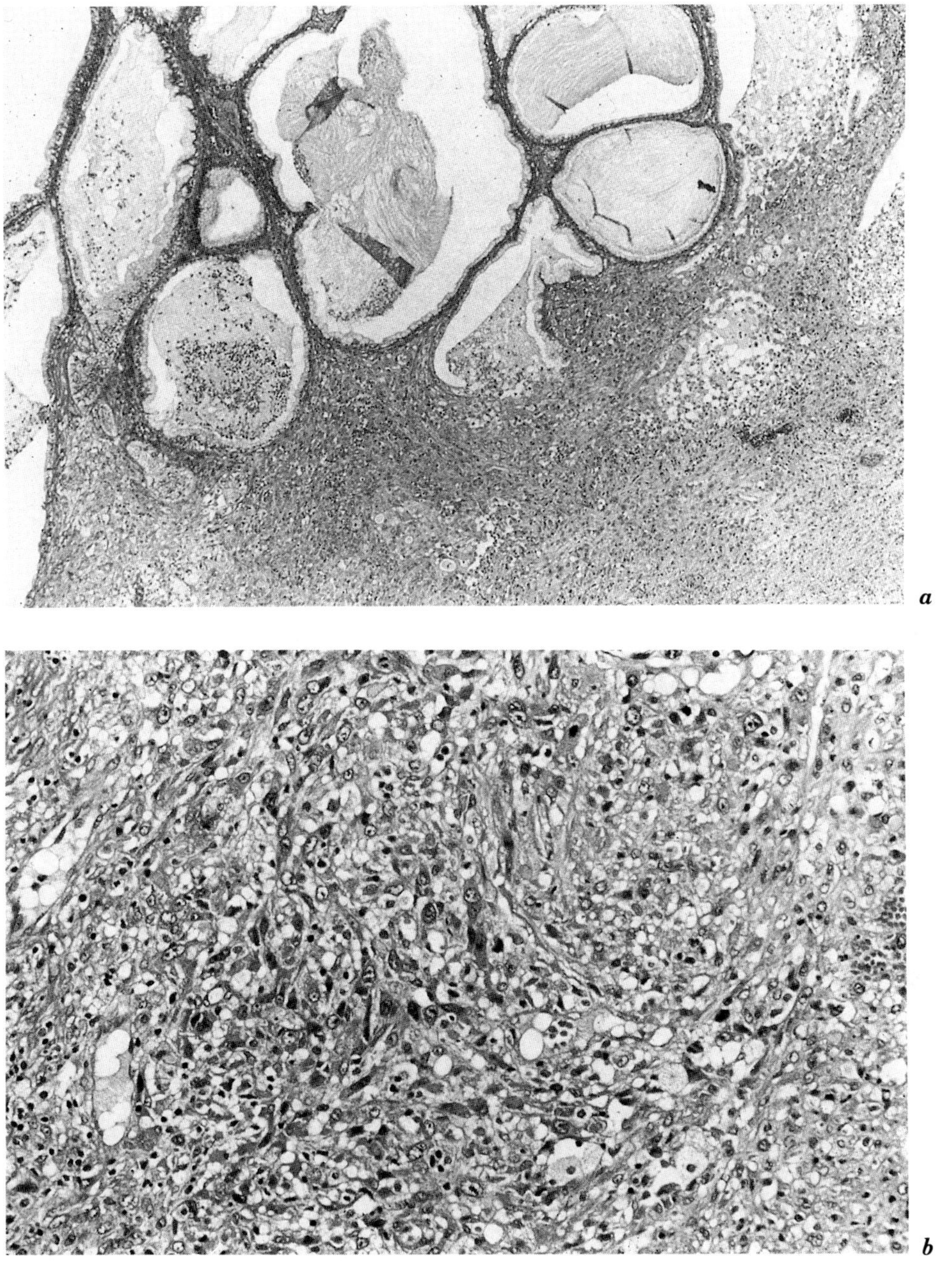

Fig. 14a,b. Mucinous cystadenocarcinoma. Stromal infiltration of carcinoma cells in the tumor of Fig. 6d. ***a*** Extensive infiltration of poorly-differentiated adenocarcinoma is observed in the fibrous septa just beneath the well-differentiated epithelial lining of the cystic cavities (H&E ×100). ***b*** High-power view of scattered carcinoma cells with no glandular formation within a thickened fibrous septum. (H&E ×400)

the multilocular structure of the cysts and irregular thickening or protrusions of cyst walls are helpful in the diagnosis of mucinous cystic tumor. However, it is sometimes difficult to distinguish this tumor from a postinflammatory pseudocyst with hemorrhage or necrotic debris. A lack of preceding history of pancreatitis or alcoholism can safely rule out pseudocyst, the most frequent cyst of the pancreas.

Histopathologically, the diagnosis of invasive or non-invasive mucinous cystic tumor can be made only after many blocks are examined from the entire specimen, especially from areas with irregular protrusions of the cyst wall, if present. The results obtained from a small biopsy can often be misleading in assessing the malignant potential as well as the neoplastic nature of the tumor, since it

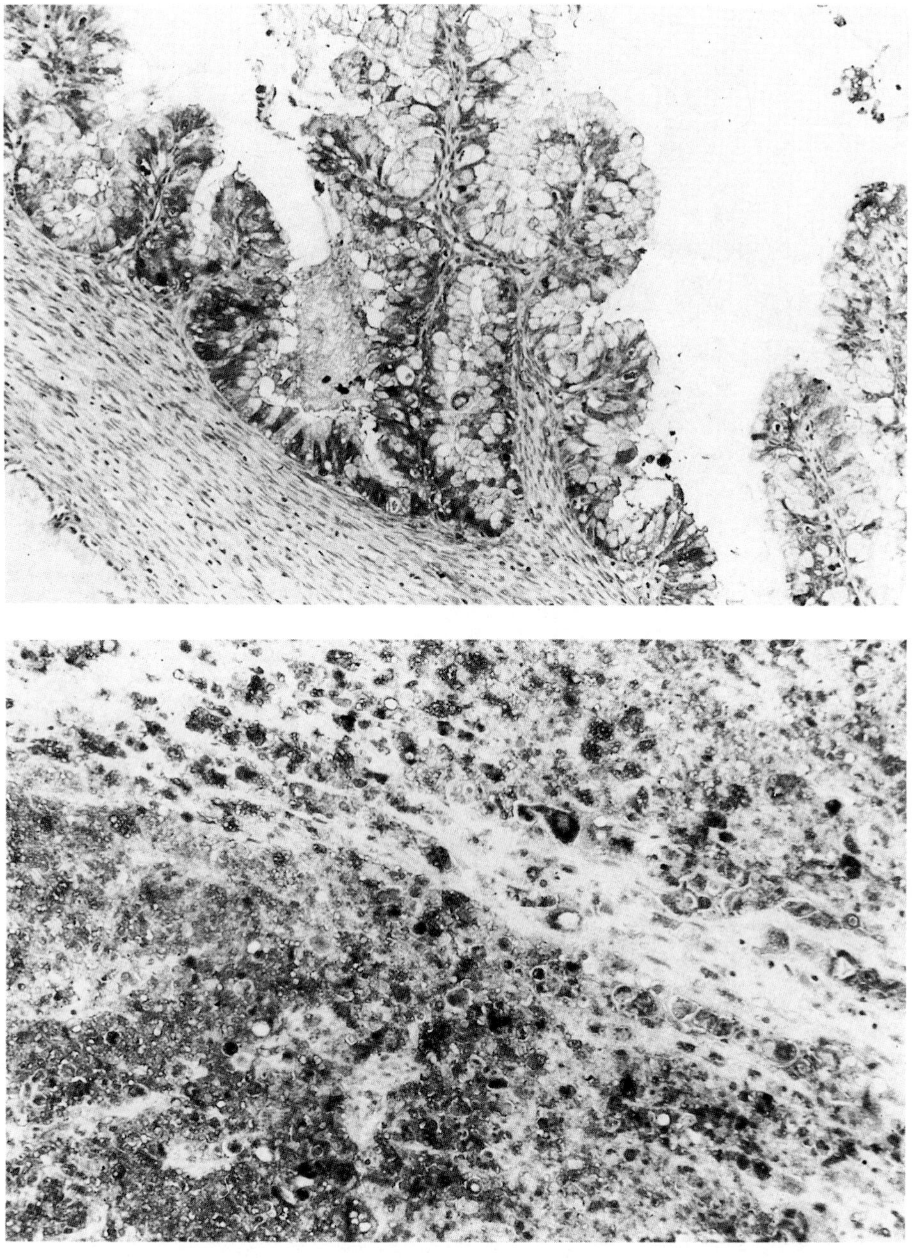

a

b

Fig. 15a,b. Mucinous cystadenocarcinoma. Immunohistochemical reaction for carcinoembryonic antigen (*CEA*) in the tumor tissue of Fig. 6d. ***a*** Intracystic well-differentiated papillary epithelium shows strong staining for CEA in the cytoplasm (×300). ***b*** A strong positive reaction for CEA is also demonstrated in the fibrous stroma, as well as in infiltrating carcinoma cells within the septum (×400)

may not provide representative epithelium needed for correct diagnosis. Additionally it should be noted that even in neoplastic cysts, the epithelial lining may be partially absent due to exfoliation related to inflammatory processes.

Biology, Treatment and Prognosis

It is generally accepted that all mucinous cystic tumors are either overtly malignant or at least potentially malignant from the standpoint of therapy. Therefore, complete removal of the tumor is recommended whenever possible. In the operative procedures used for tumor resection in previously reported cases, distal pancreatectomy has been most frequently performed (in over half of the cases), and less frequently extirpation, pancreatoduodenectomy, and total pancreatectomy in decreasing frequency [28, 29].

Formerly, patients with cystadenoma were occasionally treated by internal or external drainage of the cyst. In several documented cases, the tumor recurred as a cystadenocarcinoma [3, 27, 42]. Although this finding may support the concept of malignant transformation from benign to malignant, unrepresentative sampling and the slow growth of low-grade malignancies could also explain the clinical course. Most patients with cystadenocarcinoma not resected or incompletely resected, died of metastatic disease within a time frame similar to that of usual non-cystic pancreatic carcinomas [7, 21, 25].

I know of no instance in which a benign cystadenoma has recurred after total excision of the tumor. Many cystadenocarcinomas are resectable, with resection rates reported in reviews of the literature of 71% [29] and 78% [28]. When curative resection is performed for cystadenocarcinoma, a relatively good prognosis can be expected with reported cure rates of about 70% or greater [21, 22, 25], which is far higher than that of usual duct cell carcinoma of the pancreas. However, this cystadenocarcinoma group also contains a significant number of aggressive tumors of high-grade malignancy which may already have metastasized at the time of operation and usually have a bad prognosis. Thus, the overall results of surgical treatment will be largely related to the proportion of truly malignant tumors in the patients studied. Some series have indicated a poor prognosis of cystadenocarcinoma, and a Japanese review has also revealed an unsatisfactory result.

The author believes that the presence or absence of extracapsular invasion is not a reliable sign for determining the prognosis of this tumor. In my own five cases of definite malignant tumor, three showed no extracapsular spread macroscopically, but two of these had extensive intracapsular stromal infiltration of adenocarcinoma with poor differentiation, and subsequently died of recurrent disease, one at 3 months and the other at 2 years after radical operation.

The most important prognostic factor is the degree of stromal invasion; that is, the total area of stromal invasion, even if it is limited within the fibrous capsule or septum. The grade of differentiation of the infiltrating carcinoma cells may also influence the prognosis.

References

1. Glenner GG , Mallory GK (1956) The cystadenoma and related nonfunctional tumors of the pancreas; Pathogenesis, classification, and significance. Cancer 9:980–996
2. Campbell JA, Cruickshank AH (1962) Cystadenoma and cystadenocarcinoma of the pancreas. J Clin Pathol 15:432–437
3. Becker WF, Welsh RA, Pratt HS (1965) Cystadenoma and cystadenocarcinoma of the pancreas. Ann Surg 161:845–863
4. Marziani R (1929) Fortschreitende, polyzentrische, cystisch-papillare Adenomatosis des Pankreas. Arch Anat Pathol 271:625–638
5. Fitz RH (1900) Multilocular cystoma of the pancreas. Am J Med Sci 120:184–190
6. Lichtenstein L (1934) Papillary cystadenocarcinoma of the pancreas. Am J Cancer 21:542–553
7. Compagno J, Oertel JE (1978) Mucinous cystic neoplasms of the pancreas with overt and latent malignancy (cystadenocarcinoma and cystadenoma); A clinicopathologic study of 41 cases. Am J Clin Pathol 69:573–580
8. Hodgkinson DJ, ReMine WH, Weiland LH (1978) Pancreatic cystadenoma: A clinicopathologic study of 45 cases. Arch Surg 113:512–519
9. Cantrell BB, Cubilla AL, Erlandson RA, Fortner J, Fitzgerald PJ (1981) Acinar cell cystadenocarcinoma of human pancreas. Cancer 47:410–416
10. Stamm B, Burger H, Hollinger A (1987) Acinar cell cystadenocarcinoma of the pancreas. Cancer 60:2542–2547
11. George DH, Murphy F, Michalski R, Ulmer BG (1989) Serous cystadenocarcinoma of the pancreas: A new entity?. Am J Surg Pathol 13:61–66
12. Hartmann WH, Sobin LH (eds) (1984) Atlas of tumor pathology, 2nd series, fascicle 19. Tumors of the exocrine pancreas. Armed Forces Institute of Pathology, Washington DC, pp 98–241
13. Albores-Saavedra J, Angeles-Angeles A, Nadji M, Henson DE, Alvarez L (1987) Mucinous cystadenocarcinoma of the pancreas: Morphologic and immunocytochemical observations. Am J Surg Pathol 11:11–20
14. Klöppel G (1984) Pancreatic, non-endocrine tumours. In: Klöppel G, Heitz PU (eds) Pancreatic pathology. Churchill Livingstone, Edinburgh, pp 79–113
15. Yamaguchi K, Hirakata R, Kitamura K (1990) Mucinous cystic neoplasm of the pancreas: Estimation of grade of malignancy with imaging tech-

niques and its surgical implications. Acta Chir Scand 156:553–564
16. Morohoshi T, Kanda M, Asanuma K, Klöppel G (1989) Intraductal papillary neoplasms of the pancreas: A clinicopathologic study of six patients. Cancer 64:1329–1335
17. Rickaert F, Cremer M, Devière J, Tavares L, Lambilliotte JP, Schröder S, Wurbs D, Klöppel G (1991) Intraductal mucin-hypersecreting neoplasms of the pancreas: A clinoco-pathologic study of eight patients. Gastroenterology 101:512–519
18. Bastid C, Bernard JP, Sarles H, Payan MJ, Sahel J (1991) Mucinous ductal ectasia of the pancreas: A premalignant disease and a cause of obstructive pancreatitis. Pancreas 6:15–22
19. Itai Y, Ohhashi K, Nagai H, Murakami Y, Kokubo T, Makita K, Ohtomo K (1986) "Ductectatic" mucinous cystadenoma and cystadenocarcinoma of the pancreas. Radiology 161:697–700
20. Dabezies MA, Campana T, Friedman AC (1990) ERCP in the diagnosis of ductectatic mucinous cystadenocarcinoma of the pancreas. Gastrointest Endosc 36:410–411
21. Warshaw AL, Compton CC, Lewandrowski K, Cardenosa G, Mueller PR (1990) Cystic tumors of the pancreas: New clinical, radiologic, and pathologic observations in 67 patients. Ann Surg 212:432–445
22. Yamaguchi K, Enjoji M (1987) Cystic neoplasms of the pancreas. Gastroenterology 92:1934–1943
23. Warren KW, Athanassiades S, Frederick P, Kune GA (1966) Surgical treatment of pancreatic cysts: Review of 183 cases. Ann Surg 163:886–891
24. Hastings PR, Nance FC, Becker WF (1975) Changing patterns in the management of pancreatic pseudocysts. Ann Surg 181:546–551
25. Hodgkinson DJ, ReMine WH, Weiland LH (1978) A clinicopathologic study of 21 cases of pancreatic cystadenocarcinoma. Ann Surg 188:679–684
26. Segesser L, Rohner A (1984) Pancreatic cystadenoma and cystadenocarcinoma. Br J Surg 71: 449–451
27. ReMine SG, Frey D, Rossi RL, Munson JL, Braasch JW (1987) Cystic neoplasms of the pancreas. Arch Surg 122:443–446
28. Kasahara Y, Tanaka S, Miyamoto M, Morishita A, Ueda S, Nakao K, Takemoto M, Sonobe N, Yamada Y, Kuyama T, Ueda Y, Asakawa T (1986) Cystadenoma of the pancreas: Review of the Japanese literature. Med J Kinki Univ 11:1–9
29. Strodel WE, Eckhauser FE (1981) Cystic neoplasms of the pancreas. In: Dent TL (ed) Pancreatic disease: Diagnosis and therapy. Grune and Stratton, New York, pp 363–377
30. Pour P, Krüger WF, Althoff J, Cardesa A, Mohr U (1974) Cancer of the pancreas induced in the Syrian golden hamster. Am J Pathol 76:349–377
31. Friedman AC, Lichtenstein JE, Dachman AH (1983) Cystic neoplasms of the pancreas; Radiological-pathological correlation. Radiology 149:45–50
32. Minami M, Itai Y, Ohtomo K, Yoshida H, Yoshikawa K, Iio M (1989) Cystic neoplasms of the pancreas: Comparison of MR imaging with CT. Radiology 171:53–56
33. Ferrer JP, Hensley G, Kalser MH, Zeppa R (1978) Cystadenocarcinoma and carcinoembryonic antigen (CEA). Cancer 42:632–634
34. Tatsuta M, Iishi H, Ichii M, Noguchi S, Yamamoto R, Yamamura H, Okuda S (1986) Values of carcinoembryonic antigen, elastase 1, and carbohydrate antigen determinant in aspirated pancreatic cystic fluid in the diagnosis of cysts of the pancreas. Cancer 57:1836–1839
35. Young NA, Villani MA, Khoury P, Naryshkin S (1991) Differential diagnosis of cystic neoplasms of the pancreas by fine-needle aspiration. Arch Pathol Lab Med 115:571–577
36. Kimura K, Yamanaka T, Sakai H, Ido K, Seki H, Yoshida Y (1982) Biochemical and cytological analyses of cystic fluid aspirated by percutaneous puncture under ultrasonic guidance in cystic diseases of the pancreas. Gastroenterol Jpn 17:4–9
37. Chen J, Baithun SI, Ramsay MA (1985) Histogenesis of pancreatic carcinomas: A study based on 248 cases. J Pathol 146:65–76
38. Roberts PF, Burns J (1972) A histochemical study of mucins in normal and neoplastic human pancreatic tissue. J Pathol 107:87–94
39. Bätge B, Bosslet K, Sedlacek HH, Kern HF, Klöppel G (1986) Monclonal antibodies against CEA-related components discriminate between pancreatic duct type carcinomas and non-neoplastic duct lesions as well as nonduct type neoplasias. Virchows Arch [A] 408:361–374
40. Makovitzky J (1986) The distribution and localization of the monoclonal antibody-defined antigen 19-9 (CA19-9) in chronic pancreatitis and pancreatic carcinoma: An immunohistochemical study. Virchows Arch [B] 51:535–544
41. Ohta T, Nagakawa T, Fukushima W, Mori K, Kayahara M, Akiyama T, Kanno M, Ueno K, Miyazaki I, Terada T, Nakanuma Y (1992) Immunohistochemical study of carcinoembryonic antigen in mucinous cystc neoplasms of the pancreas. Eur Surg Res 24:37–44
42. Warren KW, Hardy KJ (1968) Cystadenocarcinoma of the pancreas. Surg Gynecol Obstet 127: 734–736

Solid Cystic Tumors

Synonyms and Related Terms

Papillary tumor of the pancreas (Frantz's tumor), papillary epithelial neoplasm, solid and papillary neoplasm, papillary-cystic tumor, solid cystic tumor of the pancreas, solid and cystic acinar cell tumor.

Incidence

More than 320 cases of solid cystic tumor (SCT) of the pancreas have been reported in the world literature [1–4]. Morohoshi et al. [5] noted a 2.7% incidence of SCT among 264 exocrine pancreatic tumors, whereas Cubilla and Fitzgerald [1] found only one case (0.2%) among 645 malignant neoplasms from the non-endocrine pancreas. The largest series is from AFIP and consists of 52 cases [6].

SCT has been reported recently with increasing frequency. This may be due to the increased awareness of the disease and improvement in the diagnostic procedures, such as ultrasonography (US), computed tomography (CT), and endoscopic retrograde pancreatography (ERCP), rather than to any significant increase in the incidence of this tumor. Some of the newly published cases of SCT include those that originally were misdiagnosed or presented unusual patterns. It is conceivable that the actual incidence of SCT is much greater than previously anticipated.

Sex

SCT of the pancreas has been described almost exclusively in young, fertile women. The tumor rarely is found in older women [7, 8] or men [9–15]. Some cases reported in men presented atypical SCT [8, 16]. The mean age of male patients with SCT is higher than that of female patients. In two young male patients, SCT within and outside the pancreas has been observed by Klöppel et al. [15].

Age

More than 90% of the patients with SCT were less than 30 years old. It is usually found in women in the second or third decade of life, but it can develop anywhere from 10 to 70 years of age.

Etiology and Pathogenesis

Because SCT occurs more often in young women, hormonal factors may be involved in its pathogenesis [17–19]. Ladanyi et al. [18] noted significant levels of estrogen receptor (ER) and progesterone receptor (PgR) in the tumor. Wrba and colleagues [19] found markedly elevated levels of PgR, but no ER. Carbone and coworkers [17] measured both type I and type II ER in two tumors, and they found a high level of type II but negligible amounts of type I ER. On the other hand, immunohistochemical examination has failed to detect nuclear ER in many cases [15, 19, 20]. Thus, results of hormone receptor analysis are conflicting probably because of the heterogeneity of assay techniques used in these studies. The availability of specific monoclonal antibodies has made it possible to localize ER and PgR immunohistochemically in tumor cells. Recently, PgR has been demonstrated immunohistochemically in the nuclei of endocrine cells of Langerhans islets [21] and in many pancreatic endocrine tumors [22]; however, ER was absent in these tissues. Immunoreactivity of PgR, but not ER, has been found in a series of SCT in women [13], and both were found in women and in a young boy [23].

Clinical Presentations

Patients normally experience a gradually enlarging mass in the upper abdomen, which is frequently in the left upper quadrant, with or without abdominal discomfort or pain. The tumor is often diagnosed incidentally by abdominal palpation or by US and CT, or when the tumor has already become a large mass. About a quarter of the patients complain of appetite loss and mild abdominal discomfort [24, 25]. A rupture of SCT, with acute hemoperitoneum and a sudden pain due to intratumoral hemorrhage [15], is another form of clinical presentation.

There are no abnormalities in the clinical laboratory tests. Serum levels of amylase and of biomarkers for pancreatic cancer, including CA19-9, carcinoembryonic antigen (CEA), and α-fetoprotein (AFP), are all within the normal range, although an atypical SCT in a 37-year-old Japanese patient has been found to produce CA19-9 [16]. Pancreatic islet hormones are also within normal limits, and no functional syndrome is associated with this tumor.

The tumor has been found mostly in the tail of the pancreas; however, recent findings indicate no predictable site of origin. Some tumors have been found in the extra-pancreatic areas, including the mesocolon or the liver [15, 26, 27]. These tumors may arise in ectopic pancreatic tissue as well.

US, CT. Abdominal plain film infrequently shows a calcified tumor (Fig. 1) [11, 18, 29]. US and CT findings have been reported extensively [9, 10, 30, 31]. US and CT project the "cut surface" of SCT and present different findings, depending on the dominant component of the tumors—cystic and mixed types. The mixed type of SCT is the most frequent. In general, abdominal US and CT show a well-demarcated "cystic" tumor with irregular septa and varying echogenicity (Figs. 2, 3). Irregular calcifications or ossifications, often in the periphery of the tumor, occur in 30% of the patients [25].

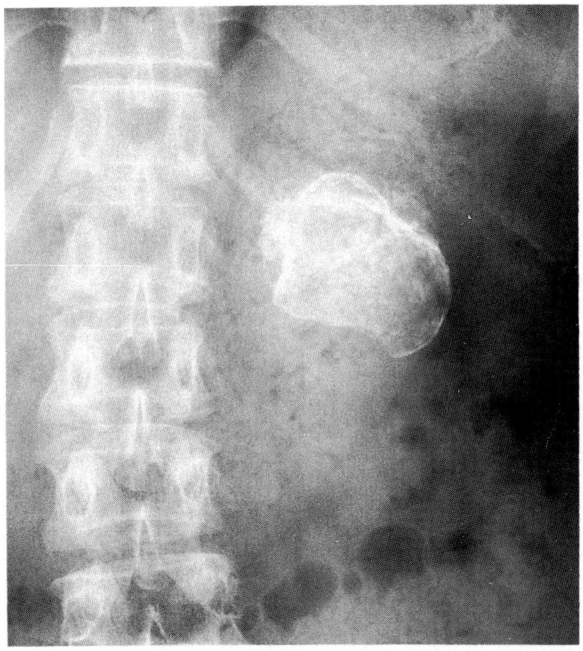

Fig. 1. A calcified abdominal mass in a 51-year-old Japanese woman (abdominal stout film). A calcified mass was noted 6 years before the present admission. The shape and size of the tumor remained unchanged. Ultrasonography and computed tomography showed a calcified cystic mass in the tail of the pancreas. Angiography showed an avascular mass displacing the splenic vessels. A distal pancreatectomy was done. The patient has been doing well 13 months after a complete resection

ERCP. The tumor is usually not connected with the pancreatic ductal system and ERCP shows displacement or stenosis of the pancreatic duct (Fig. 4). The main features on magnetic resonance imaging (MRI) are a well-demarcated rim enclosing a multiloculated mass and the presence of internal structures consistent with tumor nodules. Angiography shows a mild neovascularity and tumor staining. However, there is no encasement or stenosis of the arteries.

Cytology. The usefulness of preoperative or intraoperative cytologic examinations (fine needle aspiration cytology) has been reported [32, 33]. The aspirates are highly cellular. Fragments of papillary structures that have branching fibro-vascular stalks lined with several layers of epithelial cells are

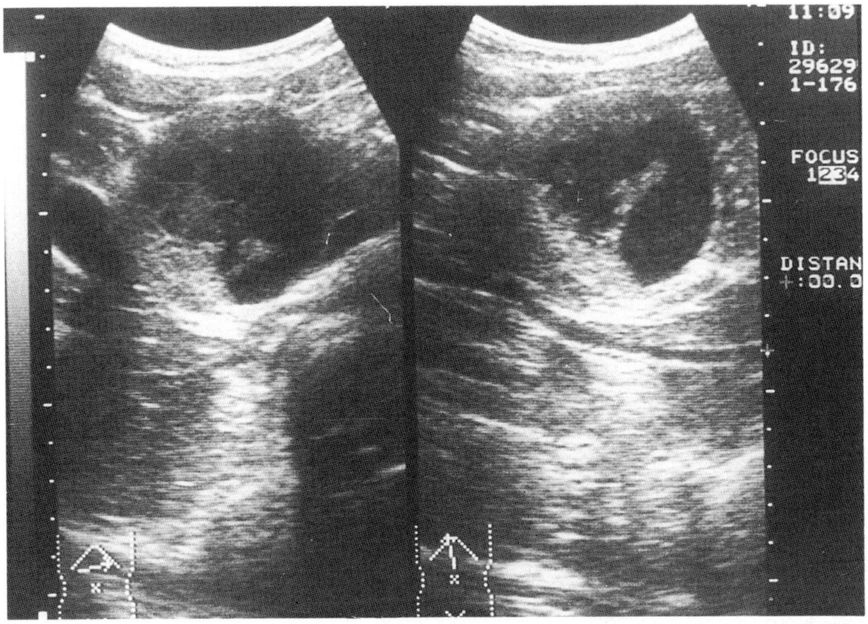

a

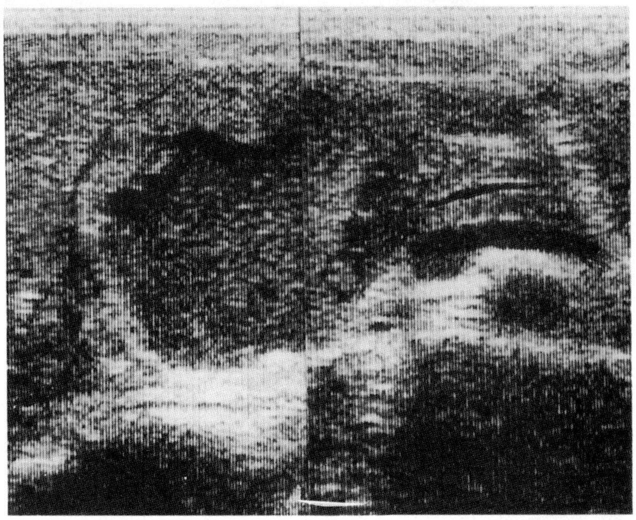

b

Fig. 2.a Abdominal ultrasonography of a 16-year-old girl showing pseudocystic lesions with irregular echogenicity in the head of the pancreas. ***b*** A pancreas head tumor with a solid and cystic pattern on ultrasonography. A dilatation of the main pancreatic duct distal to the tumor is present. A 21-year-old Japanese woman developed abdominal pain, and a mass was palpated in the right upper quadrant. Serum CEA and CA19-9 levels were within the normal limits. A pancreatoduodenectomy was done. The patient was doing well 48 months after a complete resection

prominent features of SCT (Fig. 5a). The tumor cells are monomorphic and have eccentric-to-central, round or oval nuclei with a fine chromatin distribution and one or two nucleoli; the cytoplasm is scanty to moderate (Fig. 5b). The nuclear membrane is delicate and smooth, while mitosis is rarely evident.

Gross Findings

SCTs are usually round or oval, well-circumscribed, and sometimes present as an encapsulated mass well-separated from the normal pancreatic tissue, thus easily removable. One case of incipient SCT, measuring 5 mm, was reported in a 34-year-old Japanese man who died of a brain hemorrhage [34]. The tumor tissue is usually fluctuant, and its cut surface shows a mixture of solid and cystic structures filled with red-brown necrotic debris surrounded by a thin irregular rim of solid tissues (Fig. 6). Some tumors are composed entirely of solid mass while others are purely cystic with thick walls. The cystic areas correspond to cystic change, hemorrhages, or necrosis. Cases with unusual calcifications have also been reported [28, 29]. Some SCTs show gross penetration into adjacent tissues [13, 14, 35] or are multicentric.

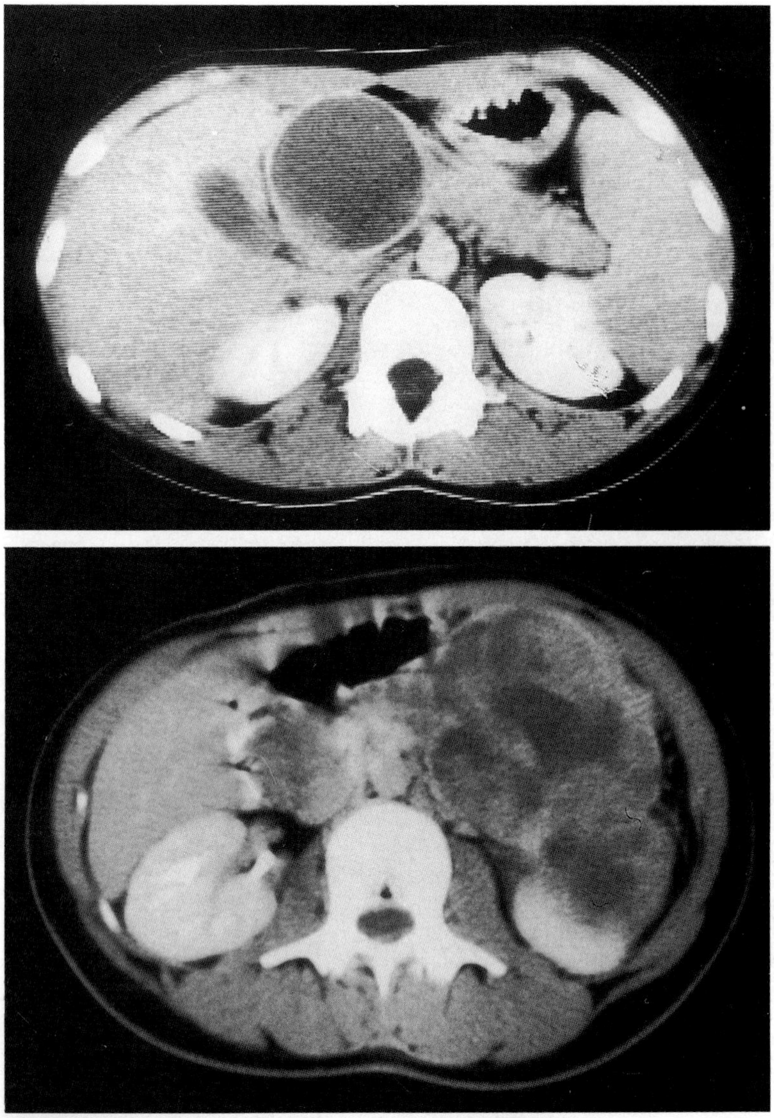

a

b

Fig. 3.a Abdominal computed tomography of the same patient in Fig. 1, showing a well-demarcated, pseudocystic lesion in the head of the pancreas. ***b*** A pancreas head tumor with a solid and cystic pattern on computed tomography (CT) of a 21-year-old woman who developed an abdominal mass. CT and ultrasonography showed a cystic mass with a solid component. A distal pancreatectomy was done. The patient was doing well 36 months after a complete resection

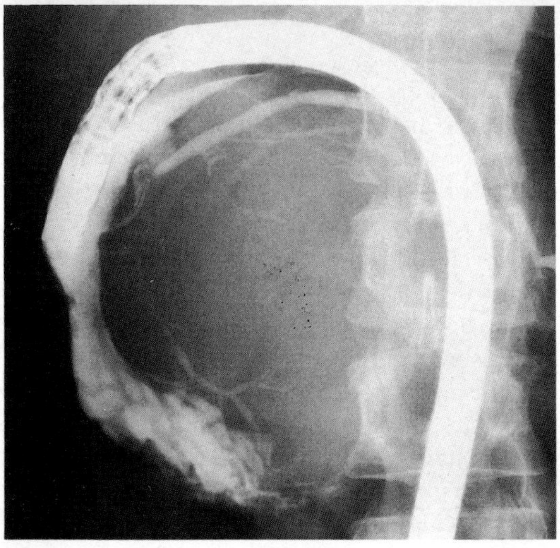

Fig. 4. Displacement of the main pancreatic duct on endoscopic retrograde pancreatography (the same case as in Fig. 2b)

Fig. 5.a Fine needle aspiration cytology. Pseudo-papillary structures overlaid by several layers of epithelial cells. (The same case as in Fig. 2b). Giemsa stain ×280. The histological pattern of this tumor is presented in Fig. 7c. ***b*** Fine needle aspiration cytology. Proliferation of monomorphic cells with round-to-oval nuclei containing fine granular chromatin and a moderate amount of cytoplasm. No mitosis is evident. (Papanicolaou's stain ×1000). (The same case as in Fig. 2b)

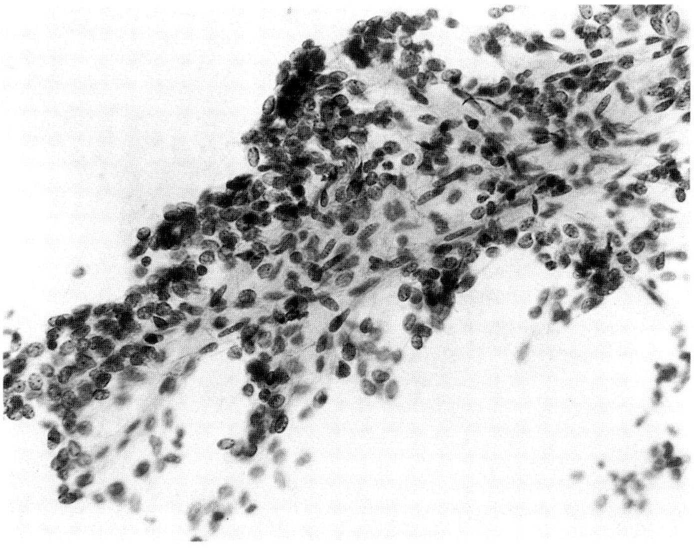

a

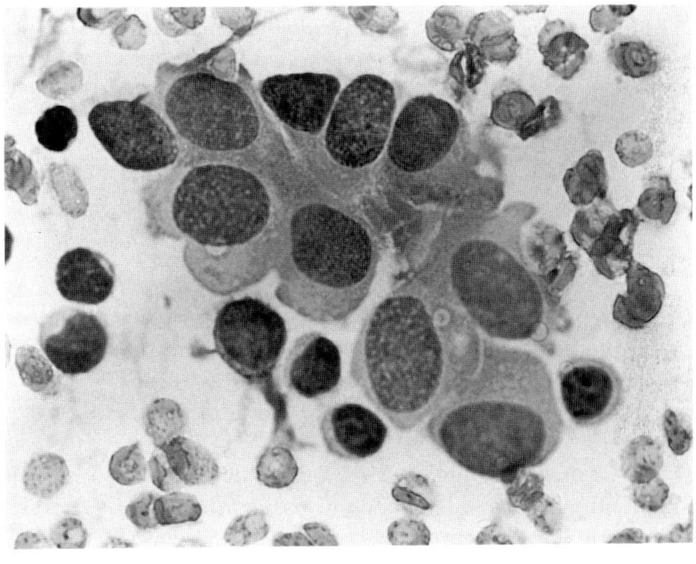

b

Microscopic Findings

Microscopically, SCT tumors usually exhibit a fibrous capsule (Fig. 7a). In some cases, however, the fibrous capsule is missing and tumor cells are directly contiguous to or invade the pancreatic parenchyma. The tumor is composed of solid and pseudo-papillary components. In solid areas, sheets of cells surround thin-walled vessels containing erythrocytes (Fig. 7b). In areas with a papillary appearance, oval cells are arranged around a fibrovascular stalk or small blood vessels (Fig. 7c). Empty spaces filled with blood are present between the pseudo-papillae (Fig. 7d). A periangiomatous arrangement is conspicuous.

Tumor cells are composed of two types: One with a round hyperchromatic nuclei and clear cytoplasm and the other with an eosinophilic granular cytoplasm. There are either very few mitotic figures or none at all, and cellular atypia, if present, is moderate.

A case with microcystic and abortive glandular patterns containing mucinous or myxoid material has been reported (Fig. 8a). In this case, a medullary arrangement of slightly pleomorphic tumor cells was seen adjacent to the cystic area (Fig. 8b).

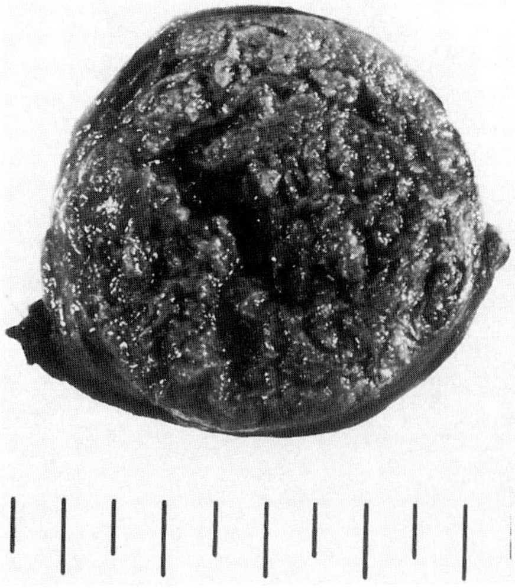

a

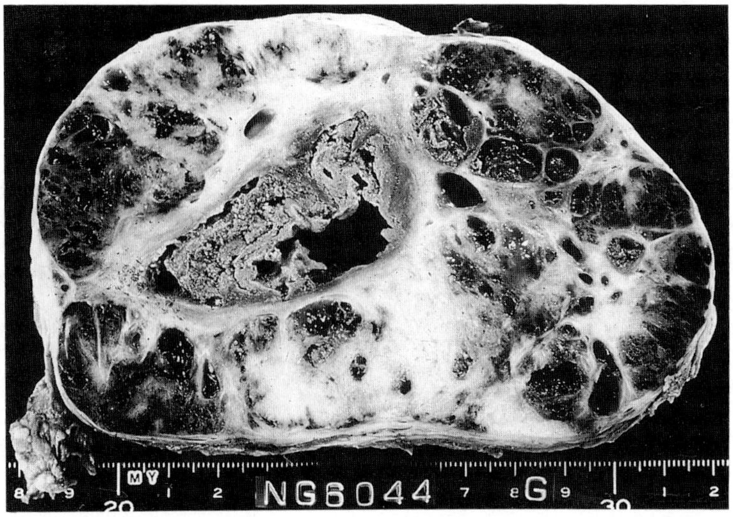

b

Fig. 6.a Cut surface of a solid cystic tumor. A 14-year-old Japanese woman developed an abdominal mass with associated pain. An upper gastrointestinal X-ray series showed a displacement of the duodenum. Ultrasonography and computed tomography showed a pancreatic head mass. An extirpation of the tumor was done. The cut surface showed a papillary growth of the tumor and cystic degeneration. The patient was doing well 104 months after a complete resection. ***b*** Well-encapsulated SCT with areas of hemorrhage and necrosis. This tumor was removed from the pancreas of a 37-year-old Japanese man who was admitted to the hospital with abdominal discomfort and abdominal mass. There were no symptoms suggestive of endocrine abnormality. (Courtesy of Dr. Kakihara [16] with permission)

Nests of vacuolated cells and collections of foamy macrophages (Fig. 9a) may be present at the periphery of the solid areas. In some cases, the tumor is almost completely necrotic and the ghost cells form papillary structures.

The stroma infrequently shows cholesterol deposits, hyalinization, calcification or ossification (Fig. 9b). In malignant cases, the tumor shows venous invasion, lymph node metastasis, or perineural infiltration. Capsular invasion of the tumor cells is seen in some cases.

Electron Microscopy

Closely packed polyhedral or cuboidal tumor cells have large nuclei sometimes with indentations and with diffusely scattered small concentrations of chromatin. The cytoplasm is sparse and of a light electron opacity. Free ribosomes, mitochondria, well-developed Golgi apparatus, desmosome-like complexes, canalicular-like structures, and microvilli projecting into the intercellular space (Fig. 10a) suggest ductal differentiation. A few granules varying in size of a slight electron opacity without a distinctive matrix are also present in a few cells [36, 37].

A few cells contain conspicuous membrane-bound, electron-dense granules (Fig. 11a), which are either similar to zymogen granules of various diameters (200–3000 nm) [3, 8, 38–41] or resemble endocrine granules [8, 16, 35–37, 42–44]. In a case reported by Kakihara et al. [16], almost all of the tumor cells had aberrant oval granules surrounded by a limiting membrane (Fig. 11a). These granules contained crystalloid needle-shaped material and highly dense round material (Fig. 11b).

Annulate lamellae (Fig. 11c) may be found in the tumor cells of SCT [36, 41]. These organells, the origin and function of which have not been clarified, are considered to be markers of immature or poorly differentiated cells.

Immunohistochemistry

Histochemical and immunohistochemical findings of SCT are not uniform and are still controversial. Some authors occasionally observe periodic acid-

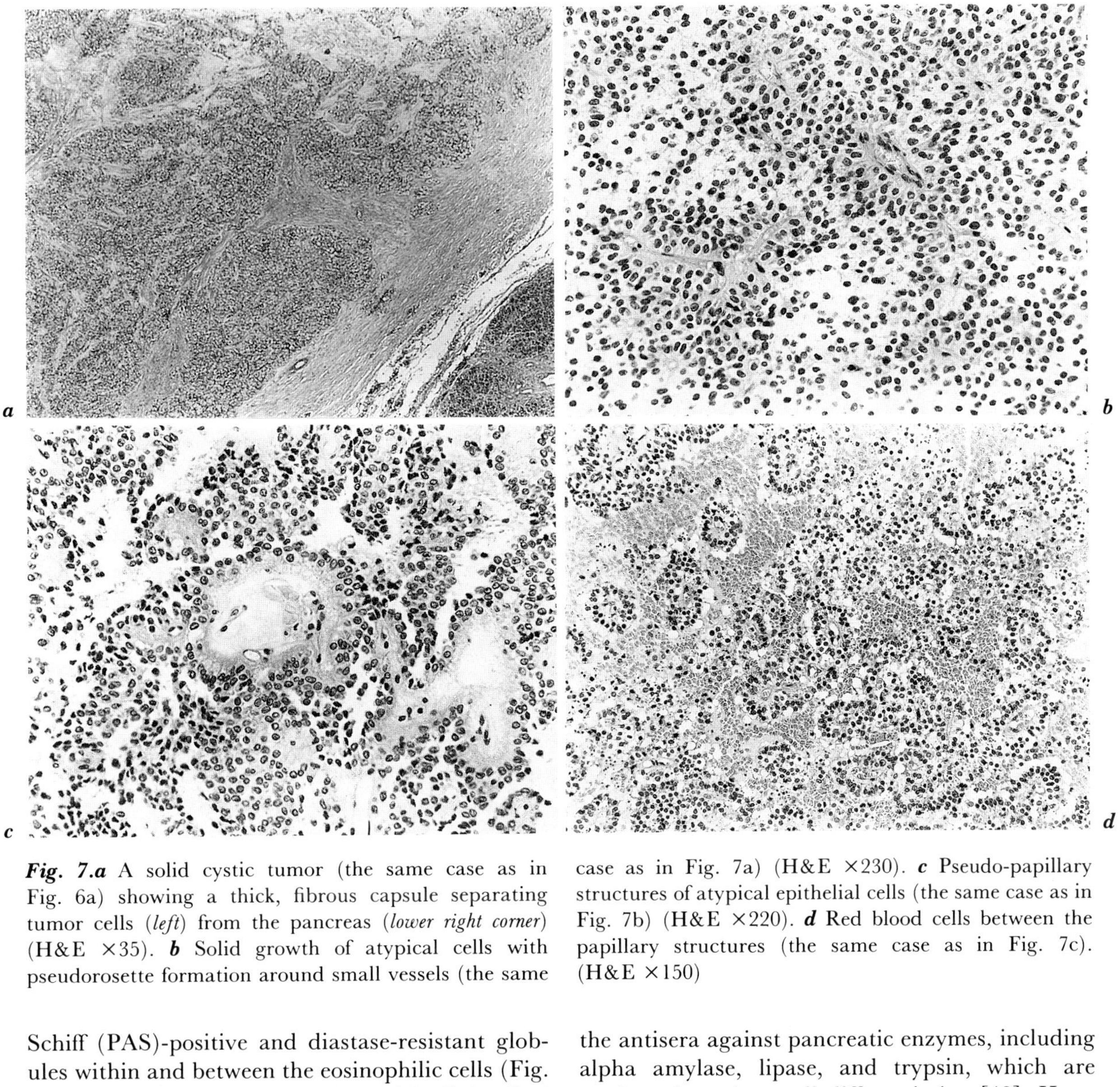

Fig. 7.a A solid cystic tumor (the same case as in Fig. 6a) showing a thick, fibrous capsule separating tumor cells (*left*) from the pancreas (*lower right corner*) (H&E ×35). ***b*** Solid growth of atypical cells with pseudorosette formation around small vessels (the same case as in Fig. 7a) (H&E ×230). ***c*** Pseudo-papillary structures of atypical epithelial cells (the same case as in Fig. 7b) (H&E ×220). ***d*** Red blood cells between the papillary structures (the same case as in Fig. 7c). (H&E ×150)

Schiff (PAS)-positive and diastase-resistant globules within and between the eosinophilic cells (Fig. 12a) or fine granules positive with Grimelius' method [16]. Others researchers have not confirmed these observations. The cytoplasm is negative for alcian blue (pH 2.5). Most authors note that the tumor cells are focally or diffusely immunoreactive for alpha-1 antitrypsin (AAT) (Fig. 12b), a marker of acinar cells. PAS-positive globules are often positive with AAT. These focal positive nests are occasionally located adjacent to microcystic structures.

Tumor cells are generally negative for pancreatic tumor markers such as CEA, pancreato-oncogenic antigen (POA) and AFP, but may express CA19-9 in unusual cases [16]. They also fail to react with the antisera against pancreatic enzymes, including alpha amylase, lipase, and trypsin, which are markers for acinar cell differentiation [40]. However, in unusual cases, a few cells may react with antichymotrypsin [16, 45].

The immunoreactivity in SCT tissue for pancreatic endocrine hormones (islet cell markers), including pancreatic polypeptide (PP), insulin, glucagon, and somatostatin, and a broad spectrum keratin marker, Lu-5 (an epithelial cell marker), is controversial. About 12% of SCT show a positive reaction with anti-neuron specific enolase (NSE) [40, 45, 46], synaptophysin, chromogranin A, and a few with anti-somatostatin, -insulin, -glucagon, and -PP [4, 16, 20, 43, 47]. According to Pettinato et al. [47], the cells reactive for islet hormones were

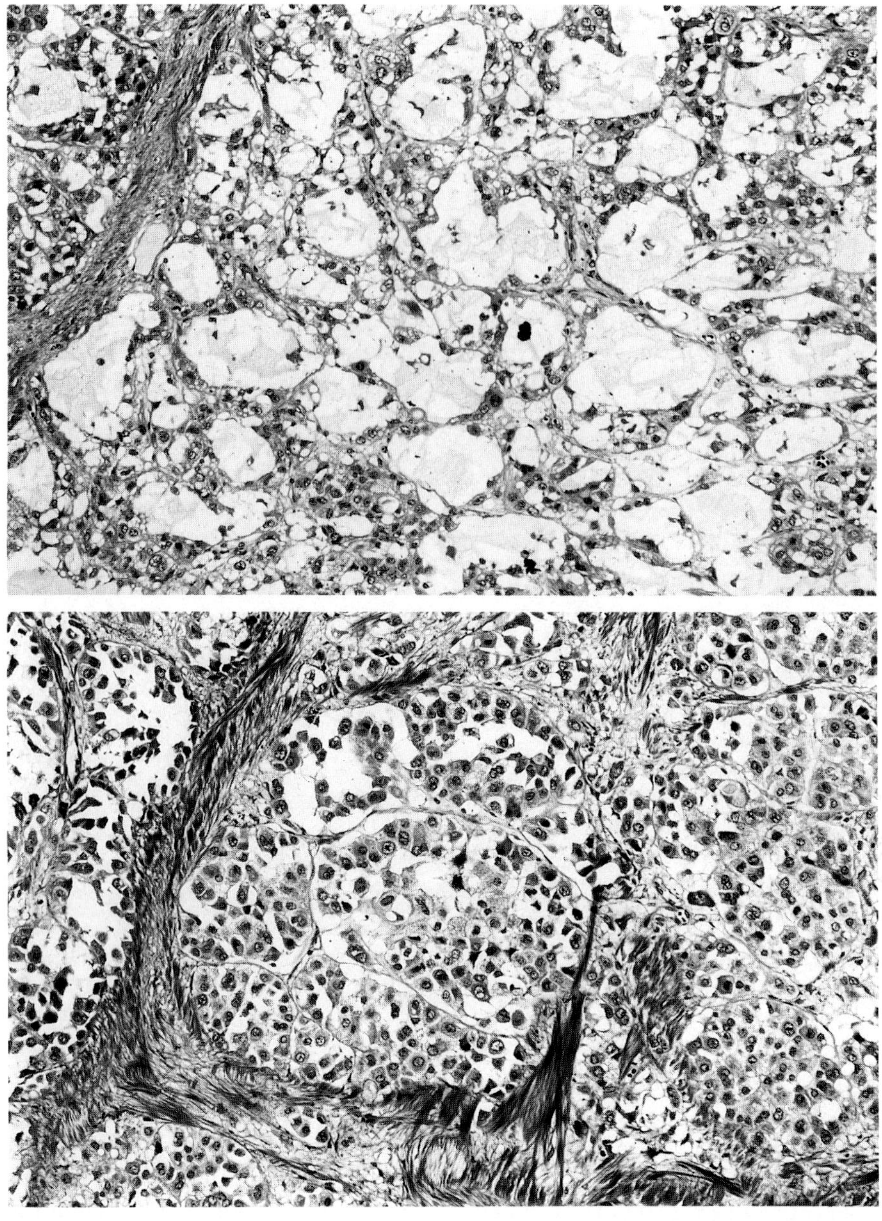

a

b

Fig. 8.a Microcystic pattern of tumor in Fig. 6b with mucinous material in cystic areas. Note focal abortive glandular pattern (*right middle field*). The appearance of the tumor cells in the *upper left corner* is shown in Fig. 8b (H&E ×200). (Courtesy of Dr. Kakihara [16] with permission). ***b*** Solid area of a solid cystic tumor adjacent to the lesion in Fig. 8a showing slightly pleomorphic tumor cells forming a medullary pattern (H&E ×400). (Courtesy of Dr. Kakihara [16] with permission)

also positive for Leu-7, synaptophysin, cytokeratin, and chromogranin A. A few cells were also immunoreactive for S-100 protein. Miettinen et al. [20], Klöppel et al. [15], Yamaguchi et al. [35], Zamboni et al. [23], and Pettinato et al. [47] have reported that tumor cells are positive for vimentin (marker of mesenchymal or undifferentiated cells).

According to studies by Zamboni et al. [23], Pettinato et al. [47], and Jorgensen et al. [45], tumor cells are reactive with keratin marker CAM 5.2, and enzymatic treatment with trypsin for 30 min seems to increase the reactivity. Keratin marker KL1 showed immunoreactivity in five out of eight cases (Fig. 13).

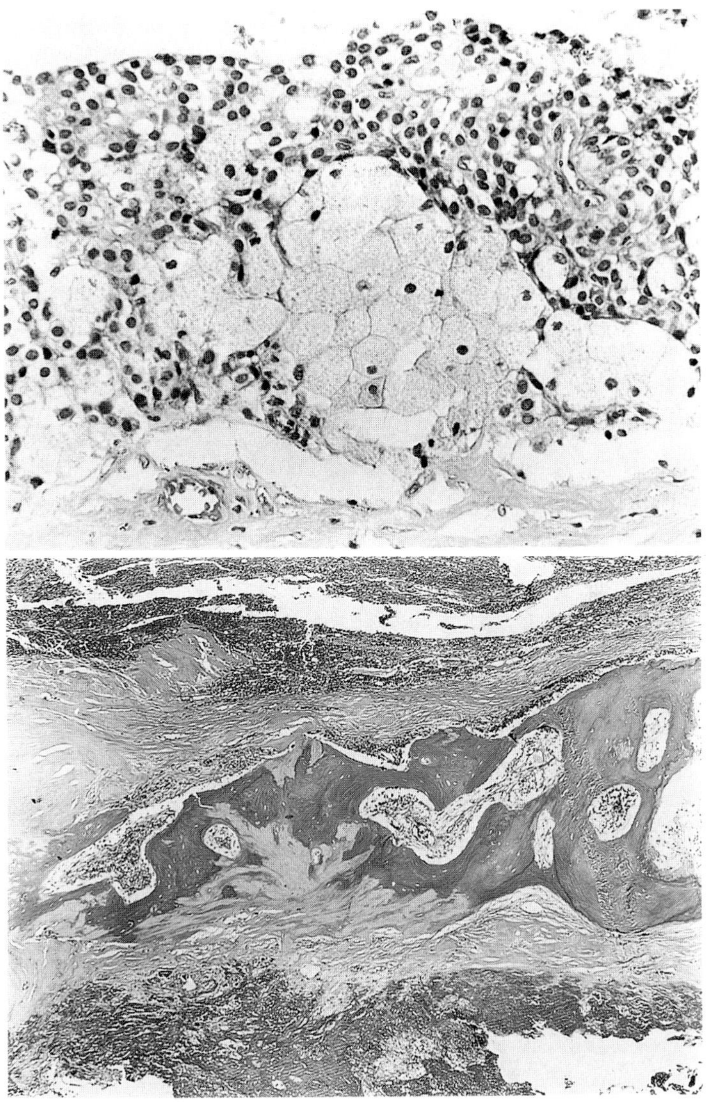

Fig. 9.a A solid cystic tumor (SCT) in a 17-year-old Japanese woman who developed right hypochondrial pain. Ultrasonography and computed tomography showed a cystic mass, measuring 3 cm, in the head of the pancreas. Angiography showed a displacement of the gastroduodenal artery and the posterior superior pancreatoduodenal artery. No encasement or tumor staining was evident. Extirpation of the tumor was done. A portion of the tumor showed collection of xanthoma cells (H&E ×250). The patient was doing well 120 months after a complete resection. ***b*** An SCT in a 34-year-old Japanese man, who noticed an abdominal mass. Abdominal plain film showed a calcified mass. A tumor measuring 11 cm in the body of the pancreas was removed. The tumor showed hyalinization and ossification of the stroma (H&E ×40). The patient was doing well 120 months after a complete resection

None of the eight tumors studied by Zamboni et al. [23] showed reactivity with antibodies against lipase or amylase, but contained PgR immunoreactive cells, ranging from 50% to almost all the neoplastic cells. As in normal islet cells, the PgR immunoreactivity was confined strictly to cell nuclei (Fig. 14). The number and distribution of the PgR positive cells in frozen tissue were similar to those in the corresponding paraffin sections. The distribution of progesterone reactive cells did not show any characteristic distribution pattern within the tumor, even though they appeared more abundant in the viable, peripheral, and solid areas. The immunocytochemical evaluation of the nuclear ER yielded negative results with either frozen or paraffin-embedded samples. However, nuclear ER was demonstrated in a tumor of a 21-year-old women [45].

PCNA (see later) immunostaining confined to the nuclei of tumor cells was detected in seven of eight cases [23]. The percentage of immunoreactive cells never exceeded 2% of the tumor cells (Fig. 15).

Flow Cytometric Findings

From nine tumors studied by Pettinato et al. [47], the coefficient variation (CV) to G_0G_1 peak was found to be <7.5% (mean CV, 5.9%; range, 4.4%–7%). Eight tumors were DNA diploid and

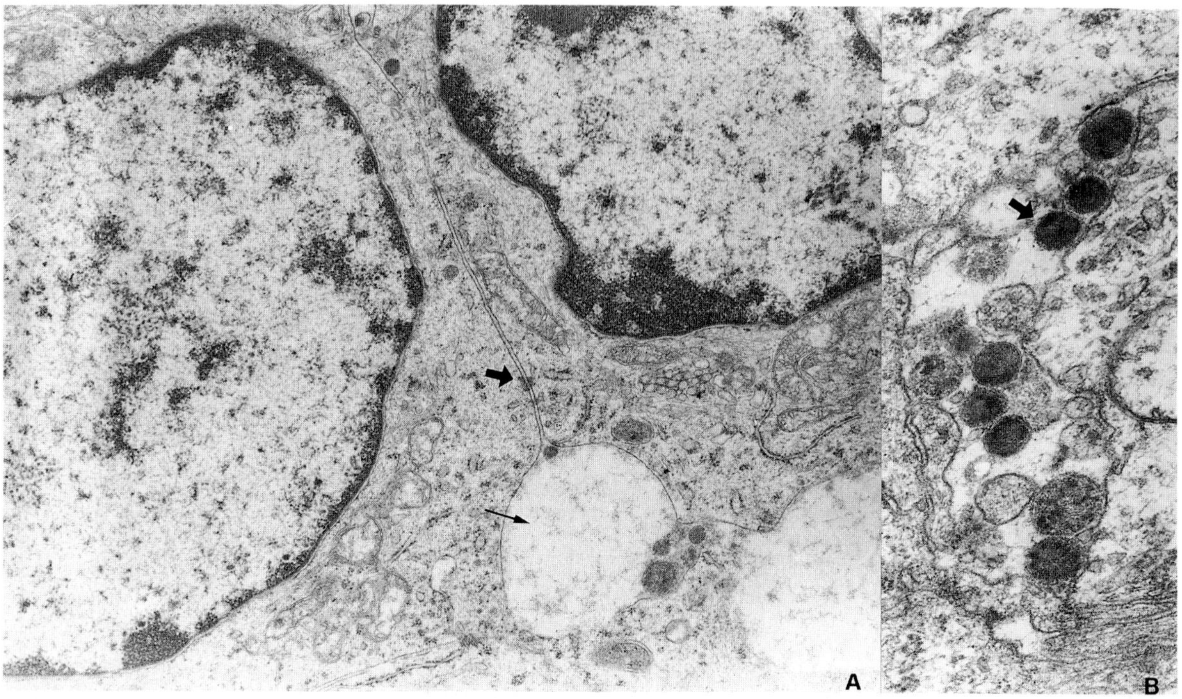

a

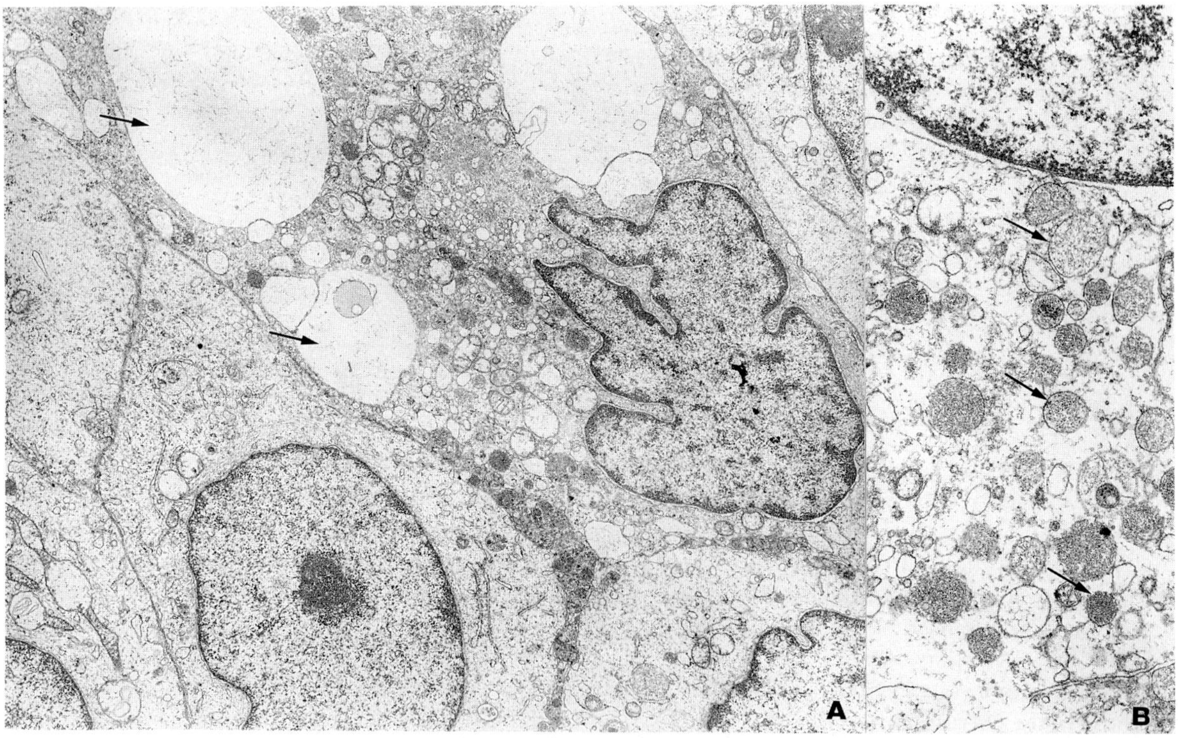

b

Fig. 10.a Intercellular spaces (*long arrow*) and an intermediate junction (*short arrow*) in *A* (×3000) and membrane-bound zymogen-like granules (*arrow*) in *B* (×15 000). A 28-year-old Japanese woman noticed a left hypochondrial mass with associated pain. Upper gastrointestinal X-ray series revealed a displacement of the stomach. A pancreas tail mass measuring 10 × 8.6 cm was removed. The cut surface was solid and cystic and contained a chocolate colored fluid. The patient was doing well 139 months after resection. ***b*** Intracytoplasmic vesicles (*arrows*) in *A* (×3280) and granules of various density (zymogen-like granules) (*arrows*) in *B* (×8200). (The same case as in Fig. 9a) tumors showed low-to-moderate proliferative activity. In one case, hyperploidy with a DNA index of 1.1 was found.

Histogenesis

The histogenesis of SCT has remained obscure because of inconsistencies in immunohistochemical and electron microscopic findings. Well-developed Golgi complexes, rough endoplasmic reticulum, zymogen-like granules, and the presence of AAT provide support for acinar cell differentiation of the tumor [3]. Immunoreactivity for neuron-specific enolase (normally present in neuroendocrine cells of the pancreas) [46], synaptophysin or chromogranin A (a marker of endocrine cells), pancreatic endocrine hormones, and the electron microscopic demonstration of neurosecretory granules in the tumor cells provide support for endocrine cell differentiation. Immunoreactivity for keratin, coexpression of vimentin and keratin, two intermediate filaments typical of mesenchymal and epithelial cells, and the electron microscopic demonstration of canaliculus-like gaps and occasional intercellular junctions support the hypothesis of small ductal cell differentiation [6]. A theory of a primitive epithelial cell capable of multidirectional differentiation [20, 35, 36] has been proposed as the cell of origin of SCT. Annulate lamellae are considered to be markers for immature cells [49]. The crystalloid structures seen in a tumor could represent aberrant zymogen granules or lysosomes [16].

The presence of PgR independent of sex or age, which has been confirmed in a number of cases, suggests a possible pathogenetic role of progesterone in SCT. The absence of ER immunoreactivity in tumor cells may imply that either: (1) the sensitivity of anti-PgR antibody is greater than the anti-ER antibody, with the result that the biochemically detectable ER cannot be immunocytochemically localized, or (2) the PgR-positive cells of SCT represent a cell population in which PgRs are constitutively synthesized in an estrogen-independent way, as in normal endocrine cells of Langerhans islets, T47D breast carcinoma cell line [50], meningioma cells [51, 52] and some gastric cancer cells [53].

In endocrine tumors of the pancreas where PgR positivity correlates with the absence of metastases and lack of tumor invasion [22], the positivity for PgR in SCT may have the same significance.

Nuclear DNA analysis by flow cytometry and by microscopical cytophotometry has been performed in some cases [48, 54, 55]. A DNA histogram shows an aneuploid pattern with a main peak between 2c and 3c, and it suggests a slow growing tumor with low proliferative activity.

The assessment of the proliferative fraction of SCT, using flow cytometry and microscopical cytometry, shows a low proliferative activity [48, 54, 55].

The immunohistochemical detection of proliferating cell nuclear antigen (PCNA), a cell-related nuclear protein that plays a fundamental role in DNA replication as an auxiliary protein of DNA polymerase delta [56, 57], agrees with the cytometry data. In all tumors tested by Zamboni et al. [23], very few (<2%) cells showed PCNA positivity. The PCNA index is considered a reliable prognostic marker in different neoplasms [58–60].

Molecular Biology

Immunohistochemically, SCT contains cells immunoreactive with an c-Ha-*ras* oncogene product (c-Ha-*ras* p21) [35]. There are as yet no data on mutations of c-Ki-*ras* or p53 in this tumor.

Diagnosis and Differential Diagnosis

A large pancreatic mass with a solid and cystic pattern in a young woman suggests SCT. A definite diagnosis depends, however, on histologic findings. The diagnosis of SCT is important because of the favorable clinical course of this tumor after complete resection. An aggressive surgical approach is mandatory, even if the tumor is huge.

Histologically, nonfunctioning islet cell tumors should be differentiated from SCT. Both lesions consist of tumor cells with round hyperchromatic nuclei and the lesions may present similar patterns. However, in reality, some SCTs have actually been diagnosed as nonfunctioning islet cell tumors [20, 35]. Endocrine tumors, as shown by immunocytochemistry and electron microscopy, exhibit some types of pancreatic islet hormone and endocrine granules in most tumor cells, even in the nonfunctioning endocrine tumors. Endocrine tumors generally exhibit a trabecular or solid pattern and not a microcystic one, although cystic endocrine

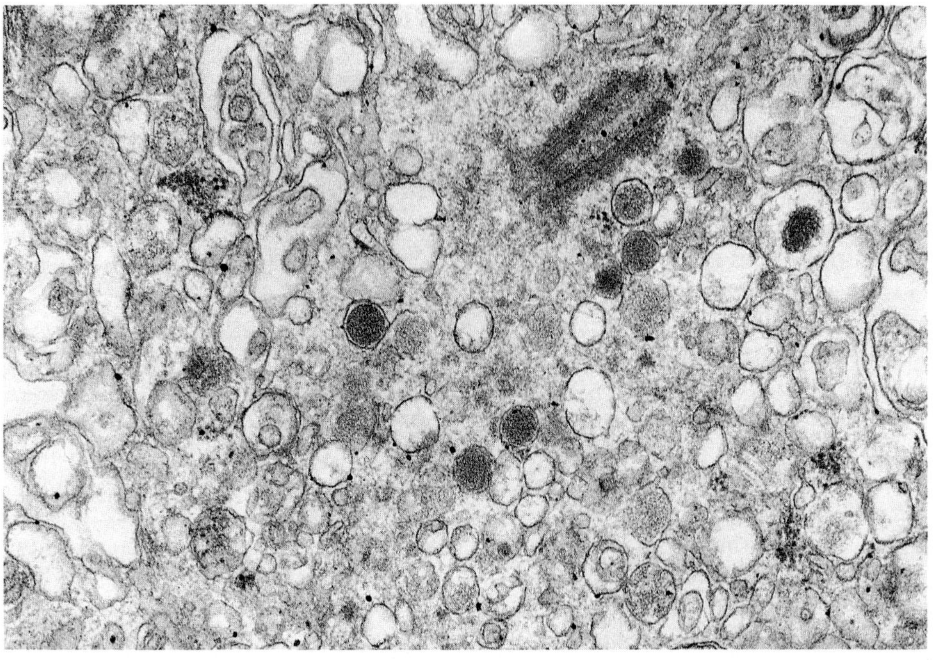

a

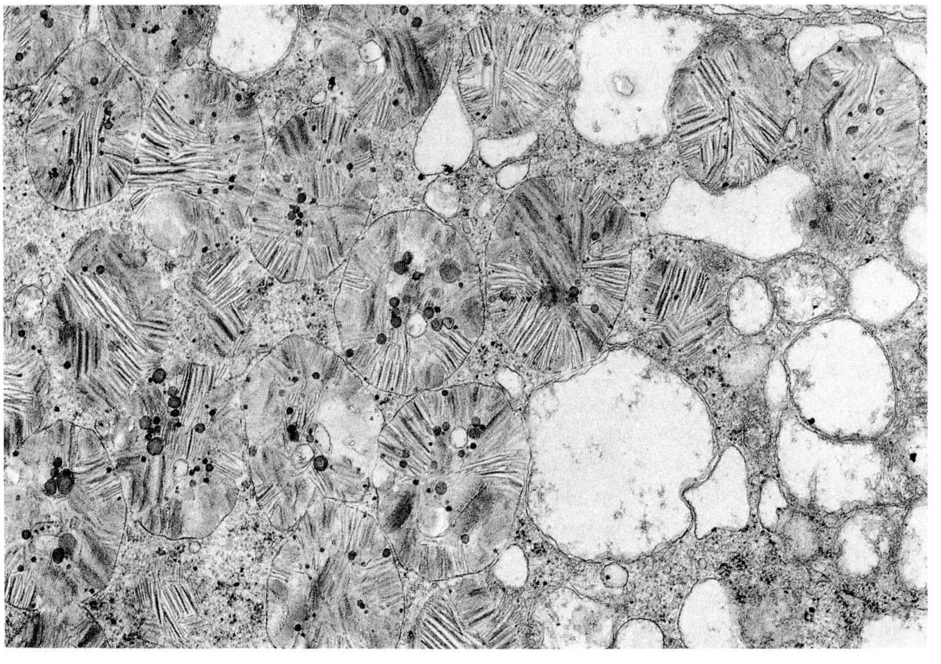

b

Fig. 11.a Ultrastructural appearance of tumor cells in Fig. 6b. Numerous vesicles, a desmosome-like structure, and a few membrane-bound granules resembling neurosecretory granules. These types of cells were positive with Grimelius staining (×30 000). ***b*** Ultrastructure appearance of the tumor in Fig. 6b. Almost all of the tumor cells had various numbers of aberrant oval granules surrounded by limiting membrane. These granules contained crystalloid, needle-shaped material, and highly dense round material (×18 000). (Courtesy of Dr. Kakihara [16] with permission). ***c*** The same tumor in Fig. 6b. Annulate lamellae in some tumor cells (×10 500). (Courtesy of Dr. Kakihara [16] with permission)

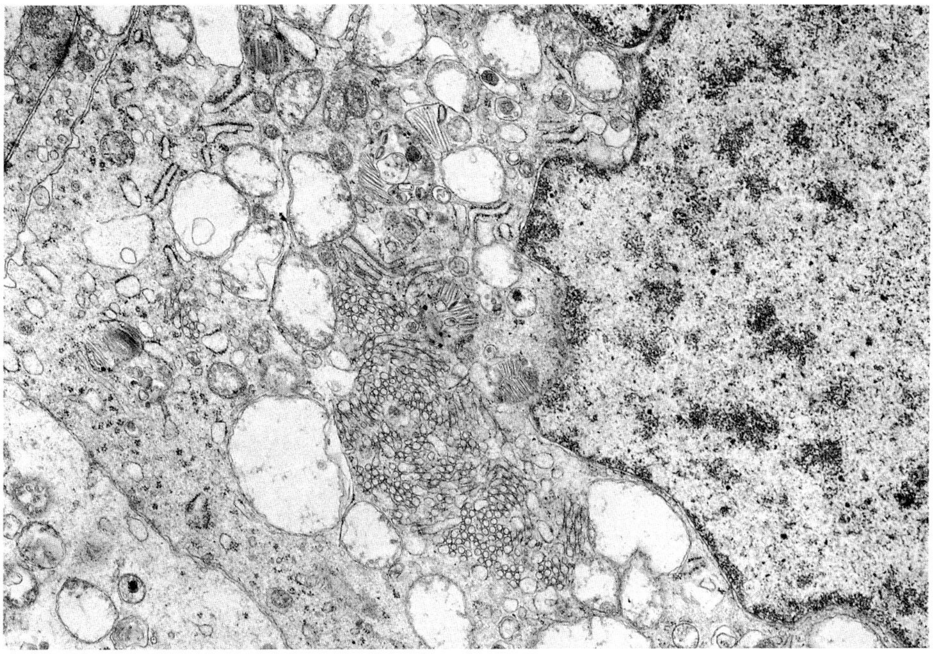

c

tumors may occur [61]. Necrosis and hemorrhage are rare in endocrine tumors and their stroma usually consist of hyaline collagen, sometimes with amyloid deposits. The demonstration of vimentin in SCT cells may be a useful differential diagnostic procedure.

Acinar cell tumors should be clearly distinguished from SCT. Acinar cell cancers occur in adults of both genders and are all malignant. Histologically, the tumor cells form acinar structures and present zymogen granules in the cytoplasm [40].

Pancreatoblastoma [62], which usually occurs in young boys in the first decade, can be differentiated from SCT by the presence of squamoid structures or mesenchymal elements and by its malignant behavior.

In some cases of SCT, CT and US show a solid and cystic pattern and, therefore, SCT may sometimes be confused with a cystic neoplasm (serous cystadenoma, mucinous cystic tumors of the pancreas [63].

Biology, Prognosis, and Survival

The clinical course of patients with SCT is favorable upon complete removal of the tumor. Even metastatic disease and local recurrence are amenable to surgical treatment with long-term results. A few patients develop a local recurrence after an incomplete resection or a distant metastasis, mainly in the liver or lung [8, 54, 64, 65]. One death due to metastasis has been reported [6]. Although most tumors appear benign or have a very low potential for metastasis, Yamaguchi et al. [31] prefer to regard them as tumors with malignant potential and believe that they should be treated by surgical extirpation until a better understanding of their biology is reached. The surgical approach depends on the location of the lesion. Tumors arising from the tail of the pancreas can be excised by a distal pancreatectomy with preservation of the spleen, an important consideration in younger patients. Proximal lesions may require a pancreatoduodenectomy. A complete removal of the entire tumor is mandatory to achieve a cure. Chemoembolization therapy was used successfully on one patient who had multiple hepatic metastases [65]. Radiation therapy was reported with a shrinkage of the tumor in one instance for which surgical excision was not feasible [66].

Evaluation of the malignant potential of SCT is difficult. The histologic infiltration of tumor cells into the peripheral fibrous capsules or extension into the adjacent parenchyma may indicate malignant potential. Cappellari et al. [54] reported that

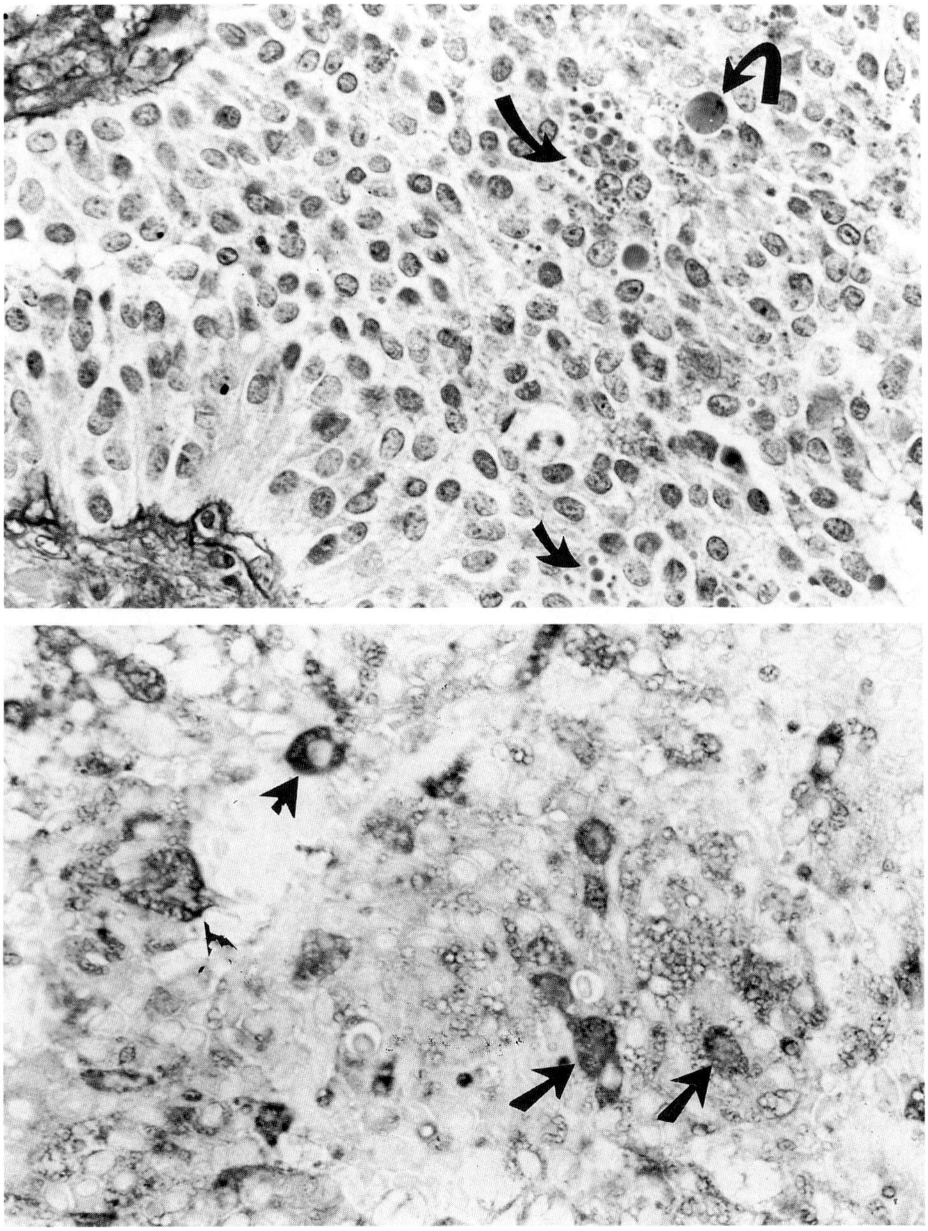

a

b

Fig. 12.a Periodic acid-Schiff (PAS)-positive granules and globules (*arrows*) scattered within and between the polygonal tumor cells (PAS-stain, ×200). ***b*** Alpha-1 antitrypsin-positive granules scattered in individual tumor cells. (PAP method ×200)

one case of malignant SCT was aneuploid according to a flow cytometric study. The assessment of the malignant potential may be warranted using such modern techniques, including immunohistochemical analysis and flow cytometric analysis of cellular DNA content and nuclear morphometry.

Acknowledgment. We wish to thank Dr. Toshio Kakihara from the Second Department of Pathology, Niigata University School of Medicine, Niigata, Japan, for the provision of some figures (specified in the Figure legends).

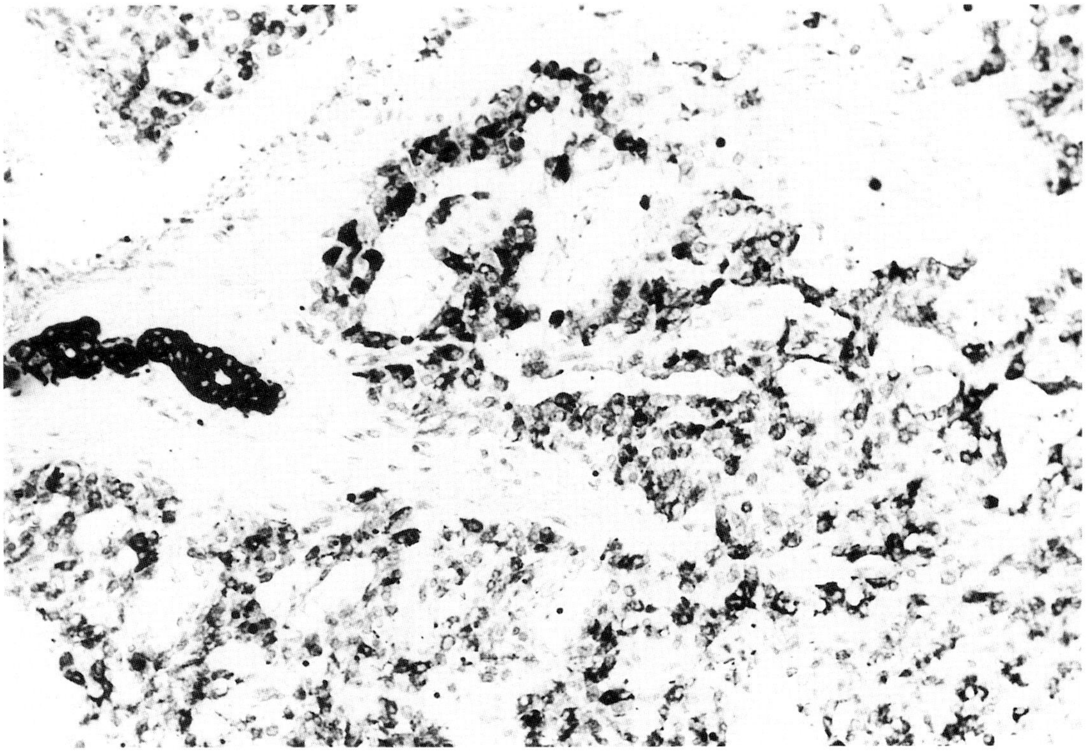

Fig. 13. KL1 immunostaining showing diffuse positivity in ductal cells (*left*) and in neoplastic cells. Undiluted antibody (Immunotech, Marseille, France) (×348)

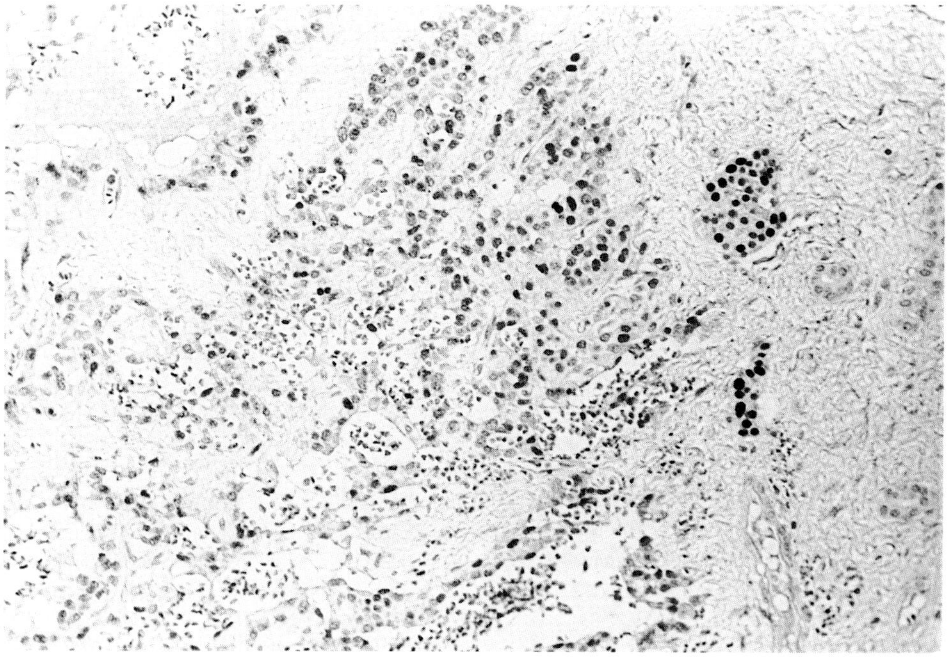

Fig. 14. Almost all the tumor cells show nuclear immunoreactivity for progesterone receptor protein. In the fibrous capsule of the tumor, an entrapped islet of Langerhans (*right upper corner*) shows strong nuclear positivity. PgR receptor antibody (Abbott Lab, Wiesbaden, Germany) in 1:5 dilution. (×348)

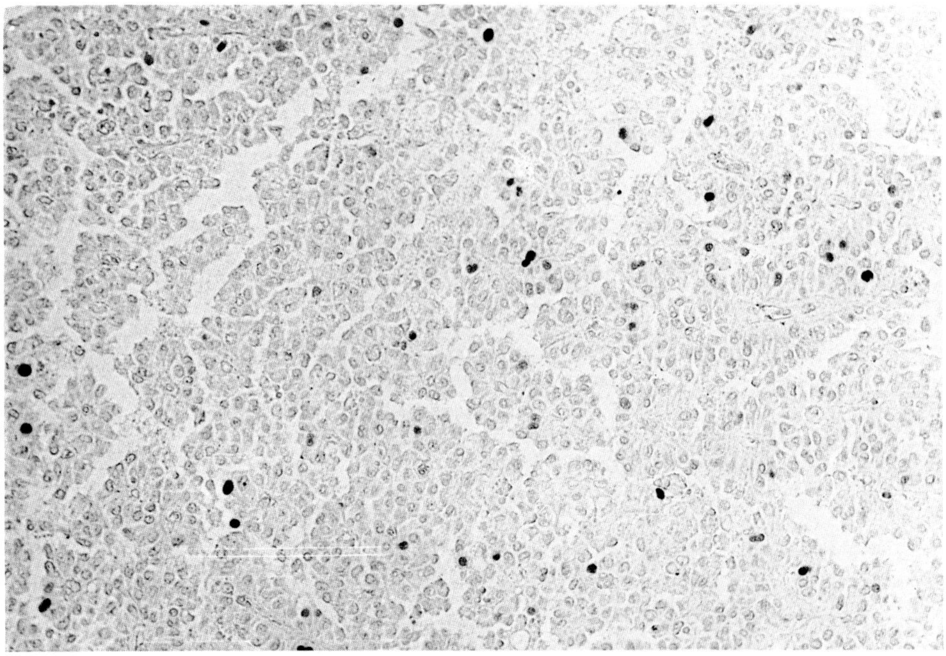

Fig. 15. Proliferating cell nuclear antigen-immunoreactivity showing nuclear positivity in a few tumor cells. 1:100 dilution of the antibody (Dakopatts, Denmark) (×348)

References

1. Cubilla AL, Fitzgerald PJ (1984) Tumor of the exocrine pancreas. In: Hartmann WH (ed) Atlas of tumor pathology. 2nd series, fascicle 19. Armed Forces Institute of Pathology, Washington DC, pp 201–207
2. Frantz VK (1959) Tumors of the pancreas. In: Frantz VK (ed) Atlas of tumor pathology. Section VII, fascicles 27 and 28, first series. Armed Forces Institute of Pathology, Washington DC, pp 32–33
3. Klöppel G, Morohoshi T, John HD, Oehmichen W, Opitz K, Angelkort A, Lietz H, Rückert K (1981) Solid and cystic acinar cell tumour of the pancreas. A tumor in young women with favourable prognosis. Virchows Arch [A] 392:171–183
4. Oertel JE, Mendelsohn G, Cameron JL (1982) Solid and papillary neoplasm of the pancreas. In: Humphrey GB (ed) Pancreatic tumors in children. Martinus Nijhoff, The Hague, pp 167–171
5. Morohoshi T, Held G, Klöppel G (1983) Exocrine pancreatic tumors and their histological classification. A study based on 167 autopsy and 97 surgical cases. Histopathology 7:645–661
6. Compagno J, Oertel JE, Kremzar M (1979) Solid and papillary epithelial neoplasm of the pancreas, probably of small duct origin: A clinicopathologic study of 52 cases. Lab Inv 40:248–249
7. Lieber MR, Lack EE, Roberts JR, Merino MJ, Patterson K, Restrepo C, Solomon D, Chandra R, Triche TJ (1987) Solid and papillary epithelial neoplasm of the pancreas. An ultrastructural and immunohistochemical study of six cases. Am J Surg Pathol 11:85–93
8. Matsunou H, Konishi F (1990) Papillary-cystic neoplasm of the pancreas. A clinicopathologic study concerning the tumor aging and malignancy of nine cases. Cancer 65:283–291
9. Friedman AC, Lichtenstein JE, Fishman EK, Oertel JE, Dachman AH, Siegelman SS (1985) Solid and papillary epithelial neoplasm of the pancreas. Radiology 154:333–337
10. Choi BI, Kim KW, Han MC, Kim YI, Kim CW (1988) Solid and papillary epithelial neoplasms of the pancreas: CT findings. Radiology 166:413–416
11. Matsunou H, Konishi F, Yamamichi N, Takayanagi N, Mukai M (1990) Solid, infiltrating variety of papillary cystic neoplasm of the pancreas. Cancer 65:2747–2757
12. Warshaw AL, Compton CC, Lewandrowski K, Cardenosa G, Mueller P (1990) Cystic tumor of the pancreas. New clinical, radiologic, and pathologic observations in 67 patients. Ann Surg 212:432–445
13. Stömmer P, Kraus J, Stolte M, Giedl J (1991) Solid and cystic pancreatic tumors. Clinical, histochemical, and electron microscopic features in ten cases. Cancer 67:1635–1641
14. Sclafani LM, Reiter VE, Coit DG, Brennan MF (1991) The malignant nature of papillary and cystic neoplasm of the pancreas. Cancer 68:153–158

15. Klöppel G, Maurer R, Hofmann E, Lüthold K, Oscarson J, Forsby N, Ihse I, Ljungberg O, Heitz PU (1991) Solid-cystic (papillary-cystic) tumours within and outside the pancreas in men: Report of two patients. Virchows Arch [A] 418:179–183
16. Kakihara T, Fukuda T, Nemoto U, Ohnishi Y, Kusama K (1991) Unusual pancreatic tumor resembling solid and cystic tumor with somatostatin production and aberrant crystalloid structures. Acta Pathol Jpn 41:629–635
17. Carbone A, Ranelletti FO, Rinelli A, Vecchio FM, Lauriola L, Piantelli M, Capelli A (1989) Type II estrogen receptors in the papillary cystic tumor of the pancreas. Am J Clin Pathol 92:572–576
18. Ladanyi M, Mulay S, Arseneau J, Bettez P (1987) Estrogen and progesterone receptor determination in the papillary cystic neoplasm of the pancreas. With immunohistochemical and ultrastructural observations. Cancer 60:1604–1611
19. Wrba F, Chott A, Ludvik B, Schratter M, Spona J, Reiner A, Schernthaner G, Krisch K (1988) Solid and cystic tumour of the pancreas: A hormonal-dependent neoplasm. Histopathology 12:338–340
20. Miettinen M, Partanen S, Fräki O, Kivilaakso E (1987) Papillary cystic tumor of the pancreas. An analysis of cellular differentiation by electron microscopy and immunohistochemistry. Am J Surg Pathol 11:855–865
21. Doglioni C, Gambacorta M, Zamboni G, Coggi G, Viale G (1990) Immunocytochemical localization of progesterone receptors in endocrine cells of the human pancreas. Am J Pathol 137:999–1005
22. Viale G, Doglioni C, Gambacorta M, Zamboni G, Coggi G, Bordi C (1992) Progesterone receptor immunoreactivity in pancreatic endocrine tumors. An immunocytochemical study of 156 neuroendocrine tumors of the pancreas, gastrointestinal respiratory tracts, and skin. Cancer 70:2268–2277
23. Zamboni G, Castelli P, Doglioni C, Iannucci A, Maran M, Pea M, Martignoni G, Bonetti F (1991) Immunohistochemical localization of progesterone receptors in papillary cystic tumor of the pancreas. Basic and Applied Histochemistry 35 [Suppl]:97
24. Fujioka T, Nakada K, Kin Y, et al (1987) Solid and cystic tumor of the pancreas in adolescent girl. Report of two cases with literature survey in Japan (in Japanese). Nippon Shouni-Geka Gakkaishi 23:1250–1257
25. Iijima T, Nitta A, Horiuchi H, et al (1988) A case of solid and cystic tumor of the pancreas with ossification. Follow-up study of 45 cases in Japan (in Japanese). Nippon Shoukakibyou Gakkaishi 85:1123–1127
26. Ishikawa O, Ishiguro S, Ohhigashi H, Sasaki Y, Yasuda T, Imaoka S, Iwanaga T, Nakaizumi A, Fujita M, Wada A (1990) Solid and papillary neoplasm arising from an ectopic pancreas in the mesocolon. Am J Gastroenterol 85:597–601
27. Kim YI, Kim ST, Lee GK, Choi BI (1990) Papillary cystic tumor of the liver. A case report with ultrastructural observation. Cancer 65:2740–2746
28. Hertzanu Y, Bar-Ziv J, Freund U (1989) Computed tomography of unusual calcified pancreatic tumors. J Comput Assist Tumogr 13:75–76
29. Sheen IS, Chang-Chien CS, Wu CS (1988) Solid and papillary neoplasm of the pancreas: A report of an unusual pattern of calcification. Am J Gastroenterol 83:789–791
30. Balthazar EJ, Subramanyam BR, Lefleur RS, Barone CM (1984) Solid and papillary epithelial neoplasm of the pancreas. Radiographic, CT, sonographic, and angiographic features. Radiology 150:39–40
31. Yamaguchi K, Hirakata R, Kitamura K (1990) Papillary cystic neoplasm of the pancreas: Radiological and pathological characteristics in 11 cases. Br J Surg 77:1000–1003
32. Jayaram G, Chaturvedi KU, Jindal RK, Venugopal S, Kapoor R (1990) Papillary cystic neoplasm of the pancreas. Report of a case diagnosed by fine needle aspiration cytology. Acta Cytologica 34:429–433
33. Katz LBK, Ehya H (1990) Aspiration cytology of papillary cystic neoplasm of the pancreas. Am J Clin Pathol 94:328–333
34. Ohshima A, Yamaguchi K, Doi R, Enjoji M (1990) Incipient papillary cystic tumor of the pancreas. Am J Gastroenterol 85:1437–1438
35. Yamaguchi K, Miyagahara T, Tsuneyoshi T, Enjoji M, Horie A, Nakayama I, Tsuda N, Fujii H, Takahara O (1989) Papillary cystic neoplasm of the pancreas. An immunohistochemical and ultrastructural study of 14 patients. Jpn J Clin Oncol 19:102–111
36. Horie A, Haratake J, Jimi A, Matsumoto M, Ishii N, Tsutsumi Y (1987) Pancreatoblastoma in Japan, with differential diagnosis from papillary cystic tumor (ductuloacinar adenoma) of the pancreas. Acta Pathol Jpn 37:47–63
37. Yagihashi S, Sato I, Kaimori M, Matsumoto J, Nagai K (1988) Papillary and cystic tumor of the pancreas. Two cases indistinguishable from islet cell tumor. Cancer 61:1241–1247
38. Arai T, Kino I, Nakamura S, Koda K (1986) Solid and cystic acinar cell tumors of the pancreas. A report of two cases with immunohistochemical and ultrastructural studies. Acta Pathol Jpn 36:1887–1896
39. Learmonth GM, Price SK, Visser A, Emms M (1985) Papillary and cystic neoplasm of the pancreas. An acinar cell tumour? Histopathology 9:63–79
40. Morohoshi T, Kanda M, Horie A, Chott A, Dreyer T, Klöppel G, Heitz PU (1987) Immunohistochemical markers of uncommon pancreatic tumors. Acinar cell carcinoma, pancreatoblastoma, and solid cystic (papillary-cystic) tumor. Cancer 59:739–747

41. Murao T, Toda K, Tomiyama Y (1983) Papillary and solid neoplasm of pancreas in a child. Report of a case in which acinar differentiation was demonstrated by immunohistochemistry and electron microscopy. Acta Pathol Jpn 33:565–575
42. Kamisawa T, Fukayama M, Koike M, Tabata I, Okamoto A (1987) So-called "papillary and cystic neoplasm of the pancreas." An immunohistochemical and ultrastructural study. Acta Pathol Jpn 37:785–794
43. Morrison DM, Jewell LD, McCaughey WTE, Danyluk J, Shnitka TK, Manickavel V (1984) Papillary cystic tumor of the pancreas. Arch Pathol Lab Med 108:723–727
44. Schlosnagle DC, Campbell WG Jr (1981) The papillary and solid neoplasm of the pancreas: A report of two cases with electron microscopy, one containing neurosecretory granules. Cancer 47:2603–2610
45. Jorgensen LJ, Hansen AB, Burcharth F, Philipsen E, Horn T (1992) Solid and papillary neoplasm of the pancreas. Ultrastruct Pathol 16:659–666
46. Chott A, Klöppel G, Buxbaum, Heitz PU (1987) Neuron specific enolase demonstration in the diagnosis of a solid-cystic (papillary cystic) tumour of the pancreas. Virchows Arch [A] 410:397–402
47. Pettinato G, Manivel JC, Ravetto C, Terracciano LM, Gould EW, DiTuoro LM, Jaszcz W, Albores-Saavedra J (1992) Papillary cystic tumor of the pancreas. A clinicopathologic study of 20 cases with cytologic, immunohistochemical, ultrastructural, and flow cytometric observations, and a review of the literature. Am J Clin Pathol, 98:478–488
48. von Herbay A, Sieg B, Otto HF (1990) Solid-cystic tumour of the pancreas. An endocrine neoplasm? Virchows Arch [A] 416:535–538
49. Ghandially FN (1985) Significance of certain ultrastructural features seen in tumors: Annulate lamellae. In: Ghandially FN (ed) Diagnostic electron microscopy of tumours, 2nd ed. Butterworths, London, pp 319–325
50. Horwitz KB, Mochus MB, Lessey BA (1982) Variant T47D human breast cancer cells with high progesterone-receptor level despite estrogen and antiestrogen resistance. Cell 28:633–642
51. Tilzer LL, Plapp FV, Evans JP, Stone D, Alward K (1982) Steroid receptor proteins in human meningiomas. Cancer 49:633–636
52. Stojkovic RR, Javancevic M, Santel DJ, Grcevic N, Gamulin S (1990) Sex steroid receptors in intracranial tumors. Cancer 65:1968–1970
53. Wu CW, Chi CW, Chang TJ, Lui WY, P'eng FK (1990) Sex hormone receptors in gastric cancer. Cancer 65:1396–1400
54. Cappellari JO, Geisinger KR, Albertson DA, Wolfman NT, Kute TE (1990) Malignant papillary cystic tumor of the pancreas. Cancer 66:193–198
55. Morohoshi T (1990) Solid and cystic (papillary-cystic) tumor of the pancreas (abstract). Proceedings of the 3rd Symposium of the International Pancreatic Cancer Study Group, Nagasaki, Japan August 20–23
56. Bravo R (1986) Synthesis of the nuclear protein cyclin (PCNA) and its relationship with DNA replication. Exp Cell Res 163:287–293
57. Bravo R, Frank R, Blundell PA, Macdonald-Bravo H (1987) Cyclin/PCNA is the auxiliary protein of DNA polymerase-d. Nature 326:515–517
58. Kamel OW, LeBrun DP, Davis RE, Berry GJ, Warnke RA (1991) Growth fraction estimation of malignant lymphomas in formalin-fixed paraffin-embedded tissue using anti-PCNA/Cyclin 19A2. Correlation with Ki67 labeling. Am J Pathol 138: 1471–1477
59. Yu CCW, Hall PA, Fletcher CDM, Camplejohn R, Waseem NH, Lane DP, Levison DA (1991) Haemangiopericytomas: The prognostic value of immunohistochemical staining with a monoclonal antibody to proliferating cell nuclear antigen (PCNA). Histopathology 19:29–33
60. Takahashi H, Strutton GM, Parsons PG (1991) Determination of proliferating fractions in malignant melanomas by anti-PCNA/cyclin monoclonal antibody. Histopathology 18:221–227
61. Nojima T, Kojima T, Kato H, Inoue K, Nagashima K (1991) Cystic endocrine tumor of the pancreas. Int J Pancreatol 10:65–72
62. Horie A, Yano Y, Kotoo Y, Miwa A (1977) Morphogenesis of pancreatoblastoma, infantile form adenocarcinoma of the pancreas. Report of two cases. Cancer 39:247–254
63. Yamaguchi K, Enjoji M (1987) Cystic neoplasm of the pancreas. Gastroenterology 92:1934–1943
64. Hernandez-Maldonado JJ, Rodriguez-Bigas MA, de Pesante AG, Vasquez-Quintana E (1989) Papillary cystic neoplasm of the pancreas. A report of a case presenting with carcinomatosis. Am Surg 55:552–559
65. Matsuda Y, Imai Y, Kawata S, Nishikawa M, Miyoshi S, Saito R, Minami Y, Tarui S (1987) Papillary-cystic neoplasm of the pancreas with multiple hepatic metastases: A case report. Gastroenterol Jpn 22:379–384
66. Fried P, Cooper J, Balthazar E, Fazzini E, Newall J (1985) A role for radiotherapy in the treatment of solid and papillary neoplasms of the pancreas. Cancer 56:2783–2785

Serous Cystadenocarcinoma

Incidence

Serous cystadenocarcinoma is extremely rare. Thus far, only four cases have been reported [1–4]. In our case [2, 5], both serous cystadenoma and cystadenocarcinoma coexisted in the same patient, which gave us an opportunity to compare the patterns of these two biologically different tumors.

Sex and Location

One of the four reported cases occurred in a man and three in women. One case was in the tail, another in the body and tail, the third in the head and body, and the fourth in the body of the pancreas.

Age

The age of the serous cystadenocarcinoma patients ranged from 63 to 72 years, the mean being 68. Thus, with respect to gender, age and anatomic localization, cystadenocarcinoma and serous cystadenoma (see Chapter "Serous Cystadenoma" in this volume) are alike.

Etiology and Pathogenesis

It appears that serous cystadenocarcinoma arises from cystadenoma. The factors responsible for this transition are unknown. In our case [2], one patient presented six tumors, 4 of which were benign and two were malignant. However, whether the malignant lesions developed de novo or whether they were secondary malignant changes of adenoma is not clear. The presence of malignant foci within the serous cystadenoma suggests an adenoma-carcinoma sequence [4].

Clinical Presentation

Because of the rare occurrence of serous cystadenocarcinomas, clinical and histopathological findings are scarce. The following descriptions are mostly from our case [2, 5] and from the case described by Yoshimi et al. (1994).

CT Findings

Serous cystadenocarcinoma, as well as its benign counterpart, serous cystadenoma, show low-density areas with clear margins. In our case [2], a honeycomb-like structure with partial calcification was observed in the low-density area (Fig. 1), and it was enhanced after intravenous contrast administration (Fig. 2). The low-density area had a necrotic appearance. The inferior vena cava was compressed and flattened by the large tumor mass (Fig. 2).

MRI Findings

The tumor showed a low-density area with a reticular septum-like structure in T-1 weighted mag-

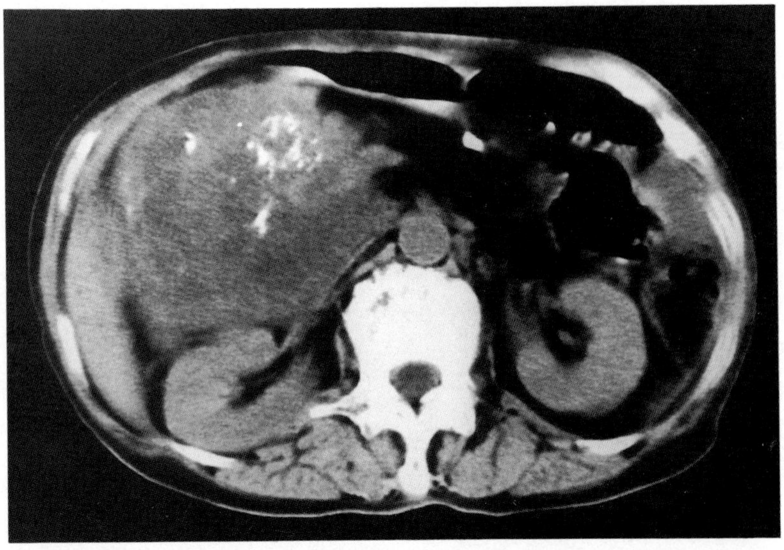

Fig. 1. Computed tomography (CT) showing a honeycomb-like structure with partial calcification in the low-density area. The patient was a 72-year-old female with multiple tumors (after [2])

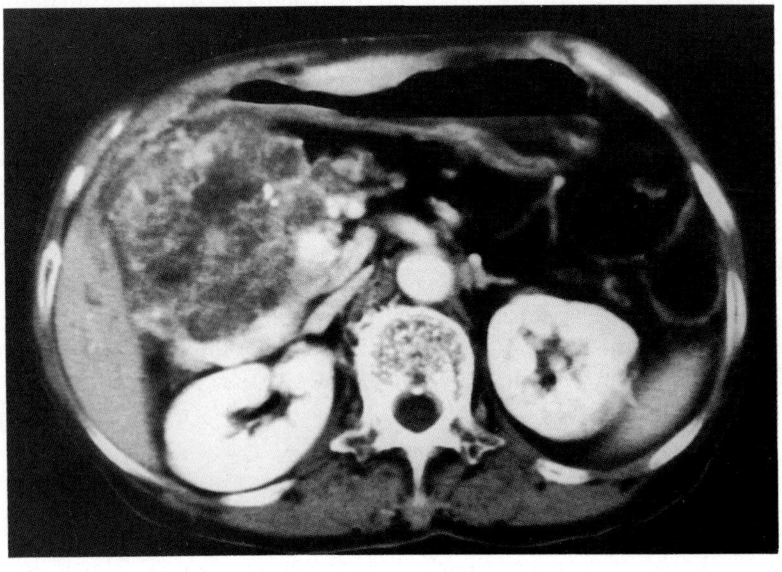

Fig. 2. The same case as in Fig. 1. A honeycomb-like structure is enhanced and is clearly evident and necrotic in appearance at the center

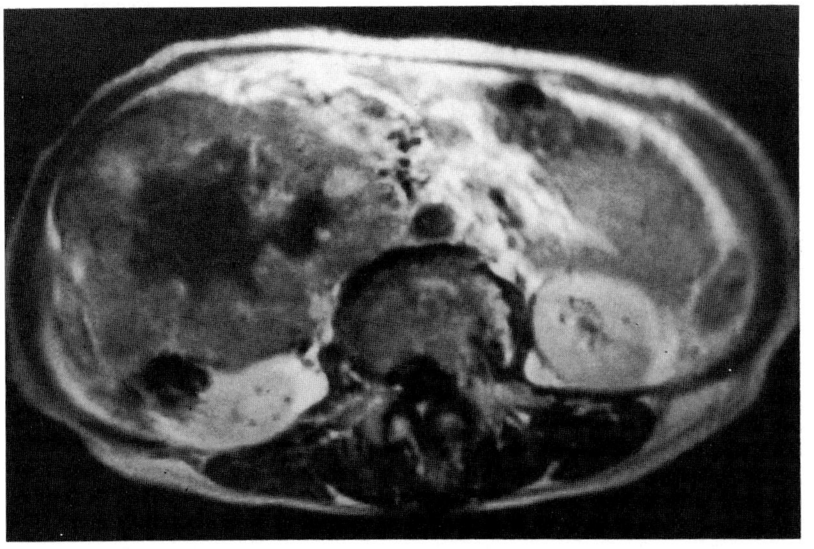

Fig. 3. The same tumor showing a low-intensity area in the T-1 weighted image using Gd-DTPA

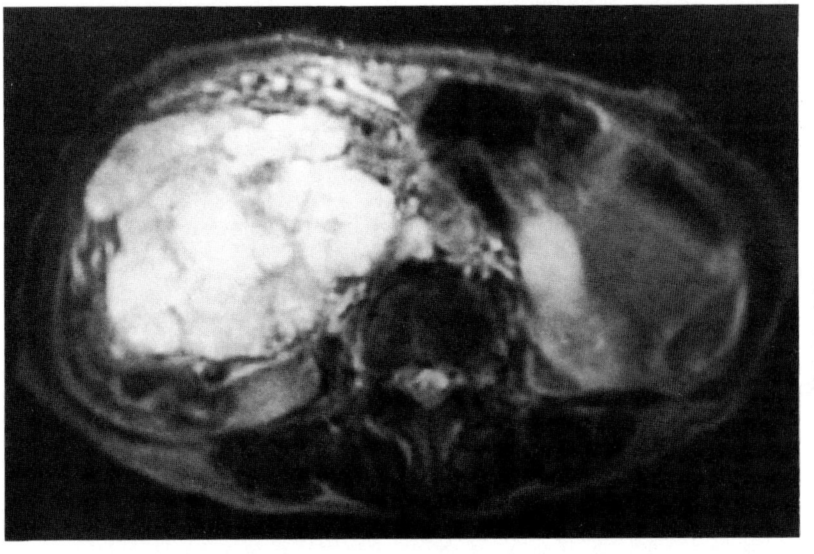

Fig. 4. Tumor showing a high intensity area in the T-2 weighted image (the same patient as in Fig. 3)

netic resonance images (Fig. 3) and a high-intensity area in T-2 weighted images (Fig. 4). The portal vein was involved and collateral vessels had developed (Fig. 5).

Angiographic Findings

Abundant "neoplastic" vessels and a remarkable pooling stain of the tumor were observed. The feeding artery and capillary vessel of the tumor were dilated, but encasement of the artery was not found (Fig. 6). At the portal phase, the main portal vein was blocked and collateral vessels were seen (Fig. 7). In Yoshimi's case [4], the tumor appeared hypervascular on celiac artery angiography, and was supplied by splenic and pancreatic dorsal arteries.

Cholangiography and Hypotonic Duodenography

Cholangiography showed obstruction of the common bile duct in the distal portion and dilation of the proximal bile duct. Bile duct obstruction has

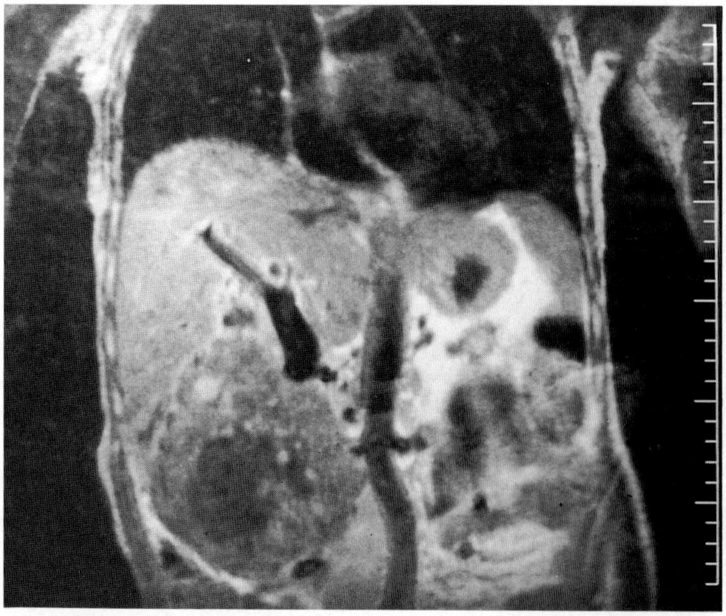

Fig. 5. Portal vein involved in the tumor (the same patient as in Fig. 3) using Gd-DTPA

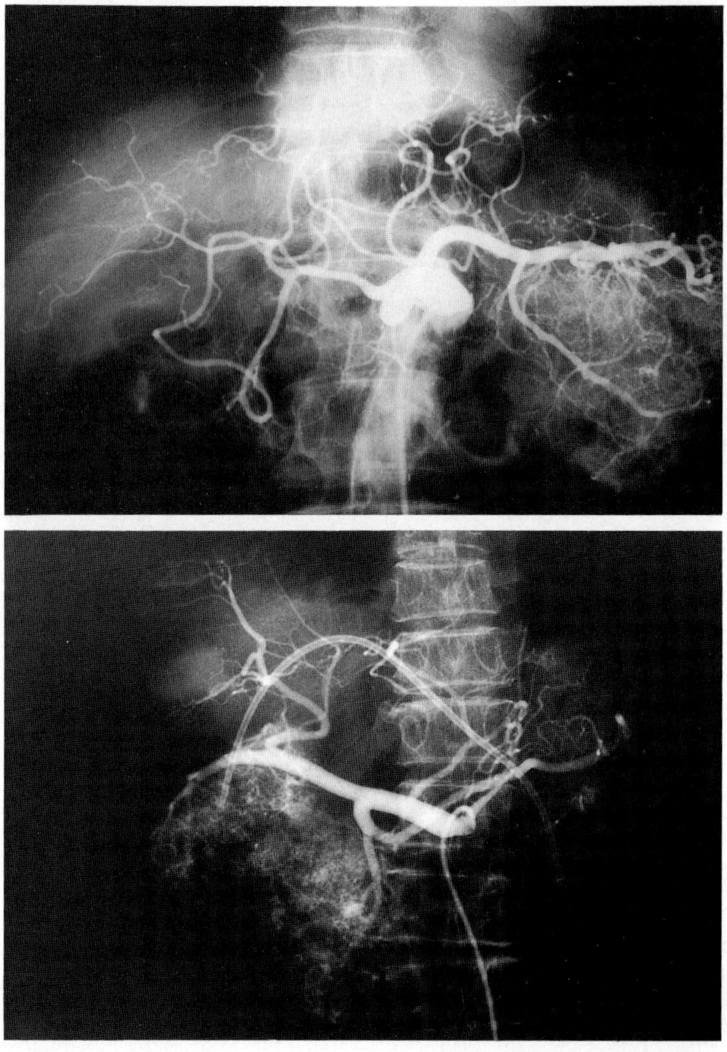

a

b

Fig. 6. ***a*** Staining of the tumor in serous cystadenoma which was, unexpectedly discovered in a 74-year-old man during an examination for sigmoid cancer, and ***b*** serous cystadenocarcinoma in the same patient

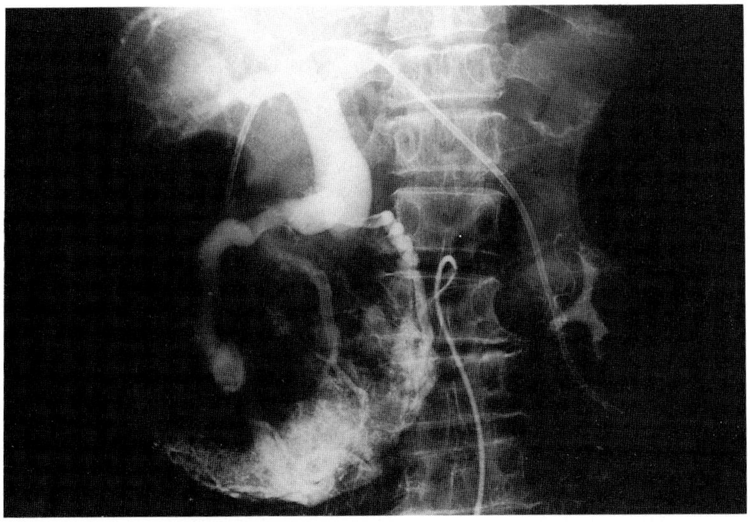

Fig. 7. Blockage at the main portal vein and development of collateral vessels in a serous cystadenocarcinoma (the same patient as in Fig. 6b)

also been reported in serous cystadenoma. Hypotonic duodenography indicated deviation of the descending portion of the duodenum to the right and dilation of the C loop (Fig. 8).

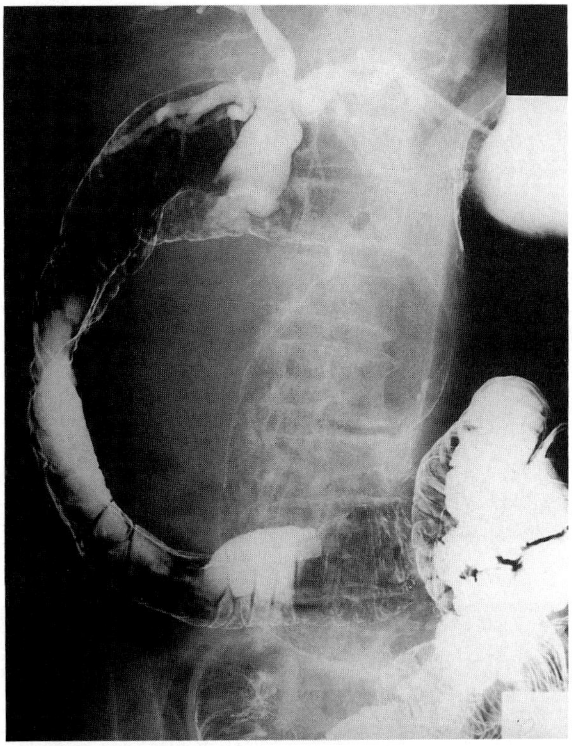

Fig. 8. Obstruction of the common bile duct and dilation of the C loop of the duodenum in a case of serous cystadenocarcinoma (the same patient as in Fig. 6b)

Gross Findings

A serous cystadenoma is usually a unifocal tumor, whereas in our case the tumor was multifocal with 1 tumor located in the head and five in the body of the pancreas. The tumor in the head and one of the five in the body were malignant. Serous cystadenocarcinomas reported by Okada et al. [3], George et al. [1] and Yoshimi et al. [4] were solid lesions, and the tumor sizes were 12 cm, 11 cm, and 12 × 10 × 10 cm, respectively. In our case [2], it was 10 cm (pancreatic head). The tumor described by George et al. [1] had multiple metastases. Similar to the serous cystadenomas, a serous cystadenocarcinoma is a spherical and well-delineated mass. A capsule may or may not be present. In both serous adenoma and carcinoma, the cut surface reveals multiple spongy cysts containing a serous fluid (but no mucin) with a little blood. The cystic spaces are segmented by white fibrous tissue. The cut surfaces of the serous cystadenocarcinomas from our case [2] were white and solid, and the margins were distinct (Fig. 9). A necrotic appearance was observed at the center of the tumor in the pancreatic head in which the common bile duct and portal vein were totally involved (Fig. 10). In the case of George et al. [1], the tumor had invaded the spleen and the gastric wall. In the case described

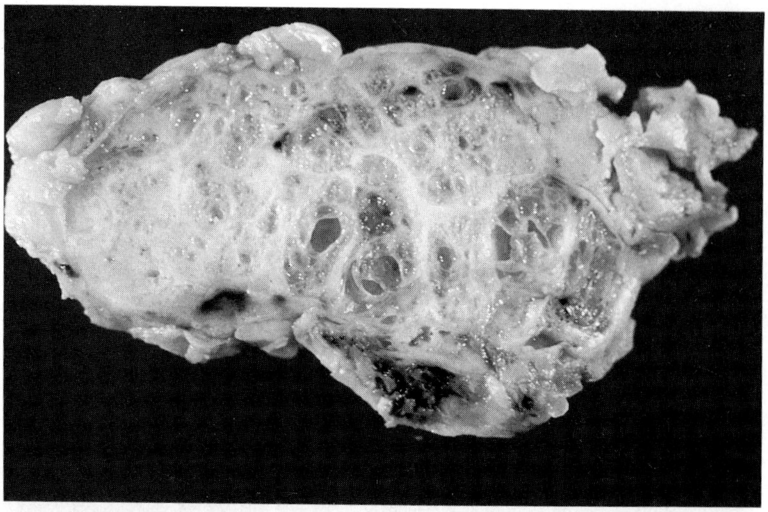

a

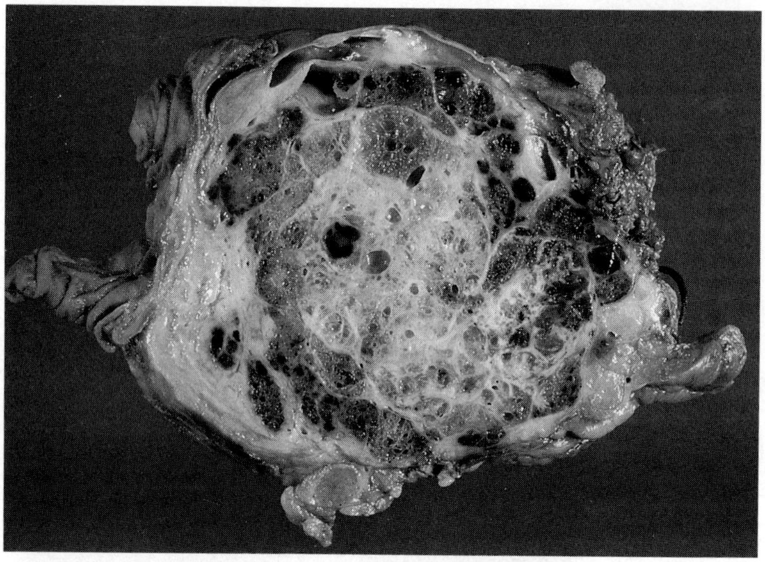

b

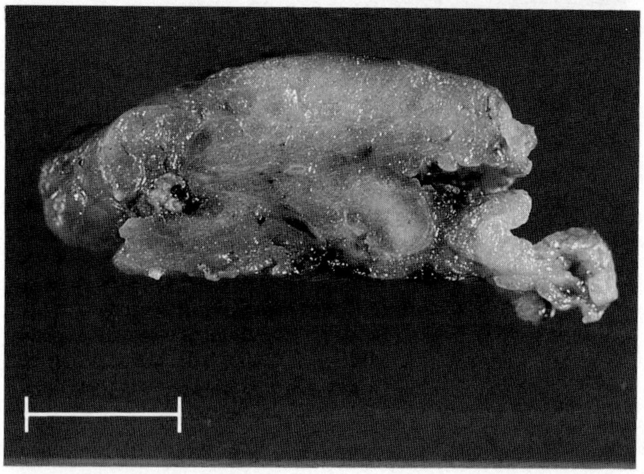

c

Fig. 9. ***a*** Multiple spongy cysts segmented by white fibrous tissue in a serous cystadenoma (the same patient in Fig. 6a), and ***b*** in a serous cystadenocarcinoma, tumor of the pancreatic head (the same patient as in Fig. 6b). ***c*** The serous cystadenocarcinoma in the pancreatic body exhibits white and solid areas (the same patient as in Fig. 6b). (*For color reproduction see color insert in the frontmatter*)

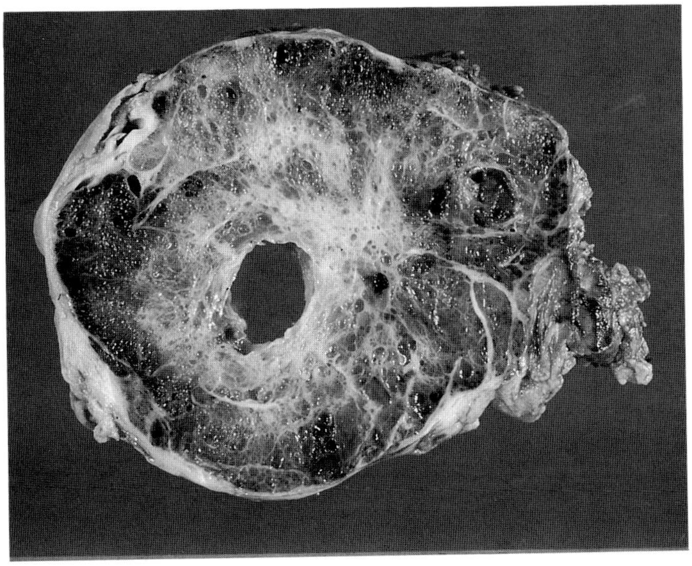

Fig. 10. A serous cystadenocarcinoma of the pancreatic head. Necrotic appearance is evident (the same patient as in Fig. 3). (*For color reproduction see color insert in the frontmatter*)

by Yoshimi et al. [4], metastases of the benign-appearing tumor were found 3 years after surgical removal of the pancreatic tumor. Both the primary and metastatic tumors showed a similar morphology.

Microscopic Findings

Like serous cystadenomas, serous cystadenocarcinomas are separated from surrounding pancreatic tissue by a layer of fibrous tissue of varying thickness, often giving rise to a cleft but without formation of a capsule. Again, like its benign counterpart, cystadenocarcinomas contain cysts of various size lined by a single layer of flat or cuboidal epithelial cells. No papillary structure is present. The cells have a clear cytoplasm with a centrally located nuclei. In Yoshimi's case [4], some areas of tubular-like structures were seen but the nuclei were uniform. Reticular collagen fibers rich in capillary vessels and focal calcification

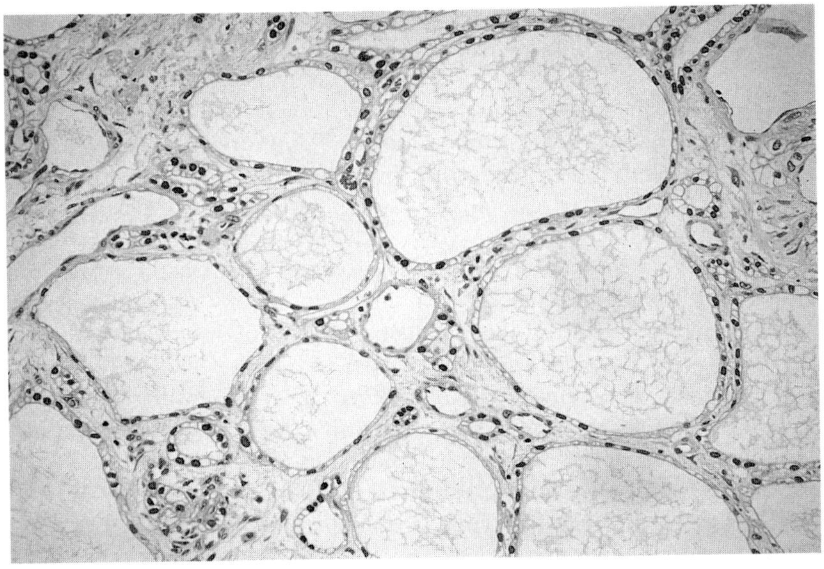

a

Fig. 11a–c. In all tumors, epithelial cells of the cysts were cuboidal or polygonal and occasionally flattened. The cytoplasm is clear and the round-to-oval dense nucleus is present at the center of the cell. H&E, ×50 (original magnification). ***a*** Serous cystadenoma (the same patient as in Fig. 1). ***b*** Serous cystadenocarcinoma in the pancreatic head. ***c*** Serous cystadenocarcinoma in the pancreatic body (the same patient)

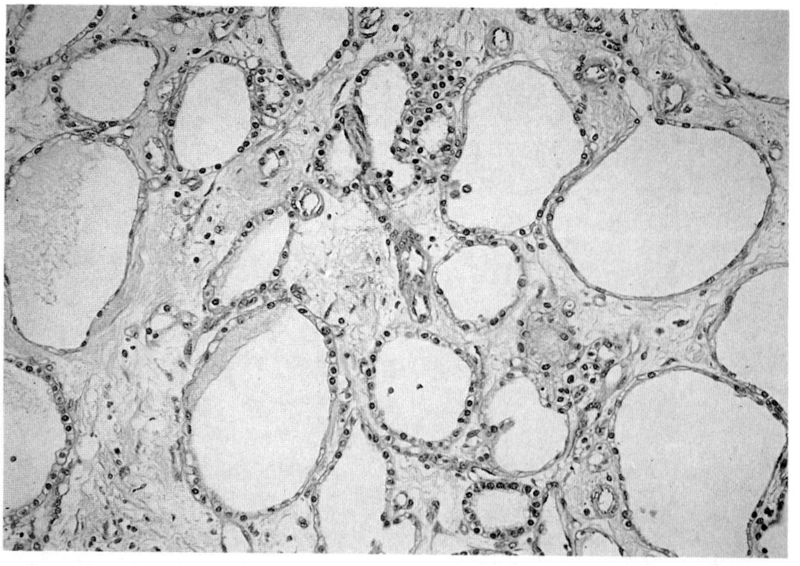

b

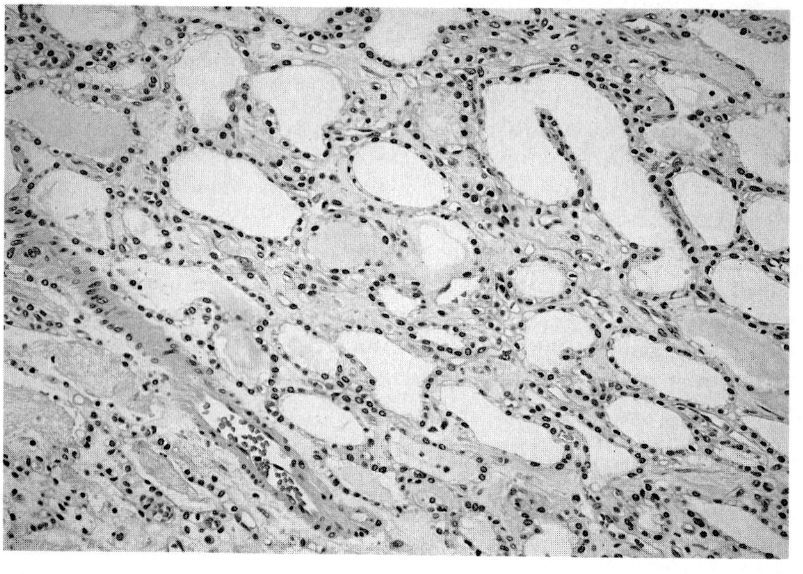

c

Fig. 11b and c. *Continued*

are observed in the interstitium (Fig. 11). Tumor cells have abundant cytoplasmic periodic Acid-Schiff (PAS)-positive granules, which are completely digested by diastase (Fig. 12). Whereas cellular atypia and mitotic figures are rarely observed in cystadenoma (Fig. 13a) there are some cellular atypia, indistinct nucleoli, and fine granular chromoplasm in cystadenocarcinoma (Fig. 13b,c). The tumor cells of the serous cystadenocarcinoma reported by Okada [3] were similar to those found in cystadenomas, and those observed by George [1] and Yoshimi [4] showed mild focal cytological atypia without mitotic activity.

In our case of a serous cystadenocarcinoma [2, 5], the tumor cells exhibited an increased nuclear/cytoplasmic ratio, irregular nuclear margins, various sized nuclei, coarse nuclear chromatin, and distinct nucleoli (Fig. 13). A few mitotic figures could also be seen, and neural invasion was evident on the margin of the tumor in the pancreatic head (Fig. 14). Necrosis was not observed, but the cyst walls were broken. In Yoshimi's case [4], both the primary tumor and its 2 metastatic foci in the liver (2.9 × 2.3 × 2.0 cm and 2.0 × 1.4 × 1.4 cm, respectively) showed a similar structure. The metastatic foci were distinctly separated from the normal liver tissue.

Fig. 12. Serous cystodenocarcinoma. Both fields stained with the periodic acid-Schiff reaction, field below was predigested with diastase (the same patient). ×100 (original magnification). (*For color reproduction see color insert in the frontmatter*)

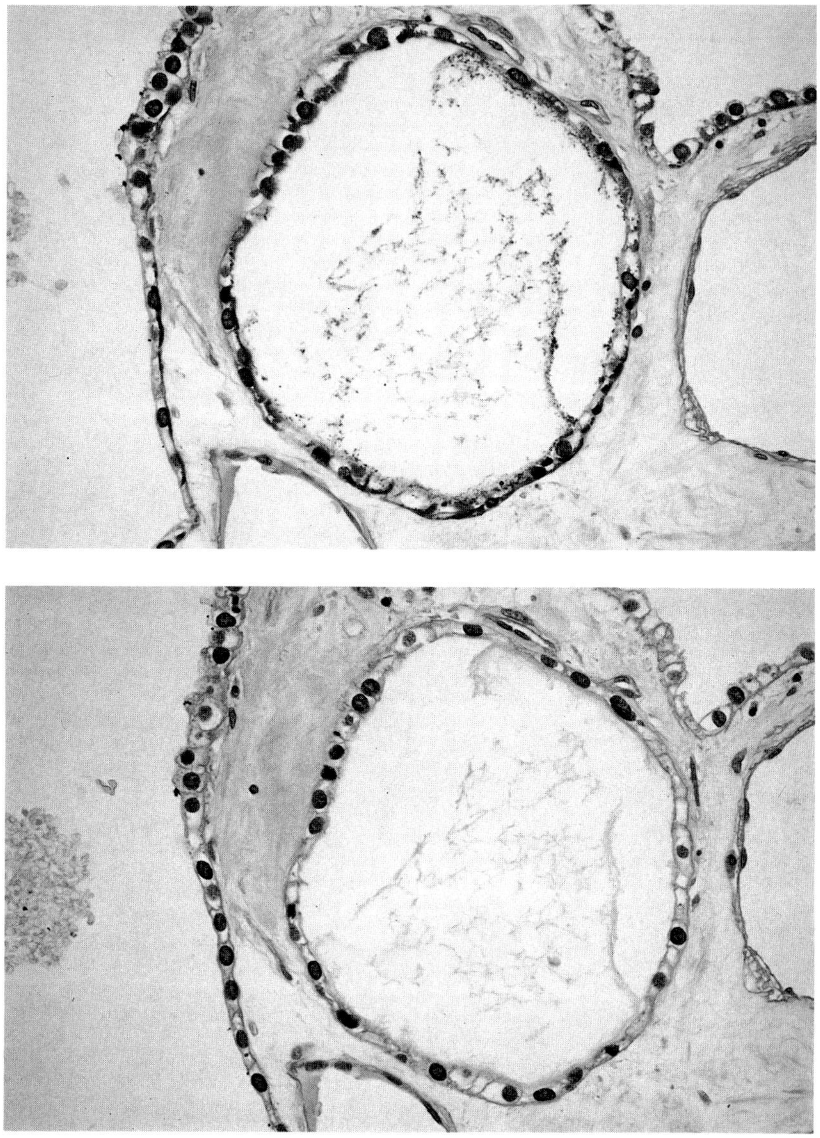

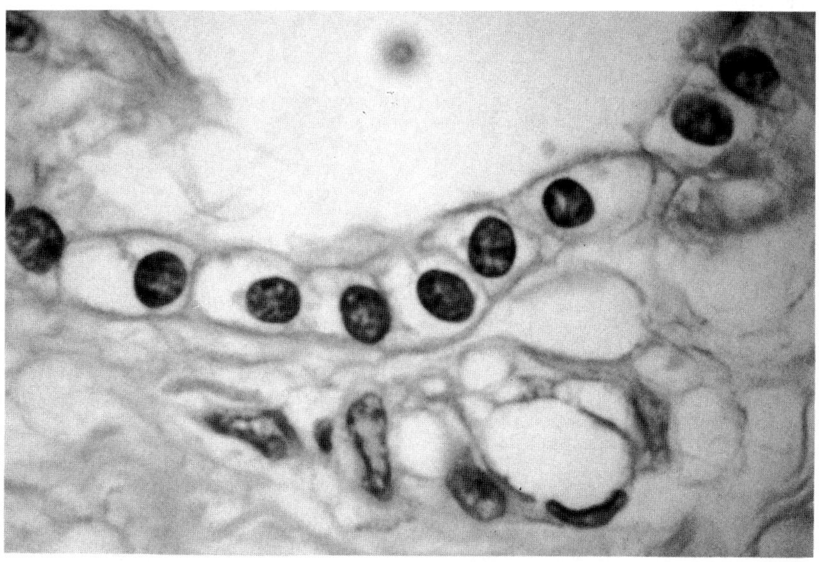

a

Fig. 13. ***a*** Cellular atypia rarely observed in serous cystadenoma, but ***b*** observed often in serous cystadenocarcinoma in a tumor of the pancreatic head, and ***c*** tumor of the pancreatic body (the same patient). H&E, ×400 (original magnification)

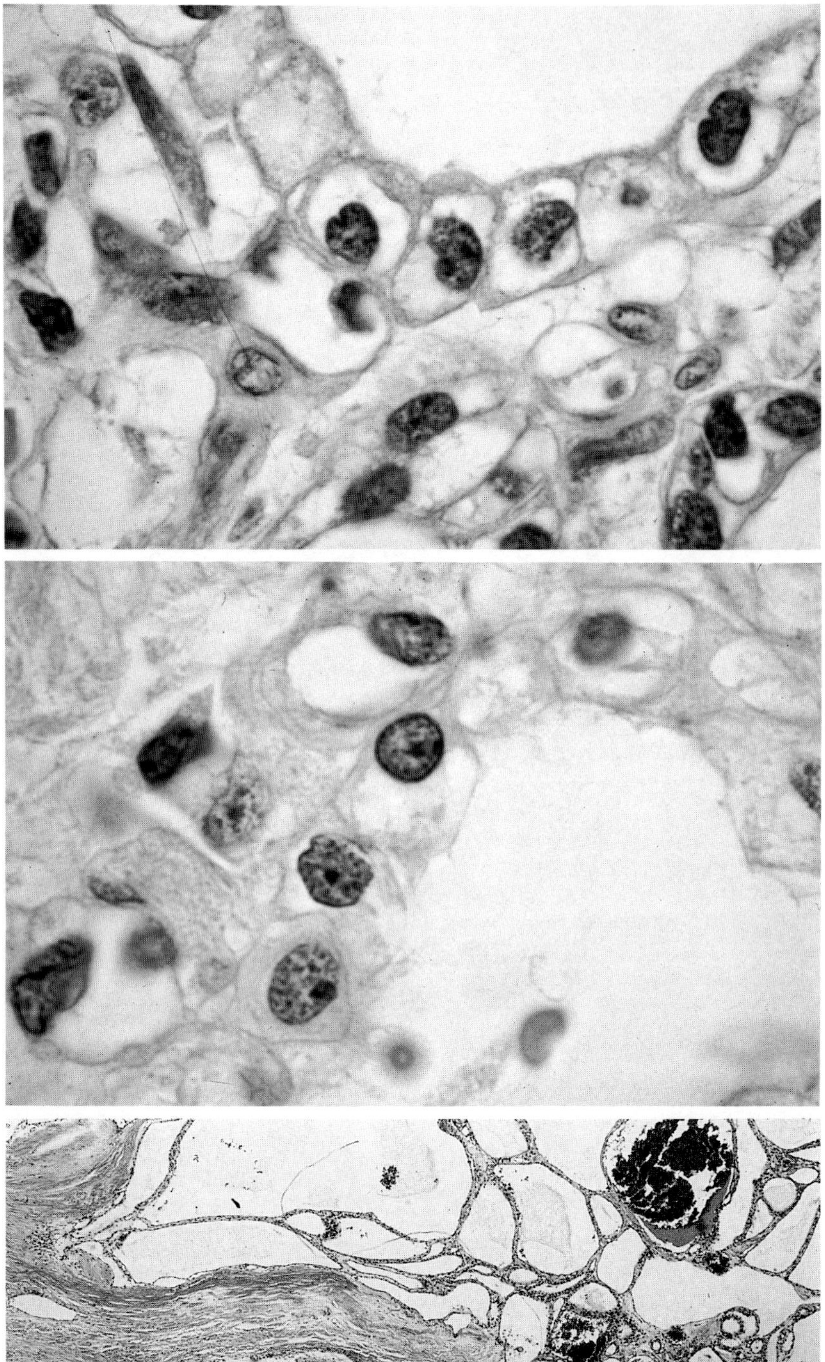

b

c

Fig. 13b and c. *Continued*

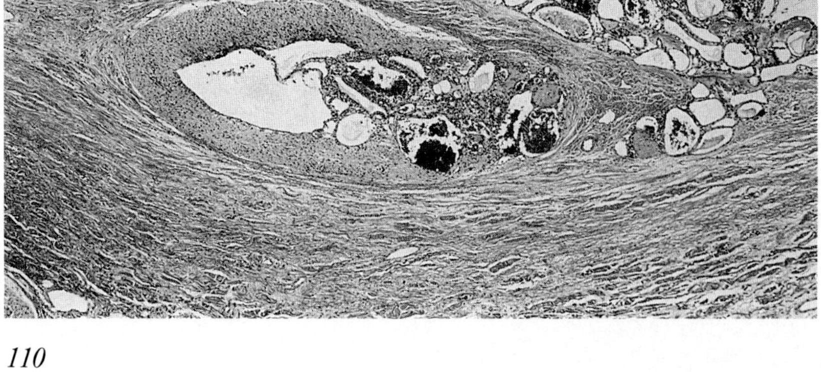

Fig. 14. Neural invasion on the margin of the serous cystadenocarcinoma (the same patient). H&E, ×50 (original magnification)

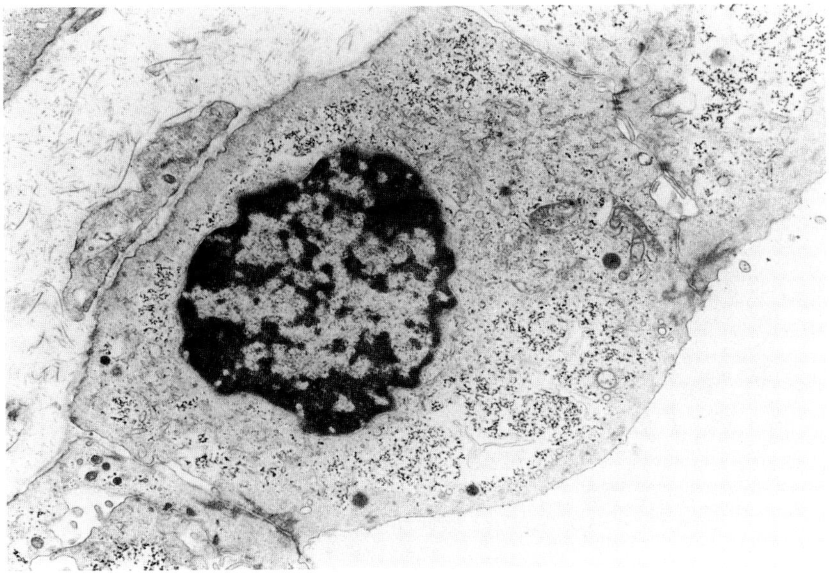

a

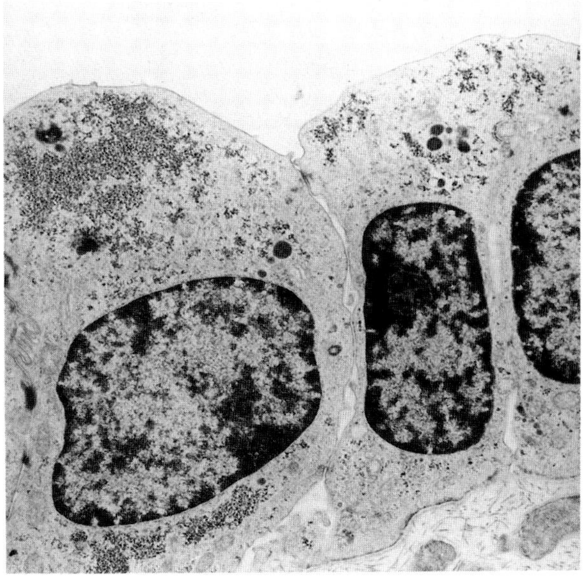

b

Fig. 15a,b. Electron micrograph showing epithelial cells including intracytoplasmic granules of glycogen. ×6000 (original magnification). ***a*** Serous cystadenocarcinoma differs from ***b*** serous cystadenoma (see text)

Electron Microscopy

The cells covering the internal wall of the cyst are typically cuboidal or flat with microvilli and desmosomes, as also seen in serous cystadenoma. Tumor cells contain massive glycogen granules within the cytoplasm. Irregular nuclei and increased heterochromatin are other features of serous cystadenocarcinomas. An increase in filaments; irregular-shaped, rough-surfaced endoplasmic reticulum; and a decrease in villi distinguish the serous cystadenocarcinoma from the serous cystadenoma. Glycogen granules are present on the apical side in the serous cystadenoma, whereas in the serous cystadenocarcinoma they are diffusely scattered within the cytoplasm (Fig. 15). Glucogen granules have been also found in liver metastases [4].

Immunohistochemistry

Neither the serous cystadenoma nor the serous cystadenocarcinoma are stained by anti carcinoembryonic antigen (CEA) [3–5]. In our case [2,

a
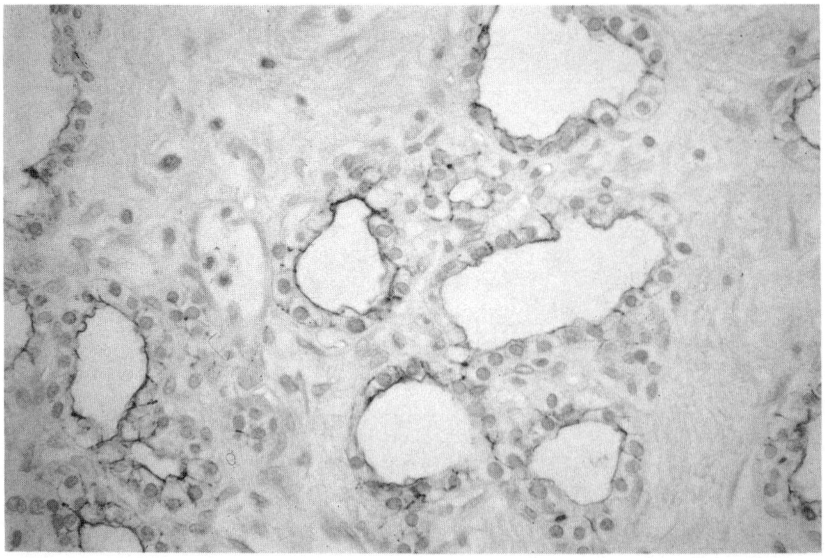

b
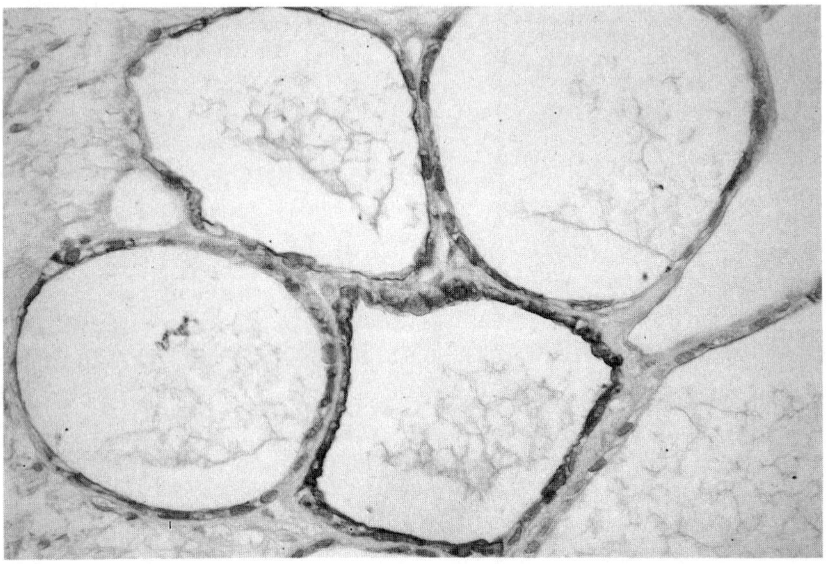

Fig. 16a,b. CA19-9 expression. ***a*** Tumor cells are stained only on the apical membrane in serous cystadenoma (the same patient). ***b*** Tumor cells are stained diffusely in serous cystadenocarcinoma (tumor of the pancreatic head, the same patient). ×100 (original magnification). (*For color reproduction see color insert in the frontmatter*)

5], the serous cystadenoma cells were stained only on the apical membrane with anti-CA19-9 antibody (Fig. 16a), whereas the tumor cells of the serous cystadenocarcinoma in the pancreatic head were diffusely stained with anti-CA19-9 (Fig. 16b). In the serous cystadenocarcinoma reported by Okada et al. [3] and Yoshimi et al. [4] no reactivity with anti-CA19-9 was found. Tumor cells of both the serous cystadenoma and serous cystadenocarcinoma were stained with anti-NCC-ST-439 on the apical membrane (Fig. 17). In the serous cystadenoma, only a few tumor cells were stained with anti-c-*erb*B-2, whereas almost all tumor cells of the serous cystadenocarcinoma were stained with this antibody (Fig. 18).

Nuclear DNA Analysis

The DNA content of our case was analyzed by flow cytometry. In all four serous cystadenomas, the tumor cells exhibited diploid nuclear DNA, with a DNA index of 1.0 and with proliferative indices between 4.9% and 20.9%, the mean being 14.4%. In the serous cystadenocarcinoma, the tumor of the head had aneuploid nuclear DNA (DNA index =

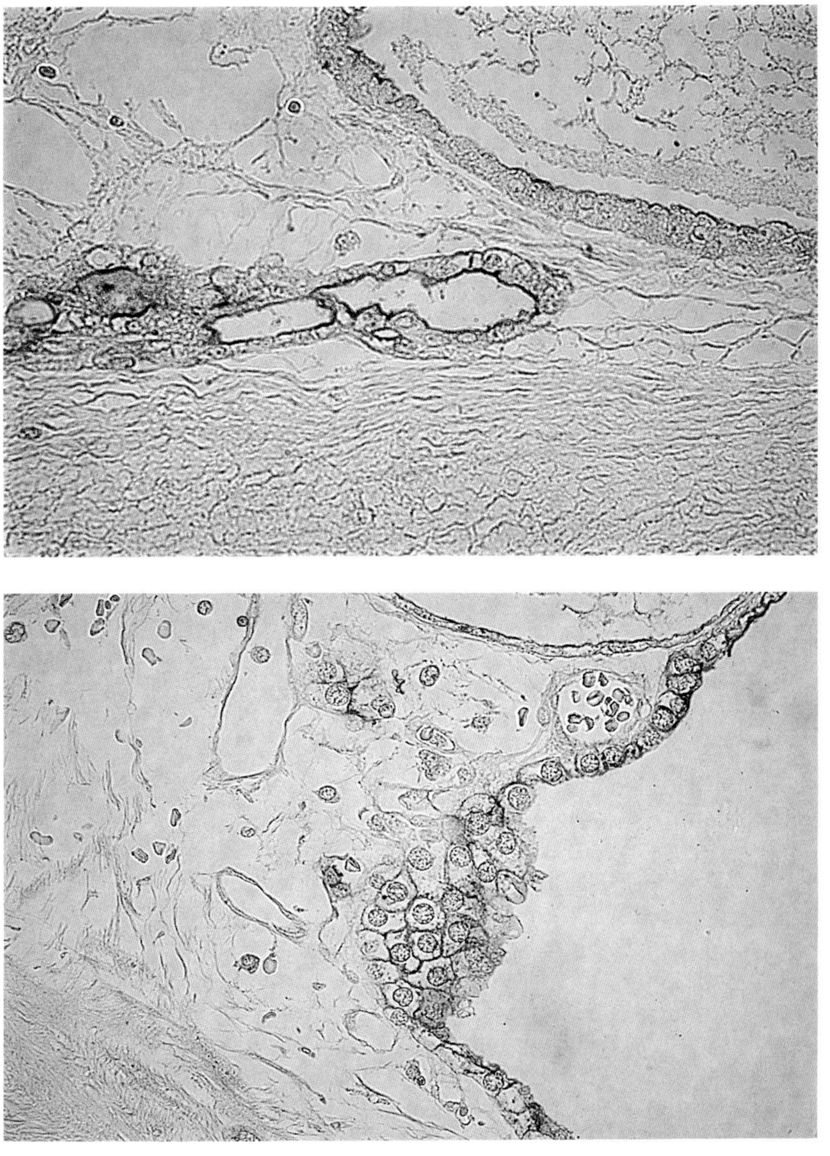

a

b

Fig. 17a,b. NCC-ST-439 expression. Tumor cells expressed on the apical membrane in ***a*** serous cystadenoma and ***b*** in all cell membrane in serous cystadenocarcinoma (the same patient). ×100 (original magnification). (*For color reproduction see color insert in the frontmatter*)

1.9) and a proliferative index of 27.8%. The tumor of the body exhibited aneuploid nuclear DNA (DNA index = 1.9) and had a proliferative index of 22.4% (Fig. 19). Thus, the serous cystadenocarcinoma differed from the serous cystadenoma by nuclear DNA analysis and had a high proliferative ability.

Ag-NORs Expression

The Ag-NORs number was defined as the mean count of black granules in the nuclei of 100 cells [2]. The average Ag-NORs number was 1.85 in serous cystadenoma cells, as compared to 3.49 in serous cystadenocarcinoma cells, 1.39 in normal pancreatic ductal cells, and 3.00 in pancreatic ductal carcinoma cells. Thus, the Ag-NORs number of serous cystadenocarcinoma cells was significantly higher than that of serous cystadenoma cells, and was comparable with that of the pancreatic ductal carcinoma cells. On the other hand, the Ag-NORs numbers of both serous cystadenoma cells and serous cystadenocarcinoma cells were significantly higher than that of the pancreatic normal ductal epithelium (Fig. 20).

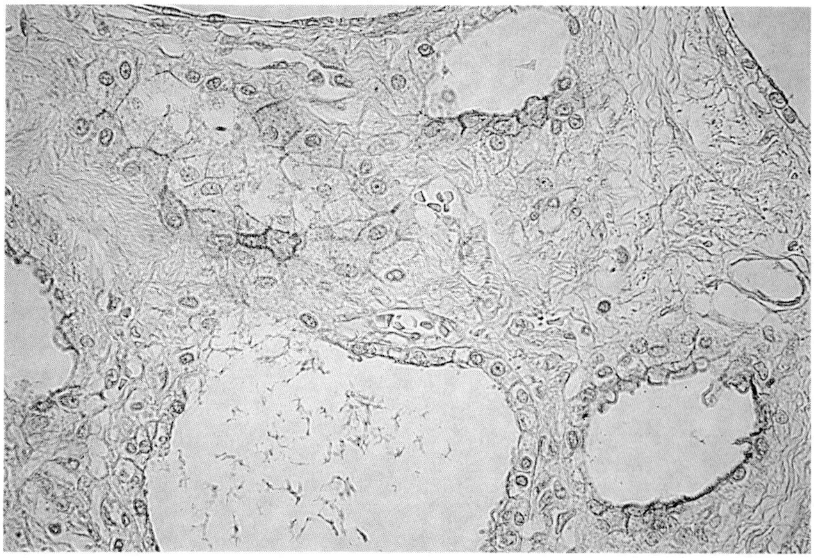

a

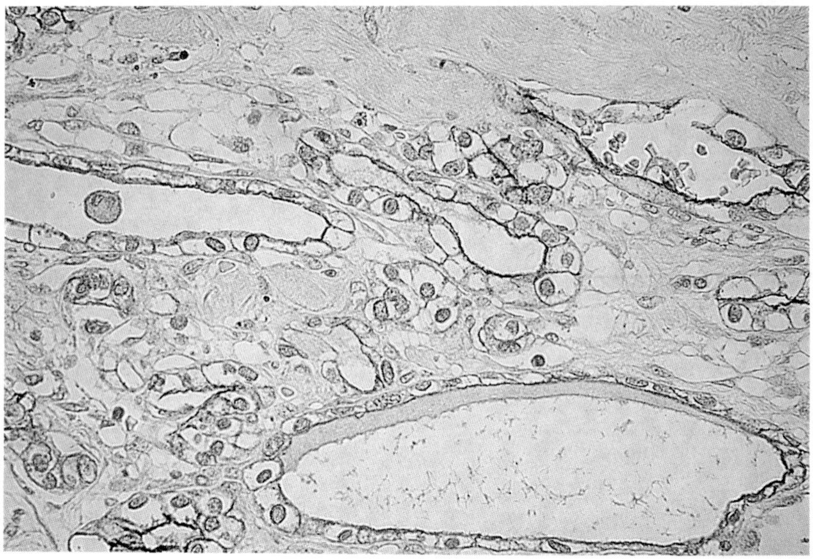

b

Fig. 18a,b. Anti c-*erb*B-2 expression (the same patient). ***a*** Only a few tumor cells are stained on the membrane in serous cystadenoma, ***b*** but in all tumor cells in serous cystadenocarcinoma ×100 (original magnification). (*For color reproduction see color insert in the frontmatter*)

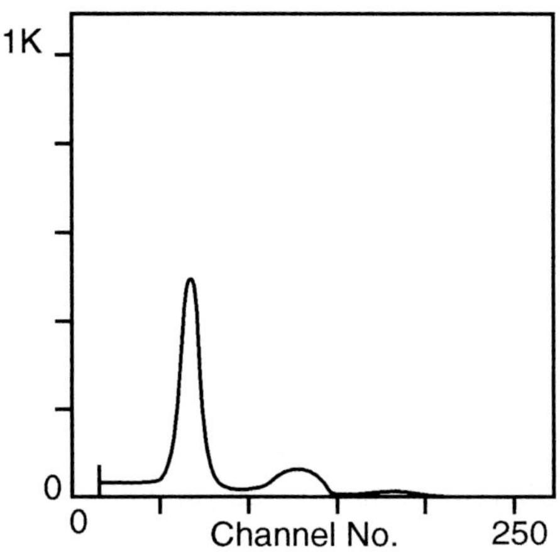

a

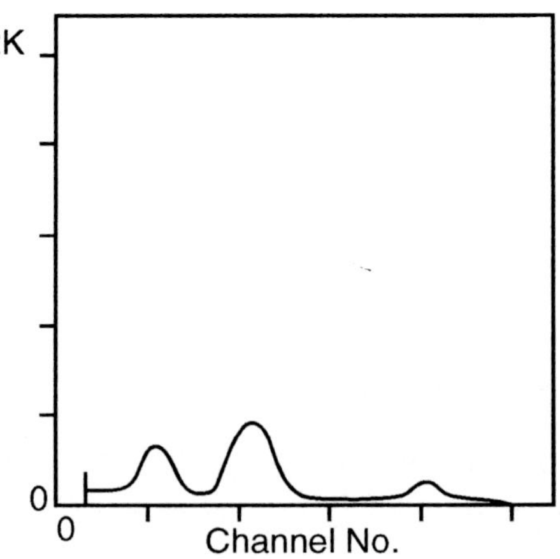

b

Fig. 20a,b. Ag-NORS expression in the same patient. Ag-NORs numbers were defined as the average number of black granules in the nucleus in ***a*** serous cystadenoma and ***b*** serous cystadenocarcinoma which contain more granules in each cell than serous cystadenoma. (*For color reproduction see color insert in the frontmatter*)

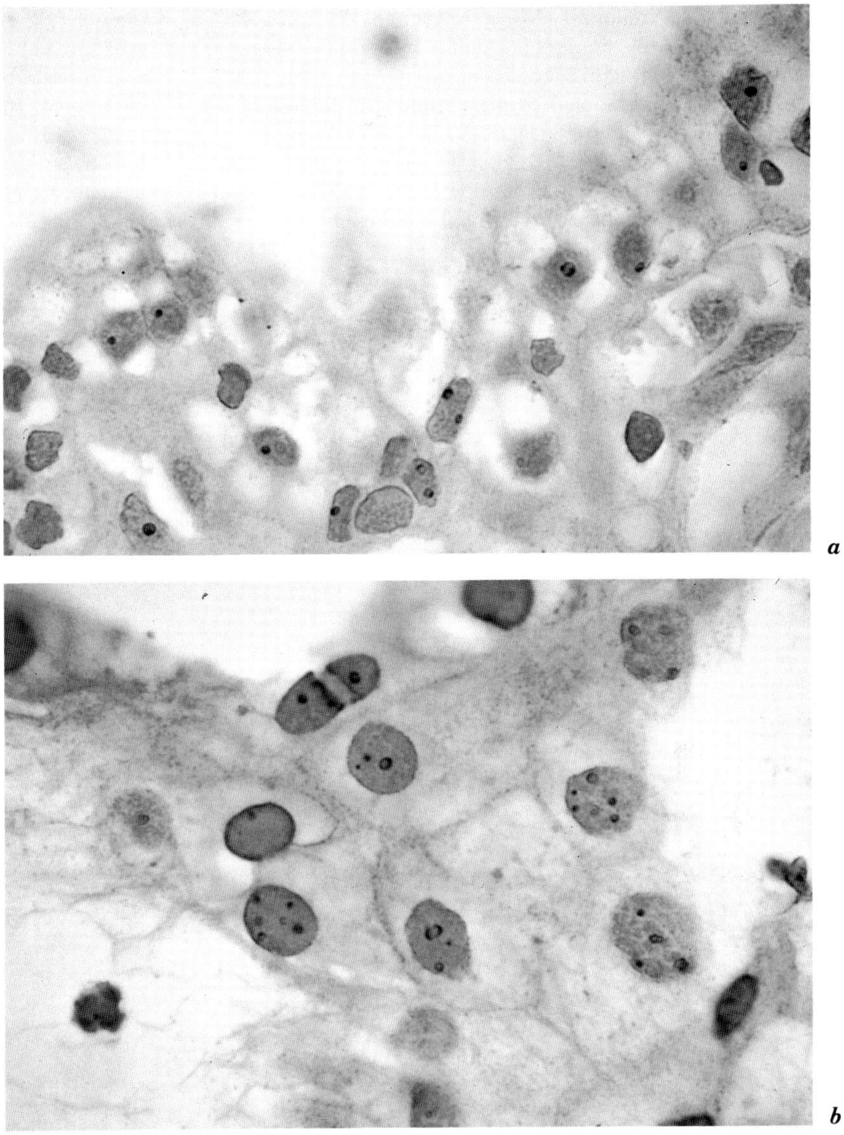

Prognosis

Two of the four reported cases died of a secondary disease in the operating room or soon following the operation. The case reported by George et al. (1989) was complicated by metastases to the liver and invasion of the stomach wall and the spleen. Okada et al. [3] and Yoshimi et al. [4] reported hepatic metastasis 4 and 3 years, respectively, after primary resection.

References

1. George DH, Murphy F, Michalski R, Ulmer BG (1989) Serous cystadenocarcinoma of the pancreas. A new entity. Am J Surg Pathol 13:61–66
2. Kamei K, Funabiki T, Ochiai M, Amano H, Kasahara M, Sakamoto T (1991) Multifocal pancreatic serous cystadenoma with atypical cells and focal perineural invasion. Int J Pancreatol 10: 161–172

Fig. 19a,b. Nuclear DNA patterns in the same patient. ***a*** Diploidy in serous cystadenoma. ***b*** Aneuploidy in serous cystadenocarcinoma

3. Okada T, Nonami T, Miwa T, Yamada F, Ando K, Tatematsu A, Sugie S, Kondo T (1991) Hepatic metastasis of serous cystadenocarcinoma resected 4 years after operation of primary tumors (in Japanese). Jpn J Gastroenterol 88:2719–2723
4. Yoshimi N, Sugie S, Tanaka T, Aijin W, Bunai Y, Tatematsu A, Okada T, Mori H (1992) A rare case of serous cystadenocarcinoma of the pancreas. Cancer 69:2449–2453
5. Kamei K, Funabiki T, Ochiai M, Amano H, Marugami Y, Kasahara M, Sakamoto T (1992) Some considerations on the biology of pancreatic serous cystadenoma. Int J Pancreatol 11:97–104
6. Katoh H, Rossi RL, Braasch JW, Munson JL, Shimozawa E, Tanabe T (1989) Cystadenoma and cystadenocarcinoma of the pancreas. Hepatogastroenteroly 36:424–430

Ductal Adenocarcinoma

Synonyms

Pancreatic cancer; adenocarcinoma of pancreas; ductal cell carcinoma; papillary adenocarcinoma; tubular adenocarcinoma

Definition

Ductal adenocarcinoma is the most common pancreatic tumor. Therefore, it is used as a general term for pancreatic exocrine malignancy. The term pancreatic ductal adenocarcinoma (PDA) should be based on pathomorphological entities. This term applies to pancreatic exocrine adenocarcinoma showing ductal differentiation. PDA shows various histological features in which tubular or focal papillotubular structures may occur. In the new Japanese pancreatic cancer classification, the term "invasive ductal carcinoma" is widely used.

According to American [1], European [2], and Japanese [3] studies, this type of malignancy accounts for about 70% to 80% of all primary exocrine tumors, and for more than 80% of all pancreatic malignancies [4]. With the recent rapid popularization of image analyzers, including ultrasonography (US) and computed tomography (CT), the relative ratio of PDA to other nonendocrine pancreatic neoplasms decreases slightly [3] because other pancreatic tumors, such as solid-cystic (papillary-cystic) tumor, mucinous cystic tumor, and serous cystic tumor are detected with increasing frequency.

Incidence

The incidence of PDA in different parts of the world ranges from 0 to 10 per 100 000 population. Although the incidence of this disease is high in Japan and presents the fifth and seventh leading causes of cancer-related death in men and women, respectively, it is rare in other Asian countries, including China and India [5]. In the United States, PDA is the fourth and fifth leading cause of death from cancer in men and women, respectively [6]. PDA is exceeded only by cancer of the lung, colon, rectum, and breast. In the United States, the number of new PDA cases is estimated to be about 27 000 (13 500 men and 14 200 women) [7]. The age-adjusted mortality rates increased from 2.9 per 100 000 in 1920 to 9 per 100 000 in 1970 and have remained nearly the same since then. The incidence in the United States is higher among blacks than in whites and all other ethnic groups except the Japanese [8]. Both American whites and blacks show a higher age-standardized incidence rates than do Africans [9]. Incidence rates among Hispanics tend to be similar to those for whites [10].

Sex and Age

According to Japanese statistics [4], more than 90% of PDA patients are older than 50 years; the mean age is 60 years. However, the disease has been seen in individuals as young as 3 months of age [11–13]. In a hospital record from 1918 to 1962, fewer than 2% of the 600 patients with pancreatic cancer were under 40 years of age [14].

In a study conducted at the Mayo Clinic from 1970 to 1985, 26 patients with PDA under the age of 40 were identified. The mean age of these patients was 34, with only one patient less than 25 years old. The aggressive behavior of the tumor and its prognosis in these patients were comparable with PDA in older patients [15].

PDA occurs with a male to female ratio between 1.1 and 2.0 to 1 [1, 2, 4]. Age modifies the relationship between PDA and gender. The male to female ratio is high (up to 2:1) in populations under 50, but decreases after the age of 70 [16]. Today, in the United States, more females develop the disease than males [7]. This situation has been suggested to be due to the androgenic control of PDA. However, the role of sex hormones on disease development is controversial. Androgens have promoted the growth of acinar cell tumors in the rat [17, 18], but not ductal cell carcinoma in the hamster [19]. Although some authors report on the presence of androgen-binding activity with a high affinity and a low capacity in pancreatic ductular adenocarcinoma and in some pancreatic cancer cell lines [20, 21], and also an increase of 5-α-reductase [21], the evidence is not convincing. Reasons for the low level of plasma testosterone in PDA patients [16] are obscure (for details see [16]). The recent dramatic increase of PDA in females could be due to increased cigarette smoking among females rather than to an androgenic influence. Furthermore, the effects of antiandrogenic substances in the treatment of pancreatic cancer have remained unsuccessful.

Etiology and Pathogenesis

The etiology of pancreatic cancer is not well understood. The epidemiological data are inconclusive and confusing. Numerous factors, including nutrition, occupation, religion, socioeconomic status, radiation exposure, infection and prior operation, (particularly gastrectomy) have been claimed to play predisposing roles. The consumption of high dietary fat, beef, coffee, alcohol, butter, red tea, certain breads, etc., has been associated with PDA. Epidemiological results and experimental data link pancreatic cancer with the consumption of a high-fat, high-protein diet [22, 23]. However, those factors may cumulatively promote the process of carcinogenesis because their individual relative risk factors are not high [24].

Several epidemiological studies have found a significant association between the incidence of PDA and cigarette smoking. However, according to Hirayama, cigarette smoking seems to be a promoting rather than an initiating factor. One of our studies in heavy smokers who died of lung cancer confirmed this. Detailed histopathological studies of the pancreas from 30 of these patients did not show any significant difference between the number of preneoplastic or neoplastic lesions found in the pancreas of these patients compared with the findings in the pancreas of nonsmokers [25]. Also, experimental studies have failed to show that cigarette smoking increases the risk of cancer of the pancreas [26].

The role of diabetes in pancreatic cancer has been questioned in recent clinical and experimental studies. In the Syrian hamster, in which pancreatic tumors similar to the human disease can be induced, streptozotocin-induced diabetes inhibits or prevents induction of pancreatic ductal adenocarcinoma [27, 28]. Moreover, clinical observations strongly suggest that development of PDA is associated with peripheral insulin resistance [29, 30], a condition that improves by the removal of pancreatic cancer [31]. It is believed that pancreatic cancer produces diabetogenic substances, such as islet amyloid polypeptide (IAPP) [32], which has been found in high levels in the sera of PDA patients [32]. This increase parallels the production of endocrine cells within the cancerous tissue (see below). However, additional studies are required to clarify the association between pancreatic cancer and diabetes.

Chemical agents may be regarded as pancreatic carcinogens, including coal gas [33] and coal tar [34, 35], β-naphtylamine, and benzidine [36]. An increased risk of PDA has also been reported in wood workers [37] and workers in coke plants, metal industries and aluminum milling, as well as among chemists [38]. However, some of these studies were not confirmed and others require further research.

Only certain carcinogenic nitrosamines have produced pancreatic cancer of the ductal type, which histologically, molecular biologically, and antigenically resembles human pancreatic cancer [39]. However, these pancreatic carcinogens have not been identified in the environment. For yet unknown reasons, the Syrian hamster is the only species known to produce this type of tumor. In other species, certain carcinogens produce acinar cell tumors, which are rare in humans. Recent studies in syngeneic mice [40–42] suggest that genetic factors may be involved in the etiology of pancreatic cancer. The frequent occurrence of PDA in certain populations (American blacks) could either be due to the exposure to some causative agents or reflect a genetic role in PDA development. Although an epidemiological study confirmed the genetic influence on the disease [43], additional epidemiological and molecular biological studies are needed for clarification.

The role of pancreatitis as an etiological factor is debatable [44, 45]. In many cases, PDAs, especially those that arise from the main duct, cause chronic obstructive pancreatitis. However, PDA tends to develop in familial pancreatitis [see 44]. Two-thirds of PDA patients who are under 40 years of age had a previous history of either pancreatitis, pseudocyst, benign cystadenoma, or choledochal cyst [15]. However, even in these cases, the development of the two abnormalities may have been incidental. Theoretically, chronic pancreatitis with ongoing degenerative and proliferative process, should predispose to PDA. However, chronic pancreatitis does not increase the rate of pancreatic cancer [44].

Finally, congenital deformities, such as anomalous arrangement of the biliary and pancreatic duct system, are also suspected risk factors for PDA [46], as well as for cancer of the biliary duct system.

Pathogenesis

Because of the frequent occurrence of PDA in the head of the pancreas, it was assumed that pancreatic tissue was exposed to bile-borne carcinogens [47]. However, several experiments have shown the blood-borne effect of the carcinogens [48, 49]. These studies have also shown a relationship between the size/volume of individual pancreatic lobes and the incidence of PDA. However, in humans, the head region is not the largest pancreatic segment and other factors appear to operate in the development of PDA in the head of the pancreas. A recent observation on the development of intraductal tumors (see Chapter "Intraductal Papillary Mucinous Tumors, Non-Invasive and Invasive" in this volume) suggests that tumors may arise in areas other than the head, progress intraductally, and manifest themselves in the head region.

The cell of origin of PDA has also remained controversial. Although many tumors, including the benign and malignant, seem to arise from the epithelium of the large duct and its branches [45, 50–54], the histogenesis of PDA arising from the periphery of the pancreas is still unclear. In the hamster and avian models of pancreatic cancer, the induced PDA arises either from large ducts or from ductules, including centroacinar cells [55–57]. In humans, however, the difficulty in the detection of early cancer obscures the site of cancer origin. Some believe that at least some tumors arise from dedifferentiated acinar cells and abnormal acinar cell foci, the presumed cancer precursors, which have been identified in the human pancreas [58–61]. However, the biological nature of these acinar cell foci has been debated [62]. During our detailed histological examination of human pancreases with or without pancreatic cancer [54], we observed a few early cancers in both duct and ductules (see Chapter "Preneoplastic Lesions of the Exocrine Pancreas" in this volume). The recent observations on the variety of cellular composition of PDA strongly suggest that the tumors derive from pancreatic undifferentiated (stem) cells, which tend to differentiate toward various epithelial components of the pancreas. In fact, all induced well-differentiated, anaplastic and sarcomatous pancreatic tumors appear to arise from ductal/ductular cells [63].

Clinical Features and Laboratory Tests

The most common symptom associated with PDA in the pancreas head is weight loss. It occurs in 75%–90% of the patients [64–66] and may be unrelated to the appetite of the patients. The average weight loss is about 25 pounds within 2 months. The weight loss could be due to anorexia, vomiting, malabsorption, depression, and increased IAPP.

Another initial symptom of pancreatic cancer is abdominal pain, which occurs in about 30% to 70% of patients, and almost all patients develop pain during the course of the disease [64–66]. It is important to note that pain may be vague and diffuse. It localizes in the epigastrium and hypochondrium in 75% of cases [64, 65, 67]. Right and left upper quadrant pain occurs in about 20% of cases. The pain radiates to the back in 25% of patients. It may be severe at night. Positions that flex the spine may bring some relief. In patients with PDA in the pancreatic body and tail, the pain is more common and occurs in 85% of the cases. In about 60% of those cases the pain radiates toward the back [65, 67].

Eighty percent to 90% of patients with pancreatic head cancer show obstructive jaundice or pancreatitis, because tumors tend to invade the common bile duct or main pancreatic (Wirsung's) duct in the early stage. The jaundice is progressive and unremitting. The development of jaundice causes detection of PDA at a relatively early course and is associated with a better prognosis. The early detection of the pancreatic tail- or uncustumor, on the other hand, is difficult because of the lack of early symptoms, and it has a grave prognosis. Tumors of this location are often discovered with massive ascites or peritonitis carcinomatosis.

Nausea, vomiting, and abnormal bowel habits are other symptoms, and these occur in 30% to 45% of patients [64, 65]. Depression and presonality changes have been reported in up to 75% of patients, particularly in those with cancer in the body and tail. Possible reasons include weight loss, anorexia, and an increase in hormones or other substances released by PDA.

Diabetes mellitus is a complication of the advanced stage. About 15% to 65% of the patients with pancreatic cancer have a past history of diabetes mellitus [29–32] and 80% of the patients show an abnormal glucose tolerance test [68]. This phenomenon may be caused by islet injury due to the tumor invasion. On the other hand, patients with diabetes often are said to be predisposed to pancreatic cancer. According to the autopsy study, however, there is no remarkable difference between the tumor incidence in diabetic and nondiabetic patients. As stated earlier, recent data suggest that the development of an abnormal glucose tolerance test and diabetes are consequences of PDA.

Elevated levels of serum bilirubin, alkaline phosphatase, lactate dehydrogenase, glutamic oxaloacetic transaminase, glutamic pyruvic transaminase, 5′ nucleotidase, and pancreatic enzymes have been found in patients with PDA [69, 70], but these abnormalities are not specific for PDA.

In the last decade, attempts were made to discover markers for pancreatic cancer (Table 1). These markers include enzymes, proteins, peptides and tumor associated/oncofetal antigens [71–103]. However, none of these markers has been found to be specific for PDA.

Alpha fetoprotein (AFP) is a poor tumor marker for PDA. Serum AFP elevation has been found in up to 25% of patients; however, only 5% of patients have levels greater than 40 ng/ml [104]. On the other hand, AFP is useful for the diagnosis of pancreatoblastoma and some type of acinar cell carcinoma. In fact, more than 60% of the patients with pancreatoblastoma have elevated serum AFP (see Chapter "Pancreatoblastoma" in this volume). The same is true for pancreatic oncofetal antigen (POA), the serum level of which increases also in patients with bronchogenic carcinoma, colon carcinoma, bile duct cancer, and in pregnancy [105].

Among the many antigens found in PDA, carcinoembryonic antigen (CEA), DU-PAN-2, CA19-9, CA50, CA125, SPan-1 and TAG-72 have been found to be useful markers. However, the lack of blood circulation of these antigens at the early stage of the disease limits their clinical value. CEA levels have been found in up to 80% of patients with PDA. Its sensitivity is 59%, specificity 63.9%, positive and negative predictive values 46.4% and 74.7%, respectively, and diagnostic accuracy 62.2%. There is no remarkable difference in the sensitivity in T_1 and T_2 cancers [106]. Increased levels of this antigen occur also in patients with other cancers (60%) and in benign pancreatic diseases (46%). Increasing the upper limit of normal from 2.5 to 10 ng/ml has not been effective in increasing the specificity of the test [104]. Also, the isomeric form of CEA, CEA-S, is not more specific than CEA [84].

CA19-9 and SPan-1 are better markers by far than the other tumor-associated antigens. Serum elevation of these two antigens has been found in over 70% of pancreatic cancers less than 4.0 cm in size, whereas DU-PAN-2, CEA, and elastase were increased in only a few of these patients [107]. The sensitivity of CA19-9 is about 80%, which is the highest among other malignant diseases, including gastric cancer (26%) and colon cancer (31%) [106]. The specificity of CA19-9 is 73%, positive predictive value 54.2%, negative predictive value 89.5%, and diagnostic accuracy 74.5% [106]. The level of CA19-9 differs according to the stage of the PDA. In T_1 cancers, its level is 52% and increases to 82% in T_2 cancers [106]. However, this marker shows a high sensitivity in diseases with jaundice including hepatoma (35%) and biliary tract cancer (64%) and is also found in relatively high levels in chronic hepatitis (30%) and liver cirrhosis (20%)

Table 1. Markers for pancreatic ductal adenocarcinoma.

Markers	Reference
Enzymes	
Pancreatic enzymes	Tournat et al. [71]
Trypsin in urine	Lake-Bakaar et al. [72]
Ribonuclease	Nakane et al. [73], Weichman, et al. [74]
Deoxyribonuclease	Douglas and Chandler [75]
Gamma-glutamyltranspeptidase	Nishida et al. [76]
Phospholipase A_2	Navalainen et al. [77]
Elastase	Hamano et al. [78]
Immunoreactive trypsin	Vezzadini et al. [79]
Glacatosyl-transferase isozyme	Douglas and Chandler [75], Podolski and Weiser [80]
Ferritin	Niitsu [81]
Protein	
Lactoferin	
Ferritin	
β_2 microglobulin	Fateh-Moghadam et al. [82]
Immunosupressive acid protein	
Peptide	
Insulin	
C-peptide	
Glucagon	
Somatostatin	
Islet amyloid polypeptide	
Calcitonin	
Gastrin	
Human chorionic gonadotropin	
Parathormone	
Tumor-associated/Oncofetal antigens	
Carcinoembryonic antigen (CEA, CEA-S)	Holyoke et al. [83], Nakamura et al. [84]
Alpha fetoprotein (AFP)	McIntire et al. [85]
Pancreatic oncofetal antigen (POA)	Banwo et al. [86]
Pancreatic oncofetal protein	Mihas [87]
α-CAP I	Klavins [88]
Fetoacinar pancreatic protein (FAP)	Fujii et al. [89]
CA19-9	Koprowski et al. [90]
CA50	Lindholm et al. [91]
CA125	Bast et al. [92]
DU-PAN-2	Metzgar et al. [93]
TAG-72	Klug et al. [94]
17-1A	Herlyn et al. [95]
Span-1	Chung et al. [96]
YPanl and YPan2	Yuan et al. [97]
Pancreatic cancer associated antigen (PCAA)	Loor et al. [98]
Pancreatic duct tissue specific antigen	Gold et al. [99]
Tumor-associated trypsin inhibitor (TAT1)	Stenman et al. [100]
Pancreas-specific antigen (PaA)	Loor et al. [98]
Sialyl SSEA-1	Lawa et al. [101]
Others	
Fucose	Wallach et al. [102]
Leucocyte adherence inhibition	Leveson et al. [103]

[106]. CA19-9 measurement is of no value for early detection of PDA. False-positive and -negative elevation can occur [108].

The sensitivity of DU-PAN-2 for PDA is low (47.7%). Biliary tract cancers show the same sensitivity (41.0%); the sensitivity in hepatoma in 27.5% and in liver cirrhosis 23.7%. The specificity of this antigen for PDA is 85.3%, its positive and negative predictive values are 57.9% and 79.4%, respectively, and its diagnostic accuracy is 74.1% (99). The sensitivity of DU-PAN-2 is almost twice as high (40%) in T_2 than in T_1 cancers (22.2%). In our study, the predictive accuracies for CA19-9, DU-PAN-2, CA125 and TAG-72 were 89%, 67%, 63%, and 61%, respectively [109]. CA19-9 was undetectable or very low in patients belonging to Le^{a-b-}, because these patients lack the Lewis gene. This disadvantage of CA19-9 could be corrected by a simultaneous measurement of serum DU-PAN-2, which was elevated in these patients [109]. Also, in another study, an elevated serum level of DU-PAN-2 was found in either the Lewis-negative or -positive groups [101]. Another disadvantage of CA19-9 in the diagnosis of pancreatic cancer is that liver dysfunction and age influence its serum level [110]. However, CA19-9 has been shown to be a relatively reliable marker for monitoring the disease; its level decreases after surgical therapy and becomes elevated after recurrence [111].

The sensitivity of SPan-1 is 81.4%, the specificity 67.5%, positive and negative predictive values 46.8% and 91.2%, respectively, and diagnostic accuracy 71.1% [106]. The sensitivity of this marker is much lower in T_1 (48.3%) than in T_2 cancers (80.9%) [106].

The combination assay of CA19-9 and SPan-1 in T_1 cancer increased the sensitivity from a single assay of 62.5% and 56.5% to 70%. In T_2 cancer, the sensitivity of the combination was 97.1% [112]. Similar results were obtained by a combination of a pancreas cancer-associated antigen (PCAA) and a pancreas-specific antigen (PaA), whereby a better specificity (85%) and sensitivity (90%) for pancreatic cancer was found than in either the PCAA or the PaA assay alone.

The sensitivity of CA50 for PDA is about 64.9%, specificity 73.2%, positive and negative predictive values 64.9% and 73.2%, respectively, and diagnostic accuracy 69.9% [106]. Elastase 1 has about the same sensitivity (51.1%), specificity (75.6%), positive and negative predictive values (70.0% and 58.0%, respectively) and diagnostic accuracy (62.7%) as CA50. Its sensitivity is almost the same in T_1 and T_2 cancers [106].

Fetoacinar pancreatic protein (FAP) has shown a sensitivity for PDA of 86% and specificity of 66%, compared to 74% and 88% for CA19-9 [89].

Alteration of pancreatic juice has also been used as marker. Using a microcomputer to analyze the isoelectric focusing pattern, researchers have found that a pancreatic secretory protein profile differs significantly between patients with chronic pancreatitis and PDA [113, 114]. In another study, the analysis of protein contained in pancreatic juice by two-dimensional isoelectric focusing/sodium dodecyl sulfate gel electrophoresis showed a number of additional proteins not observed in the pancreatic juice obtained from the normal pancreas [115].

The ratio of renal clearance of immunoreactive trypsin relative to renal clearance of creatinine was found to be raised in pancreatic cancer patients but not in chronic pancreatitis cases [72]. However, conclusive data are missing.

Diagnostic Procedures

An upper gastrointestinal series rarely helps in the diagnosis of PDA. Two classical findings are an enlarged duodenal sweep and the reversed or inverted figure 3, which occurs due to the adherence and fixing of ampulla and duodenum with the indentation of the concave border of the duodenum. However, these findings occur in fewer than 10% of PDA patients [64, 65]. Hypotonic duodenography allows a more detailed evaluation of duodenal contour and mucosa in patients with PDA in the head of the pancreas, but it's useless in patients with tumors in the body or tail of the pancreas [116, 117].

Pancreatic Scanning

Ultrasonography. Ultrasonography (US) is a relatively reliable technique to detect pancreatic tumors. Solid and cystic masses can be distinguished and atypical echo patterns have been defined for benign and malignant tumors [118–120]. The accuracy of diagnosis is reportedly between 67% [62] to 86% [121] with a false-positive value of 28% and a false-negative value of 33% [69]. Positive and negative predictive values of

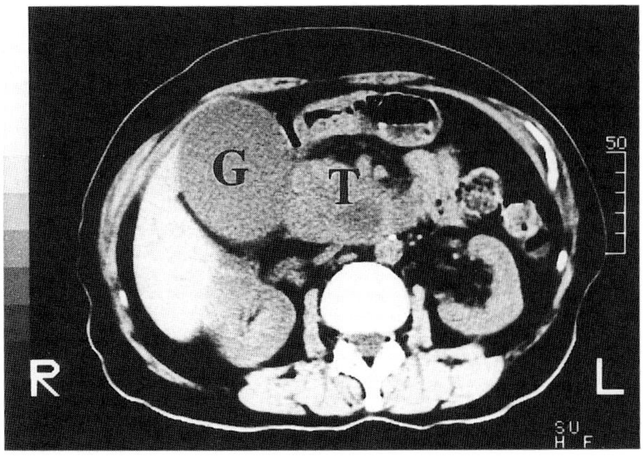

Fig. 1. Computed tomography of PDA showing a dilated gall bladder (*G*) and a low-density tumor (*T*) occupying the pancreas head (T, 1a). The patient was a 75-year-old woman who was admitted to the hospital with a 3-month history of abdominal fullness and back pain. Clinical examination showed a mass of the right hypochondral region, which seemed to be the gall bladder. The liver and pancreatic tumor were not palpable. Initial laboratory data were within the normal range. Endoscopic retrograde cholangiopancreatography (ERCP) showed complete obstruction of the pancreatic duct. At laparotomy, a 4.2 × 3.3 cm mass in the pancreas head with obstruction of the common bile duct was found

78% and 79%, respectively, have also been reported [121]. Other investigators have found similar results [118–120, 122]. In Japan, US detects about 40% of the patients [4].

Computed Tomography. Computed tomography (CT) can be used to detect deformities of the contour of the gland and shows a lower density for PDA than for the normal gland [123]. Correct diagnosis of PDA has been made in 79% to 94% of cases [69, 70, 104]. However, a false-positive value of 40% has been found in patients without cancer [69]. According to the Japanese Pancreatic Cancer Registration [4], 20% of PDA have been found by CT, a value that for some unknown reason is much lower than that of US (see above). Others have found similar diagnostic accuracies with US and CT. As with US, CT usually reveals the tumor as an irregular echoic low density region (Fig. 1). Irregular dilation of pancreatic ducts at the periphery is also important circumstantial evidence for detection. Incremental bolus-dynamic CT appears to be the single test modality for diagnosis and staging of PDA [124].

Magnetic Resonance Imaging. The use of magnetic resonance imaging (MRI) is of no additional aid in detecting pancreatic cancer.

Pancreatic Function Tests

Pancreatic function abnormalities occur in pancreatic cancer patients. After hormonal stimulation, abnormal output in patients with PDA involving the head, body, and tail was 90% to 95%, 70% to 83%, and 81%, respectively [125]. However, these abnormalities are mostly due to damage to pancreatic tissue by stenosis of the duct and pancreatitis rather than to the tumor itself.

Cytological Examination

The presence of malignant cells in the pancreatic juice has been found in 16% to 23% of the patients [126]. In other studies, after stimulation with secretin or CCK, a 68% sensitivity and 99% specificity of the cytological test has been reported [104, 127]. Positive results are far better for PDA in the pancreas head (70.6%), than in those in the pancreas body and tail (37.5%) [127]. However, cytological findings generally do not discriminate between types of pancreatic cancer.

Aspiration cytology with endoscopic cannulation of the pancreas duct leads to tumor diagnosis in 79% of the patients [128, 129]. A combination of CEA level determination and cytology increases the diagnostic accuracy to 86% [130].

Endoscopic Retrograde Cholangiopancreatography

The diagnostic accuracy of endoscopic retrograde cholangiopancreatography (ERCP) has been reported variously between 73% and 95% [96, 104, 131–133], with a predictive value of 90% [121], a 94% sensitivity, and a 97% specificity [134].

Compared with US and CT, ERCP is a sensitive and invasive test for the diagnosis of PDA. In Japan, ERP or ERCP detects about 10% of the pancreatic cancers [4] with unusual findings of the pancreatic duct system, such as irregular shift, stenosis, obstruction, or suppression (Fig. 2a). Endoscopic examination of the pancreatic duct is especially useful for the detection of intraductal tumors, and ERCP with brush cytology improves the diagnostic accuracy.

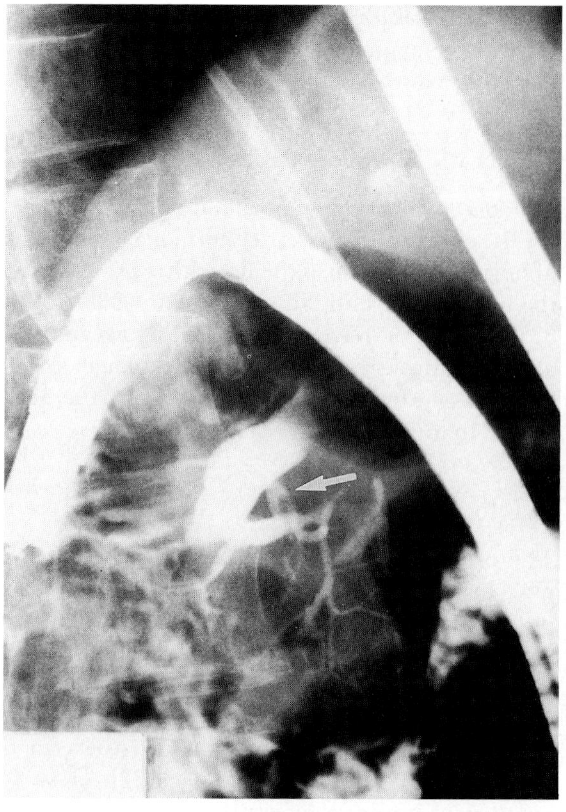

a

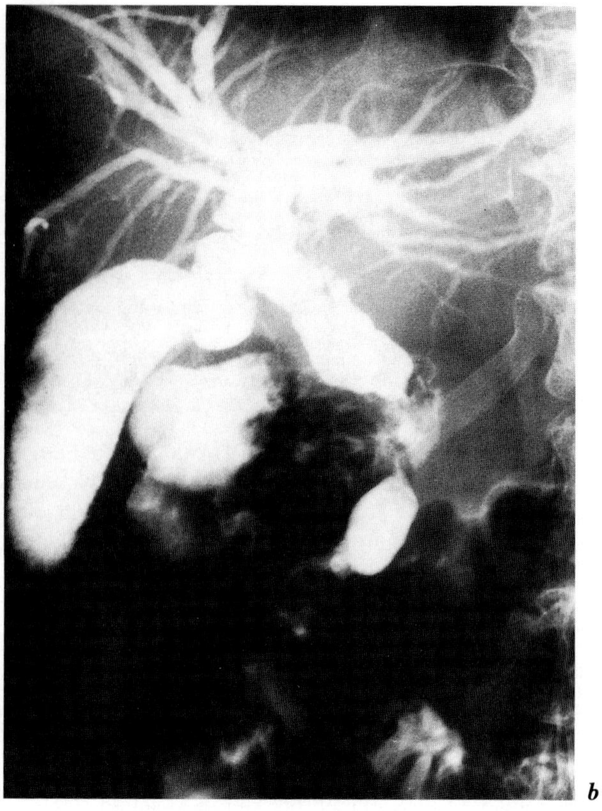

b

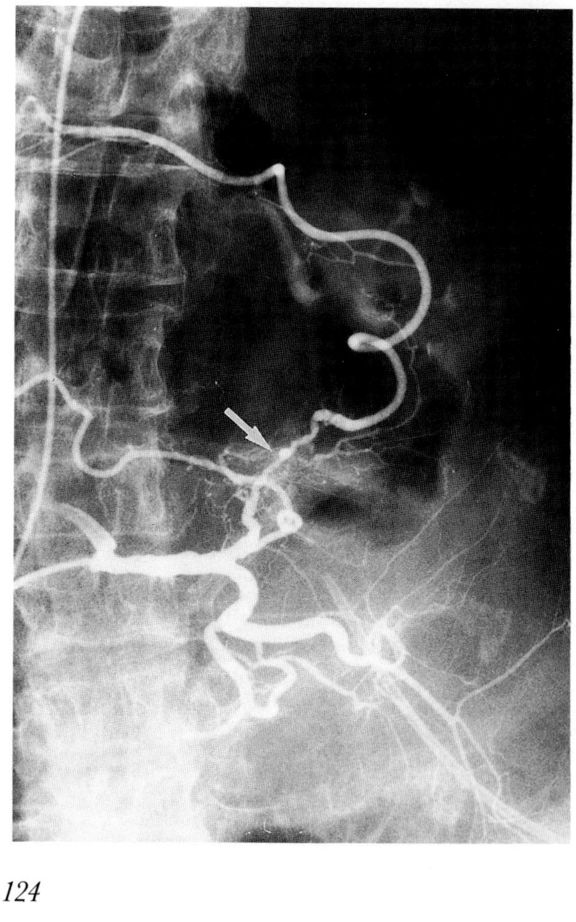

c

Fig. 2. ***a*** ERCP of a 76-year-old woman with a PDA shows the obstruction of the main pancreatic duct in the pancreas head. Santorini was intact (*arrow*). The patient was admitted to the hospital with 1 month of general fatigue and epigastralgia. ***b*** Percutaneous transhepatic cholangiography (PTC) of the same patient showing prominent bile duct dilatation and stenotic changes in the intrapancreatic common bile duct. ***c*** Selective celiac angiography of the same case. Serrated encasement of gastroduodenal artery (*arrow*). ***d*** Shift and encasement of posterior pancreaticoduodenal artery and stenosis of the portal vein in venous phase (*arrow*) of the same case. ***e*** Gross appearance of the tumor, which had invaded the wall of the portal vein. The cut surface of the 3.5 × 3.0 × 5.5 cm tumor shows stenotic common bile duct (*CD*), pancreatic duct (*PD*), and lymph node metastasis (*LN*). (*For color reproduction of **e** see color insert in the frontmatter*)

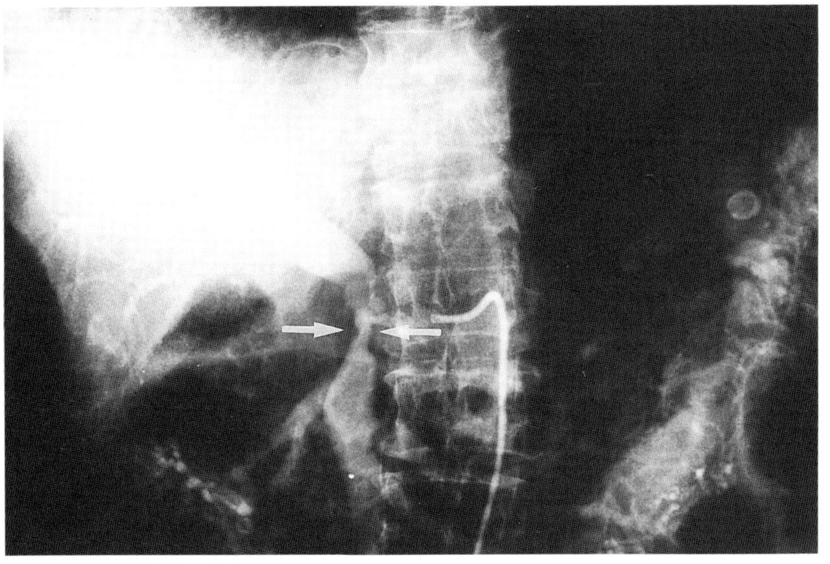

d

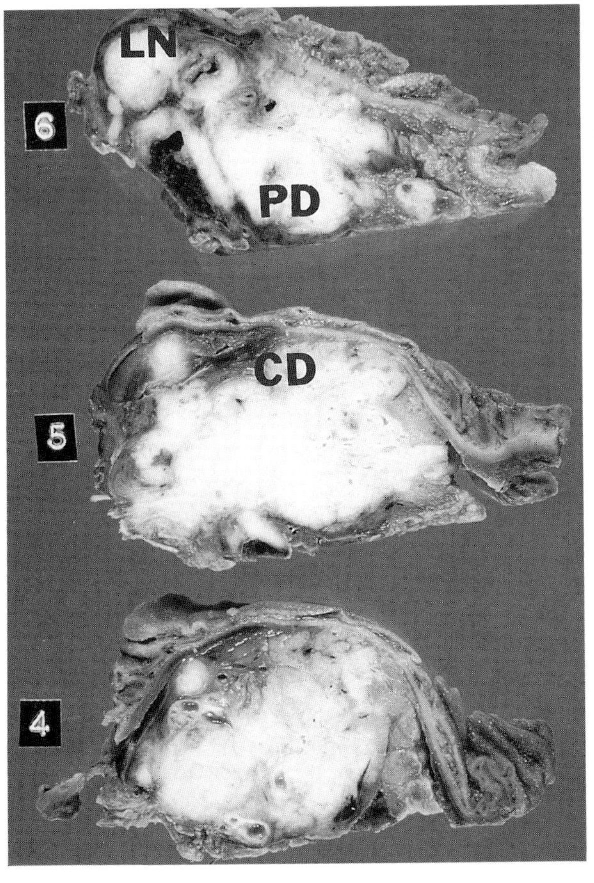

e

Fig. 2. *Continued*

Recently, a new method of intraoperative cytodiagnosis for accurate location of occult PDA has been described [135]. With this method, a catheter is inserted in both the caudal and cranial opening of the duct in the pancreatic neck that is dissected at a right angle. After intravenous injection of secretin, pure pancreatic juice is collected and cytologically examined.

Percutaneous transhepatic cholangiography gives a diagnostic accuracy of 100% and a specificity of 96% [134, 136–138]. With this technique, abnormalities in the pancreatic and common bile duct can be visualized (Fig. 2b).

Percutaneous Needle Biopsy

Advances in noninvasive imaging techniques have encouraged a more accurate pancreatic needle biopsy with accuracy. Most investigators have found an 85% to 100% diagnostic accuracy [139–142] with no false-positive results [126, 142–144] but with a 12% false-negative rate [142]. However, the cells of well-differentiated PDA, benign conditions, and neuroendocrine tumors could not be distinguished by cytology [142]. The danger of abdominal wall implantation may have been exaggerated, because in over 5000 needle aspirations possible abdominal wall implantation of tumors was seen in only two cases [145, 146].

Quantitative nuclear DNA content measurement in fine needle aspirates of PDA seems to give information on biological behavior of tumors and on survival [147]. It is also claimed that cytology allows cystic pancreatic tumors to be differentiated [148]. Determination of the c-Ki-ras mutation in aspirates is an advance technique for accurate diagnosis (see later).

Laparoscopy

In difficult-to-diagnose cases, laparoscopy with visually directed biopsies are used [149, 150]. With this technique, the stage of the disease can be determined and the correct diagnosis can be made in 32% of PDA in the pancreas head and in 88% of PDA in the body and tail [149]. The positive biopsy rate is about 75% for head cancer and 85% for body/tail cancers.

Angiography

Angiography is an important examination to reconfirm the tumorous lesions, which are generally revealed as avascular or hypervascular areas with encasement, obstruction, angulation, and serration of blood vessels (Fig. 2c–e). However, tumors smaller than 2 cm can be missed. The diagnostic accuracy reportedly ranges between 40% and 100% [151–154]. A characteristic feature is localized invasion of arteries with serpiginous, irregular or serrated encasement. Neovascularity is seen in 50% of cases [134, 152]. Alteration in parenchymal blush during the capillary phase and in the major peripancreatic venous trunks during the venous phase can be seen [152]. Selective arteriography gives a diagnostic accuracy of 73%–83%, a false-negative rate of 17% [69, 104], a sensitivity of 70%, and a specificity of 96% with predictive values of 85% and 80% for positive and negative tests, respectively [121]. Superselective pharmacoangiography gives a diagnostic sensitivity of 93.7% and 100% [134, 156]. Phlebography in 18 patients with obstructive jaundice resulted in the diagnosis of 15 PDA and 3 cholangiocarcinoma [156].

Radioimmunodiagnosis

Immunoscintigraphic demonstration of PDA has proven difficult. A clinical study with ^{131}I-labeled CA19-9 and CEA and SPECT in 21 patients showed that localization of primary tumors and metastases in the upper abdomen was more difficult than in colorectal cancer in the lower abdomen because of relatively high tracer accumulation in the kidneys, liver, and spleen [157]. Thus, this technique for the diagnosis of PDA is of no value and improvement of the technique is required.

Macroscopic Findings

Side of PDA

About 60% to 70% of PDA occur in the head of the pancreas. Of these, about 45% arise around the intrapancreatic part of the common bile duct, i.e., the upper half of the dorsal portion of pancreatic head [158]. Other tumors are found in the central area of the pancreas head behind the ampulla of Vater or in the uncinate process. Cancers in the upper dorsal area obstruct the bile duct, whereas those occurring in the other head region obstruct the main pancreatic duct and often cause severe stenotic or obstructive signs such as obstructive jaundice and obstructive (secondary) pancreatitis. In cases of severe secondary pancreatitis, the peripheral pancreatic ducts show marked irregular dilation with marked parenchymal atrophy.

Size of PDA

Pancreatic head tumors are relatively smaller than the body-and-tail tumors. The size of tumors in surgical specimens ranges from 1.5 to 10 cm, with a median diameter of about 2.5 [2] to 3.5 cm [1]. The minimum size of pancreatic cancers preoperatively detected by US or CT and surgically removed is more than 1 cm. Even so, such a minimal tumor is already invasive. The average size of body-and-tail tumors is between 5 and 7 cm.

Gross Appearance

Grossly, the tumor is recognized as irregular infiltrative lesions, which are relatively hard with sclerotic or fibrotic changes, and are grayish-white (Figs. 2e, 3). They may show hemorrhagic or necrotic change and often form pseudocysts. Some type of tumors produce mucin.

Pancreatic head tumors directly invade the common bile duct and pancreatic duct (Figs. 2a,3). Fibrosis and occasionally acute change, such as fatty necrosis or hemorrhagic change, may be seen.

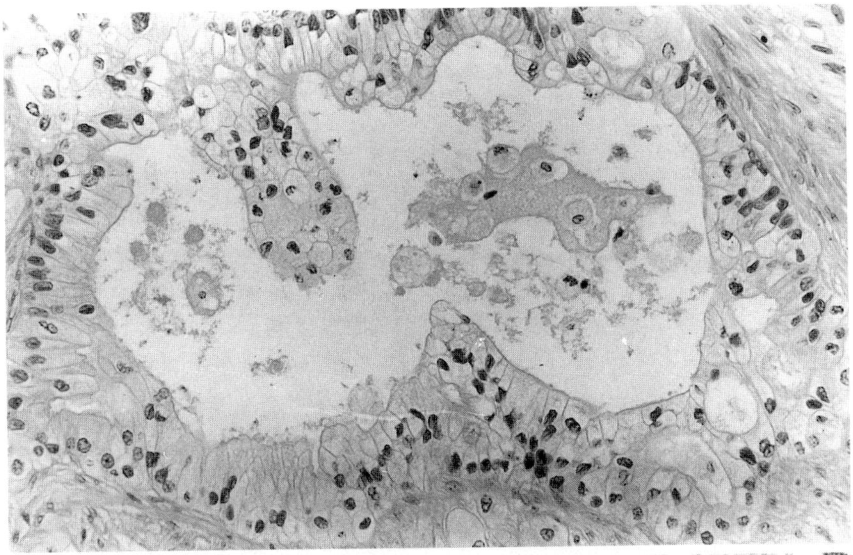

e

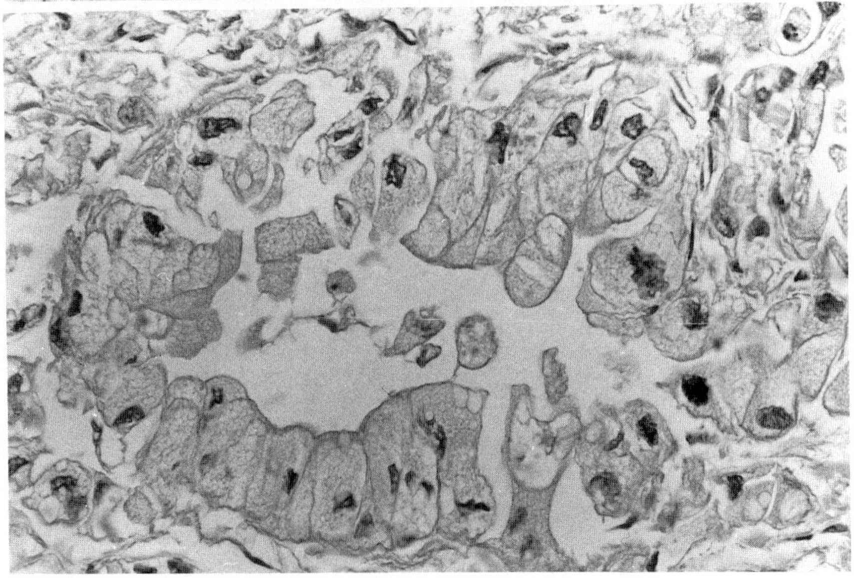

f

Fig. 5a–f. Well-differentiated PDA showing tubular structures formed by cells of different morphology. ***a*** Tubular structures with focal intratubular papillary arrangement (*top*). ***b*** Ductal structures resembling normal pancreatic ducts. ***c*** The same tumor as in ***b***, showing tubular structures formed by cylindrical cells. Note the focal crowded nuclei. ***d*** Cylindrical cells with vesicular nuclei form a glandular pattern. Note the presence of many mitotic figures and focal multi layering of tumor cells. ***e*** A malignant gland composed of tall cylindrical clear cells. ***f*** A PDA with focal formation of glands lined by clear hobs-nail cells. Note the marked abnormalities of the nuclei. Moderate fibrotic change of the stroma in ***a–d***. H&E, ×200 (***a***), ×300 (***a–d***), ×350 (***e***, ***f***)

negative for Sudan II, or oncocytic cells is rare [160, 161]. The nuclei tend to be situated at the base of the cell. Some glands may contain aberrant cells which occur in the intestinal epithelium such as pyloric glandular cells and Paneth cells. These variations in the structure are due to differences in the differentiation degree of the cells in different areas of the tumors and reflect the enormous potency of the cancer precursor cells for differentiation. Usually, cells lose polarity with increasing malignant changes. In large tubular structures and small (microcystic) glands, a papillary configuration can be seen. However, this structure does not warrant the diagnosis of papillary or tubulopapillary terminology, if the papillary formation is not a predominant feature; the prognosis and the growth of PDA with tubular structures, with or without papillary structures, are the same.

Moderately differentiated PDA differs from the well-differentiated type by the presence of less dif-

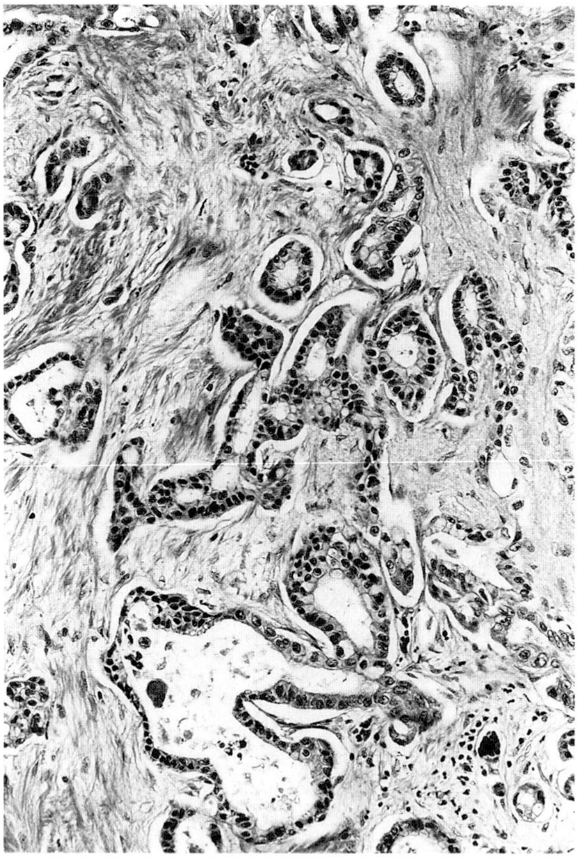

Fig. 6. A moderately differentiated PDA forming irregular glandular structures in a fibrotic stroma. H&E, ×200

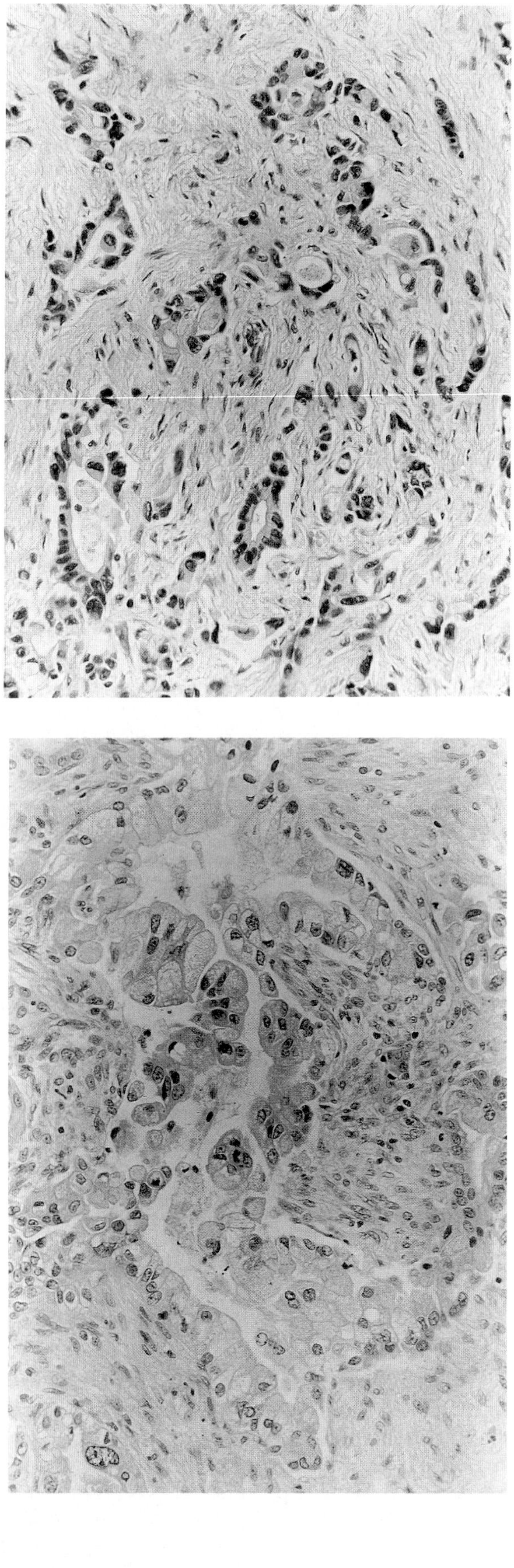

a

b

Fig. 7a–j. Poorly differentiated PDA showing various structures. ***a*** Small and abortive glands interchange with undifferentiated areas. ***b*** Abnormal glands in a tumor that showed a well-differentiated patterns in another area of the tumor shown in Fig. 5b,c. ***c*** Abortive small glandular structure (*arrows*) surrounded by pleomorphic cells. This tumor was found in a vicinity of the well-differentiated PDA depicted in Fig. 5e. The tumor invades the peripancreatic fatty tissue. ***d*** Cord-like pattern of a poorly differentiated PDA. ***e*** Poorly differentiated area of the well-differentiated PDA depicted in Fig. 5b,c. Note the pleomorphism of the cells and many mitotic figures. ***f*** Poorly differentiated region of a PDA showing multinucleated giant cells and intracytoplasmic lumens. (*Continued*)

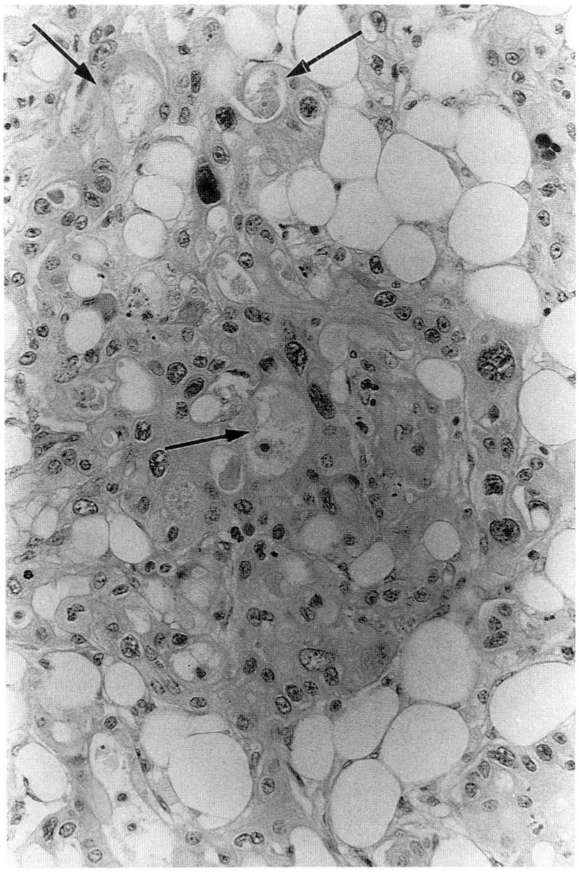

c

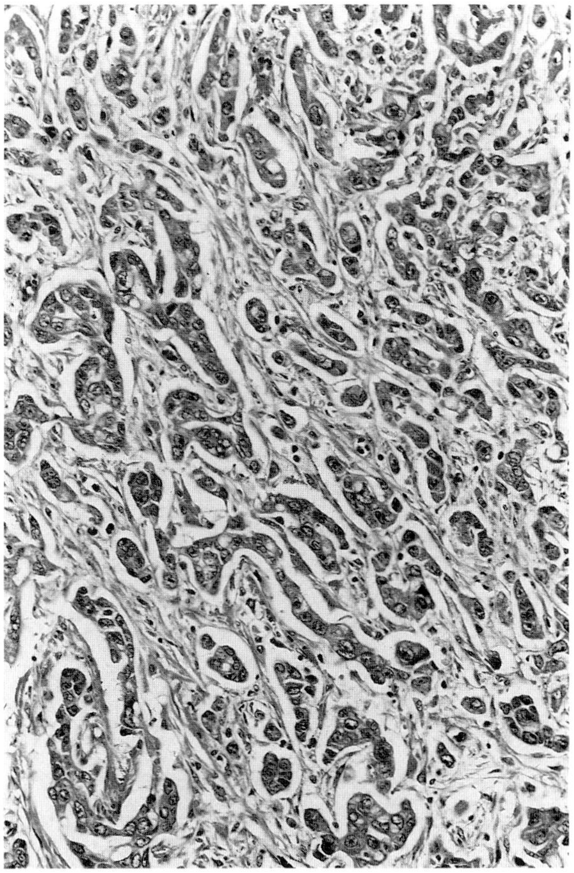

d

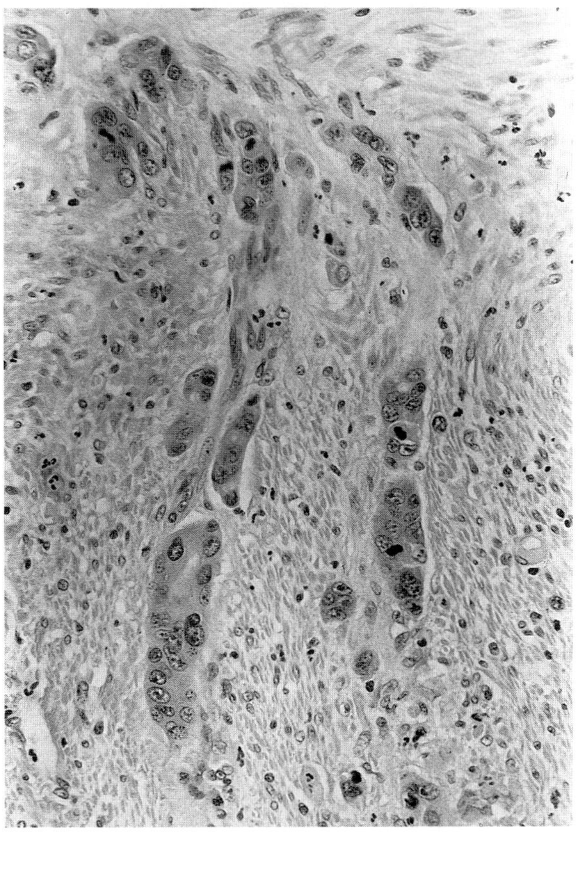

e

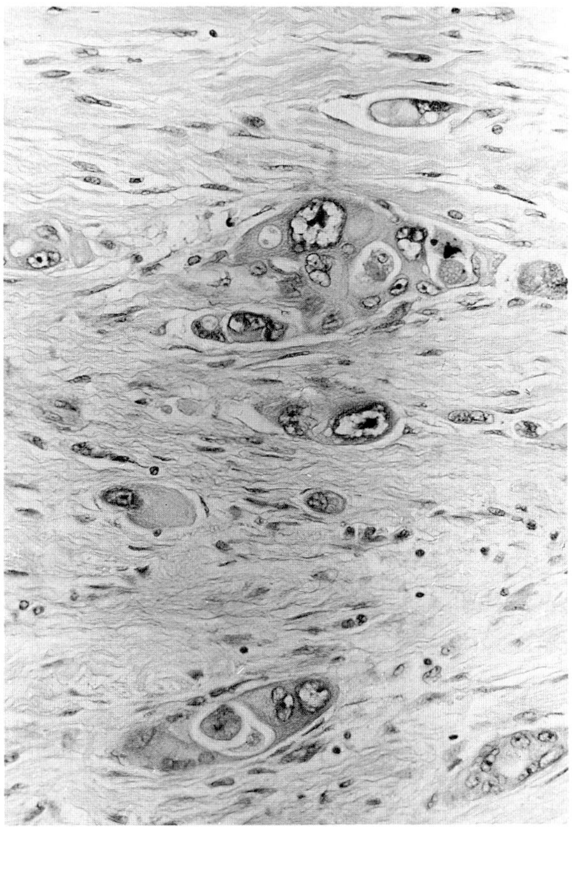

f

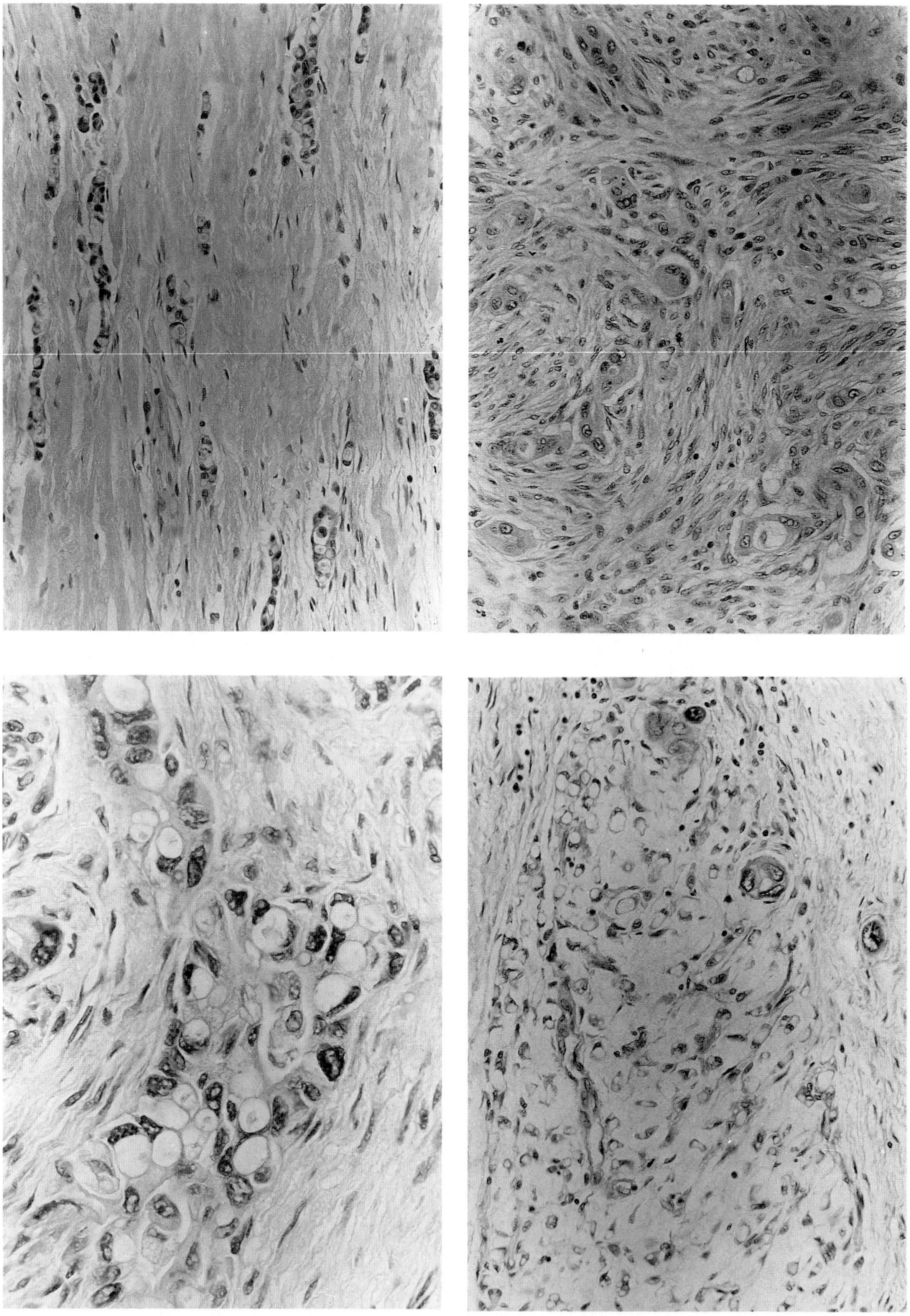

g h i j

Fig. 8. Perineural (*N*) invasion of a well-differentiated PDA. H&E, ×200

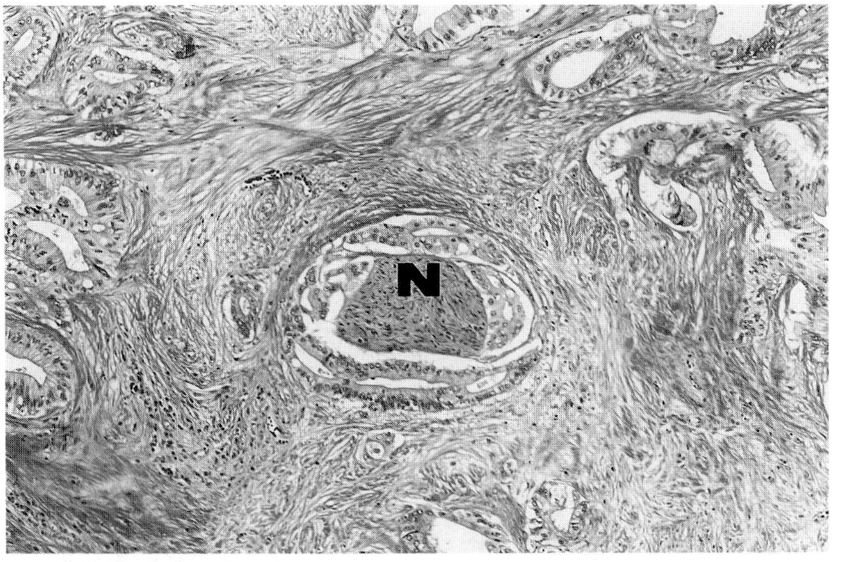

ferentiated glandular structures, which show variation in size and shape of the glands embedded in a dense connective tissue (Fig. 6).

Poorly differentiated adenocarcinoma is characterized by a cord-like pattern or diffuse proliferation (Fig. 7). The cellular patterns of the cords or tongues can vary considerably from giant cells to sarcomatous patterns (Fig. 7f–h). Foci of signet-ring formation can also be seen (Fig. 7i and j). Intracytoplasmic lumens can be seen (Fig. 7f).

Pancreatic ductal carcinoma usually produces more or less mucin, which is a neutral or acidophilic mucopolysaccharide, and is histologically positive for PAS and alcian blue stain. Massive mucin producing PDA forms characteristic "muconodular" or "mucocellular" pattern with numerous signet-rings or goblet cells. These carcinomas are difficult to distinguish from non-cystic mucinous adenocarcinoma (see Chapter "Mucinous (Non-Cystic) Adenocarcinoma, Including Signet-Ring Carcinoma" in this volume).

It must be recognized that even within the same tumor, the histological type of PDA can vary considerably (Figs. 5a–d, 7b,c,e,h). The well-differentiated glands are usually accompanied by small poorly formed glands, and poorly differentiated areas may be found in the vicinity. According to the Japanese General Rules for Cancer Classification [148], histological diagnosis is based on the most predominant histology. On this point, Japanese rules differ from American [1] and European [2] rules. We recommend that tumors should be diagnosed according to the predominant structure with phrases such as "with focal poor differentiation" as additional terms. However, as stated above, a limited number of sections taken for histology may not adequately represent the differentiation degree and the grade of malignancy. Therefore, the examination of several sections from different areas of the tumor is essential for adequate judgment on the differentiation degree of PDA.

Compared with other carcinomas, most PDAs are already in an advanced stage and are associated with characteristic infiltrations of lymphatic and neural tissue when they are diagnosed (Fig. 8). In fact, these invasive features are found more frequently in surgically resected cancer than in other invasive patterns, including venous invasion (splenic vein and portal vein) and peripancreatic neural plexus-infiltration. The venous and peripancreatic neural invasion seems to follow the lymphatic and intrapancreatic neural infiltrations. Well-differentiated PDA shows more perineural invasion than the poorly differentiated types. Intraductal spreading is often seen.

◀

Fig. 7g. Scirrhous pancreatic carcinoma with Indian-file pattern. ***h*** Abortive glandular and sarcomatous pattern in a PDA depicted in Fig. 5d. ***i*** Focal signet-ring formation in an invasive area of an otherwise well-to-moderately differentiated carcinoma. ***j*** A few abortive glands surrounded by loosely arranged signet-ring cells. PAS staining showed mucin between the tumor cells. H&E, ×210

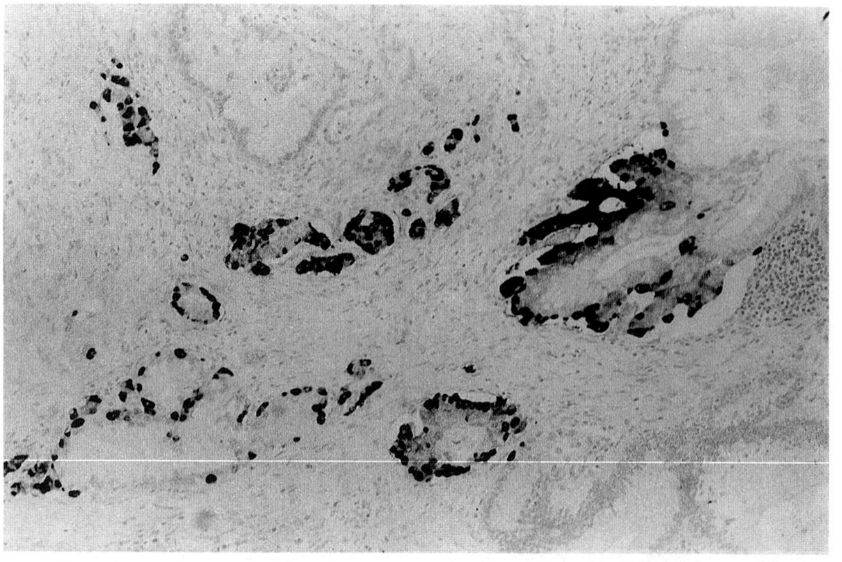

Fig. 9. A well-differentiated PDA containing many endocrine cells. Avidin-biotin complex (ABC) method with anti-insulin antibody ×90

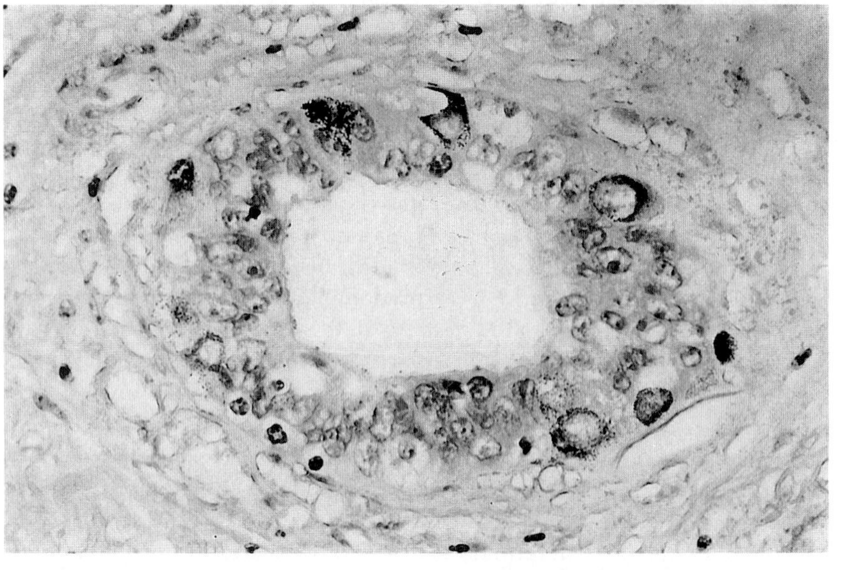

Fig. 10. A malignant gland with at least 10 argyrophilic cells. Grimelius stain, ×300

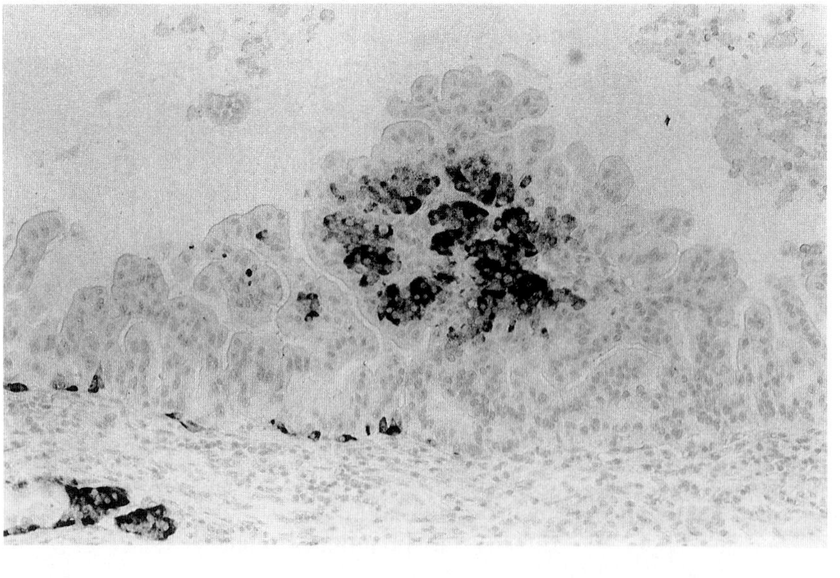

Fig. 11. Intraductal papillary configuration with many endocrine cells at the base of the malignant epithelium and in the papillary projection. Chromogranin A, ABC method, ×160

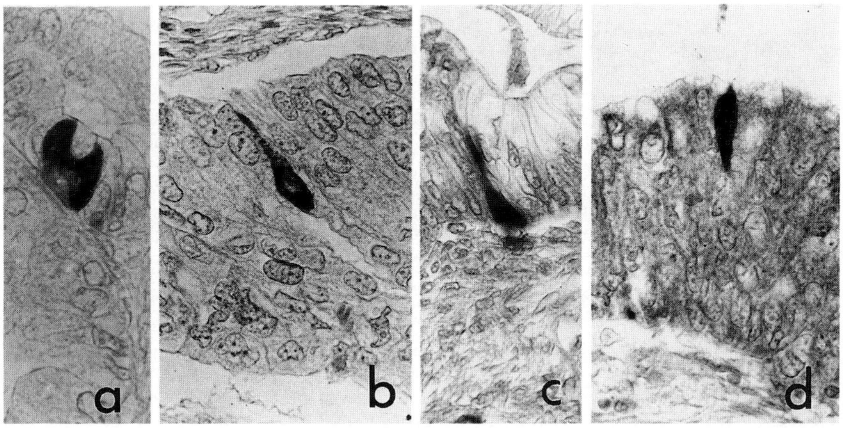

Fig. 12a–d. The "open" form of endocrine cells in PDA. ***a*** A U-shaped cell immunoreactive with chromogranin A, ***b*** somatostatin cell, ***c*** Pancreastatin cell, ***d*** somatostatin cell. ABC method, ×210

Several investigators have demonstrated the presence of endocrine cells within PDA. According to our study, most, if not all PDAs, contain a few or many endocrine cells. Serial sectioning of relatively large surgical specimens was examined by the multilabeling technique [162] with antibodies against insulin, glucagon, somatostatin, pancreatic polypeptide (PP), serotonin, pancreastatin, chromogranin A, and neuron-specific enolase (NSE). Cells immunoreactive with all of the antibodies were found in all 9 cases in which the reactivity with chromogranin A, insulin, NSE, and serotonin was predominant. The number and distribution of the immunoreactive cells differed in each case and in different areas of the same specimen. Many endocrine cells were found in well-differentiated carcinomas but less frequently in poorly differentiated areas. In some tumor areas, the number of endocrine cells was so high (Figs. 9, 10) that the term mixed ductal-insular cells could be used [1]. However, it seems that the production of endocrine cells is part of the natural history of PDA, and the presence of endocrine cells within the cancer does not justify their subclassification, unless further studies demonstrate a better prognosis of tumors with many endocrine cells. It seems more appropriate to diagnose the cancer according to its differentiation degree and to add a phrase such as "with a few or many endocrine cell components" as a subterm.

Although most endocrine cells are located within the basal layer of malignant glands, some were intraepithelial and presented features typical of intestinal endocrine cells (Figs. 11–14). Although many endocrine cells had a typical appearance, some had atypical shapes and granular patterns

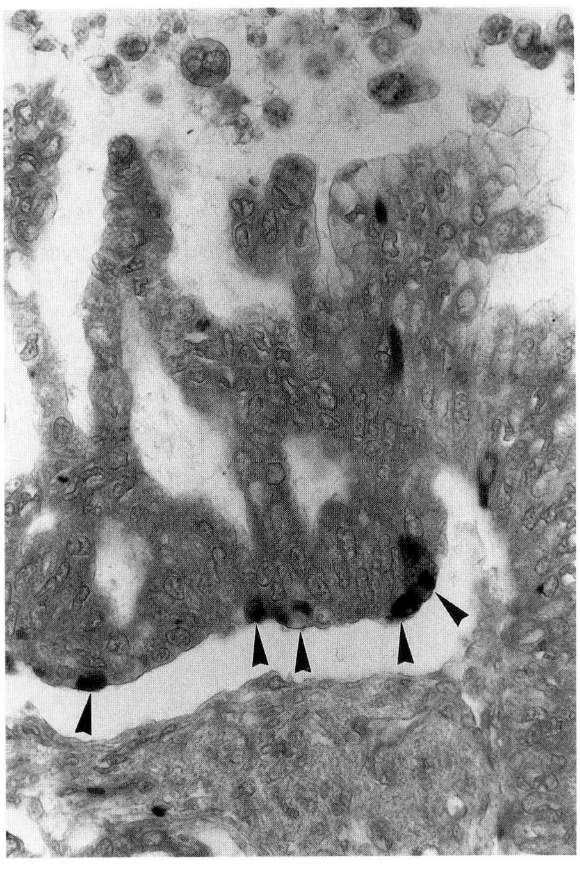

Fig. 13. Insulin (*arrowheads*) and somatostatin cells in a well-differentiated PDA. Note the presence of somatostatin cells at different heights of the malignant epithelium. ABC method, ×210. (*For color reproduction see color insert in the frontmatter*)

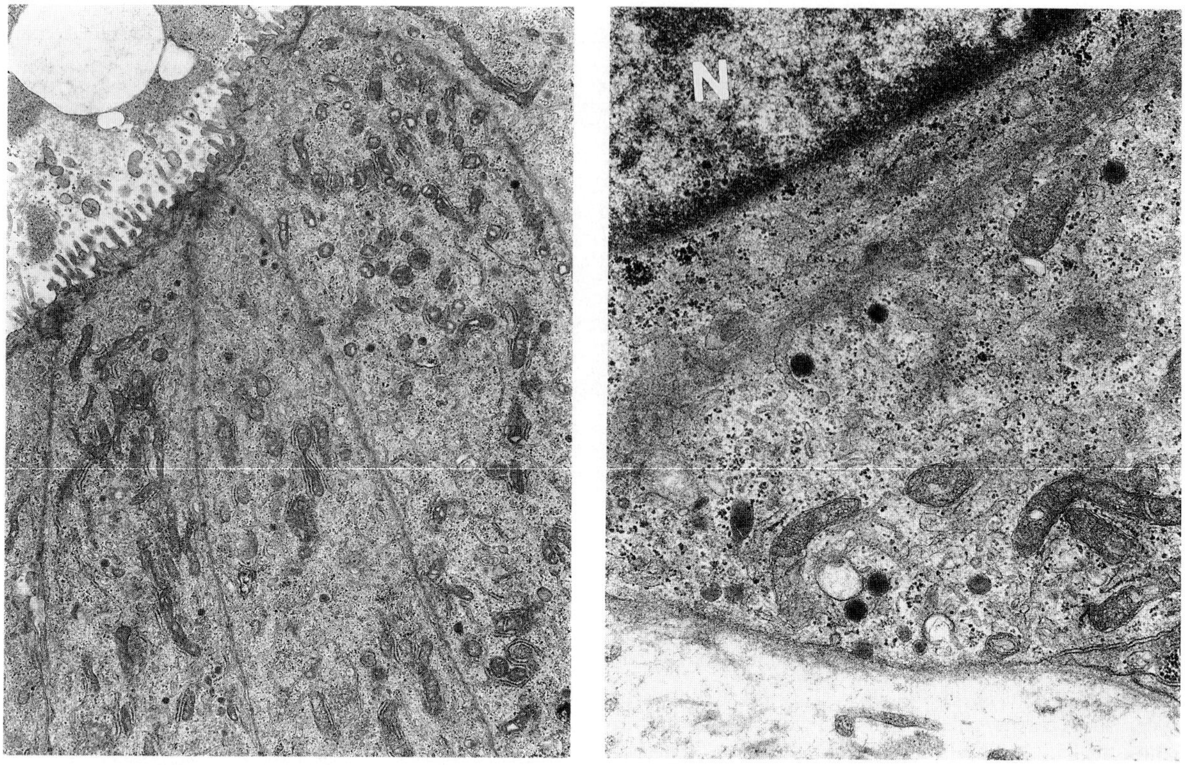

a b

Fig. 14. Electron microscopical findings of the endocrine cells in PDA. ***a*** Numerous microvilli at the luminal side and intercellular attachment of endocrine cells within a ductal cancer. ×12 000. ***b*** Basal lamina at the interstitial side and dense core granules of neurosecretory type, 100–200 nm in size. *N*, nucleus. ×21 000

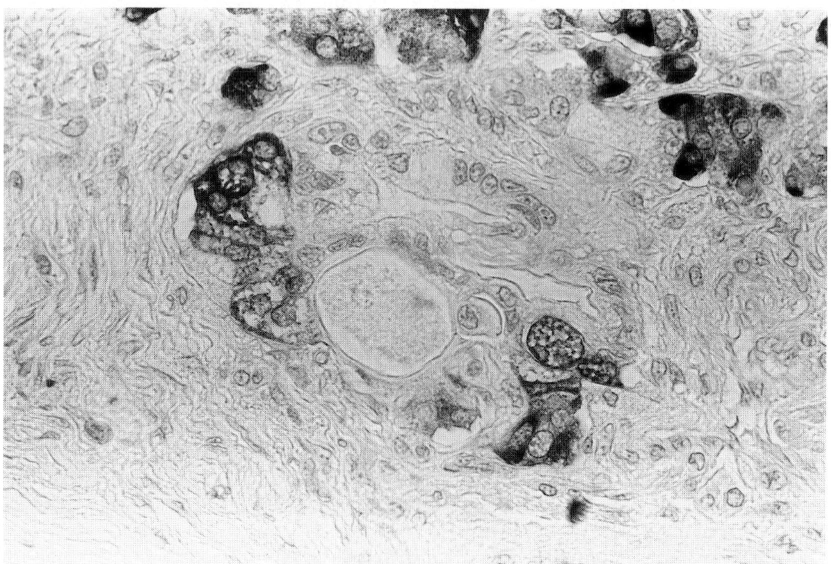

Fig. 15. Atypical endocrine cells in a moderately differentiated PDA. Note the irregular size and granular content of the endocrine cells, some with cytoplasmic "vacuoles". Chromogranin A, ABC, ×300

Fig. 16a–d. A PDA containing many endocrine cells. ***a*** A mixture of glandular structures and pleomorphic cells with foamy cytoplasm. H&E, ×200. ***b*** Tumor cells around the ductular structures were positive for neuron-specific enolase (NSE). PAP method, ×200. ***c*** An area of the tumor showing two types of cells: small dark cells forming gland and large foamy cells representing endocrine cells. H&E, ×200. ***d*** Vascular invasion of endocrine cell components. H&E, ×150. (Courtesy of Dr. Kanji Kashiwabara [163], with permission)

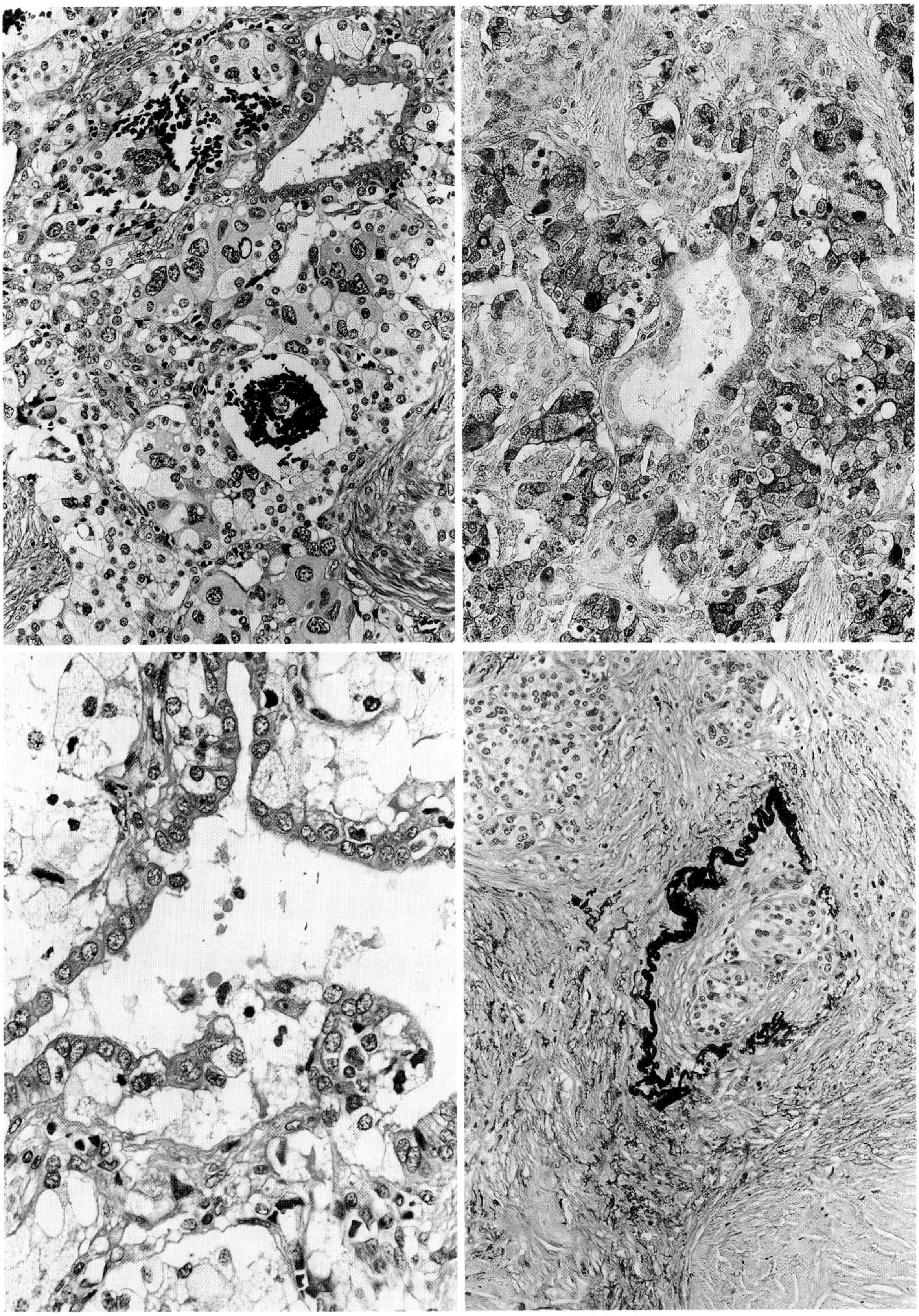

a b c d

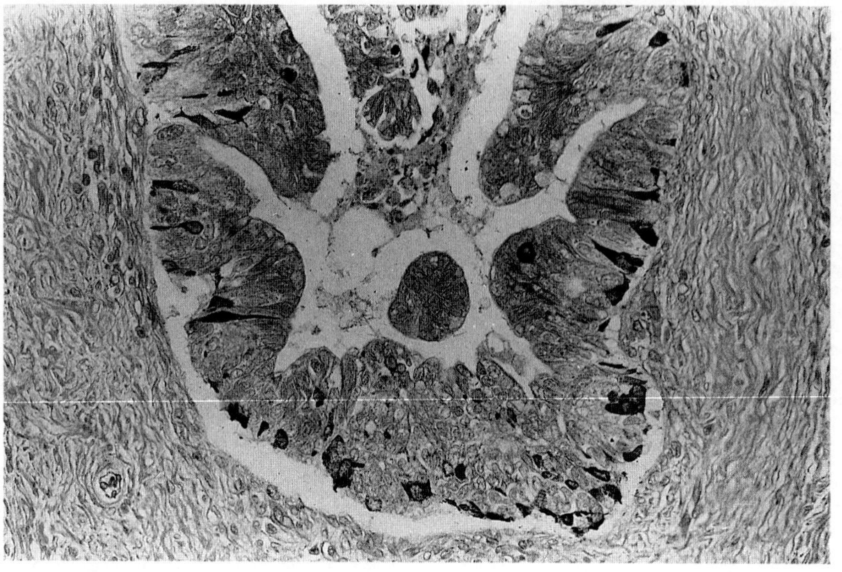

Fig. 17. Atypical ductal cell hyperplasia in a 52-year-old man with chronic pancreatitis. Note the presence of many argyrophilic cells, some of "open" form. Grimelius stain, ×130

(Fig. 15). Most endocrine cell types were also found in the invasive regions of the cancers, including perineural spaces, which indicated the malignant nature of these endocrine cells. In fact, a case with a mixture of malignant ductal and islet cells with invasion and metastases has been reported [163]. This 1.9 × 1.3 cm tumor in the pancreas head was composed of a mixture of malignant islet and ductal cells (Fig. 16). Both cell components of the tumor had invaded the vessels and perineural spaces (Fig. 16d). The results of cytofluorometry and AgNOR counts (see later) were consistent with the malignant nature of both cell components.

The above finding reflects the multipotential nature of the cell of origin in pancreatic cancers. However, it must be pointed out that some islet cell tumors may contain neoplastic ducts [164], and a proliferation of endocrine cells is not restricted to ductal neoplasms and can occur in benign pancreatic diseases (Fig. 17). Endocrine cell proliferation has also been observed in experimentally induced PDA [55, 56, 165]. In fact, in the hamster model of pancreatic cancer, endocrine cells were seen from the earliest induced ductal/ductular lesions [55, 56]. Although in our material, we did not observe ductal-acinar or acinar-insular tumors in either human or experimental tumors, they seemed to occur sporadically [1].

In the vicinity of tumors and occasionally also in the areas distal to the tumor, malignant cells can be observed within islets. Characteristically, cancer cells occupy the peripheral region of the islets and are confined within the islet boundary (Fig. 18). Tumor cells merge imperceptibly into islet cells and there are no signs of islet cell degeneration. These findings have been interpreted differently. Some believe that cancer cells invade the islets directly. Our step-sectioning techniques did not show any evidence for that. Tumor cells were strictly confined within the islet, and islet cells did not show any signs of degeneration, which would be expected if tumor cells had invaded the islets. Tumor invasion of islets through the peri-insular ductules is a possibility; however, based on the above-mentioned association between cancer cells and islet cells, we believe that tumor cells arise per se from undifferentiated cells within the islet. However, this has yet to be confirmed.

One of our findings of conceptual and clinical interest was an abnormality in the production of the peptide not only in the endocrine cells of PDA but also in the islets near the cancers. Of particular note was the dissociation of IAPP and insulin. Contrary to the normal beta cells, most insulin-containing cells near the cancer lacked IAPP, possibly because of their rapid release [162]. Moreover, many islet cells close to the cancer expressed CA19-9 (Fig. 19). Thus, the overall data suggested that abnormalities of endocrine cells in tumors and in the preexisting islets may contribute to the glucose metabolic alteration observed frequently in PDA patients.

The incidence of PDA multiplicity is controversial and reportedly occurs in 15% to 40% of patients. Recent molecular biological findings

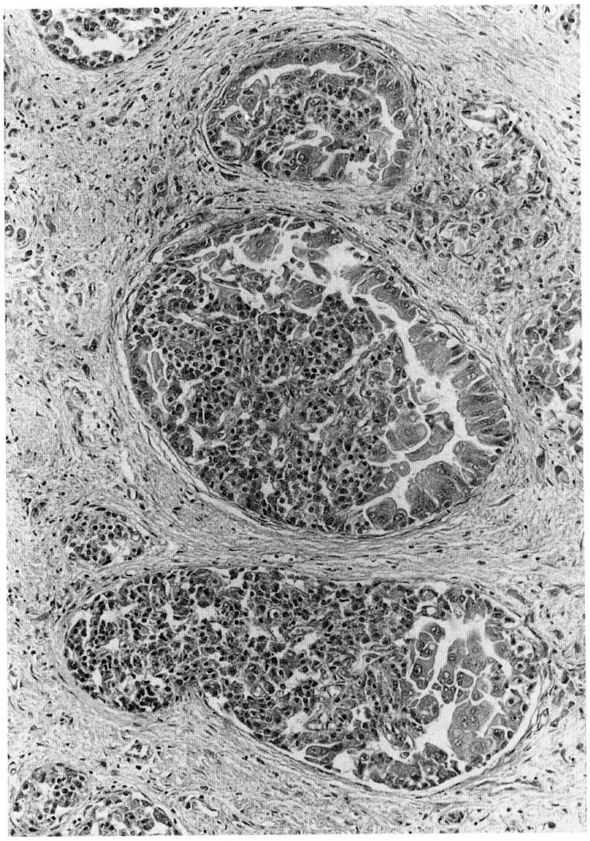

a

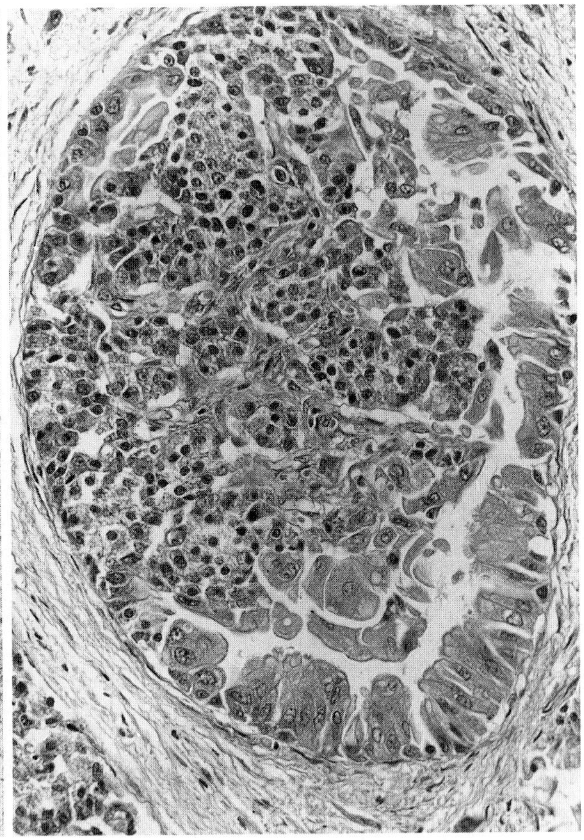

b

Fig. 18a–b. In the atrophic tail of the pancreas of a 60-year-old man with pancreatic head PDA. ***a*** Many enlarged and small islets contained malignant epithelial cells in the islet periphery. H&E, ×120. ***b*** High-power view of one of the islets showing arrangement of cylindrical tumor cells in the periphery of the islet. There is no degeneration of the islet cells. H&E, ×210

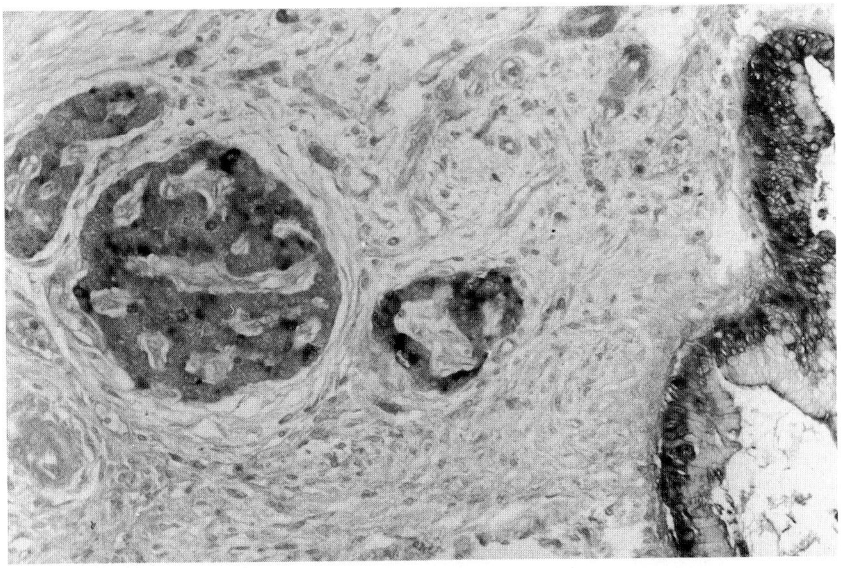

Fig. 19. Expression of CA19-9 antigen in the islets of a 64-year-old woman with a well-to-moderately differentiated PDA. CO19-9, ABC, ×210. (*For color reproduction see color insert in the frontmatter*)

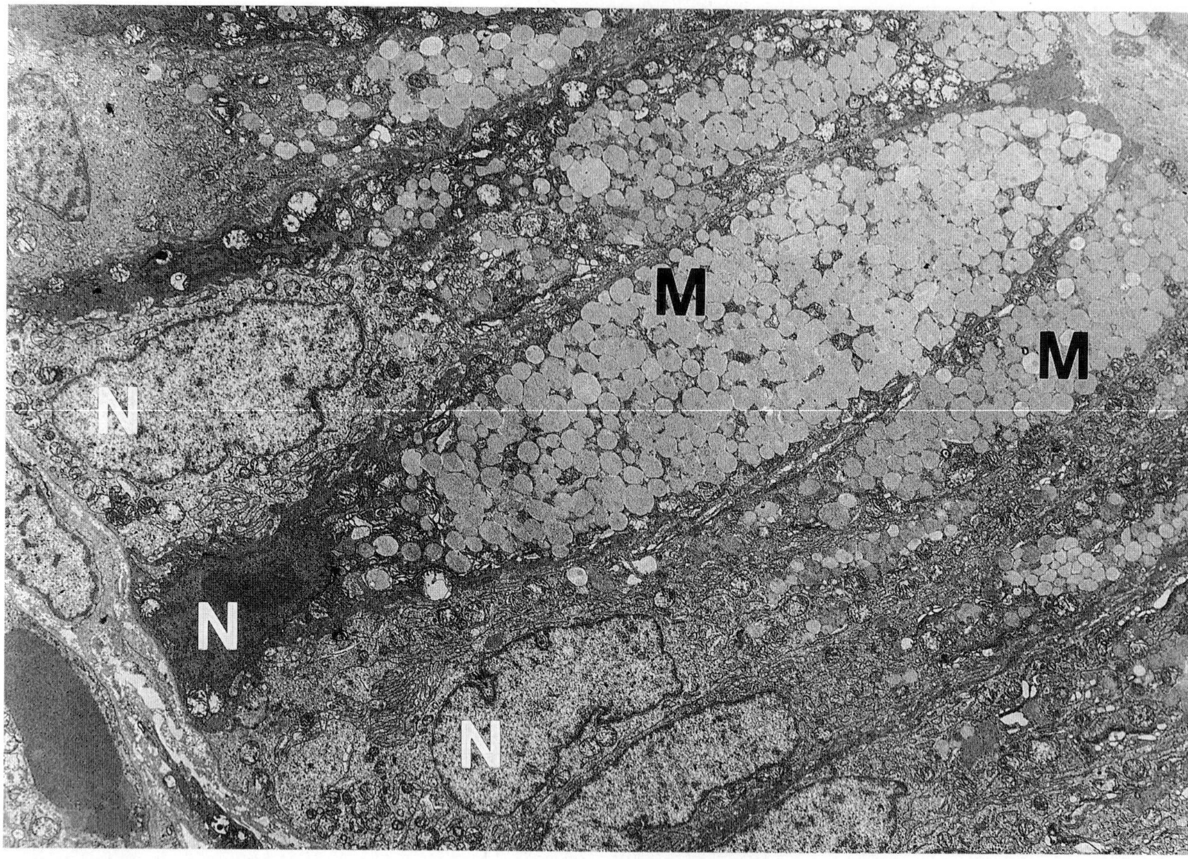

Fig. 20. Electron microscopical findings of a well-differentiated PDA. Most cancer cells showed mucus production and goblet-like figure. *M*, mucus; *N*, nucleus. ×1500

suggest that the rate of multiplicity is no more than 6% (see below).

Electron Microscopy

The tumor cells lined the basement membrane, are connected with each other by junctional complexes, and form luminal spaces with microvilli (Figs. 20, 21). Round or oval nuclei with marked cleavings are situated at the basal side, and well-developed mitochondria and sparce rough endoplasmic reticulum are scattered in the cytoplasm. Numerous secretory granules may be revealed at the apical region (Fig. 20). Some tumors may show many mucinous granules (Fig. 20) and intracellular microcysts, whereas others may not. The poorly developed intracellular organelles and abundant microvilli suggest their origin from ductular cells [166]. Zymogen-like granules have been described in a single tumor [166]. In another study [167], three different cell types were observed in tumors, which were diagnosed as PDA. Two cell types had a ductal cell character and the third had swollen mitochondria and well-developed RER with a different distribution of zymogen granules, suggesting that these cells originated from acinar cells. However, the origin of cancer cells from multipotent pancreatic cells makes the presence of acinar cells, as well as of islet cells within the PDA, not surprising. Similar findings have been observed in the experimental model of PDA in hamsters [168]. (For a further description of the fine structure of PDA see [169].)

Histochemical Findings

The positive reactivity with PAS, alcian blue and the iron diamine method indicates the presence of mucin with sulfated glycoprotein (sulfomucin), which also occurs in the normal ductal cells. However, malignant ductal cells, contrary to the normal ductal cells, contain carboxylated non-sulfated glycoprotein rich in sialic acid (sialomucin) [1]. A significant decrease in the amount of mucin

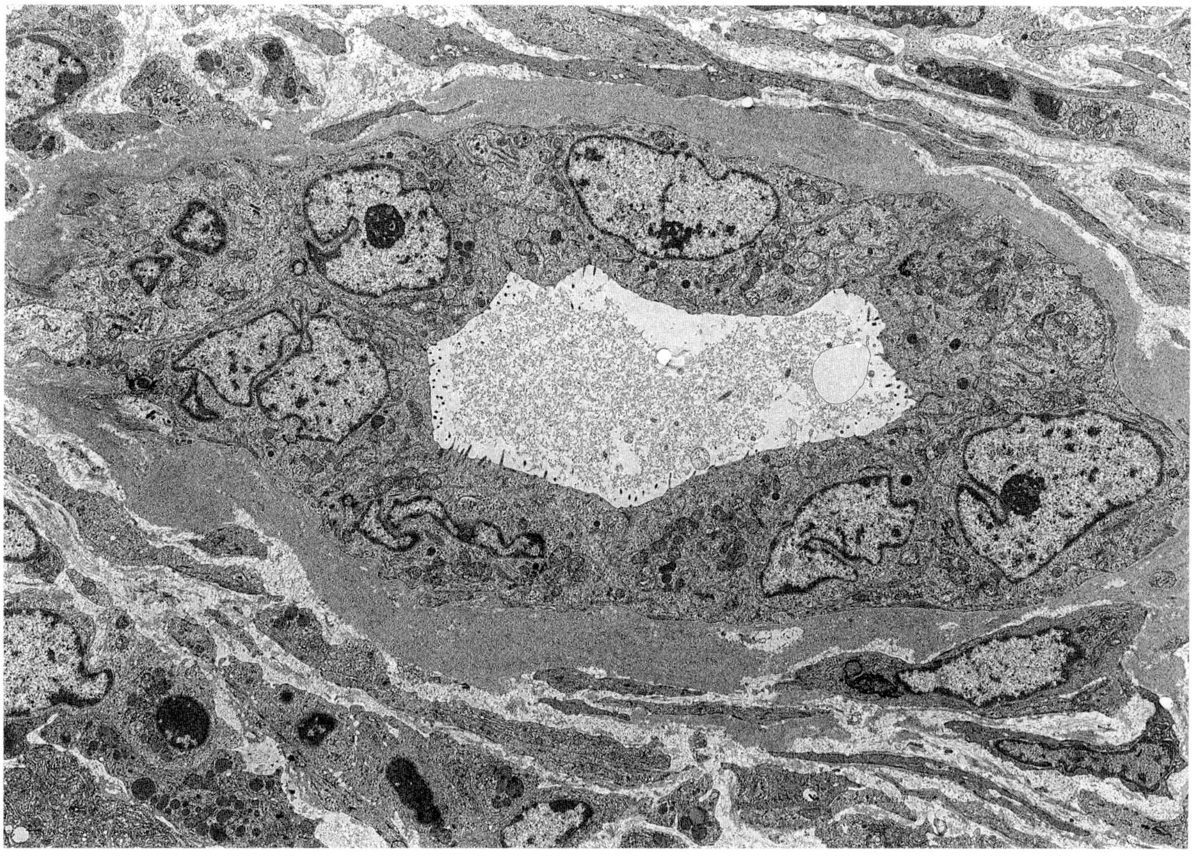

Fig. 21. Ultrastructure appearance of a moderately differentiated PDA. ×1000

was found in invasive lesions, and this was associated with a shift toward production of neutral mucins and especially sialomucins [170].

Among the lectins examined, reactivity has been seen with peanut lectin, *Ulex europeaus*, *Helix pomatia*, wheat germ, and *Dolichus biflorus*. The latter two lectins do not show any reactivity with the normal ductal cells but react strongly with hyperplastic ductal cells [171]. The reactivity of PDA with lectins is consistent with findings in experimentally induced PDA [172].

Immunohistochemistry

Well-differentiated tubular structures are surrounded by a distinct layer of laminin-positive material [169]. In the less differentiated areas, the laminin distribution is rather spotty [169]. The integrity of the basal membrane seems to correlate with the degree of malignancy in PDA, but this is not the case for mucinous cystic neoplasms or for islet cell tumors [173].

Blood group antigens, CEA, CA19-9, DU-PAN-2, and TAG-72, are common antigens expressed by PDA cells (Figs. 22–24).

Blood group antigens, A, B, O, Le^a, Le^b, Le^x, and Le^y, are expressed in PDA in a high frequency. In our study, compatible antigen expression was found in 82%, 75%, and 50% of tumors from patients with A, B, amd O blood types, respectively [174]. Deletion of the compatible antigen was found in 10 (33%) of the cases, mostly in patients of blood group O, and incompatible expression (of B antigen only) occured in 4 (13%). In a similar study, deletion of A, B, H, or Le^b antigen occurred in about 25% of cases, particularly in poorly differentiated tumors, and an incompatible expression on an expected A or B antigen in 33% of cases, regardless of the degree of differentiation [163]. Metastatic cancers also exhibited blood group antigen deletion. Interestingly, in both primary and metastatic cancers the incidence of incompatible A or B expression was higher in cancers from the United States than in those from Japan, but the incidence of blood group antigen deletion was similar between the two countries [175].

We found Le^a expression in 87%, Le^b in 90%, Le^x in 30%, and Le^y in 43% of the cases, regardless of the ABO and Lewis phenotype of the patients [174]. Coexpression of Le^a and Le^b was found in 40% of the cases. The overall results indicated that blood group antigen expression in PDA differs from that of other gastrointestinal cancers [174]. However, because blood group antigens are also expressed in the normal pancreas (although with a much lower incidence and to a much lesser extent) and in acute and chronic pancreatitis [176], their value for tumor diagnosis is limited, although the deletion and the inappropriate expression of blood group antigens, found also in other studies [175, 177], can be used to discriminate between benign and malignant cells.

Although Le^y occurs in the normal pancreas, benign pancreatic diseases and PDA, Le^x is not expressed in the normal pancreas, but is expressed in 10%–20% of chronic pancreatitis and in 50%–70% of PDA. It is expressed more in well-differentiated than in poorly differentiated tumors [178]. It appears that Le^x-related antigens are cancer-associated determinants in the human pancreas [178]. In most specimens from patients with PDA, the 2–3 sialylated Le^a antigen was strongly expressed, whereas 2–6 sialylated Le^a antigen was less frequently expressed [179]. A marked expression of sialosyl Tn has also been found in PDA. The lower expression of the T antigen in these tissues suggests that with malignant transformation there is a selective usage of the glycosyltransferase enzymes involved in mucin oligosaccharide synthesis [177]. In another study, the following alterations in the expression of blood-group antigens in PDA were found: (1) enhanced expression of Le^x, Tn and sialylated Tn; (2) enhanced expression of precursor type 1, independent of secretory status of the patients; (3) loss of regulation of Le^b by the secretor gene; and (4) decreased expression of Le^y [180].

CA19-9 is one of the most common antigens produced by PDA (Figs. 22–24). In our study [174, 181], this antigen was found to be expressed in 80% of PDA. This value is comparable with the serological findings [106]. We found a correlation between the Lewis phenotype of the patients and the expression of this antigen. It was expressed in 21 of 22 patients with Le^{a-b+} and all 4 patients from Le^{a+b-}, but none of the 4 patients from Le^{a-b-} phenotype ($P < 0.01$) [174, 181]. This is apparently because individuals lacking the Lewis gene, which is required for the synthesis of CA19-9 (a sialylated Le^a), are unable to produce this antigen. Unlike the other markers, a fairly good correlation exists between the incidence of the expression of this antigen in PDA and in the serum of patients.

DU-PAN-2 is another common antigen in PDA cells (Figs. 22–24). Our comparative studies with antibodies against CA19-9 and DU-PAN-2, the epitopes of which are distinct and non-cross-reactive [182], showed that 82% and 87% of tumors expressed these antigens [181]. Because in a serological test the sensitivity of DU-PAN-2 is low (47.7%) [106], it follows that there is a poor correlation between the incidence of the expression of this antigen in tumor tissue and in serum. The combination of DU-PAN-2 and CA19-9 reacted with tumor cells of 97% of the cases. Six CA19-9 negative cases were DU-PAN-2-positive and four DU-PAN-2-negative cases expressed CA19-9. The reactivity of cancer cells with each antibody varied from case to case and even within the same tumor. The number of antigen-expressing cells was much greater in well-differentiated than in poorly differentiated areas [181].

TAG-72 is as common a PDA antigen as CA19-9 and DU-PAN-2 [181] (Figs. 22–24). However, it is expressed in fewer normal ductal/ductular cells

Fig. 22. Expression of CA19-9, DU-PAN-2 and TAG-72 antigens in a poorly differentiated area of a PDA. Some cells (for example that shown by an *arrow*) express two antigens. ABC method, ×210

Fig. 23. A well-differentiated PDA, the cells of which express either CA19-9, DU-PAN-2 and/or TAG-72. Because of different cellular localization of each antigen, expression of two or three antigens can be found in some tumor cells. *Arrow* points to a cell expressing all of the three antigens. ABC method, ×210

Fig. 24. Heterogeneity of antigen expression in a well-differentiated PDA. Only a few cells express CA19-9, DU-PAN-2 or/and TAG-72. ABC method, ×210

Figs. 22–24. *For color reproduction see color insert in the frontmatter*

Fig. 25. A moderately differentiated PAD expressing carcinoembryonic antigen. ABC method, ×200

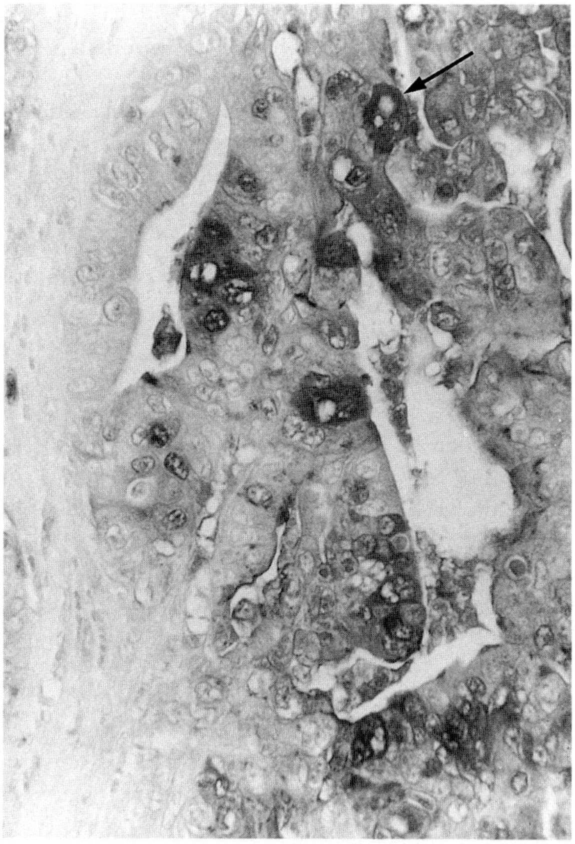

22

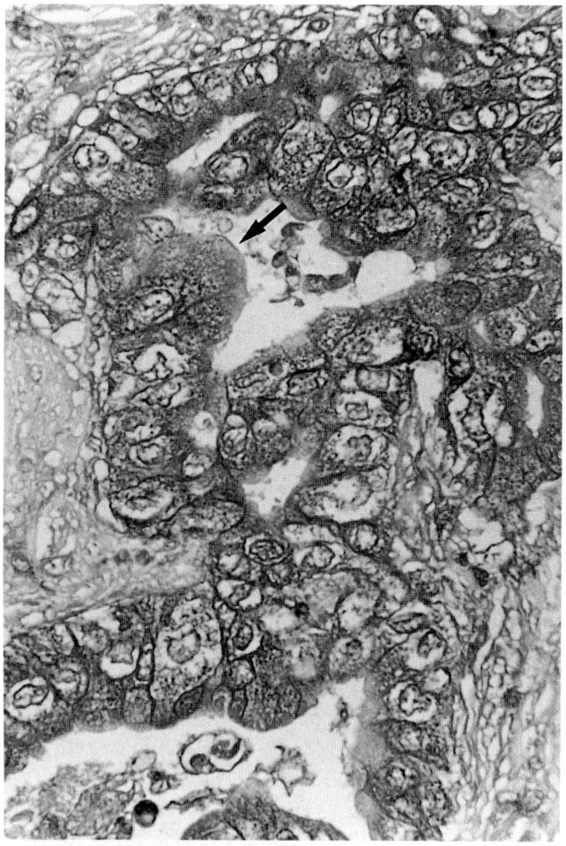

23

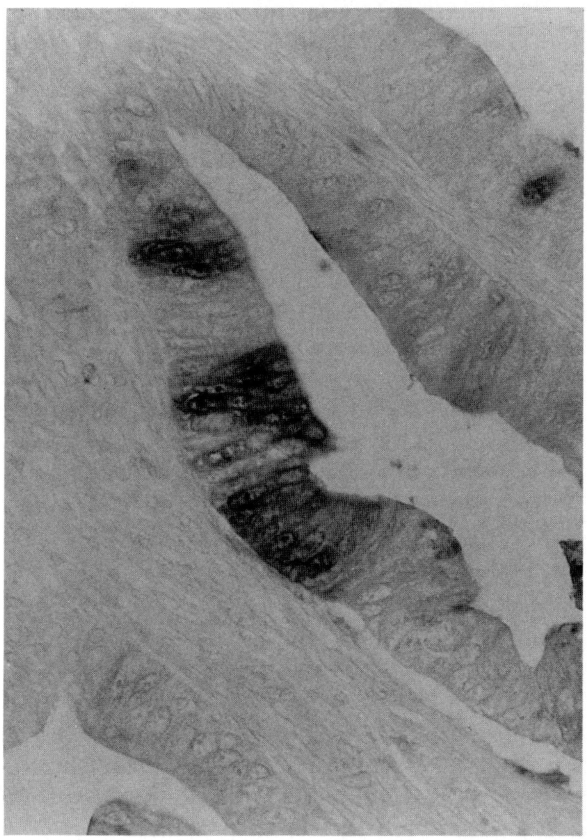

24

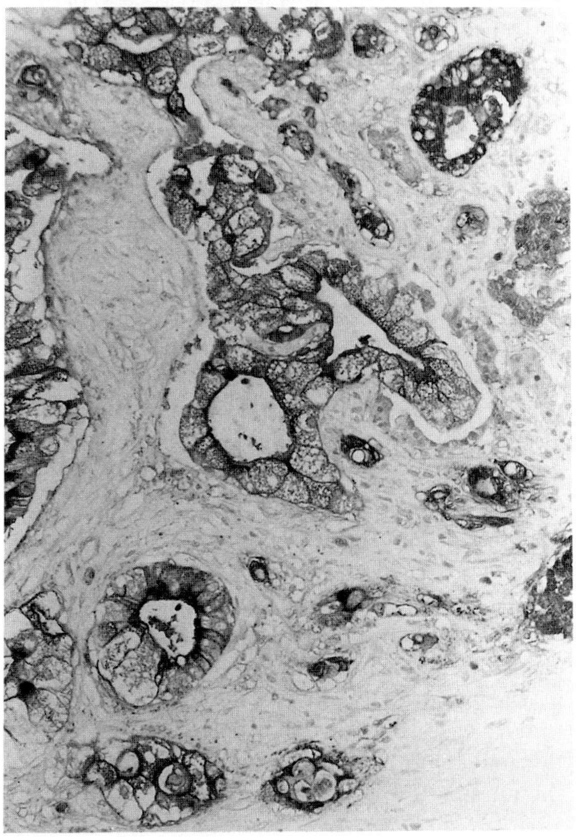

25

than CA19-9 ($P < 0.05$) and DU-PAN-2 ($P < 0.01$). In chronic pancreatitis, however, all three antigens were expressed, but their cellular localization differed: CA19-9 showed mostly a glycocalyx pattern, DU-PAN-2 showed an intracytoplasmic and glycocalyx pattern, but TAG-72 mostly showed a Golgi pattern [181]. According to these comparative studies, it appears that TAG-72 can be used to distinguish PDA from normal pancreatic ductal cells better than CA19-9 or DU-PAN-2.

Using a multilabeling technique [183] for simultaneous demonstration of CA19-9, DU-PAN-2 and TAG-72, we found that the combination of these antibodies reacted with the PDA cells of all 31 tumors (Figs. 22–24). However, with these combinations, not all tumor cells of a given tumor could be stained. A marked heterogeneity of antigen expression was observed between different cases and even within the same tumor (Figs. 22–24). All three antigens were coexpressed in ten tumors: CA 19-9 and DU-PAN-2 in 16 cases, TAG-72 and CA19-9 in 10 cases, and TAG-72 and DU-PAN-2 in 8 cases. About 2% of cancer cells coexpressed all three antigens (Fig. 23), 9% of them coexpressed TAG-72 and DU-PAN-2, 11% TAG-72 and CA19-9, and 22% CA19-9 and DU-PAN-2. About 8% of cancer cells did not express any of these antigens [183]. Hence, it appears that a combination of antibodies produces better differential diagnosis of PDA.

Monoclonal antibodies against CEA-related antigens (e.g., NCA) react with PDA cells (Fig. 25), and seem to distinguish between ductal and carcinoma cells [171, 184]. Moreover, other types of exocrine tumors (acinar cells, serous cystic adenomas and solid-cystic tumors) are not stained with these antibodies. However, these antibodies are useless for differential diagnosis between PDA and other gastrointestinal cancers [185].

CA125, although a good marker for ovarian tumors, has a limited value for the demonstration of PDA. The reactivity of CA50 is similar to that of CA19-9 with the advantage that it does not discriminate between the Le^{a+} and Le^{b-} individuals.

POA is a good marker for PDA [186], but it also lacks specificity. Epithelial membrane antigen (EMA) and keratin are also revealed in the tumor tissues of most cases. The reactivity is usually seen in the cytoplasm and plasma membrane of the tumor cells and in the peripheral stroma of the malignant glands, possibly by the leakage of the antigen.

Phospholipase A_2 has been demonstrated in 83% of PDA [187]. Although immunoreactivity was seen in the normal pancreas and in chronic pancreatitis cases, the staining patterns differed significantly from that in cancer cells. The incidence of expression was significantly higher in infiltrative cancers than in localized tumors. Further, the expression was significantly higher in tumors with abundant interstitial tissue than in those with a small amount of fibrotic tissue (187).

Cell Proliferation Markers

The nuclear organizer region (NOR), which represents loops of DNA that encode the genes for ribosomal RNA, was investigated in PDA and other types of exocrine pancreatic tumors by the argyrophilic technique (AgNOR). It was found that the mean number of AgNOR was significantly higher in PDA than in the normal pancreas and benign pancreatic lesions. The mean number increased stepwise in the following order: normal pancreatic duct (1.26), serous cystadenoma (1.27), mucinous cystadenoma (1.65), mucinous cystadenocarcinoma (2.29), noninvasive mucin-producing intraductal tumor (3.16), and PDA (3.78). Hence, the pattern of AgNOR seems to reflect the grade of malignancy [188].

DNA Content and Cell Cycle Analysis

Analysis of DNA content and ploidy in paraffin-embedded material has led to conflicting results relative to the relationship between ploidy and survival. In one study, the aneuploid DNA content was boserved in 15% of the tumors. Compared to the non-neoplastic tissue of the pancreas, the S + G2M fraction was significantly higher in PDA and was an independent prognostic factor, whereas ploidy was of no prognostic value [189]. Aneuploidy was restricted to tumors in advanced stages. Yoshimura et al. [190], on the other hand, found that of 86 PDA patients, DNA aneuploidy occured in 42.9% of well-differentiated, 52.3% of moderately differentiated, and of 71.4% of poorly differentiated tumors. The DNA ploidy showed a statistically significant positive correlation with the T category. The prognosis for patients with retroperitoneal invasion and DNA aneuploidy was significantly worse than those with DNA ploidy or those without retroperitoneal invasion. These controversial results indicate that DNA ploidy alone does not predict the prognosis. In another study [191], 40% of PDA were diploid and 60% aneuploid. The median survival of patients with diploid tumors was significantly longer (25 months) than in those with aneuploid tumors (10.5 months). Similar results were observed by other studies [192, 193], but disputed by some investigators, who reported that the value of the detection of aneuploidy is limited and that diploid pancreatic cancers are also generally fetal [194, 195]. The volume-corrected mitotic index (M/v index) was considered to be better than histological grade or clinical stage in predicting survival of PDA patients [196].

Growth Hormones and Growth Hormone Receptors

In the normal human pancreas, the epidermal growth factor (EGF), epidermal growth factor receptor (EGFR) and transforming growth factor alpha (TGF-α) are expressed in ductal, acinar, and islet cells [197]. However, in PDA cells and in cultured human pancreatic cancer cells, overexpression of EGF, EGFR, and TGF-α are seen [197–201]. In our study of 30 PDA, 4 normal and 8 chronic pancreatitis cases, TGF-α and EGFR were found in the normal ducts, islet cells, and acinar cells. In chronic pancreatitis and pancreatic cancer cells, their expression was higher than in the normal pancreas; however, no differences in expression were found between the ducts and ductules in chronic pancreatitis and pancreatic cancer cells. Contrary to the previous reports, the expression of EGFR and TGF-α in islet cells was found not in β cells, but in α cells. For more detail about the growth hormones, see Chapter "Molecular Biology" in this volume.

Molecular Biology

The mutation of c-Ki-*ras* oncogene is a predominant finding in PDA (see Chapter "Molecular Biology" in this volume), but not in acinar cell carcinoma [202]. C-Ki-*ras* mRNA in PDA was found to be expressed up to sixfold more than in normal tissues. C-*fos* mRNA was also overexpressed up to tenfold in 4 of 5 PDA. In contrast, c-*myc* mRNA levels varied and did not differ significantly between tumors and normal tissues [203].

Because the mutation of the c-Ki-*ras* oncogene is a clonal marker [204], examination of this mutation could be used to detect the multicentricity of PDA. In a recent study, the c-Ki-*ras* mutation was found in 46 out of 53 tumors. Two of these 46 tumors had two different mutations to aspartic acid (GAT) and to valine (GTT) in c-Ki-*ras* codon 12. Another isolate had an additional mutation in codon 13. These findings may point to the multicentricity of PDA, which seems to occur in 6% of the cases [206]. However, the result may also point to tumor cell heterogeneity and polyclonality. Moreover, different tumors in the same tissue may present the same mutation and hence cause the incidence of multiplicity to be underestimated.

On the other hand, the same c-Ki-*ras* point mutation is found both in carcinoma and in the coexisting adenoma components [205], suggesting an adenoma-carcinoma sequence.

Thirty-three percent of noninvasive intraductal papillary tumors and 88% of invasive PDA demonstrated a strong binding of the *ras*-p21 antibody [170]. No obvious differences in the expression of c-*erb*B-2 were evident between hyperplastic, benign, and malignant cells [170].

Diagnosis and Differential Diagnosis

PDA should be initially differentiated from ampullary carcinoma (which has a favorable prognosis) and duodenal carcinoma. Conversely, PDA may simulate duodenal carcinoma, when a cancer of the uncinate process infiltrates the duodenum and produces a large tumor with central ulceration [207]. Histopathologically, PDA should also be distinguished from other types of pancreatic carcinoma, such as adenosquamous cell carcinoma, noncystic mucinous carcinoma, and anaplastic carcinoma because PDA can present various morphological patterns within the same tumor. Difficulties in differential diagnosis can be overcome by studying different regions of the tumors. Immunohistochemical, histochemical, and electron microscopic examination may not be of help in differentiating tumors that derive from ductal epithelium.

The differentiation of PDA from advanced intraductal carcinoma and mucinous cystic carcinoma may also pose difficulties. Both tumors can exhibit similar histomorphology at the invasive portions.

Thus, only extensive histological examination can lead to a correct diagnosis.

PDA should also be differentiated from tumors of other gastrointestinal cancers and lung cancers that invade or, respectively, metastasize into the pancreas. Clinical information is essential for adequate diagnosis.

Some histological patterns of ductal changes in chronic pancreatitis may mimic neoplastic cells. This is especially true for groove pancreatitis [208]. Groove pancreatitis can present symptoms and radiological findings similar to PDA, including pain and jaundice, duodenal stricture, biliary and pancreatic duct stenosis, and even encasement of vessel and hypovascular mass (206). In difficult cases, examination of the c-Ki-*ras* mutation may be helpful, although according to a report, 62.5% of ductal hyperplasia in chronic pancreatitis shows the mutation of this oncogene (209). However, this finding requires information.

Prognosis and Survival

The prognosis of PDA is extremely bleak. According to the Japanese Pancreatic Cancer Registration [4], the 1-year survival rate of all cases reported to date (total: 3244 surgical and autopsy cases) was about 30%, and the 3-year survival rate did not exceed 10%. In the surgical cases, the 1-year survival rate was about 40% and the 3-year rate was 15%. Similar results are seen in other countries. In the United States, the median survival time, regardless of therapy, is 2–3 months after diagnosis. The 1-year survival rate is about 8%, and the 5-year rate is about 2% [210]. The rates were similar in patients whose tumors were diagnosed earlier, and there was no relationship between survival and tumor size, histological grade of differentiation, age, and sex [211]. The grave prognosis of the disease is related to its silent growth and the high metastatic and invasive behavior of even small tumors. According to other reports, the determining factors of the prognosis include the size of the tumor, the degree of metastasis (including lymph node infiltrations), the direct invasion into the peripheral tissues, and the histological degree of differentiation, although small well-differentiated tumors are also lethal. DNA ploidy appears to be an independent factor of poor prognosis [190, 202]. For details, see Chapter "Tumor Spread and the Factors Influencing Prognosis in Patients with Resected Pancreatic Carcinoma" in this volume.

References

1. Cubilla AI, Fizgerald PJ (1984) Malignant neoplasms in tumors of the exocrine pancreas. Atlas of tumor pathology, Second Series Fascicle 19. AFIP, Washington DC, pp 109–233
2. Klöppel G (1984) Pancreatic non-endocrine tumours in pancreatic pathology. In: Klöppel G, Heitz PU (eds) Churchill Livingstone, Edinburgh, pp 79–113
3. Morohoshi T, Shimizu K, Kanda M (1991) Pancreatic tumors—their pathology and morphogenesis. Jpn J Cancer Dig Org 1:556–562
4. Saito Y (1990) Annual report of pancreatic cancers registered at Japan Pancreatic Society. Japanese Pancreatic Cancer Registration
5. Watanabe, S (1992) Epidemiology of pancreatic cancer in pancreatic tumor. In: Takeuchi M, Honnma T (eds) Nakayama-Shoten, Tokyo, pp 39–52
6. National Center for Health Statistics, U.S. Department of Health, Education, and Welfare (HSM72-1101), 1968
7. Boring CC, Squires TS, Tong T (1993) Cancer statistics. J Am Cancer Soc 43:7–26
8. Fraumeni JF (1975) Cancer of the pancreas and biliary tract: Epidemiological considerations. Cancer Res 35:3437–3446
9. Kovi J, Heshmat MY (1973) Incidence of cancer in Negroes in Washington DC and selected African cities. Am J Epidemiol 95:401–413
10. Mack TM, Paganini-Hill A (1981) Epidemiology of pancreatic cancer in Los Angeles. Cancer 47:1474–1484
11. Moynan RW, Neerhour R, Johnson TS (1964) Pancreatic carcinoma in children: Case-report and review. J Pediatr 65:711–720
12. Taxy JB (1976) Adenonarcinoma of the pancreas in childhood. Cancer 37:1508–1518
13. Tsukimoto I, Watanabe K, Lin JB, Nakajima T (1973) Pancreatic carcinoma in children in Japan. Cancer 31:1203–1207
14. Smith PE, Krementz ET, Reid RJ, Bufkin WJ (1967) An analysis of 600 with carcinoma of the pancreas. Surg Gynecol Obstet 124:1288–1290
15. Ivy EJ, Sarr MG, Reiman HM (1990) Nonendocrine cancer of the pancreas in patients under age forty years. Surgery 108:481–487
16. Andrén-Sandberg Å (1989) Androgen influence on exocrine pancreatic cancer. Int J Pancreatol 7: 167–176
17. Longnecker DS, Roebuck BD, Yager JD Jr, Lilja HS, Siegmund B (1981) Pancreatic carcinoma in azaserine-treated rats: induction, classification and dietary modulation of incidence. Cancer 1562–1572
18. Lhoste F, Roebuck BD, Brinck-Johansen T,

Longnecker DS (1987). Effect of castration and hormone replacement on azaserine-induced pancreatic carcinogenesis in male and female Fischer rats. Carcinogenesis 8:699–703

19. Meijers M, Visser CJT, Klijn JGM, Lamberts SWJ, Garderen-Hoetmer FH, de Jong JA, Foeskens, Woutersen RA (1992) Effect of orchiectomy alone or in combination with testosterone and cyproterone acetate on exocrine pancreatic carcinogenesis in rats and hamsters. Int J Pancreatol 137–164
20. Corishley TP, Iqbal MJ, Wilkinson ML, Williams RS (1986) Androgen receptor in human normal and malignant pancreatic tissue and cell lines. Cancer 57:1992–1995
21. Greenway BA, Iqbal MJ, Johnson PJ, Williams RS (1982) Estrogen receptor proteins in malignant and fetal pancreas. Br J Surg 69:293–296
22. Birt DF, Salmasi S, Pour PM (1981) Enhancement of experimental pancreatic cancer in Syrian golden hamsters by dietary fat. J Natl Cancer Inst 67: 1327–1332
23. Hirayama T (1981) A large-scale cohort study on the relationship between diet and selected cancers of digestive organs. In: WB Bruce, P Correa, M Lipkin, SR Tannenbaum, TD Wilkins (eds) Banbury Report 7. Gastrointestinal cancer: endogenous factors. Cold Spring Harbor Laboratory, pp 409–429
24. Mack TM, Yu MC, Hanisch R, Henderson BE (1986) Pancreas cancer and smoking, beverage consumption and past medical history. J Natl Cancer Inst 76:49–60
25. Tomioka T, Andrén-Sandberg Å, Fujii H, Egami H, Takiyama Y, Pour PM (1990) Comparative histopathological findings in the pancreas of cigarette smokers and non-smokers. Cancer Lett 55:121–128
26. Feron VJ, Kuper CF, Spit BJ, Reuzel PG, Woutersen RA (1985) Glass fibers and vapor phase components of cigarette smoke as cofactors in experimental respiratory tract carcinogenesis. Carcinog Compr Surv 8:93–118
27. Pour PM, Kazakoff K, Carlson K (1990) Inhibition of Streptozotocin-induced islet cell tumors and BOP-induced exogenous pancreatic tumors in Syrian hamsters. Cancer Res 50:1634–1639
28. Bell RH, Strayer DS (1983) Streptozotocin prevents development of nitrosamine-induced pancreatic cancer in the Syrian hamster. J Surg Oncol 24: 258–262
29. Cerosimo E, Pisters P, Pesola G, McDermot K, Bajorunas D, Brenann MF (1991) Insulin secretion and action in patient with pancreatic cancer. Cancer 67:468–493
30. Permert J, Ihse I, Jorfeldt L, von Schenk H, Arnqvist HJ, Larsson J (1993) Pancreatic cancer is associated with impaired glucose metabolism. Eur J Surg 159:101–107
31. Permert J, Larsson J, Ihse I, Pour PM (1991) Diagnosis of pancreatic cancer. Alteration of glucose metabolism. Int J Pancreatol 9:113–117
32. Permert J, Adrian TE, Jacobsson P, Jorfeld L, Fruin B, Larsson J (1993) Is profound peripheral insulin resistance in patients with pancreatic cancer caused by a tumor-associated factor. Am J Surg 16:119–124
33. The Registrar General's Decennial Supplement (1985) England and Wales, 1951, Part II, Occupational Mortality. Her Majesty's Stationary Office, London 20
34. Doerken H (1964) Einige Daten bei 280 Patienten mit Pankreaskrebs. Gastroenterologia 10:47–77
35. Turner HM, Grace HG (1938) An investigation into cancer mortality among males in certain Sheffield trades. J Hyg 38:90–103
36. Mancuso TF, El-Attar AA (1967) Cohort study of workers exposed to betanaphtylamine and benzidine. J Occup Med 9:277–285
37. Anonymous (1974) Study finds cancer-woodworking tie. Eng News Rec 195:15
38. Li FP, Fraumeni JF, Mantel N, Miller RW (1969) Cancer mortality among chemists. J Natl Cancer Inst 43:1159–1164
39. Pour PM, Runge RG, Birt D, Gingell R, Lawson T, Nagel D, Wallcave L (1981) Current knowledge of pancreatic carcinogenesis in the hamster and its relevance to the human disease. Cancer 47: 1573–1587
40. Palmiter RD, Chen HY, Messing A, Brinster RL (1985) SV40 enhancer and large-T antigen are instrumental in development of choroid plexus tumors in transgenic mice. Nature 316:457–460
41. Sandgren EP, Quaife CL, Paulovich AG, Palmiter RD (1991) Pancreatic tumor pathogenesis reflects the causative genetic lesion. Proc Natl Acad Sci USA 88:93–97
42. Ceci JD, Kovattch RM, Swing DA, Jones JM, Snow CM, Rosenberg MP, Jenkins NA, Copeland NG, Meisler MH (1991) Transgenic mice carrying a murine amylase 2.2/SV40 T antigen fusion gene develop pancreatic acinar cell and stomach carcinomas. Oncogene 6:323–332
43. Ghadirian P, Boyle P, Simard J, Baillargeon J, Maisonneuve P, Perret C (1991) Reported family aggregation of pancreatic cancer with a population-based case-control study in the francophone community in Montreal, Canada. Int J Pancreatol 10:183–196
44. Pour PM (1990) Is there a link between chronic pancreatitis and pancreatic cancer. In: Beger H, Büchler M (eds) Chronic pancreatitis. Springer, Berlin Heidelberg New York, pp 106–112
45. Mizumoto K, Tsutsumi M, Kitazawa S, Tsujita S, Nakayama M, Tsujii T, Kanehiro H, Nakajima Y, Nakano H, Konishi Y (1990) Intraductal carcinoma

in a surgically resected pancreas with chronic pancreatitis. Int J Pancreatol 6:279–285
46. Morohoshi T, Kunimura T, Kanda M, Takahasi H, Yagi H, Shimizu K, Nakayoshi A, Asanuma K (1990) Multiple carcinomata associated with anomalous arrangement of the biliary and pancreatic duct system. Acta Pathol Jpn 40:755–763
47. Wynder EL, Mabuchi K, Maruchi N, Fortner JG (1973) Epidemiology of cancer of the pancreas. J Natl Cancer Inst 50:645–667
48. Pour PM, Donnelly T (1978) The effect of cholecystoduodenostomy and choledochostomy in pancreatic carcinogenesis. Cancer Res 38:2048–2051
49. Pour PM, Donnelly T, Stepan K (1983) Modification of pancreatic carcinogenesis in the hamster model. 5. Effect of partial pancreatico-colostomy. Carcinogenesis 10:1327–1331
50. Konishi Y, Mizumoto K, Kitazawa S, Tsujiuchi T, Tsutsumi M, Kamano T (1990) Early ductal lesions of pancreatic carcinogenesis in animals and humans. Int J Pancreatol 7:83–89
51. Mizumoto K, Inagaki T, Koizumi M, Uemura M, Ogawa M, Kitazawa S, Tsutsumi M, Toyokawa M, Konishi Y (1988) Early pancreatic duct adenocarcinoma. Human Pathology 19:242–244
52. Mukada T, Yamada S (1982) Dysplasia and carcinoma in situ of the exocrine pancreas. Tohoku J Exp Med 137:115–124
53. Nakao A, Ichihara T, Nonami T, Harada A, Koshikawa T, Nakashima N, Nagura H, Takagi H (1989) Clinicohistopathologic and immunohistochemical studies of intrapancreatic development of carcinoma of the head of the pancreas. Ann Surg 209:181–187
54. Pour PM, Sayed S, Sayed G, Wolf GL (1982) Hyperplastic, preneoplastic, and neoplastic lesions found in 83 human pancreases. Am J Clin Path 77:137–152
55. Pour PM (1984) Histogenesis of exocrine pancreatic cancer in the hamster model. Eviron Health Perspect 56:229–243
56. Pour PM (1988) Mechanism of pseudoductular (tubular) formation during pancreatic carcinogenesis in the hamster model. Am J Pathol 130: 335–344
57. Toshkov I, Kirev T, Bannasch P (1991) Virus-induced pancreatic cancer in Guinea Fowl: An electron microscopic study. Int J Pancreatol 10: 51–64
58. Longnecker DS, Shinozuka H, Dekker A (1988) Focal acinar cell dysplasia in human pancreas. Cancer 45:534–540
59. Longnecker DS, Hashida Y, Shinozuka H (1980) Relationship of age to prevalence of focal acinar cell dysplasia in the human pancreas. J Natl Cancer Inst 65:63–66
60. Shinozuka H, Lee R, Dunn JL, Longneckaer DS (1980) Multiple atypical acinar cell nodules of the exocrine pancreas. Hum Pathol 11:389–391
61. Tanaka T, Mori H, Williams GM (1988) Atypical and neoplastic acinar cell lesions of the pancreas in an autopsy study of Japanese patients. Cancer 61:2278–2285
62. Kodama T, Mori W (1983) Atypical acinar cell nodules of the human pancreas. Acta Pathol Jpn 33:701–714
63. Pour PM (1985) Induction of unusual pancreatic neoplasms with morphologic similarity to human tumors and evidence for their ductal/ductular cell origin. Cancer 55:2411–2416
64. Howard JM, Jordan GL Jr (1977) Cancer of the pancreas. Curr Probl Cancer 2:5:52
65. McDonald JS, Wilderlite L, Schein PS (1977) Biology, diagnosis and chemotherapeutic management of pancreatic malignancy. Adv Pharmacol Chemother 14:107–142
66. Moertel CG (1973) Exocrine pancreas. In: Holland JF, Frei E III (eds) Cancer medicine. Lea and Febiger, Philadelphia
67. Gambill EE (1970) Pancreatic and ampullary carcinoma: Diagnosis and prognosis in relation to symptoms, physical findings, and elapse of time as observed in 255 patients. South Med J 63:1119–1122
68. Moossa AR, Lewis MH, Bowie JD (1980) Clinical features and diagnosis of pancreatic cancer. In: Moossa AR (ed) Tumors of the pancreas. Williams and Wilkins, Baltimore, pp 429–442
69. Fitzgerald PJ, Fortner JG, Watson RC, Schwartz MK, Sherlock P, Benua RS, Cubilla AL, Shottenfeld D, Miller D, Winawer SL, Lightdale CJ, Leidner SD, Nisselbaum JS, Menendez-Botet CJ, Poleski MM (1978) The value of diagnostic aids in detecting pancreas cancer. Cancer 41:868–879
70. Go VL, Taylor WF, DiMagno EP (1981) Efforts at early diagnosis of pancreatic cancer: The Mayo Clinic experience. Cancer 3:1698–1703
71. Tournat R, Allan BJ, White TT (1978) Cancer, pancreatitis, and detection of isoenzymes of DNASE, RNASE, and amylase. Clin Chem Acta 88:345–353
72. Lake-Bakaar G, McKavnagh S, Summerfield JA (1979) Urinary immunoreactive trypsin excretion: a non-invasive screening test for pancreatic cancer. Lancet 2:878–880
73. Nakane H, Yoshida M Murakami T (1979) Assessment of the clinical usefulness of serum ribonuclease assays: an indicator for the detection of pancreatic cancer. J Jpn Soc Gastroenterol 14:55–62
74. Weickmann JL, Olson EM, Glitz DG (1984) Immunological assay of pancreatic ribonuclease in serum as an indicator of pancreatic cancer. Cancer Res 44:1682–1687

75. Douglas AP, Chandler C (1978) Galactosyl transferase isoenzymes for screening of patients with cancer and gluten-sensitive enteropathy. Gastroenterology 74:1120
76. Nishida K, Sugiura M, Yoshikawa T, Kondo M (1981) Enzyme immunoassay of pancreatic oncofetal antigen (POA) as a marker of pancreatic cancer. Gut 26:450–455
77. Nevalainen TJ, Eskola JU, Aho AJ, Havia VT, Lövgren TN-E, Näntö V (1985) Immunoreactive phospholipase A_2 in serum in acute pancreatitis and pancreatic cancer. Clin Chem 31:1116–1120
78. Hamano H, Hayakawa T, Kondo T (1987) Serum immunoreactive elastase in diagnosis of pancreatic diseases. A sensitive marker for pancreatic cancer. Dig Dis Sci 32:50–56
79. Vezzadini P, Sterwiwi C, Gullo L, Bonora G, Campione O, Marrano P, Labo G (1984) Effect of secretin stimulation upon serum immunoreactive trypsin in patients with carcinoma of the pancreas. Surg Gynecol Obstet 158:319–321
80. Podolsky DK, Weiser MM (1978) Galactosyl transferase isozyme II: Correlation with extent of gastrointestinal malignancy and prediction of recurrence. Gastroenterology 74:1140
81. Niitsu Y (1980) Serum ferritin and malignancy. Rinsho Ketsueki (Clin Hematol) 21:1135–1143
82. Fateh-Moghadam A, Matel W, Nejmeier D, Hannig C, Kristin M, Otte M (1978) The significance of beta 2-microglobulin and carcinoembryonic antigen in the diagnosis of the carcinoma of the pancreas. Klin Wochenschr 56:267–270
83. Holyoke ED, Douglass HO, Goldrosen MH, Chu TM (1979) Tumor markers in pancreatic cancer. Semin Oncol 6:347–356
84. Nakamura RM, Plow EF, Edington TS (1978) Current status of carcinoembryonic antigen (CEA) and CEA-S assays in the evaluation of neoplasms of the gastrointestinal tract. Ann Clin Lab Sci 8:4–10
85. McIntire KR, Waldmann TA, Moertel GG, Go VLW (1975) Serum fetoprotein in pateints with neoplasm of the gastrointestinal tract. Cancer Res 35:991–996
86. Banwo O, Versey J, Hobbs JR (1974) New oncofetal antigen for human pancreas. Lancet 643–645
87. Mihas AA (1978) Immunologic studies on a pancreatic oncofetal protein. J Natl Cancer Inst 60: 1439–1444
88. Klavins JV (1981) Tumor markers of pancreatic carcinoma. Cancer 47:1597–1601
89. Fujii Y, Albers GHR, Carre-Llopis A, Escribano MJ (1987) The diagnostic value of the foetoacinar pancreatic (FAP) protein in cancer of the pancreas; a comparative study with CA19-9. Br J Cancer 56:495–500
90. Koprowski H, Steplewski Z, Mitchell K, Herlyn M, Herlyn D, Fuhrer JP (1974) Colorectal carcinoma antigen detected by hybridoma antibodies. Som Cell Genet 5:957–972
91. Lindholm L, Holmgren J, Svennerholm L, Fredman P, Nilsson O, Persson B, Myrvold H, Lagergrad T (1983) Monoclonal antibodies against gastrointestinal tumor-associated antigens isolated as monosialogangliosides. Int Arch Allergy Appl Immun 71:178–181
92. Bast RC, Freeny M, Lazarus H, Nadler LM, Colvin RB, Knall RC (1981) Reactivity of a monoclonal antibody with human ovarian carcinoma. J Clin Invest 68:1331–1337
93. Metzgar RS, Rodriguez N, Fin OJ, Lan MS, Daasch VN, Fernsten PD, Meyers WC, Sindelar WF, Sandler RS, Seigler HF (1984) Detection of a pancreatic cancer-associated antigen (DU-PAN-2 antigen) in serum and ascites of patients with adenocarcinoma. Proc Natl Acad Sci USA 81: 5242–5246
94. Klug TL, Sattler MA, Colcher D, Schlom J (1986) Monoclonal antibody immunoradiometric assay for an antigenic determinant (CA72) on a novel pancarcinoma antigen (TAG-72) Int J Cancer 38: 661–669
95. Herlyn M, Steplewski Z, Herlyn D, Koprowski H (1979) Colorectal carcinoma-specific antigen: Detection by means of monoclonal antibodies. Proc Natl Acad Sci USA 76:1438–1442
96. Chung YS, Ho JJ, Kim YS, Tanaka H, Nakata B, Hiura A, Motoyoshi H, Satake K, Umeyama K (1987) The detection of human pancreatic cancer-associated antigen in the serum of cancer patients. Cancer 60:1636–1643
97. Yuan SZ, Ho JJ, Yuan M, Kim YS (1985) Human pancreatic cancer-associated antigens detected by murine monoclonal antibodies. Cancer Res 45: 6179–6187
98. Loor R, Kuriyama M, Bodziak MLM, Inaji H, Douglass HO Jr, Berjian R, Nicolai JJ, Tytgat GN, Chu TM (1984) Simultaneous evaluation of a pancreas-specific antigen and a pancreatic cancer-associated antigen in pancreatic carcinoma. Cancer Res 44:3604–3607
99. Gold DV, Hollingsworth P, Kremer T, Nelson D (1983) Identification of a human pancreatic duct tissue-specific antigen. Cancer Res 43:235–238
100. Stenman UH, Huhtala ML, Koistinen R, Seppälä M (1982) Immunochemical demonstration of an ovarian cancer-associated urinary peptide. Int J Cancer 30:53–57
101. Kawa S, Oguchi H, Kobayashi T, Tokoo M, Furuta S, Kanai M, Homma T (1991) Elevated serum levels of Dupan-2 in pancreatic cancer patients

negative for Lewis blood group phenotype. Br J Cancer 64:899–902
102. Wallach MK, Brown AS, Rosato EF (1978) Serum fucose as a monitor for recurrent malignancy. J Surg Oncol 10:39–44
103. Leveson SH, Russo AJ, Douglas HO, Goldrosen MR, Holyoke ED (1978) Diagnosis of pancreatic carcinoma using the leucocyte adherence inhibition microassay. Br J Surg 65:360
104. Moossa AR, Levin B (1981) The diagnosis of "early" pancreatic cancer. The University of Chicago experience. Cancer 47:1688–1697
105. Gelder FB, Reese CJ, Moossa AR, Hall T, Hunter R (1978) Studies on the oncofetal antigen, POA. Cancer 42:1635–1645
106. Satake K (1991) Diagnosis of pancreatic cancer. Serological markers. Int J Pancreatol 9:93–98
107. Satake K, Chung Y-S, Umeyama K, Takeuchi T, Kim YS (1991) The possibility of diagnosing small pancreatic cancer (less than 4.0 cm) by measuring various serum tumor markers. Cancer 68:149–152
108. Frebourg T, Bercoff E, Manchon N, Senant J, Basuyau J-P, Breton P, Janvresse A, Brunelle P, Bourreille J (1988) The evaluation of CA 19-9 antigen level in the early detection of pancreatic cancer. Cancer 62:2287–2290
109. Tempero M, Takasaki H, Uchida E, Takiyama Y, Colcher D, Metzgar RS, Pour PM (1989) Co-expression of CA 19-9, DU-PAN-2, CA125, and TAG-72 in pancreatic adenocarcinoma. Am J Surg Pathol 13:89–95
110. Del Favero G, Fabris C, Panucci A, Basso D, Plebani M, Baccaglini U, Leandro G, Burlina A, Naccarato R (1986) Carbohydrate antigen 19-9 (CA19-9) and carcinoembryonic antigen (CEA) in pancreatic cancer. Bull Cancer (Paris) 73:251–255
111. Satake K, Chung Y-S, Yokomatsu H, Nakata B, Sawada T, Nishiwaki H, Umeyama K (1991) Various tumor markers for small pancreatic cancer with special reference to the present status of pancreatic cancer in Japan and our experience over the past 2 years. Pancreas 6:234–241
112. Beretta E, Malesci A, Zerbi A, Mariani A, Carlucci M, Bonato C, Ferrari AM, Di Carlo V (1987) Serum CA19-9 in the postsurgical follow-up of patients with pancreatic cancer. Cancer 60: 2428–2431
113. White TT, Allan BJ, Schilling JJ, Miyashita H (1985) Human pancreatic secretory protein profiles in pancreas cancer and chronic pancreatitis. Dig Dis Sci 30:200–203
114. White TT, Allan BJ, Schilling JJ, Miyashita H (1983) Human pancreatic secretory protein profiles in the search for tumor markers. Dig Dis Sci 28: 792–800
115. Scheele GA (1981) Human pancreatic cancer: analysis of proteins contained in pancreatic juice by two-dimensional isoelectric focusing/sodium dodecyl sulfate gel electrophoresis. Cancer 47: 1513–1515
116. Rennel CL (1974) Diagnostic value of hypotonic duodenography. Am J Roentgenol Radium Ther Nuc Med 121:256–263
117. Shirley DV (1974) Hypotonic duodenography in suspected pancreatic disease. Br J Radiol 47: 437–443
118. Pollock D, Taylor KJ (1981) Ultrasound scanning in patients with clinical suspicion of pancreatic cancer. Cancer 47:1662–1665
119. Robbens AH, Gerzof SG, Pugatch RS (1979) Newer imaging techniques for diagnosis of pancreatic cancer. Semin Oncol 6:332–343
120. Taylor KJ, Buchen PJ, Viscomi GN (1981) Ultrasonographic scanning of the pancreas: Prospective study of clinical results. Radiology 138:211–213
121. DiMagno EP, Malagelada JR, Taylor WF, Go VLW (1977) A prospective comparison of current diagnostic tests for pancreatic cancer. N Engl J Med 297:737–742
122. Savarino V, Mansi C, Bistofi L, Rentilin P, Celle G (1983) Failure of new diagnostic aids in improving detection of pancreatic cancer at a resectable stage. Dig Dis Sci 28:1078–1082
123. Redman HC (1981) Standard radiologic diagnosis and CT scanning in pancreatic cancer. Cancer 47:1656–1661
124. Freeny PC (1989) Radiologic diagnosis and staging of pancreatic ductal adenocarcinoma. Radiol Clin North Am 27:121–128
125. Dreiling DA (1970) The early diagnosis of pancreatic cancer. Scand J Gastroenterol 6 [Suppl]: 115–122
126. Endo Y, Mori T, Tamuta H (1974) Cytodiagnosis of pancreatic malignant tumors by aspiration under direct vision, using duodenal fiberscope. Gastroenterology 67:944–951
127. Kameya S, Kuno N, Kasugai T (1981) The diagnosis of pancreatic cancer by pancreatic juice cytology. Acta Cytol 25:354–360
128. Yamada T, Murohisa B, Muto Y, Okamato K, Doi K, Tsuchiya R (1984) Cytologic detection of small pancreaticoduodenal and biliary cancers in the early developmental stage. Acta Cytol 28:435–442
129. Mithchell MK, Carney CN (1985) Cytologic criteria for the diagnosis of pancreatic carcinoma. Am J Clin Pathol 83:171–176
130. Tatsuta M, Yamamura H, Yamamoto R, Okano Y, Takeshi M, Okuda S, Tamura H (1983) Significance of carcinoembryonic antigen levels and cytology of pure pancreatic juice in diagnosis of pancreatic cancer. Cancer 52:1880–1885
131. Clouse ME, Gregg JA, Sedgwick CE (1975) Angiography vs pancreatography in diagnosis of carcinoma of the pancreas. Radiology 144:605–610

132. Feinberg SB, Screiber DR, Goodale R (1977) Comparison of ultrasound pancreatic scanning and endoscopic retrograde cholangiopancreatograms: A retrospective study. J Clin Ultrasound 5:96–100
133. Nakano S, Horiguchi Y, Takeda T (1974) Comparative diagnostic value of endoscopic pancreatography and pancreatic function tests. Scan J Gastroenterol 9:383–389
134. Freeny PC, Ball TJ (1981) ERCP and PTC in evaluation of suspected pancreatic carcinoma—Diagnostic limitations and contemporary roles. Cancer 47:1666–1678
135. Ishikawa O, Imaoka S, Ohigashi H, Nakaizumi A, Uehara H, Wada A, Nagumo CT, Yamamoto R, Sasaki Y, Iwanaga T (1992) A new method of intraoperative cytodiagnosis for more precisely locating the occult neoplasms of the pancreas. Surgery 111:294–300
136. Ferrucci JT, Wittenberg T, Sarno RH, Dreyfuss JR (1976) Fine needle transhepatic cholangiography: New approach to obstructive jaundice. AJR 127: 403–407
137. Okuda K, Tanikawa K, Emura T (1974) Nonsurgical percutaneous transhepatic cholangiography diagnostic significance in medical problems of the liver. Am J Dig Dis 19:21–36
138. Pereiras R, Chiprut RO, Greenwald RA (1977) Percutaneous transhepatic cholangiography with the "skinny" needle. Ann Intern Med 562–568
139. Ferrucci JT, Wittenberg J (1978) CT biopsy of abdominal tumors. Aids for lesion localization. Radiology 129:739–744
140. Kline TS, Neal MS (1978) Needle aspiration biopsy: A critical appraisal-eight years and 3267 specimens later. JAMA 239:36–39
141. Yeh H (1981) Percutaneous fine needle aspiration biopsy of intraabdominal lesions with ultrasound guidance. Am J Gastroenterol 75:148–152
142. Kocjan G, Rode J, Lees WR (1989) Percutaneous fine needle aspiration cytology of the pancreas: advantages and pitfalls. J Clin Pathol 42:341–347
143. Goodale RL, Gajl Peczalska K, Dressel T, Samuelson J (1981) Cytologic studies for the diagnosis of pancreatic cancer. Cancer 47:1652–1655
144. Hovdenak N, Lees WR, Pereira J, Beilby JDW, Cotton PB (1982) Ultrasound-guided percutaneous fine needle aspiration cytology in pancreatic cancer. Br Med J 285:1183–1184
145. Ferrucci JF Jr, Wittenberg J, Margolies MN, Carry RW (1979) Malignant seeding of the tract after thin-needle aspiration biopsy. Radiology 130: 345–356
146. Smith FP, MacDonald JS, Schein PS (1980) Continuous seeding of pancreatic cancer by skinny-needle aspiration biopsy. Arch Intern Med 140:855
147. Weger AR, Glaser KS, Schwab G, Oefner D, Bodner E, Auer GU, Mikuz G (1991) Quantitative nuclear DNA content in fine needle aspirates of pancreatic cancer. Gut 32:325–328
148. Young NA, Villani MA, Khoury P, Naryshkin S (1991) Differential diagnosis of cystic neoplasms of the pancreas by fine-needle aspiration. Arch Pathol Lab Med 115:571–577
149. Ishida M (1983) Peritoneoscopy and pancreas biopsy in the diagnosis of pancreatic diseases. Gastrointest Endosc 29:211–218
150. Ishida H, Domzono T, Furukawa Y (1984) Laparoscopy and biopsy in the diagnosis of malignant intra-abdominal tumors. Endoscopy 16: 140–142
151. Goldstein HM, Neiman HL, Bookstein JJ (1974) Angiography evaluation of pancreatic disease—A further appraisal. Radiology 112:275–282
152. Rosch J, Keller FS (1981) Pancreatic arteriography, transhepatic pancreatic venography and pancreatic venous sampling in diagnosis of pancreatic cancer. Cancer 47:1679–1684
153. Tylen V, Arnesjo B (1973) Resectability and prognosis of carcinoma of the pancreas evaluated by angiography. Scand J Gastroenterol 8:691–697
154. Uden R (1976) Secretin and epinephrine combined in celiac angiography. Acta Radiol Diag 17:17–40
155. MacGregor AHC, Hawkins IF Jr (1973) Selective pharmacodynamic angiography in the diagnosis of carcinoma of the pancreas. Surg Gynecol Obstet 137:917–920
156. Reichardt E, Lunderquist A, Tylen U (1978) Selective phlebography in carcinoma of the pancreas. Acta Radiol Diagn 19:305–315
157. Montz R, Klapdor R, Kremer B, Rothe B (1985) Immunoszintigraphie und SPECT bei Patienten mit Pankreaskarzinom. Nucl Med 24:232–237
158. Klöppel G (1986) Pathomorphology of pancreatic cancer: classification, histogenesis, localization, multifocal development, prognosis and differential diagnosis. In: Malfertheiner P, Ditschuneit H (eds) Diagnostic procedures in pancreatic disease. Springer Berlin Heidelberg New York
159. Japan Pancreatic Society (to be published) General rules for cancer of the pancreas, 4th edn. Mizumoto R (ed) Kanchara Shuppan, Tokyo
160. Kanai N, Nagaki S, Tanaka T (1987) Clear cell carcinoma of the pancreas. Acta Pathol Jpn 37: 1521–1526
161. Hunterkoon M (1983) Oncocytic carcinoma of the pancreas. Cancer 51:332–336
162. Pour PM, Permert J, Mogaki M, Kazakoff K. Endocrine aspects of exocrine cancer of the pancreas. Their patterns and suggested biological significance. Am J Clin Pathol 100:223–230
163. Kashiwabara K, Nakajima T, Shinkai H, Fukuda T, Oono Y, Kurabayashi Y, Kojima T, Nagamachi Y (1991) A case of malignant duct-islet cell tumor of the pancreas. Immunohistochemical and cyto-

fluorometric study. Acta Pathol Jpn 41:636–641

164. Frantz VK. Tumours of the pancreas (1959) Atlas of tumor pathology, Section VII-Fascicles 27 and 28. Armed Forces Institute of Pathology, Washington DC, pp 96–141
165. Dawiskiba S, Pour PM, Stenram U, Sundler F, Andén-Sandberg Å (1992) Immunohistochemical characterization of endocrine cells in experimental exocrine pancreatic cancer in the Syrian golden hamster. Int J Pancreatol 11:97–104
166. Satake K, Shim K, Sowa M, Umeyama K (1985) Electron microscopic studies of human pancreatic adenocarcinoma. Eur J Surg Oncol 11:125–135
167. Sim K, Satake K, Sowa M, Umeyama K (1984) Ultrastructural observations of human pancreatic duct cell carcinoma. Nippon Geka Gakkai Zasshi 85:338–345
168. Pour PM, Parsa I, Hauser R (1987) Evidence for partial exocrine acinar differentiation in experimentally induced pancreatic ductal/ductular cell tumors. Int J Pancreatol 2:47–58
169. Kern HF, Rausch U, Mollenhauer J (1986) Fine structure of human pancreatic adenocarcinoma. In: Go VLW, Gardner JD, Brooks FP, Lebenthal E, DiMagno EP, Scheele GA (eds) The exocrine pancreas: Biology, pathobiology, and diseases. Raven, New York, pp 637–647
170. Yamao K, Nakazawa S, Fujimoto M, Tsuda H, Matsumoto K, Iwase T (1993) A mucous histochemical and immunohistochemical study of precancerous and neoplastic lesions in the human pancreas. Int J Pancreatol 14:37–44
171. Klöppel G, Dreyer T, Lampe V, Kalthoff H, Schmiegel WH, von Bülow M, Kern HF, Heitz PU (1984) Immunozytochemische Typisierung von exokrinen Pankreastumoren und ihren Metastasen. Verh Dtsch Ges Pathol 68:104–107
172. Pour PM, Burnett D. Uchida E (1985) Lectin binding affinities of induced pancreatic lesions in the hamster model. Carcinogenesis 6:1775–1780
173. Haglund C, Roberts PJ, Nordling S, Ekblom P (1984) Expression of laminin in pancreatic neoplasms and in chronic pancreatitis. Am J Surg Pathol 8:669–676
174. Pour PM, Tempero MA, Takasaki H, Uchida E, Takiyama Y, Burnett DA, Steplewski Z (1988) Expression of blood-group related antigens ABH, Lewis A, Lewis B, Lewis X, Lewis Y and CA19-9 in pancreatic cancer cells in comparison with the patient's blood group type. Cancer Res 48: 5422–5426
175. Itzkowitz SH, Yuan M, Ferrell LD, Ratcliffe RM, Chung Y-S, Satake K, Umeyama K, Jones RT, Kim YS (1987) Cancer-associated alterations of blood group antigen expression in the human pancreas. J NCI 79:425–433
176. Pour PM, Takasaki H, Büchler M (1987) Immunologic aspects of acute and chronic pancreatitis. Verh Dtsch Ges Path 71:255–265
177. Itzkowitz S, Kjeldsen T, Friera A, Hakomori S-I, Yang U-S, Kim YS (1991) Expression of Tn, sialosyl Tn, and T antigens in human pancreas. Gastroenterology 100:1691–1700
178. Kim YS, Itzkowitz SH, Yuan M, Chung Y-S, Satake K, Umeyama K, Hakomori S-I (1988) Le^x and Le^y antigen expression in human pancreatic cancer. Cancer Res 48:475–482
179. Itai S, Nishikata J, Yoneda T, Ohmori K, Yamabe H, Arii S, Tobe T, Kannagi R (1991) Tissue distribution of 2–3 and 2–6 sialyl Lewis A antigens and significance of the ratio of two antigens for the differential diagnosis of malignant and benign disorders of the digestive tract. Cancer 67:1576–1587
180. Schuessler MH, Pintado S, Welt S, Real FX, Xu M, Melamed MR, Lloyd KO, Oettgen HF (1991) Blood group and blood group-related antigens in normal pancreas and pancreas cancer: enhanced expression of precursor type 1, Tn and sialyl-Tn in pancreas cancer. Int J Cancer 47:180–187
181. Takasaki H, Tempero MA, Uchida E, Büchler M, Ness MJ, Burnett DA, Metzgar RS, Colcher D, Schlom J, Pour PM (1988) Comparative studies on the expression of tumor-associated glycoprotein (TAG-72), CA19-9 and UD-PAN-2 in normal, benign and malignant pancreatic tissue. Int J Cancer 42:681–686
182. Lan MS, Bast RC Jr, Colnaghi MI, Knapp RC, Colcher D, Schlom J, Metzgar RS (1987) Coexpression of human cancer-associated epitopes on mucin molecules. Int J Cancer 39:68–72
183. Pour PM, Kazakoff K, Dulany K (1993) A new multilabeling technique for simultaneous demonstration of different islet cells in permanent slides. Int J Pancreatol 13:139–142
184. Klöppel G, Bosslet K, von Bülow M, Kern HF (1984) Detection of different CEA epitopes in ductal adenocarcinoma of the pancreas by monoclonal antibodies (abstract) Dig Dis Sci 29:956
185. Klöppel G, Fitzgerald PJ (1986) Pathology of nonendocrine pancreatic tumors. In: Go VLW, Gardner JD, Brooks FP, Lebenthal E, DiMagno EP, Scheele GA (eds) The exocrine pancreas: Biology, pathobiology, and diseases. Raven, New York, pp 649–674
186. Morohoshi T, Kanda M, Horle A, et al. (1987) Immunocytochemical markers of uncommon pancreatic tumors. Cancer 59:739–747
187. Kiyohara H, Egami H, Kako H, Shibata Y, Murata K, Ohshima S, Sei K, Suko S, Kurano R, Ogawa M (1993) Immunohistochemical localization of Group II phospholipase A_2 in human pancreatic carcinoma. Int J Pancreatol 13:49–57
188. Ohta T, Nagakawa T, Tsukioka Y, Mori K, Kayahara M, Kanno M, Ueno K, Miyazaki I,

Terada T, Nakanuma Y (1992) Argyrophilic nuclear organizer region counts in exocrine pancreatic tumors. Int J Pancreatol 12:201–209

189. Baisch H, Klöppel G, Reinke B (1990) DNA ploidy and cell-cycle analysis in pancreatic and ampullary carcinoma. Flow cytometric study of formalin-fixed paraffin-embedded tissue. Virchows Arch [A] 417:145–150
190. Yoshimura T, Manabe T, Suwa H, Imamura T, Wang Z, Ohshio G, Yamabe H, Matsumoto M, Ogasahara K, Takasan H (1993) Nuclear content as a prognostic predictor in carcinoma of the pancreas. Int J Pancreatol 14:29–36
191. Sciallero S, Giaretti W, Geido E, Bonelli L, Zhankui L, Saccomanno S, Zeraschi E, Pugliese V (1993) DNA aneuploidy is an independent factor of poor prognosis in pancreatic and peripancreatic cancer. Int J Pancreatol 14:21–28
192. Allison DC, Bose KK, Hruban RH, Piantadosi S, Dooley WC, Boitnott JK, Cameron JL (1991) Pancreatic cancer cell DNA constant correlates with long-term survival after pancreaticoduodenectomy. Ann Surg 214:648–656
193. Alanen KA, Joensuu H, Klemi PJ (1991) Letters to the editors, Virchows Arch [A] 419:255–256
194. Eskelinen M, Lipponen P, Collan Y, Marin S, Alhava E, Nordling S (1991) Relationship between DNA ploidy and survival in patients with exocrine pancreatic cancer. Pancreas 6:90–95
195. Herrera M, van Heerden JA, Katzmann JA, Weiland LH, Nagorney DM, Ilstrup D (1992) Evaluation of DNA nuclear pattern as a prognostic determinant in resected pancreatic ductal adenocarcinoma. Ann Surg 215:120–124
196. Lipponen PK, Eskelinen MJ, Collan Y, Marin S, Alhava E (1990) Volume correlated mitotic index in human pancreatic cancer. Relation to histologic grade, clinical stage, and prognosis. Scan J Gastroenterol 251:548–554
197. Korc M, Chandrasekar B, Yamanaka Y, Friess H, Büchler M, Beger HG (1992) Overexpression of the epidermal growth factor receptor in human pancreatic cancer is associated with concomitant increases in the levels of epidermal growth factor and transforming growth factor alpha. J Clin Invest 90:1352–1360
198. Ro J, North SM, Gallick GE, Hortobagyi GN, Gutterman JU, Blick M (1987) Amplified and overexpressed epidermal growth factor receptor gene in uncultured primary human breast carcinoma. Cancer Res 48:161–164
199. Sainsbury JRC, Sherbet GV, Farndon JR, Harris AL (1985) Epidermal growth factor receptors in human brain tumors. Lancet i:364–366
200. Yamanaka Y, Onda M, Uchida E, Kobayashi T, Sasajima K, Tokunaga A, Yajiri T, Egami K, Asano G (1990) Immunohistochemical study on epidermal growth factor and its receptor in human pancreatic carcinoma. Jpn J Gastroenterol 87: 1544–1550
201. Hoorens A, Lemoine N, McLellan E, Morohoshi T, Kamisawa T, Heitz PU, Stamm B, Rüschoft J, Wiedenmann B, Klöppel G (1993) Pancreatic tumors with acinar cell differentiation: their histologic, immunocytochemical, ultrastructural and molecular biological spectrum. Am J Pathol 143: 685–698
202. Barton CM, Hall PA, Hughes CM, Gullick WJ, Lemoine NR (1991) Transforming growth factor alpha and epidermal growth factor in human pancreatic cancer. J Pathol 163:111–116
203. Wakita K, Ohyanagi H, Yamamoto K, Tokuhisa T, Saitoh Y (1992) Overexpression of c-Ki-*ras* and c-*fos* in human pancreatic carcinoma. Int J Pancreatol 11:43–47
204. Smit THBMV, Boot JMA, Bos LJ (1988) K-*ras* codon 12 mutations occurs very frequently in pancreatic adenocarcinomas. Nucl Acids Res 10: 7773–7782
205. Yanagisawa A, Kato Y, Ohtake K, Kitagawa T, Ohashi K, Hori M, Takagi K, Sugano H (1991) c-Ki-*ras* point mutations in ductectatic-type mucinous cystic neoplasms of the pancreas. Jpn J Cancer Res 82:1057–1060
206. Motojima K, Urano T, Nagata Y, Shiku H, Tsurifune T, Kanematsu T (1993) Detection of point mutations in the Kirsten-*ras* oncogene provides evidenace for the multicentricity of pancreatic carcinoma. Ann Surg 217:138–143
207. Kato O, Kuno N, Kasugai T (1979) Pancreatic carcinoma difficult to differentiate from duodenal carcinoma. Am J Gastroenterol 71:74–77
208. Yamaguchi K, Tanaka M (1992) Groove pancreatitis masquerading as pancreatic carcinoma. Am J Surg 163:312–316
209. Yanagisawa, A Ohtake K, Ohashi K, Hori M, Kitagawa T, Sugano H, Kato Y (1993) Frequent c-Ki-*ras* oncogene activation in mucous cell hyperplasias of pancreas suffering from chronic inflammation. Cancer Res 53:953–956
210. Baylor SM, Berg JW (1973) Cross-classification and survival characteristics of 5000 cases of cancer of the pancreas. J Surg Oncol 5:335–358
211. Tannapfel A, Wittekind C, Hünefeld G (1992) Ductal adenocarcinoma of the pancreas. Histopathological features and prognosis. Int J Pancreatol 12:145–152

Mucinous (Noncystic) Adenocarcinoma, Including Signet-Ring Carcinoma

Synonyms

Colloid carcinoma, gelatinous carcinoma.

Definition

This malignant epithelial tumor is a variant of ductal adenocarcinoma. It is characterized by the presence of excessive amounts of extracellular mucin in the tumor tissue. Sometimes the tumor may be entirely composed of signet-ring cells.

Incidence

Mucinous adenocarcinoma is uncommon. It comprises between 1% and 3% of all carcinomas of the pancreas [1, 2].

Sex and Age

Sex distribution and median age are similar to those of ductal adenocarcinoma. Thus, it occurs predominately in men, and the peak incidence occurs between 60 and 70 years of age.

Etiology and Pathogenesis

Mucinous noncystic adenocarcinomas are considered to be variants of ductal carcinoma [2]. They share the same etiology and pathogenesis. The invasive components of some of the intraductal papillary tumors may show features similar to that of mucinous noncystic adenocarcinoma [3].

Gross Findings

Similar to the usual ductal adenocarcinomas, mucinous noncystic carcinomas occur predominantly in the head of the pancreas. The tumors are usually larger (3–6 cm in diameter) than ductal adenocarcinomas. Due to the production of excessive amounts of mucin, the tumors have a relatively soft consistency and a gelatinous appearance on the cut surface (Fig. 1). In the case of a pure signet-ring cell carcinoma, the pancreas may be diffusely enlarged because of the markedly infiltrative spread of the tumor.

Microscopic Findings

Microscopically, the mucinous adenocarcinomas show large mucin pools, the walls of which are lined either by flattened mucin-producing cuboidal cells or connective tissue (Figs. 2, 3). Often clumps or strands of tall columnar tumor cells are found floating free in the mucin lakes (Figs. 4, 5). Some floating cells may be of the signet-ring cell type (Fig. 4). Tumors, which are exclusively composed of signet-ring cells, show marked infiltrative spread and usually involve almost the entire pancreas.

Immunohistochemistry

The periodic acid-Schiff (PAS)-positive tumor cells stain for the same tumor markers [carcinoembryonic antigen (CEA), DU-PAN-2, TAG-72, and others] as do the usual ductal adenocarcinoma. Particularly intense staining for CEA is found in signet-ring cells.

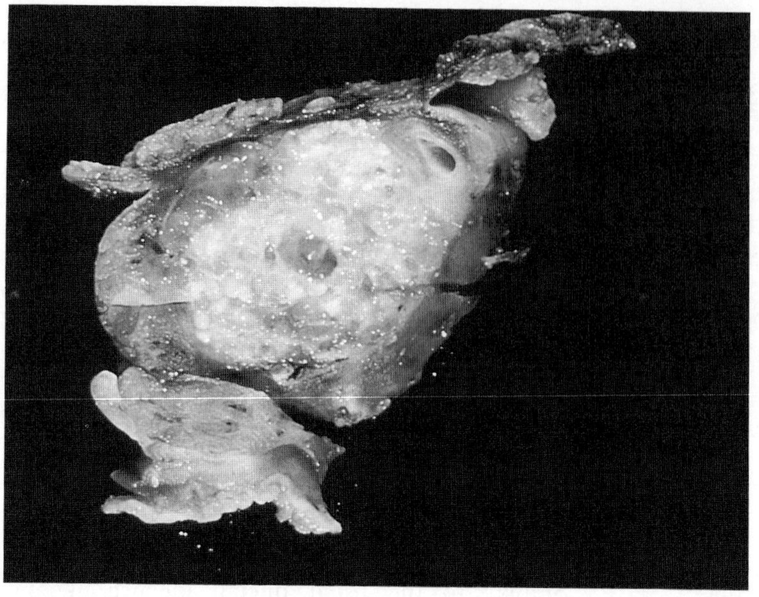

Fig. 1. Gross appearance of a mucinous (noncystic) carcinoma. Pools of mucous are visible. The tumor occurred in the tail of the pancreas. (*For color reproduction see color insert in the frontmatter*)

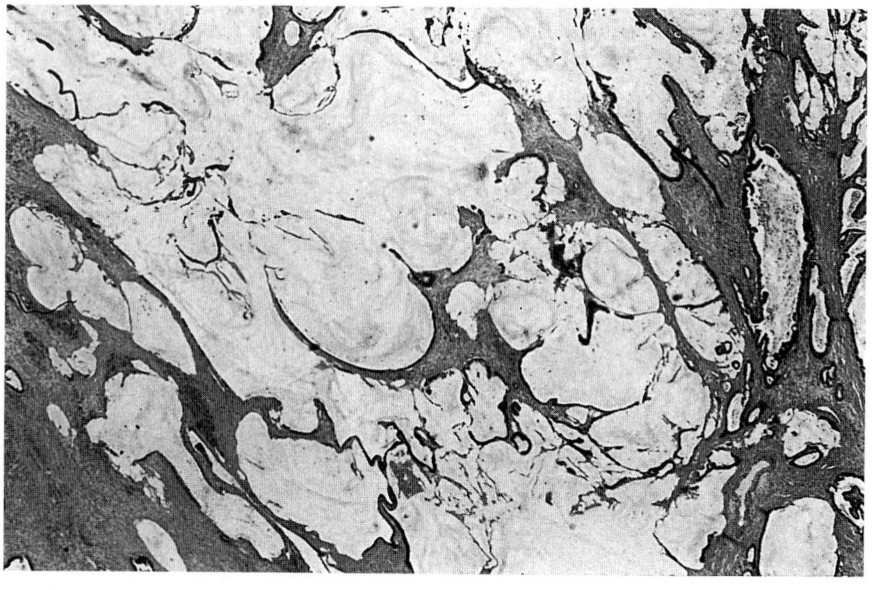

Fig. 2. A multilobulated tumor is composed of mucin-containing "lakes", which are divided by fibrous septa

Differential Diagnosis

The mucinous noncystic adenocarcinoma has to be differentiated from ductal adenocarcinoma, which may also produce considerable mucin. By definition, more than 50% of the tumor tissue of mucinous noncystic adenocarcinoma consists of mucin. Mucinous noncystic carcinomas should not be confused with mucinous cystic tumors because of the much better prognosis of the latter. Mucinous cystic tumor shows a grossly visible cyst, which is absent in mucinous noncystic adenocarcinoma.

Biology and Prognosis

The prognosis of mucinous noncystic adenocarcinomas depends on the differentiation of the tumor cells. Tumors that contain many signet-ring cells or are composed entirely of signet-ring cells have a distinctly worse prognosis than those mucinous noncystic carcinomas that only show differentiated columnar cells.

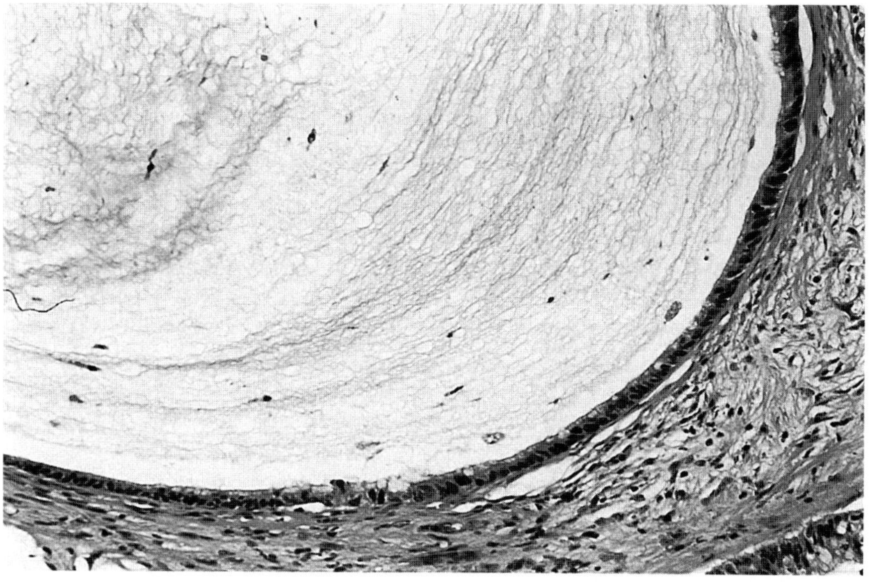

Fig. 3. A well-differentiated mucinous noncystic carcinoma. The walls of mucous lakes are lined by a single layer of columnar cancer cells

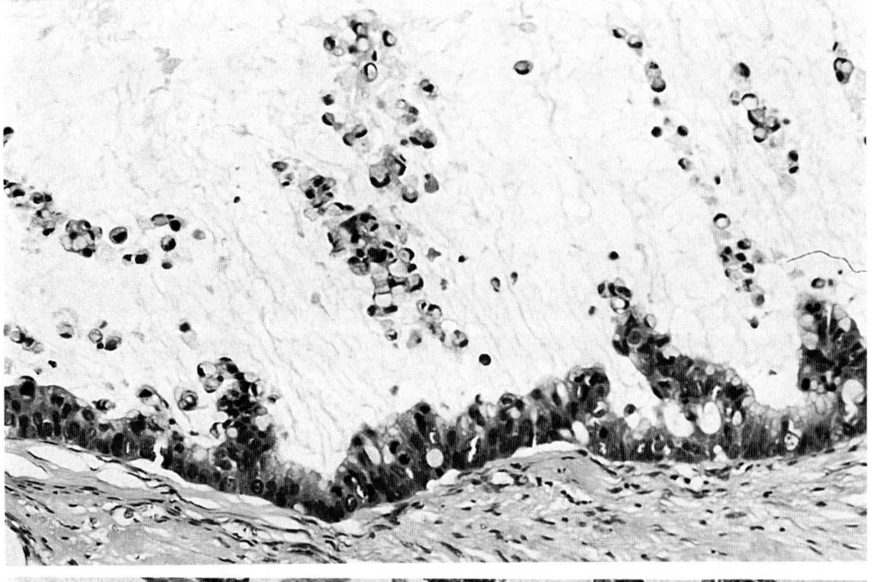

Fig. 4. A well-differentiated mucinous noncystic carcinoma. Mucous lakes are lined by a single layer of mucous epithelium. Cancer cells with signet-ring morphology are floating in mucous lake

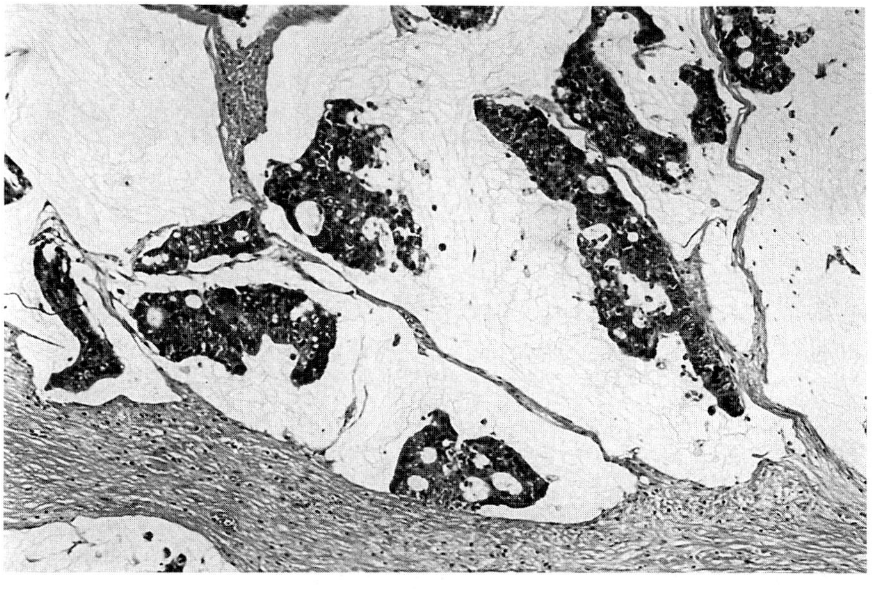

Fig. 5. A moderately differentiated noncystic mucinous carcinoma. Cancer cell nests with cribriform morphology were floating in mucous lake

References

1. Cubilla AL, Fitzgerald PJ (1984) In: Firminger HI (ed) Tumors of the exocrine pancreas. 2nd Series, Fascicle 19 Atlas of tumor pathology, 2nd Series, Fascicle 19. Armed Forces Institute of Pathology, Washington DC, 177–180
2. Klöppel G (1984) Pancreatic and non-endocrine tumours in pancreatic pathology. In: Klöppel G, Heitz PU (eds) Churchill Livingstone, Edinburgh, pp 79–113
3. Yamada M, Kozuka S, Yamao K, Nakazawa S, Naitoh Y, Tsukamoto Y (1991) Mucin-producing tumor of the pancreas. Cancer 68:159–168

Adenosquamous Cell Carcinoma

Synonyms and Related Terms

Adenoacanthoma; mucoepidermoid carcinoma

Definition

Adenosquamous carcinoma is characterized by the presence of two components: the glandular and squamous cell components. Differentiation in the glandular areas may vary from well to moderate. The squamous cell component consists of epidermoid cell nests, which show intercellular bridges, individual cell keratinization, and keratohyalin pearls. Poorly differentiated squamous cell foci may occur. The atypical patterns of the squamous cell element could be slight and be consistent with the term adenoacanthoma. Some tumors may present themselves as pure squamous cell carcinomas when the squamous cell component predominates. Therefore, a diagnosis of pure squamous cell carcinoma should only be made after extensive histological examination of the tumor (see Chapter "Squamous Cell Carcinoma" in this volume).

Incidence

According to the Pancreatic Cancer Registry of the Japan Pancreas Society, 1981–1990, the incidence of adenosquamous carcinoma was 2.3% of the 3534 cases of pancreatic cancer examined. In other series of pancreatic carcinoma, 4 out of 205 (1.95%) [1]; 5 of 142 (3.5%) [2]; 5 of 120 (4.1%) [3]; 4 of 90 (4.4%) [4]; 3 of 123 (2.4%) [5]; 1 of 239 (0.4%) [5]; 20 of 821 (2.4%) [6]; 13 of 387 (3.4%) [7]; 12 of 264 (4.1%) [8]; and 8 of 89 (9.0%) [9] had pancreatic adenosquamous carcinoma. The highest reported incidence was 11.1% [10]. The apparent regional differences in the occurrence of this tumor may be related to the method of histological examination, as demonstrated by Ishikawa et al. [10] and Yamaguchi and Enjoji [9].

Age and Sex

The age and sex of patients with adenosquamous carcinoma do not differ from those with the more common pancreatic ductal adenocarcinoma. According to the Pancreatic Cancer Registry of the Japan Pancreas Society (1993), men are more affected than women (Table 1). The age ranges between 41–86 years with an average age of 66.7 [5, 7].

Etiology

The experience in atomic bomb victims in Japan suggests that exposure to radiation is a factor in its pathogenesis [6]. Other possible causes of the disease are unknown.

Pathogenesis

The origin of the squamous cell component in adenosquamous carcinoma is still unclear. The following hypotheses are offered: (1) heterotropic or metaplastic theory: metaplastic changes in

Table 1. Age and sex distribution in pancreatic carcinomas.

Type of tumor	No. of cases	Peak age (year)	M/F ratio
Ductal adenocarcinoma	4180	61.1 ± 18.5	1.7
Adenosquamous carcinoma	118	64.0 ± 11.4	1.8
Squamous cell carcinoma	26	61.8 ± 10.8	3.3

an adenocarcinoma; (2) transformation theory: partial malignant transformation of an adenocarcinoma into squamous cell carcinoma; (3) collision theory: collision of two separate tumors; and (4) stem cell theory: differentiation of the tumor progenitor cells into both glandular and squamous cell components. However, the existence of pure squamous cell carcinoma, the presence of both glandular and squamous components in metastatic sites, and particularly the occurrence of mucin within squamous cells [11] favor the fourth possibility. Mucoepidermoid carcinoma of the salivary glands, which shows morphologic architecture similar to pancreatic adenosquamous carcinoma, has been regarded as intercalated ductal cell in origin [12, 13].

Case reports on pancreatic adenoacanthoma are rare. Because the clinical manifestations, site of metastases, gross pathology and survival are similar between adenoacanthoma and adenosquamous cell carcinoma, they seem to represent the same entity. Further, the metastatic components of these tumors are generally similar and present either a mixture of both cell types, of pure squamous or pure adenocarcinoma elements [5]. It has been found that although the atypical features of the squamous cell component are slight, its metastatic potential is high in many cases.

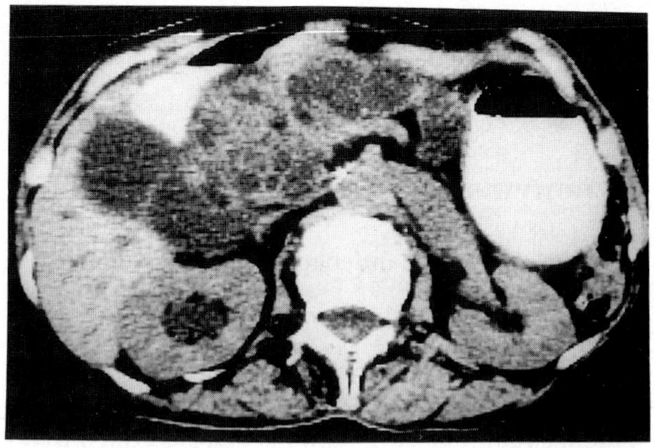

Fig. 1. Adenosquamous carcinoma of the pancreas. A 74-year-old woman with a 3-year history of diabetes mellitus was admitted to hospital due to an abdominal tumor. A cystic tumor with a focal solid area in the head of the pancreas was found by ultrasonography (US). Angiography showed a patent superior mesenteric artery and vein. Endoscopic retrograde cholangiopancreatography (ERCP) revealed the proximal main pancreatic duct and cystic space in the tumor but no distal duct. At operation, the tumor, located in the head of the pancreas, was adhered to the mesocolon of the transverse colon. Massive retroperitoneal invasion had caused hydronephrosis of the right kidney. The total pancreas, right kidney, stomach, and regional lymph nodes were resected. Computed tomography (CT) shows a large mass in the head of the pancreas with some small "cysts" on CT scan

Clinical Presentation

There may be no characteristic preoperative finding of adenosquamous carcinoma compared with the common types of duct cell carcinoma of the pancreas. It is usually diagnosed first by pathological examination of surgically excised materials. The predominantly glandular and desmoplastic tumors show the same radiological and CT scan patterns as ductal cell carcinomas. Tumors in which the squamous cell component predominates tend to become necrotic and present a cystic region on CT scan (Figs. 1, 2) [14]. One case with cavitation into the main pancreatic duct, abscess formation, and minimal calcification has been demonstrated by endoscopic retrograde cholangiopancreatography (ERCP) and CT [15]. Hepatomegaly, jaundice, and metastatic foci may be present, and serum carcinoembryonic antigen (CEA) may be increased [11]. Alpha-fetoprotein was negative in a case described by Ohtsuki et al. [11]. Also, an adenosquamous cell carcinoma in a 43-year-old Japanese man with marked leukocytosis and hypercalcemia, possibly due to the production of a colony stimulating factor by the tumor cells, is reported [16].

Diabetes mellitus was roughly four times as common among the patients with carcinoma of the pancreas as in the general population [17]. However, diabetes in these patients could be a sequela of pancreatic cancer (see chapter "Ductal Adenocarcinoma").

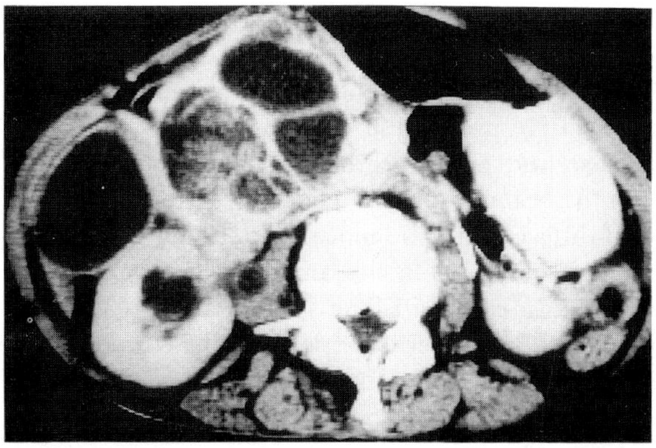

Fig. 2. A deeper slice of the CT of the same tumor in Fig. 1, shows multilocular cysts and hydronephrosis

Gross Findings

Adenosquamous carcinomas present ill-defined, indurated, firm or partially necrotic masses (Fig. 3). The cut surface of the tumor is usually yellowish to grayish-white with mottling lines of red to brown color. The appearance of the cut surface depends on the microscopical pattern of the tumor. It is firm when the tumor consists predominantly of glandular and desmoplastic components, and it is likely to be necrotic when there is a large squamous cell component. Fibrous connective tissue may be seen in many sites of the tumor. Focal calcification of the stroma has been found in one case [15]. The tumors generally show no clear demarcation with the surrounding parenchyma, which may exhibit various degrees of compressive and obstructive pancreatitis. The main pancreatic duct may be free. However, communication of the main duct with the cavity was observed in one case [15].

The tumors could measure up to 10 cm in diameter and could be located anywhere in the pancreas, but like the ductal adenocarcinoma, they are more likely to occur in the pancreas head. According to the registration of the Pancreatic Cancer Registry of the Japan Pancreas Society (1993), 63.3% of the tumors occurred in the head, 16.7% in the body, and 3.3% in the tail (Table 2).

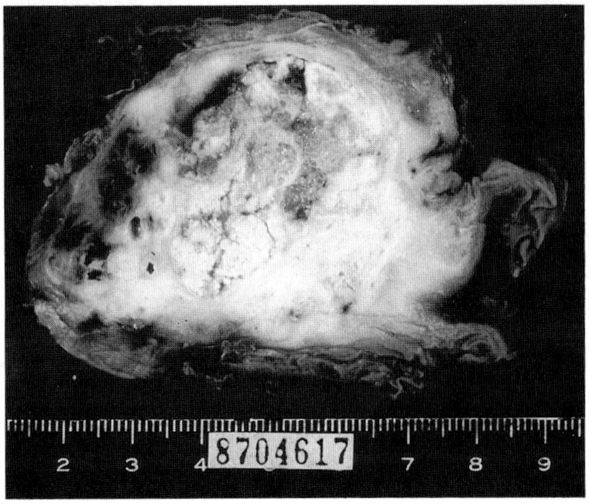

Fig. 3. Cut surface of the tumor in Fig. 1. The tumor was grayish-white, somewhat brittle, and formed an irregular space inside the capsule wall. Degenerative changes and caseous-like focus in the center of the tumor

Of the 13 tumors examined by Chen and Baithun [7], 6 were in the head or neck, 1 was in the body, 4 were in the tail, and 2 were in the body and tail.

Table 2. Original site of pancreatic carcinoma within the pancreas.

Type of cancer	No. of cases	Head	Body	Tail	Body and Tail	≥2 loci	Whole
Ductal adenocarcinoma	3618	2508	—	—	861	90	159
Adenosquamous cell carcinoma	60	38	10	2	—	8	2
Squamous cell carcinoma	12	5	3	2	—	2	0

Microscopic Findings

Tumors are composed of two cell components, and the relative proportion of each can vary from case to case and even within the same tumor (Figs. 4 and 5). Some tumors consist predominantly of well-differentiated adenocarcinoma with abundant fibrous stroma. The squamous cell component is either admixed with the glandular structures or is in the peripheral region of the tumor. The squamous cells show intercellular bridges, keratohyalin granules, and occasionally pearl formations (Fig. 6). In the areas where the two components are in contact, glandular structures blend gradually into the squamous cell elements (Figs. 4, 5, 7). The tumor cells have nuclei that vary in size and shape. Malignant cells may have giant, bizarre hyperchromatic nuclei, some exhibiting prominent nucleoli. Mitotic figures are frequent. In a few neoplastic cells, PAS-positive, diastase-sensitive material can be found [18]. In a case described by Ohtsuki et al. [11], squamous cells showed intracytoplasmic lumina, which contained mucin. The mucin had a positive reactivity with PAS, alcian blue, and mucicarmine.

Electron Microscopic Findings

Different areas of tumors may exhibit neoplastic cells with varying ultrastructural characteristics. In some areas, tumor cell clusters are separated from connective tissue by a thin basal lamina. The basal lamina may display irregular discontinuities through which cytoplasmic processes bulge into the surrounding connective tissue [18]. The cell nuclei are of various shapes and irregularity, and the nuclei are usually prominent. The cytoplasm contains many rough endoplasmic reticulum (RER), fine granular material, and well-developed Golgi complexes. In other areas of the tumor, basal lamina can be missed and the RER and Golgi apparatus may be scanty. Electron-dense glycogen particles and tonofibrils are found in the perinuclear region [18].

In the mucoepidermoid tumor reported by Ohtsuki et al. [11], three kinds of cells were found: squamous cells with intracytoplasmic lumina containing mucin (Fig. 8), undifferentiated epithelial cells and those intermingled with transitional cells. Most cells had well-developed desmosomes and bundles of tonofilaments, which surrounded intracytoplasmic lumina covered by microvilli (Fig. 7). Many of these tumor cells contained mucin.

Immunohistochemistry

The presence of mucinous material in tumor cells has been mentioned above. Antisera to keratin, epithelial membrane antigen (EMA), and CEA have been shown to react with tumor cells, whereas no reactivity was seen with anti-alpha-fetoprotein and S-100 protein [11]. Immunoreactivity of

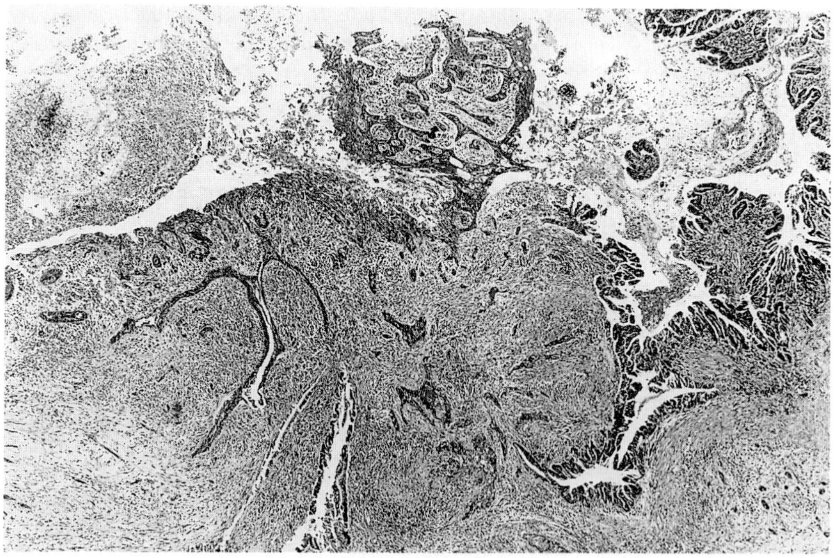

Fig. 4. Microscopic appearance of the same tumor as in Fig. 3. Adenocarcinoma component (*right*) and squamous cell carcinoma (*left*) merge into each other (*middle*). Both cell components seem to cover a cyst wall. Note the infiltrative patterns of the squamous cell component. H&E, ×30

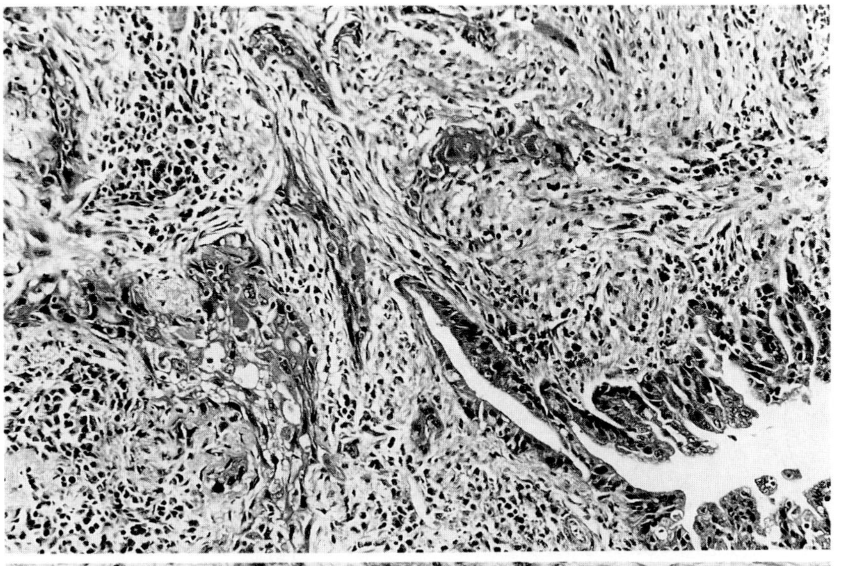

Fig. 5. A high-power view of the tumor in Fig. 4, depicting adenocarcinoma (*right*) and squamous cell carcinoma components. Marked desmoplasia in squamous cell carcinoma component. H&E, ×150

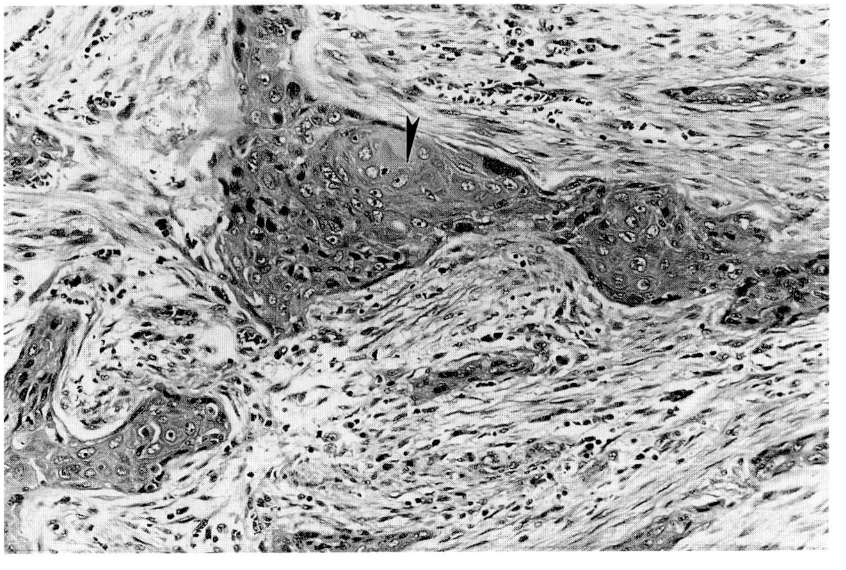

Fig. 6. Another area of the tumor in Fig. 5. Squamous carcinoma is composed of pleomorphic cells with tendency for keratinization and intracellular bridge formation (*arrowhead*). H&E, ×150

malignant glandular cells but not of squamous cells has been found with the antibody 35βH11, corresponding to Gown's antigen. The squamous and poorly differentiated cells reacted with the antibody 34βE12, and adenocarcinoma and squamous cell carcinoma were clearly counterstained with 34βE12 and alcian blue [9].

No information is available about the genetic abnormalities of the cells of adenosquamous carcinoma.

Diagnosis and Differential Diagnosis

The differential diagnosis between adenosquamous cell carcinoma and "pure" squamous cell carcinoma requires extensive sampling of the tumor. In some cases, the well-differentiated squamous cells are difficult to separate from squamous cell metaplasia and well-differentiated squamous cell carcinoma. There may also be cases in which the squamous cell components are minute compared to the adenocarcinoma component. In a series of adenosquamous carcinoma reported by Cihak et al. [4], two cases, which had originally been diagnosed as pure squamous cell carcinoma, were found to contain adenocarcinoma components after

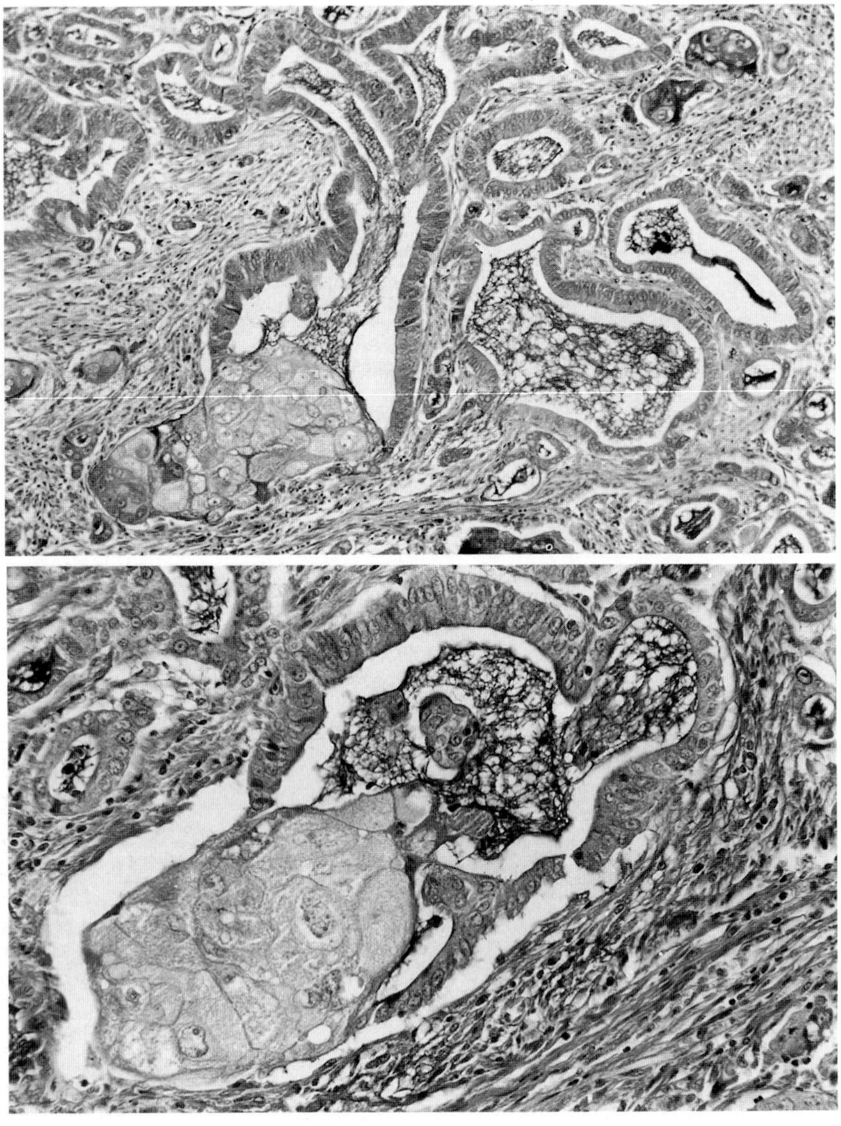

Fig. 7a,b. Adenosquamous cell carcinoma in a 61-year-old man who had an episode of intermittent epigastria within the last 3 months and increasing jaundice of 1-month duration. A hen's egg-sized mass and the enlarged gall bladder were palpated in the right hypogastrium. US and ERCP indicated the presence of a carcinoma in the head of the pancreas. At surgery, a 5 cm mass in diameter involving the superior mesenteric vein and the duodenal wall was found. The patient died on peritoneal dissemination 12 months after a pancreatoduodenectomy. ***a*** Histological examination showed typical features of ductal adenocarcinoma with foci of malignant squamous cells, which blended into the glandular elements. H&E, ×200. ***b*** A high-power view of the glandular-squamous cell contact. H&E, ×300. (Courtesy of Dr. Osamu Ishikawa)

microscopic examination of additional sections. Similarly, close examination enabled Ishikawa et al. [10] to detect a very small focus of squamous cell carcinoma on the periphery of the adenocarcinoma components. This careful examination is important because of the poor prognosis of adenosquamous cell carcinoma (see below). The grade of cellular atypia in squamous cell carcinoma is different in each case. When the squamous element is evident in a tumor, even when adenocarcinoma predominates, the diagnosis of adenosquamous cell carcinoma should be given.

The clinical significance of adenosquamous cell carcinoma of the pancreas lies in the variety of its

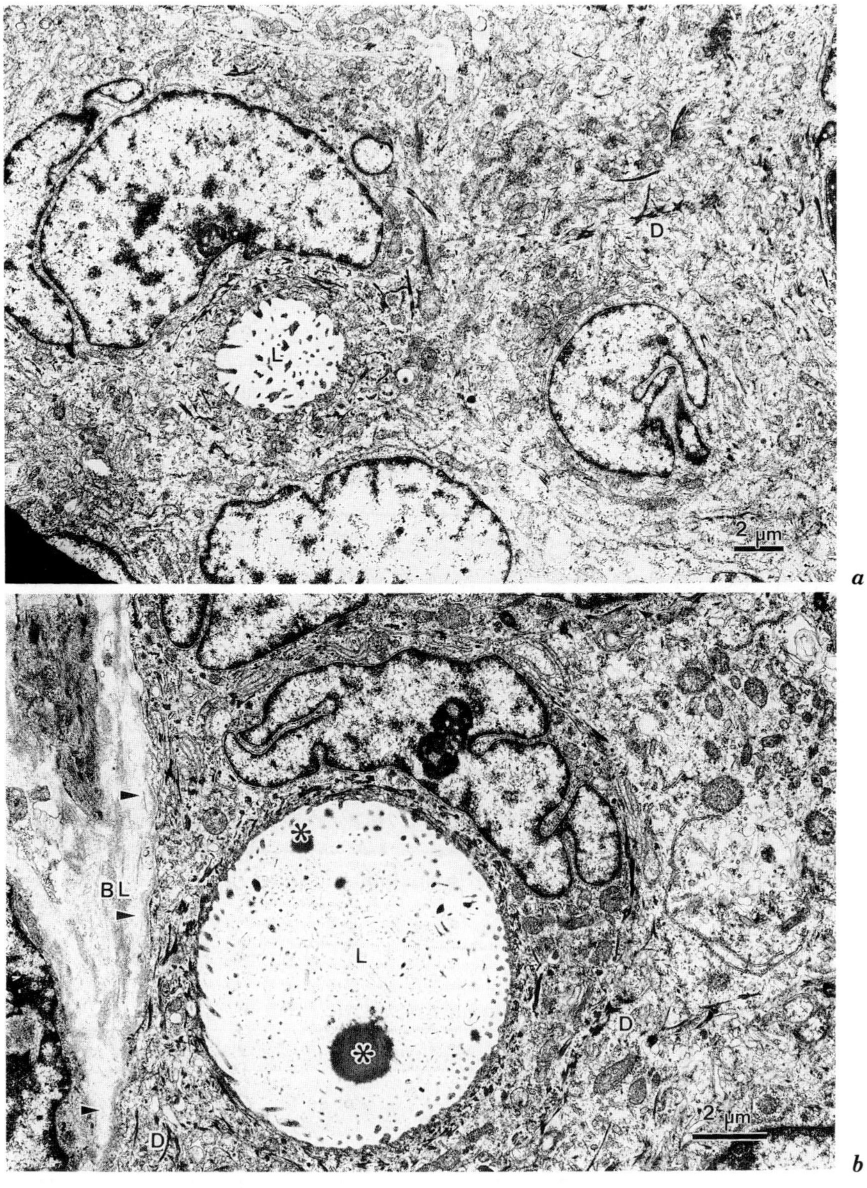

Fig. 8a,b. Electron microscopic findings of an adenosquamous cell carcinoma in a 58-year-old man, who complained of lumbago, loss of appetite, fever, and upper abdominal pain during the last 12 months. Physical examination revealed hepatomegaly, leukocytosis, slight elevation of total bilirubin and increased carcinoembryonic antigen (CEA) (5–7 ng/ml). Alpha-fetoprotein was negative. CT showed a large cystic tumor in pancreas tail with tumor nodules in the liver. ***a*** Cancer cells show well-developed desmosomal junctional complexes associated with tonofilament bundles (*D*) and intracytoplasmic lumen (*L*). ***b*** The cytoplasmic lumen (*L*) containing electron-dense homogenous material (*asterisk*) is surrounded by bundles of tonofilaments. *D*, desmosomes; *BL*, basal lamina (*arrowhead*) Uranyl acetate and lead citrate. ***a*** ×3900; ***b*** ×5400 (Courtesy Dr. Y. Ohtsuki with permission)

metastases. There is no significant difference between the rate of lymph node metastasis of ductal adenocarcinoma, adenosquamous cell carcinoma, and squamous cell carcinoma at the time of operation. However the frequency and grade of lymphatic invasion, venous invasion, and neural invasion are significantly higher in squamous cell carcinoma (Tables 3–6). This may explain the poor prognosis of squamous cell carcinoma. This finding indicates that vascular invasion is one of

Table 3. Lymph node involvement of pancreatic cancers.

Type of cancer	No. of cases	n0	n1	n2	n3	Ratio
Ductal adenocarcinoma	2507	857	1082	341	227	65.8%
Adenosquamous cell carcinoma	62	21	27	6	8	66.1%
Squamous cell carcinoma	11	4	2	1	4	63.6%

n0, no nodal involvement; n1, a few nodal metastases; n2, moderate involvement; n3, extensive involvement.

Table 4. Lymphatic invasion of pancreatic cancers.

Type of cancer	No. of cases	ly0	ly1	ly2	ly3	Ratio
Ductal adenocarcinoma	2419	282	773	918	446	88.3%
Adenosquamous cell carcinoma	60	9	18	22	11	85.0%
Squamous cell carcinoma	8	0	4	2	2	100.0%

ly0, no lymphatic invasion; ly1, minimal invasion; ly2, moderate invasion; ly3, extensive invasion.

Table 5. Venous invasion of pancreatic cancers.

Type of cancer	No. of cases	v0	v1	v2	v3	Ratio
Ductal adenocarcinoma	2399	887	732	529	251	63.0%
Adenosquamous cell carcinoma	63	21	20	14	8	66.7%
Squamous cell carcinoma	9	2	2	3	2	77.8%

v0, no venous invasion; v1, minimal invasion; v2, moderate invasion; v3, extensive invasion.

Table 6. Neural or perineural invasion of pancreatic cancers.

Type of cancer	No. of cases	ne0	ne1	ne2	ne3	Ratio
Ductal adenocarcinoma	1169	226	294	390	259	77.8%
Adenosquamous cell carcinoma	25	8	4	11	2	68.0%
Squamous cell carcinoma	4	0	1	1	2	100.0%

ne0, no neural/perineural invasion; ne1, minimal invasion; ne2, moderate invasion; ne3, extensive invasion.

the most important factors affecting the prognosis.

The diagnosis of pancreatic adenosquamous cell carcinoma should be included in patients who have an unknown primary but have a metastasis of squamous carcinoma or an admixture of squamous and glandular elements. Adenosquamous cell carcinoma of the pancreas might also be suspected in patients with different metastases consisting of pure squamous carcinoma and pure adenocarcinoma [5].

Biological Behavior, Prognosis

Adenosquamous cell carcinoma shows a high metastatic potential. According to Ishikawa et al. [10], invasion into lymphatic and vascular vessels occurs more frequently in adenocarcinoma components than in squamous cell components; of 25 metastases to the lymph node, these authors found squamous cell elements in only one, in which adenocarcinoma components were also found

Table 7. Survival of patients with pancreatic cancers.

Type of cancer	No. of cases	1yr	2yr	3yr	4yr	5yr
Ductal adenocarcinoma	4180	30.8%	14.1%	9.7%	7.2%	6.1%
Adenosquamous cell carcinoma	118	19.8%	12.9%	12.9%	12.9%	0%
Squamous cell carcinoma	26	10.5%	5.3%	0%	0%	0%

independently. Numerous metastatic foci in the liver, lungs and kidneys have been observed in many patients [5, 10]. Because of the highly metastatic nature of adenosquamous cell carcinoma, the prognosis of this tumor is worse than that of the usual ductal adenocarcinoma. The average survival after the onset of symptoms has been 7.75 months (range 6 weeks to 13 months) [5], 12 months [10], and 3–7 months [9]. The 0% 1-year survival of patients with adenosquamous cell carcinoma contrasts with a 17% 1-year survival of patients with ductal cell carcinoma [7, 15]. According to the Pancreatic Cancer Registry of the Japan Pancreas Society (1993), the 1-year survival rate of patients with ductal adenocarcinoma, adenosquamous cell carcinoma, and squamous cell carcinoma are 30.8%, 19.8%, and 10.5%, respectively. The survival rates of the patients with adenosquamous cell carcinoma fell to 0% at 5 years and in patients with squamous cell carcinoma, it fell to 0% already at 3 years (Table 7).

In another study, the cumulative 1-year survival rates of the patients with adenosquamous cell carcinoma, well-differentiated adenocarcinoma, moderately differentiated adenocarcinoma, and poorly differentiated adenocarcinoma were 21.4%, 42.12%, 61.2%, 24.6%, and 11.1% respectively. The difference in the survival rate between patients with well-differentiated adenocarcinoma and adenosquamous cell carcinoma was statistically significant [9]. The survival rates for pancreatic cancer patients with no venous invasion and no lymph node metastases were significantly more favorable than those with venous invasion and/or lymph node metastases [19].

References

1. Kissane JM (1975) Carcinoma of the exocrine pancreas: Pathologic aspects. J Surg Oncol 7:167
2. Sommers SC, Meissner WA (1954) Unusual carcinomas of the Pancreas Arch Pathol 58:101
3. Halpert B, Mark L, Jordan GL Jr (1965) A retrospective study of 120 patients with carcinoma of the pancreas. Surg Gynecol Obstet 121:91
4. Cihak RW, Kawashima T, Steer A (1972) Adenoacanthoma (adenosquamous carcinoma) of the pancreas. Cancer 29:1133
5. Weitzner S (1978) Adenoacanthoma of the pancreas. Report of four cases and literature review. Am J Surg 44:206–209
6. Cubilla AL, Fitzgerald PJ (1984) Tumors of the exocrine pancreas. Fascicle 19, second series, atlas of tumor pathology. Armed Forces Institute of Pathology, Washington DC pp 168–173
7. Chen J, Baithun SI (1985) Morphological study of 391 cases of exocrine pancreatic tumors with special reference to the classification of exocrine pancreatic carcinoma. J Pathol 146:17–29
8. Klöppel G, Maillet B (1989) Classification and staging of pancreatic nonendocrine tumors. Radiol Clin North Am 27:105–119
9. Yamaguchi K, Enjoji M (1991) Adenosquamous carcinoma of the pancreas: a clinicopathologic study. J Surg Oncol 47:109–116
10. Ishikawa O, Matsui Y, Aoki I, Iwanaga T, Terasawa T, Wada A (1980) Adenosquamous carcinoma of the pancreas: A clinicopathologic study and report of three cases. Cancer 46:1192–1196
11. Ohtsuki Y, Yoshino T, Takahashi K, Sonobe H, Kohno K, Akagi T (1987) Electron microscopic study of mucoepidermoid carcinoma in the pancreas. Acta Pathol Jpn 37:1175–1182
12. Healey WV, Perzin KH, Smith L (1970) Mucoepidermoid carcinoma of salivary gland origin. Cancer 26:368–388
13. Thackray AC, Lucas RB (1974) Tumors of the major salivary glands. Fascicle 10, Series 2, atlas of tumor pathology. Armed Forces Institute of Pathology, Washington DC pp 69–80
14. Friedman AC (1987) Radiology of the liver, biliary tract, pancreas and spleen. Williams and Wilkins, Baltimore, pp 837–860
15. Wilczynski SP, Valente PT, Atkinson BF (1984) Cytodiagnosis of adenosquamous carcinoma of the pancreas. User of fine-needle aspiration. Acta Cytol 18:733–736
16. Fujii H, Yamamoto Y, Yoshioka M, Matsuda H, Yoshida T, Suda K, Matsumoto Y (1993) Adeno-

squamous carcinoma of the pancreas accompanied by marked leukocytosis and hypercalcemia: a case report. J Jpn Pancreas Soc 8:176–183

17. Andersson A, Bergdahl L (1976) Carcinoma of the pancreas. Am Surg 42:173–177
18. Kovi J (1982) Adenosquamous carcinoma of the pancreas. A light and electron microscopic study. Ultrastruct Pathol 3:17–23
19. Yamaguchi K, Enjoji M (1989) Carcinoma of the pancreas: a clinicopathologic study of 96 cases with immunohistochemical observations. Jpn J Clin Oncol 19:14–22
20. Motojima K, et al. (1992) Immunohistochemical characteristics of adenosquamous carcinoma of the pancreas. J Surg Oncol 49:58–62
21. Sprayregen S, Schoenbaum SW, Messinger NH (1975) Angiographic features of squamous cell carcinoma of the pancreas. J Can Assoc Radiol 26: 122–124

Squamous Cell Carcinoma

Definition

Squamous carcinoma of the pancreas consists entirely of squamous cell elements and lacks any ductal component. The diagnosis of squamous cell carcinoma should only be made after extensive sampling of the tumor to exclude adenosquamous cell carcinoma (see Chapter "Adenosquamous Cell Carcinoma" in this volume).

Incidence

Pure squamous cell carcinoma is rare. In a large series of 5075 patients from eight cancer registry systems, 25 (0.5%) had squamous cell cancers [1]. According to other reports, the incidence ranges between 0% and 1.9% [2–6]. The highest incidence of 5.0% has been reported by Halpert et al. [7]. According to the Pancreatic Cancer Registry of the Japan Pancreas Society, from 1981 to 1990, 13 cases of squamous cell carcinoma were recorded out of 3534 cases, which corresponds to 0.37% of all carcinomas of the pancreas and 0.8% of all duct cell carcinomas (see also Table 1, Chapter "Adenosquamous Cell Carcinoma" in this volume).

Age and Sex

Like the common pancreatic ductal adenocarcinoma, squamous cell carcinoma generally affects individuals older than 50 years. The youngest patient reported was a 33-year-old woman [8]. According to the registration of the Pancreatic Cancer Registry of the Japan Pancreas Society, men are about 3.3 times more likely to develop squamous cell carcinoma than women (see Table 1, chapter "Adenosquamous Cell Carcinoma" in this volume).

Etiology

It is believed that cases of pure squamous cell carcinoma of the pancreas are the result of malignant transformation of areas of squamous metaplasia of ductal epithelium. We observed the presence of squamous cell metaplasia of ductal epithelium in a squamous cell carcinoma (see below). However, the high incidence of squamous cell metaplasia and the very low frequency of squamous cell carcinoma indicate that other unknown factors are involved.

Clinical Presentation

The clinical presentation of squamous cell carcinoma of the pancreas is indistinguishable from that of ductal adenocarcinoma (Fig. 1) and no diagnostic test is specific for this type of tumor. Beyer et al. [8] described an unusual case of cystic squamous cell carcinoma that communicated with the pancreatic duct. Sprayregen et al. [9] reported new vessel formation and a tumor blush pattern on angiography in a squamous cell carcinoma. However, these findings have also been reported in other exocrine and endocrine tumors of the pancreas [9–13]. Additionally, squamous cell carcinoma of the pancreas associated with hypercalcemia has been reported in a 57-year-old black man [14].

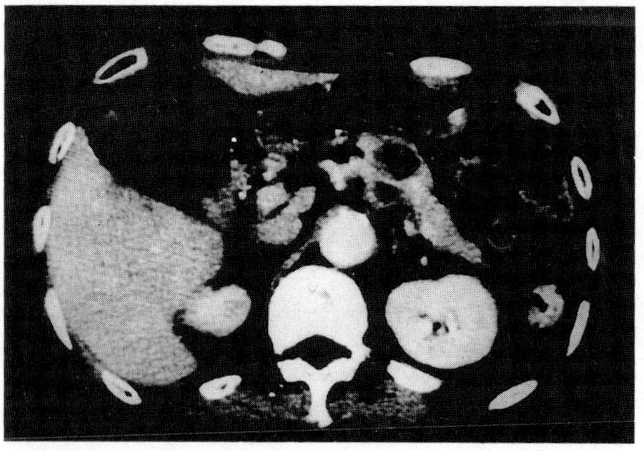

Fig. 1. "Pure" squamous cell carcinoma of the pancreas. A computed tomography (CT) scan shows a tumor with an irregular margin and a central cystic space. The patient was a 73-year-old man with a 23-year history of diabetes mellitus. He was admitted to the hospital with poor control of blood glucose levels. A tumor in the body of the pancreas was detected by both ultrasound (US) and CT scan. Endoscopic retrograde cholangiopancreatography (ERCP) showed no abnormality of the main pancreatic duct, but celiac angiography showed encasement of the left gastric artery. CT scan showed a tumor with an irregular margin and a central cyst. At operation, the tumor was adherent to the surrounding tissues by dense connective tissue. The distal two-thirds of the pancreas, spleen, and regional lymph nodes were removed

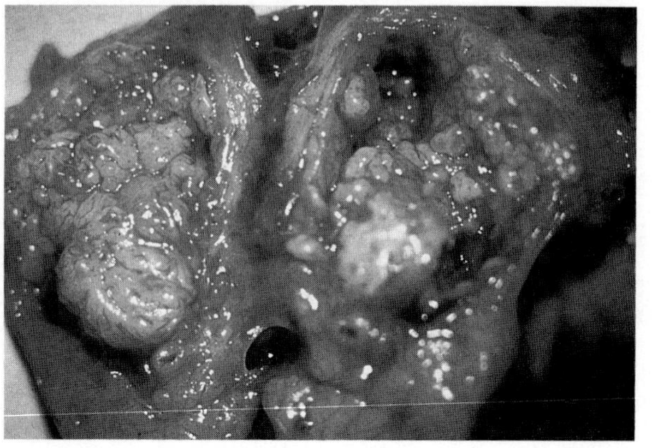

Fig. 2. The cut surface of a squamous cell carcinoma of the pancreas (same case as in Fig. 1). The tumor was adherent to the surrounding tissues by dense connective tissue. (*For color reproduction see color insert in the frontmatter*)

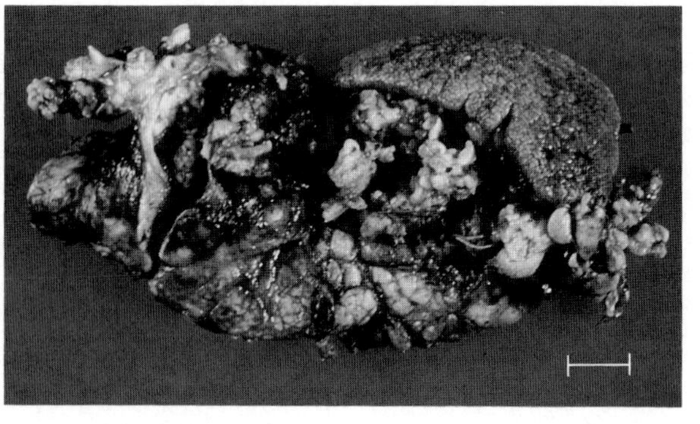

Fig. 3. The same case as in Fig. 2. The protruding tumor located in the pancreatic body was well-circumscribed with a fibrous capsule, measuring 3.2 × 2.8 × 3 cm, situated in the pancreas body and about 2.5 cm from the proximal stump. (*For color reproduction see color insert in the frontmatter*)

Macroscopic Findings

The macroscopic appearance of squamous cell carcinoma resembles that of ductal cell carcinoma. Some tumors present with a well-circumscribed fibrous capsule. Tumors occur in the head (73%), body (45%), and tail (23%); about 95% of patients show evidence of disseminated or locally metastatic disease [8]. The cut surface is often grainy, grayish-white, and resembles squamous cell carcinoma of other tissues. Some tumors show a fibrous connective tissue and multiple septa with a thick cheesy content, possibly representing keratinaceous debris. The main pancreatic duct is generally preserved, but communication of the duct with the central cavity of the tumors has been seen in one case [8]. Calcified areas were seen in a case of cystic squamous cell carcinoma [8]. We observed a tumor in which the cut surface of the tumor showed papillary growth along the inner surface of the irregular central cavity (Figs. 2–4).

In squamous cell carcinoma, the central area of the tumor tends to become necrotic; there are many cases of the tumor forming central cavitation (Figs. 2, 4).

Microscopic Findings

"Pure" squamous cell carcinoma is composed of malignant squamous cells that are usually well-differentiated. No adenocarcinoma element can

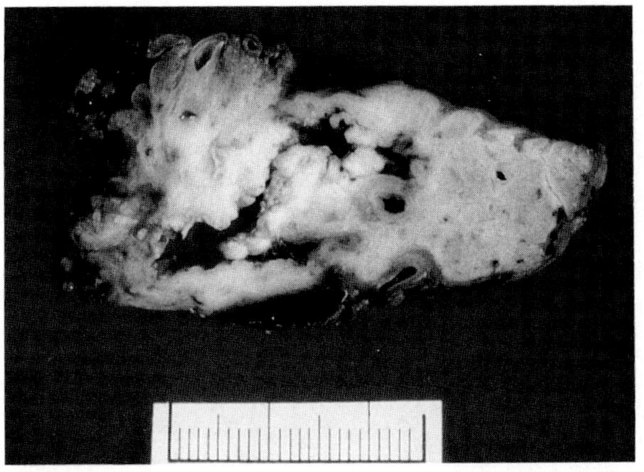

Fig. 4. Cut section of the tumor in Fig. 3 after fixation in formalin. Nodules protruding from the inner surface of the irregular central cavity

be found even with complete examination of the tumor by serial sectioning. No mucin can be found within the tumor. The necrotic areas may form cavities, the wall of which can show focal squamous lining and abundant keratinaceous debris in the presumed lumen (Fig. 5). The fibrous wall is infiltrated by malignant epithelial cells and shows tongues and nests with central keratinization (Fig. 6). The cells are oval or spindle-shaped with eosinophilic cytoplasm, hyperchromatic nuclei, and prominent nucleoli. Loss of differentiation can be seen in some areas (Fig. 7) and desquamation of malignant epithelium lining the cavity may also be seen (Fig. 8). Focal calcification of the stroma has been found in an unusual case of squamous cell carcinoma [8]. Capsular, lymphatic, and venous invasions are usually present. The main pancreatic duct is free or shows communication with the cavity of some tumors. Several foci of squamous metaplasia and hyperplastic epithelium in some of the intralobular ducts in the surrounding lobules may be present.

Immunohistochemistry

Tumor cells react with antikeratin antibody (Fig. 9). There are no detailed reports on immunohistochemical staining of this tumor or on its molecular biology.

Diagnosis and Differential Diagnosis

A careful histological examination of the tumor is essential to differentiate squamous cell carcinoma from adenosquamous cell carcinoma. This differentiation is important because of the poorer prognosis of squamous cell carcinoma (see Chapter "Adenosquamous Cell Carcinoma" in this volume). Some cases of well-differentiated squamous cell carcinoma may present problems in distinguishing the malignant cells from squamous cell metaplasia. The cavitation in these tumors is thought to be a relatively frequent complication. Its pathogenesis

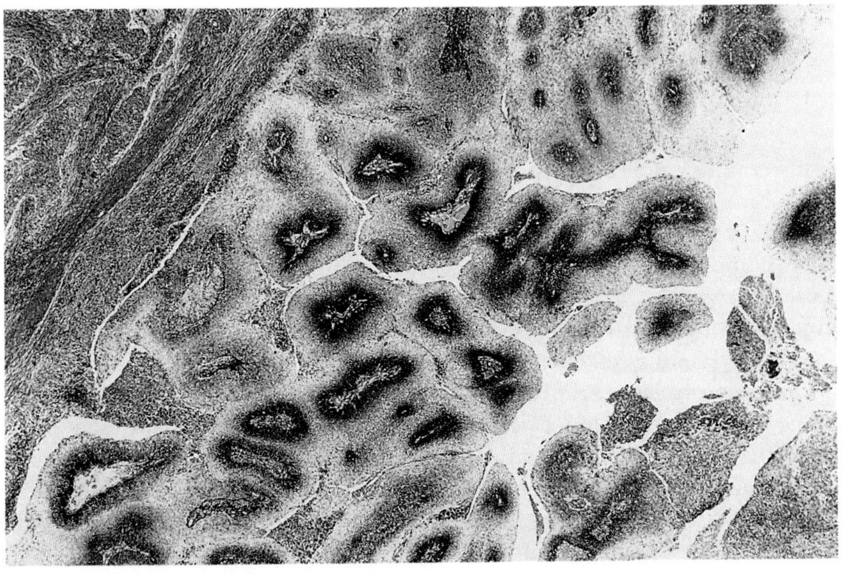

Fig. 5. Microscopic appearance of the same tumor in Fig. 4. Carcinoma cells form a papillary structure and line an irregularly shaped cavity. Marked lymphocytic reaction is seen (*left*) H&E, ×15

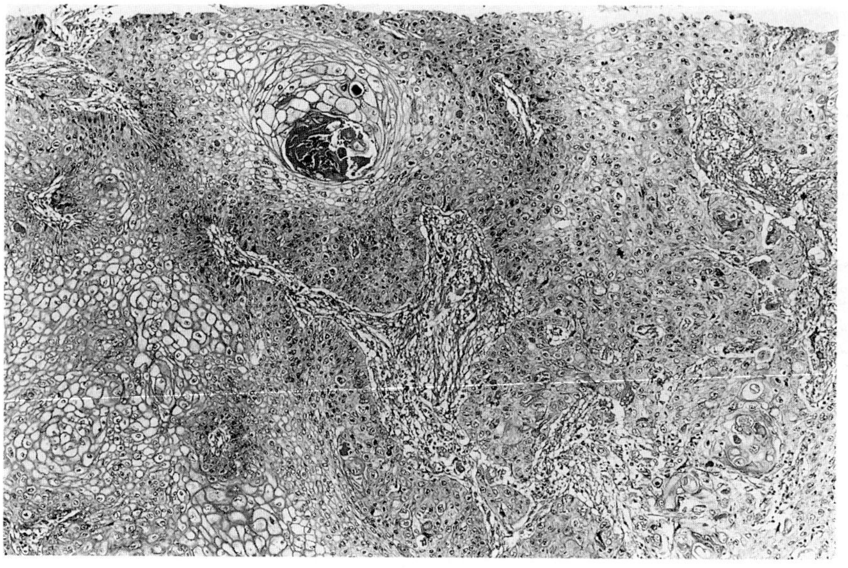

Fig. 6. Another area of the same tumor in Fig. 5. Keratinizing well-differentiated squamous cell carcinoma. There is no glandular differentiation or mucus production. No Alcian blue or periodic acid Schiff (PAS) positivity appears in any part of the tumor. H&E, ×120

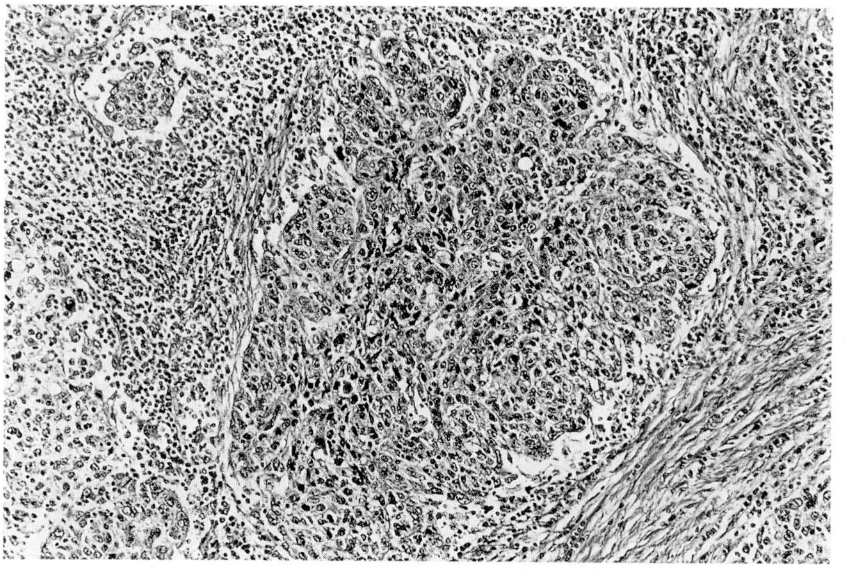

Fig. 7. Another region of the tumor in Fig. 5 depicting a poorly differentiated area of squamous cell carcinoma surrounded by a heavy inflammatory reaction. No intraductal spread was observed in the remaining pancreatic tissue. H&E, ×120

still remains unclear, but there are three possibilities. First, the tumor may develop within a preexisting pseudocyst wall. Second, the degeneration of squamous cell carcinoma may have resulted in cyst formation, and the immunohistochemical finding of cytokeratin suggests that the degeneration of squamous cell carcinoma can cause marked granulation of the capsule. Third, the tumor may have primarily developed as a cystic tumor, with growth due to the combination of proliferation of tumor cells and development of granulation tissue. There are some cases of pure squamous cell carcinoma of the pancreas with papillary growth associated with cavity formation, and many of these are thought to represent the development of carcinoma within a pseudocyst. In these cases, the coexistence of pure squamous cell carcinoma and cyst formation does not seem to be an incidental finding. Differential diagnosis may be important with cyst-forming carcinomas and other cystic lesions (see Chapter "Serous Cystadenoma" in this volume). Metastases of squamous cell carcinoma of other tissues, particularly of the lung, and primary squamous cell carcinoma of the pancreas could present some difficulties and require clinical information.

Fig. 8. In places, the carcinoma cells are detached from the cavity wall, and associated with granuloma formation containing numerous foreign body giant cells. The same tumor as in Fig. 5. H&E, ×15

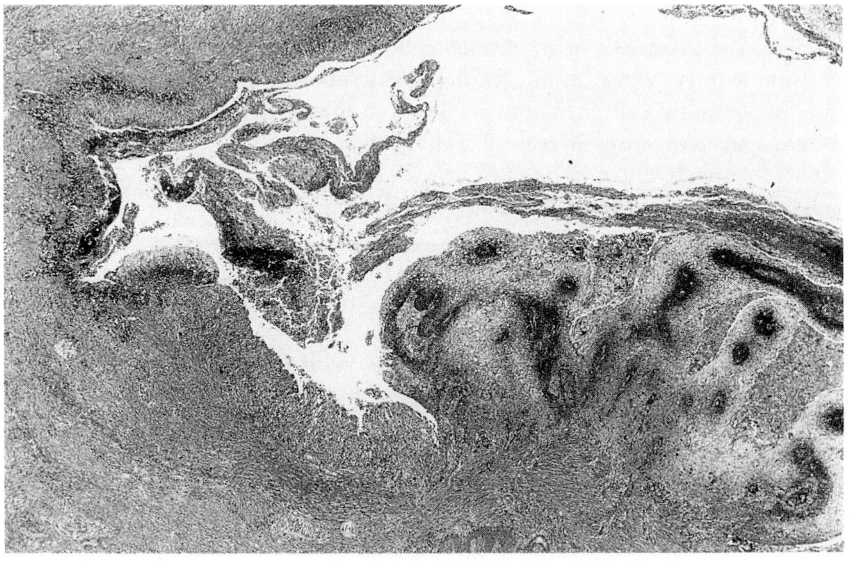

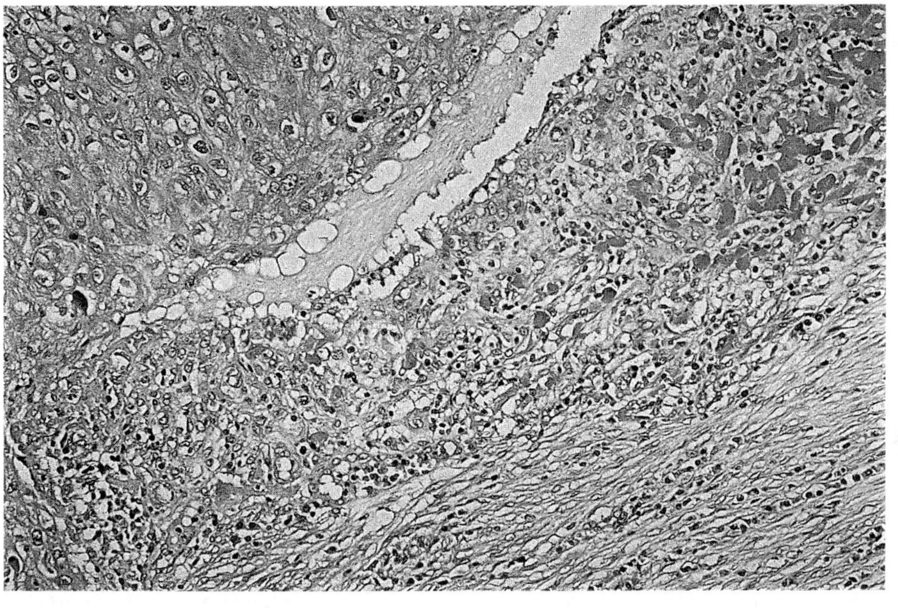

Fig. 9. Immunohistochemistry for cytokeratin revealed a positive reaction in squamous cell carcinoma cells, in the remaining keratinocytes, and in the breakdown products of keratohyalin in the surrounding granulation tissue. This may indicate that the granulation tissue developed secondary to the degeneration of squamous cell carcinoma. Immunohistochemistry with anti-cytokeratin antibody, ×120. (*For color reproduction see color insert in the frontmatter*)

Biology, Prognosis, and Survival

Biological behavior of squamous cell carcinoma of the pancreas is worse than the more common ductal adenocarcinoma. Squamous cell carcinoma metastasizes primarily to regional lymph nodes, the liver, and the lung [7, 15], with a mean survival from the time of diagnosis similar to that for pancreatic adenocarcinoma [15]. About 95% of the patients show evidence of disseminated or locally metastatic disease during the initial evaluation or at laparotomy. According to the registration of the

Pancreatic Cancer Registry of the Japan Pancreas Society, the prognosis of squamous cell carcinoma is significantly worse than those of ductal and adenosquamous cell carcinomas. The cumulative 1-year survival rates were 10.5%, 19.8%, and 30.8%, respectively, and no patient with squamous cell carcinoma survived 3 years (see Table 7 in Chapter "Adenosquamous Cell Carcinoma" in this volume). This may be due to a high prevalence of lymphatic invasion (100%), venous invasion (77.8%), and neural-perineural invasion (100%), Neither chemotherapy nor radiation has been of benefit, although an objective response to bleomycin has been seen in one patient [16]. As defined by Ravry et al. [16], the criteria for an objective response are: (a) a decrease of at least 50% in the size of the longest perpendicular diameters of the most clearly measurable area of known malignant disease or, if malignant hepatomegaly is the indicator, a decrease of 30% in the sum of measurements below the xyphoid process and both costal margins at the midclavicular lines during quiet respiration; (b) no increase in the size of other areas; and (c) no new areas of disease.

References

1. Baylor SM, Berg JW (1973) Cross-classification and survival characteristics of 5000 cases of cancer of the pancreas. J Surg Oncol 5:335–358
2. Chen J, Baithun SI (1985) Morphological study of 391 cases of exocrine pancreatic tumors with special reference to the classification of exocrine pancreatic carcinoma. J Pathol 146:17–29
3. Cubilla AL, Fitzgerald PJ (1979) Cancer of the pancreas (nonendocrine): A suggested morphological classification. Semin Oncol 6:285–297
4. Mikal S, Campbell AJA (1950) Carcinoma of the pancreas. Diagnostic and operative criteria based on 100 consecutive autopsies. Surgery 28:963–969
5. Miller JR, Baggenstoss AH, Comfort MW (1951) Carcinoma of the pancreas: Effect of histological type and grade of malignancy on its behavior. Cancer 4:233–241
6. Morohoshi T, Held G, Klöppel G (1983) Exocrine pancreatic tumours and their histological classification: A study based on 167 autopsy and 97 surgical cases. Histopathology 7:645–661
7. Halpert B, Makk L, Jordan GL Jr (1965) A retrospective study of 120 patients with carcinoma of the pancreas. Surg Gynecol Obstet 121:91–96
8. Beyer KL, Marshall JB, Metzler MH, Poulter JS, Seger RM, Diza-Arias AA (1992) Squamous cell carcinoma of the pancreas: Report of an unusual case and review of the literature. Dig Dis Sci 37: 312–318
9. Sprayregen S, Scoenbaum SW, Messinger NH (1975) Angiographic features of squamous cell carcinoma of the pancreas. J Can Assoc Radiol 26:122–124
10. Gray RK, Rösch J, Grollman JH Jr (1970) Arteriography in the diagnosis of islet-cell tumor. Radiology 97:39–44
11. Abrams RM, Beranbaum ER, Beranbaum SL (1967) Angiographic studies of benign and malignant cystadenoma of the pancreas. Radiology 89:1028–1032
12. Rösch J, Bret J (1965) Angiography of the pancreas. Am J Roentgenol 94:182–193
13. Meaney TF, Buonocore E (1965) Arteriographic manifestation of pancreatic neoplasm. Am J Roentgenol 95:720–726
14. Brayko CM, Doll DC (1982) Squamous cell carcinoma of the pancreas associated with hypercalcemia. Gastroenterology 83:1297–1299
15. Sears HF, Kim Y, Strawitz J (1980) Squamous cell carcinoma of the pancreas. J Surg Oncol 14:261–265
16. Ravry M, Moertel CG, Schutt AJ (1973) Treatment of advanced squamous cell carcinoma of the gastrointestinal tract with bleomycin. Cancer Chemother Rep 57:493–495
17. Shariff S, Thomas JA (1989) Adenosquamous carcinoma of the pancreas: A case report with literature review. Indian J Pathol Microbiol 32:62–65

Anaplastic (Undifferentiated) Carcinoma

Synonyms and Related Terms

Pleomorphic carcinoma, giant cell carcinoma, osteoclastoma, spindle cell carcinoma, sarcomatoid carcinoma, carcinosarcoma, anaplastic carcinoma, undifferentiated carcinoma.

Definition

Anaplastic carcinoma is a relatively rare pancreatic neoplasm. It was first described in 1954 [1], and about 100 cases have been reported. Pleomorphic giant cell carcinoma is composed of pleomorphic giant cells and/or undifferentiated spindle cells. Some histomorphological and immunohistochemical findings point to their origin from ductal cells. Giant cell tumors are often divided into pleomorphic and osteoclastic types. A few cases containing a mixture of both pleomorphic and osteoclastic giant cells have been reported [2–7].

Incidence, Age, and Sex

Data from Japanese and American literature relative to the tumor incidence, age, and sex of the patients are listed in Table 1. There are no significant differences in these parameters between the two countries. These neoplasms usually occur in elderly people. In the United States, giant cell tumors account for 2%–13% of all nonendocrine pancreatic carcinomas, with the osteoclastic type being rarer than the pleomorphic type [8]. The mean age of the U.S. patients with pancreatic giant cell tumors is 67 years (range 43 to 82 years), with males affected more than females.

Clinical Presentation

Presenting symptoms are nonspecific and include abdominal pain, back pain, weight loss, nausea, vomiting, jaundice, and occasional recent onset of diabetes mellitus. In a 72-year-old male patient with mixed pleomorphic and osteoclastic giant cells, episodes of acute cholangitis with jaundice, fever, and chills were additional complaints [5]. In this patient, a mass could be palpated in the epigastrium. Pathological laboratory findings included increased serum titer of transaminase (twofold), alkaline phosphatase (twofold), and gammaglutamyl transpeptidase (sixfold). The serum concentrations of carcinoembryonic antigen (CEA), CA19-9, and CA50 were all within the normal range [5] as were amylase and lipase levels.

Clinical Diagnosis

Radiologic, computed tomographic (CT), ultrasound (US), or angiographic findings are similar to those seen in ductal cell carcinoma. Both US and CT usually show a mass in the pancreatic head. Dilatation of the biliary tract may be present. Endoscopic retrograde cholangiopancreatography (ERCP) may demonstrate gross enlargement and irregularity of Vater's papilla. Selective angiography usually does not show any abnormalities, but laparotomy may disclose lymphatic and hepatic metastases.

Table 1. Anaplastic carcinoma of the pancreas.

	No. of cases	Age median (years)	Sex (no.)	M/F ratio	Site (%)	Size median (cm)	Survival median (months)	Survival 1-year
Japan[a]	16	64	M: 11 F: 5	2.2	H: 50 BT: 50	6	4	18
U.S.A.[b]	27	62	M: 16[c] F: 11	1.5	H: 50 BT: 50	11	2	0

[a] Japan cases: 1981–1990 in Showa University School of Medicine.
[b] U.S.A. cases: 1949–1978 in Memorial Hospital, New York (see [3]).
[c] For giant cell tumor the ratio is 4:1.
H, head; B, body; T, tail.

Gross Findings

Anaplastic carcinomas are generally large, ranging from 3 to 18 cm [3] and are often associated with hemorrhagic necrosis. Hemorrhagic cyst formation is often observed in the tumor. The anatomic location of the tumors is listed in Table 1.

Histological Findings

The microscopic appearance of anaplastic tumors is striking. They may be composed of pleomorphic mononucleated and multinucleated cells and often with bizarre giant cells (Fig. 1). Histologically, two types of giant cell tumors are distinguished: pleomorphic and osteoclastic. In the pleomorphic type, the giant cells exhibit bizarre cytologic features (Figs. 1, 2), with marked cellular pleomorphism, hyperchromatic nuclei, coarsely clumped chromatin, and prominent nucleoli. There may be cannibalism of tumor cells (Fig. 3) and abnormal mitoses. The cytoplasm of the tumor cell is abundant, dense, eosinophilic, and sometimes contains vacuoles. Hemosiderin and erythrocytes are sometimes seen in the cytoplasm of the giant cells. Spindle cells and small round cells with little cytoplasm are often observed in this tumor, but the number of these cells is few. However, in some cases, major components show spindle and sarcomatous cells (Fig. 4). This type of carcinoma is sometimes called carcinosarcoma. Connective tissue is generally scant in this type of tumor, and tumor cells usually form solid nests and show invasion into the surrounding tissue. The formation of irregular-shaped ducts suggests that this

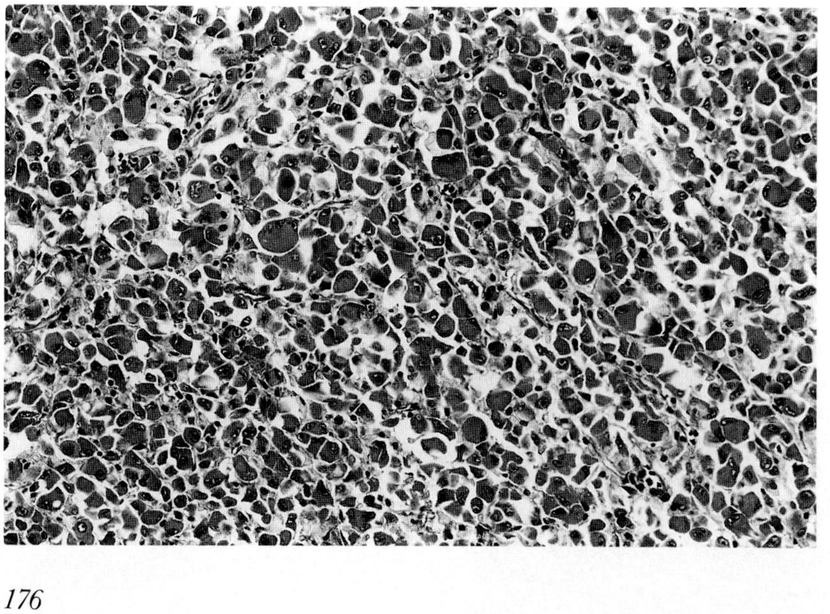

Fig. 1. Tumor cells with mono- or multinucleated cells with hyperchromatic nuclei and abundant cytoplasm. No evidence of ductal differentiation is present in this area. (H&E ×200)

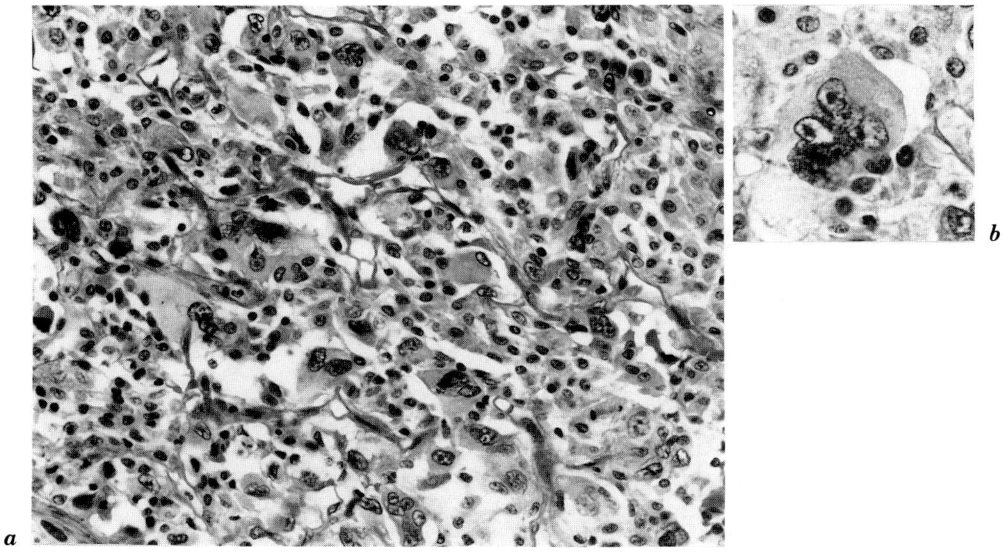

Fig. 2. ***a*** A pleomorphic giant cell carcinoma composed of giant cells and monomorphic stromal cells (H&E ×250). ***b*** High-power view of a multinucleated giant cell showing abundant foamy cytoplasm, irregular nuclei, and prominent nucleoli. (H&E ×400)

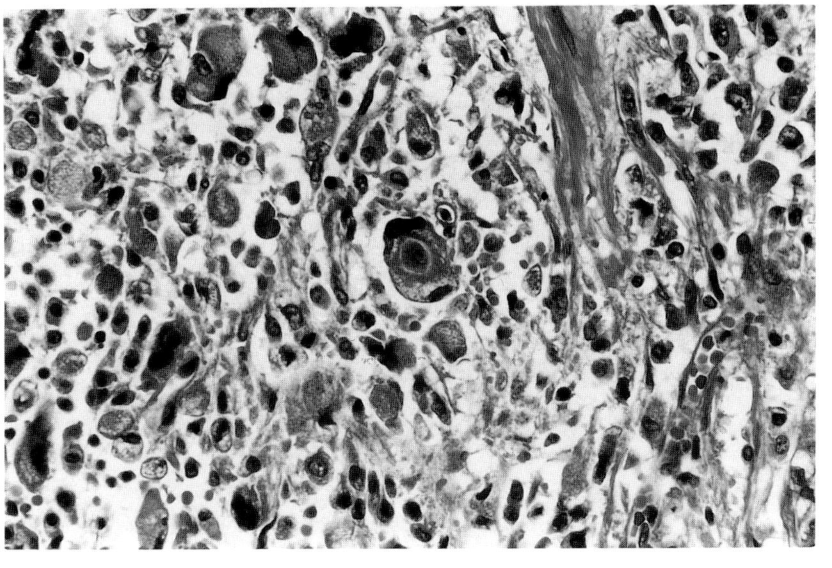

Fig. 3. A pleomorphic giant cell carcinoma depicting a giant cell with an engulfed cell in its cytoplasm (*center*). (H&E ×300)

tumor arises from pancreatic ductal epithelium. Cytological examination of fine needle aspirates reveals multinucleated giant cells with clustered, overlapping, and uniform nuclei that show prominent nucleoli [8, 9].

The histological features of osteoclast-like giant cells are identical to giant cell tumors of bone (Fig. 5). The giant tumor cells have irregular nuclei with large prominent nucleoli and course granular chromatin. The multinucleated giant cells may contain up to 100 nuclei, which are oval, vesicular, and bland in appearance and may contain one to two nucleoli. The nuclei of the stromal cells resemble those of the osteoclast-like giant cells. In some osteoclastic giant cell carcinomas, osteoid formation in the stroma can be found and the mononuclear cells contain osteonectin, a noncollagenous protein that is characteristic of osteoblasts [10–12].

A few reported tumors contained both pleomorphic and osteoclast-like giant cells. Such a tumor was recently reported in a 72-year-old man and was composed of three cell types: large pleomorphic anaplastic cells, giant osteoclast-like ele-

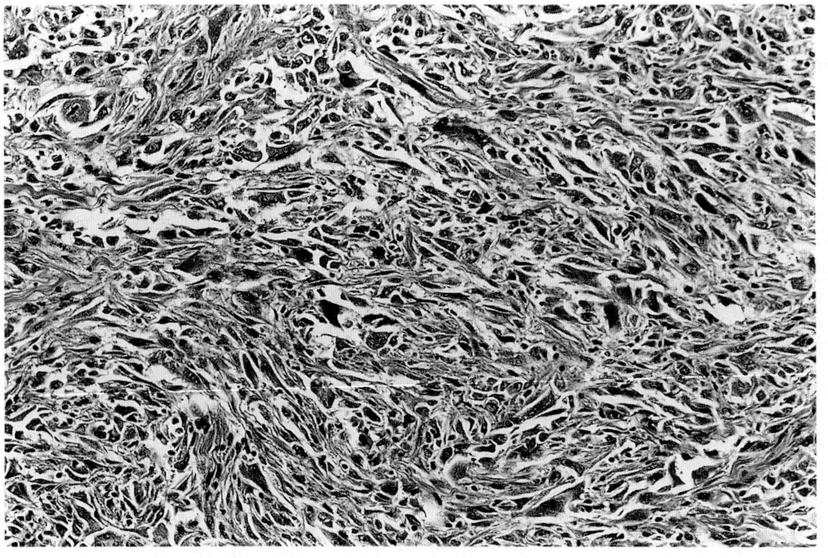

Fig. 4. A pleomorphic giant cell carcinoma with interlacing cells forming sarcomatous pattern. (H&E ×200)

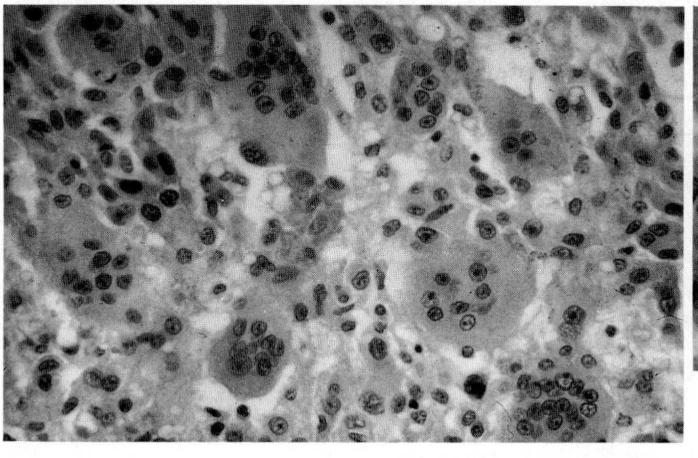

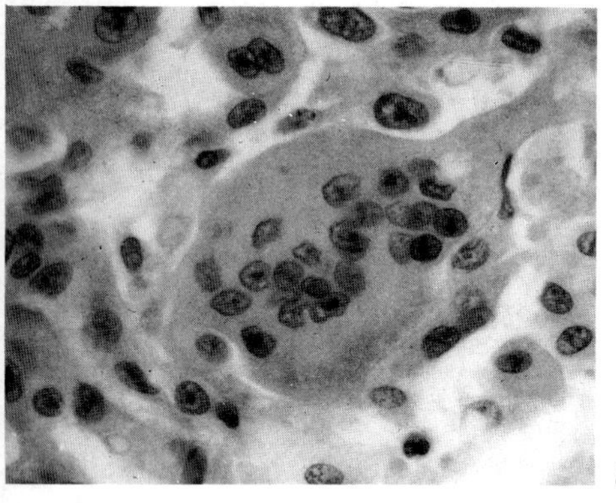

Fig. 5. a Osteoclastic giant cell tumor is composed of multinucleated giant cells in a mononuclear stroma (H&E ×400). ***b*** High-power view of a giant cell with more than 20 nuclei. (H&E ×500)

ments, and mononucleated spindle, fibroblast-like cells. The pleomorphic giant cells had multiple irregular and often vacuolated nuclei and abundant cytoplasm containing hemosiderin or engulfed erythrocytes. They frequently showed mitosis with many abnormal forms. The osteoclastic giant cells were either interspersed between the giant anaplastic cells (Fig. 6) or formed cell aggregates around foci of osteoid-osseous tissue (Fig. 7). The mononucleated spindle cells were arranged in nodular areas or were admixed with the osteoclastic cells. In numerous step sections from the block, a few glandular structures could be detected but only in one microscopic field.

In two recently reported pleomorphic-osteoclastic giant cell carcinomas [6], the osteoclast-like giant cells were frequently found around the necrotic and hemorrhagic areas admixed with mononuclear macrophages; no mitoses were found in these cells, many of which had phagocytized debris in their cytoplasm (Fig. 8). In some areas of both tumors, glandular structures in varying degrees of differentiation were present (Fig. 9). No foci of osteoid or bone formation were identified, but blood vessel invasion was seen in both cases. Lymph node metastases in one of the cases showed the same histological pattern.

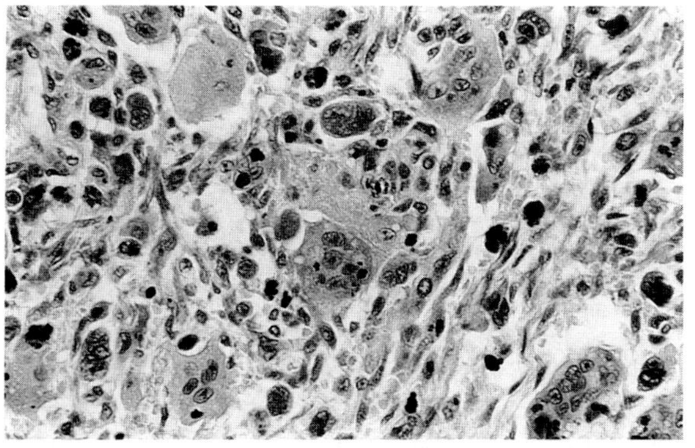

Fig. 6. Osteoclast-like giant cells interspersed between anaplastic cells (H&E ×400). This tumor was found in a 72-year-old man. The 6 × 4 × 5 cm reddish, multilobulated soft neoplasm in the pancreas head had invaded the surrounding tissues. The tumor showed necrotic and hemorrhagic areas

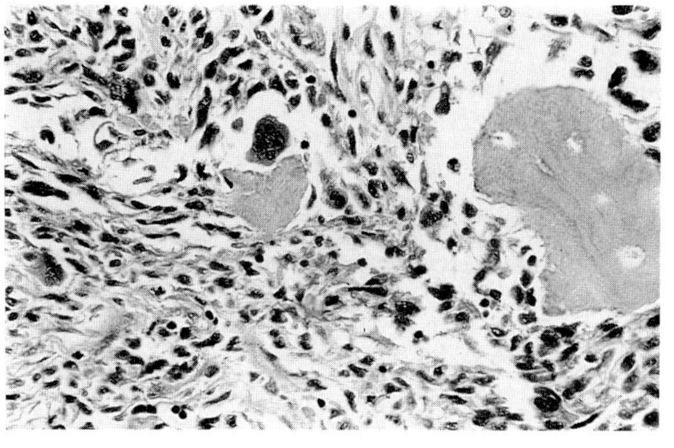

Fig. 7. Foci of osseous metaplastic material surrounded by spindle cells and giant cells (H&E ×400). The same tumor as in Fig. 6

Electron Microscopic Findings

The electron microscopic features of osteoclast-like giant cell carcinomas of the pancreas were first reported by Rosai in 1968 [13]. Microvilli were observed on giant cell surfaces and desmosomes between mononuclear stromal cells, features suggestive of an epithelial origin. In addition, the presence of abundant rough endoplasmic reticulum with intracisternal dense granules suggested an acinar cell origin. However, rough endoplasmic reticulum with dense condensations, and junctions have been reported in mesenchymal tumors and both microvilli and desmosomes may occur in giant cell tumors of bone. Others have reported abundant mitochondria, surface ruffling, filopodia and occasionally desmosomes, findings similar to those in mesenchymal bone osteoclasts [14]. Well-developed Golgi apparatus, scattered lysosomes, and intracytoplasmic aggregates of intermediate filaments were found in two cases with benign-appearing osteoclast-like cells [6]. In the latter giant cells, no junctional complexes or desmosomes were found. Their cytoplasmic membrane was irregular, and scanty filopodia were observed (Fig. 10).

The mononuclear stromal cells of osteoclast-like giant cell carcinomas have been divided into A and B type cells [14]. Type A cells are polygonal with abundant mitochondria, whereas type B cells are elongated, resembling fibroblasts, and exhibit dilated cisternae of rough endoplasmic reticulum filled with fine granular material. Both type A and B cells have extensive filopodia.

Immunohistochemical Findings

The results of immunohistochemical studies of giant cell tumors of the pancreas have been conflicting. The presence of keratin and epithelial membrane antigen (Fig. 11) in the tumor giant cells suggests an epithelial origin. Although vimentin has been found in some cases (Fig. 11), keratin or epithelial membrane antigen was missing in others [7]. Lysozyme, α_1-antitrypsin, α_1-antichymotrypsin, leucocyte common antigen, CD 68, CEA, and CA19-9 may be present in some cases. In other instances, most cancer cells were stained negatively with anti-CEA antibody or anti-CA19-9 antibody, but a few cells showed immunoreactivity with these antibodies. Amylase was negative.

The immunohistochemical findings of a case with a mixed pleomorphic-osteoclast-like giant cell tumor are summarized in Table 2 and illustrated in Fig. 11. Those observed in two cases with benign-appearing osteoclast-like cells are summarized in Table 3. In the latter two cases, the osteoclast-like cells did not react with epithelial cell markers, CA 19-9 or CEA, but showed a strong reactivity with mesenchymal cell markers (Fig. 12), as did the surrounding macrophages; none of the cells expressed chromogranin A, lipase, trypsin, α_1-antitrypsin, lysozyme, or S-100 protein [6].

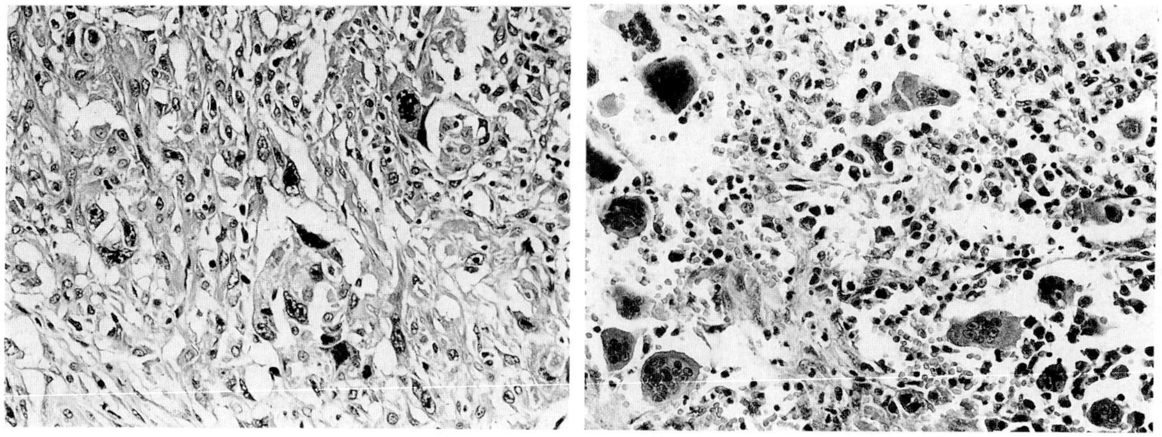

Fig. 8. A mixed pleomorphic/osteoclast-like giant cell carcinoma of the pancreas in a 70-year-old man, who was admitted to the hospital because of epigastric pain of 1 month duration. Computed tomography (CT) and ultrasound (US) showed a large mass (5.5 × 6.5 × 4.5 cm) in the pancreatic head. Carcinoembryonic antigen (CEA), CA 19-9, amylase and lipase levels were normal. Grossly, the cut surface of the tumor was soft, reddish-brown, and hemorrhagic with focally whitish-grey and solid areas at the periphery. The tumor had invaded the surrounding pancreatic parenchyma and obliterated the common bile duct. ***a*** Histologically, the tumor was composed of mononuclear and multinucleated cells simulating sarcoma (H&E ×87). ***b*** A tumor from a 72-year-old Japanese man with a 7.0 × 5.0 × 4.0 cm tumor in the pancreatic head. The laboratory finding was similar to the case in Fig. 8***a***. Microscopically, numerous benign-appearing multinucleated giant cells with many nuclei and prominent small nucleoli were seen (H&E ×100). From [6] with permission

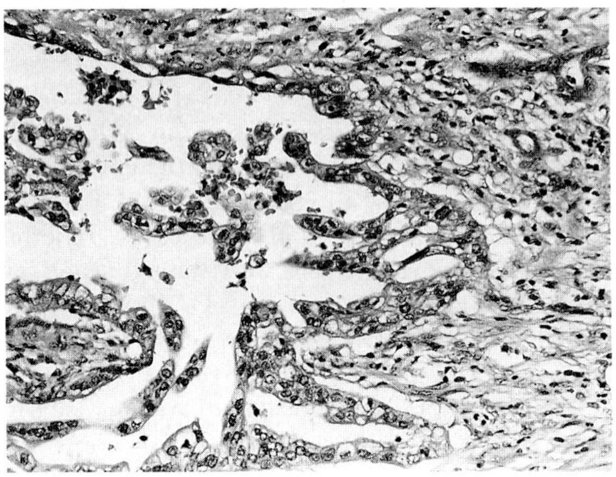

Fig. 9. The same case as in Fig. 8***b***. Tumor cells form glandular structures with papillary patterns (H&E ×87). From [6] with permission

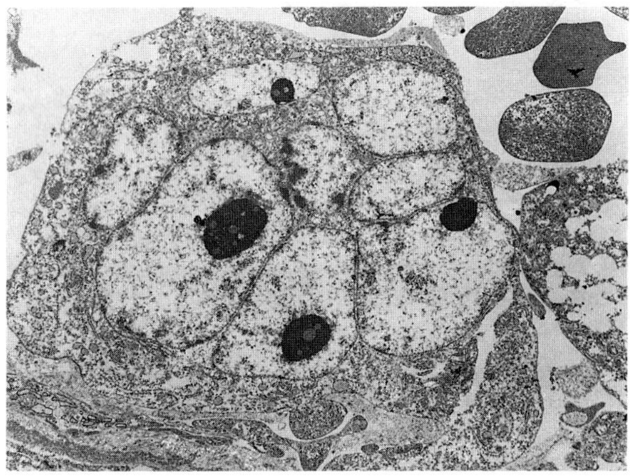

Fig. 10. Electron microscopic finding of an osteoclast-like giant cell tumor. The giant cell has eight nuclei with prominent nucleoli. The cytoplasm is rich in mitochondria and rough endoplasmic reticulum. The same case as in Fig. 8***a*** (×1827). From [6] with permission

Histogenesis

Pleomorphic giant cell carcinoma of the pancreas is generally thought to arise from ductal epithelium and is frequently associated with conventional adenocarcinoma. While pleomorphic giant cell carcinoma may demonstrate mucin production and glandular structures consistent with a ductal epithelial origin [15, 16], the histogenesis of osteoclast-like giant cell tumor of the pancreas is controversial. Most authors favor an epithelial origin based on a combination of microscopic (adenoid differentiation), ultrastructural, and immunohistochemical findings [9, 14–21]. In 1977, Robinson reported a case with cells having ultrastructural

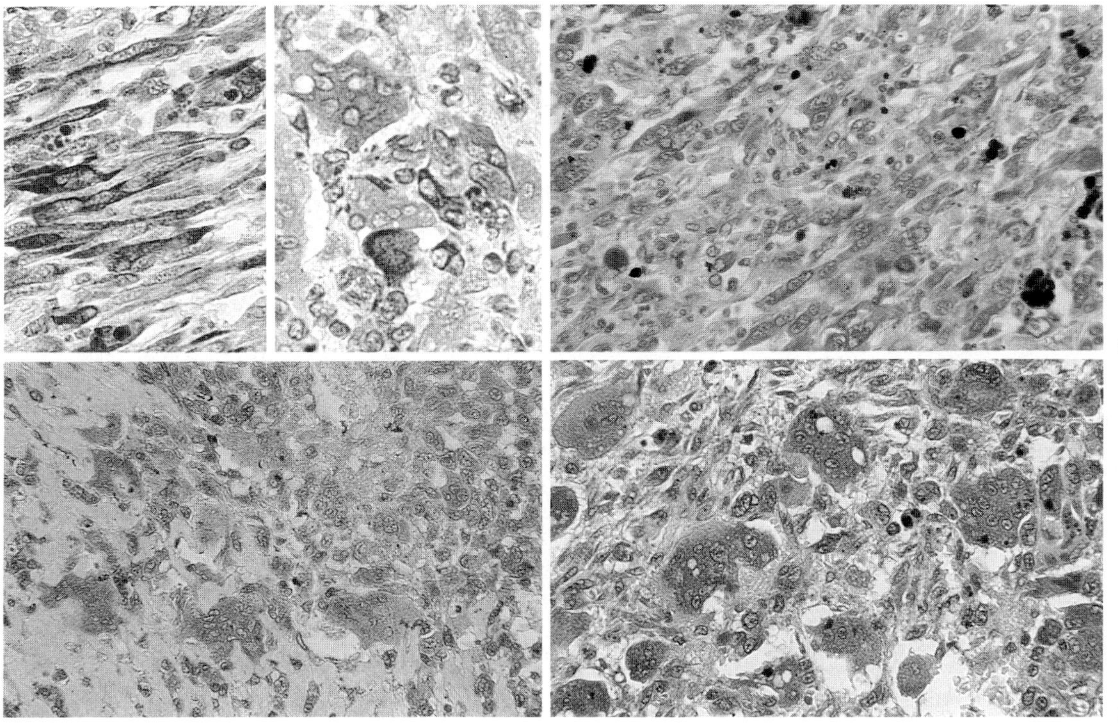

Fig. 11a–d. Immunohistochemical pattern of a mixed giant cell tumor of the pancreas. ***a*** A strong immunoreactivity of osteoclast-like and spindle cells with anti-vimentin; ***b*** a weak reactivity of tumor cells with HMFG2 antibody; ***c*** reactivity of some anaplastic cells with CAM 5.2 antibody; ***d*** NSE positivity in anaplastic and osteoclast-like cells. See also Table 2. The same tumor as in Figs. 5 and 7

features of bone osteoclasts, but suggested that these findings could be an expression of a lesser degree of cellular differentiation rather than an indication of a mesenchymal origin [14]. Berendt et al. [22] described positive staining for CEA (polyclonal) and low molecular weight keratin, but were unable to demonstrate any staining for histiocytic markers. On the other hand, Fisher et al. [23], Goldberg et al. [24] and Nojima et al. [6] observed a strong reactivity of giant cells with anti-vimentin or other mesenchymal cell markers but not with epithelial cell markers. Consequently, Berendt et al. concluded an epithelial origin, whereas the other three groups favored mesenchymal differentiation.

Pleomorphic giant cell tumors of the pancreas may be best regarded as arising from a precursor cell capable of differentiating along divergent lines and giving rise to a spectrum of morphologic, immunohistochemical, and ultrastructural phenotypes [5, 7]. Experimental data strongly support this. Among the induced pancreatic ductal/ductular cancers in Syrian hamsters, both pleomorphic and osteoclast-like giant cell carcinomas could be observed occasionally [25]. Both cell types expressed blood group A antigen which is expressed in altered pancreatic ductal/ductular cells [25]. Cubilla and Fitzgerald have suggested that both types of giant cell tumors may represent opposite ends of the biologic spectrum of a single type of neoplasm, the latter being more biologically aggressive [3]. This theory is further supported by reports of mixed osteoclastic and pleomorphic giant cell tumors [2–5, 7] and immunohistochemical findings. The positive reactivity of pleomorphic and osteoclast-like giant cells and stromal cells in some tumors with anti-NSE suggests also a neuroendocrine differentiation. Moreover, the absence of reactivity with lysozyme and LCA argues against a macrophagic origin of the osteoclast-like cells. However, some reports have indicated positive staining for leucocyte common antigen and CD68 consistent with either bone osteoclasts or histiocytes. Based on these and other findings, it appears that in some tumors the osteoclast-like cells are of histiocytic-macrophage lineage.

Table 2. Immunophenotype of mixed giant cell tumor of the pancreas.

Primary antibody	Antigen specificity	Anaplastic giant cells[a]	Osteoclastic-like giant cells[a]	Spindle cells[a]
CAM 5.2	Keratin polypeptides 39-43-50 Kd	++/+	−	++
AE1/AE3	KP 50-56, 5-58-65-67 Kd	+	−	++
34BB4	KP68 Kd	−	−	−
CEA 85 A 12	CEA	−		−
HMFG2		++	+/−	++
Vimentin V9	Vimentin	+++	+++	+++
Desmin D33	Desmin	+/− focal	+/− focal −	−
HHF35	Actin 42 Kd isotype α and γ	−	−	−
vWf	FVIII	−	−	−
LCA PD7/26 and2B11	Human leukocyte common antigen	−	−	−
Antihuman lysozyme	Lysozyme	−	−	−
α-fetoprotein 946:11	α-fetoprotein	−	−	−
Antihuman hCG	Chorionic gonadotropin	−	−	−
Anticow S100	S100 protein	−	−	−
MAS346c MIG-N3	Neuron-specific γ enolase	++	++	+ focal
Synaptophysin SY 38	Synaptophysin	++	++	++

[a] +++, strong positivity; ++, middle positivity; +, weak positivity; hCG, human chorionic gonadotropin.

Table 3. Immunohistochemical reactivity of mixed pleomorphic-osteoclast-like giant cell carcinoma of the pancreas.

	Case 1			Case 2		
Antibody	PC	EP	OGC	PC	EP	OGC
Keratin wide	+++	+++	−	+++	+++	−
Keratin AE1	+++	+++	−	+++	+++	−
CEA	−	−	−	−	+	−
CA 19-9	−	−	−	−	+	−
Vimentin	+++	+	+++	++	+	+++
KPI	−	−	+++	−	−	+++
PG-M1	−	−	+++	−	−	+++

PC, pleomorphic mononuclear and multinuclear tumor cells; EP, epithelial tumor cells; OGC, osteoclast-like giant cells; −, negative; +, slightly positive; ++, moderate immunoreactivity (20%–50% of cells stained); +++, intense immunoreactivity (>50% of cells stained); KPI, CD68 (Dako), 1:50; PG-M1, CD68 (Dako), 1:100.
From Nojima et al. [6].

Differential Diagnosis

Anaplastic carcinomas should be differentiated histologically from other mesenchymal or epithelial tumors containing giant and spindle cells such as rhabdomyosarcoma, undifferentiated sarcoma, malignant melanoma, choriocarcinoma, and metastatic giant cell carcinoma of the lung, thyroid, kidney, or other organs. The presence of melanin pigment, melanosomes, or melanocyte immunohistochemical markers in melanoma is helpful for diagnosis. In rhabdomyosarcoma, the presence of striations is important and immunohistochemical staining for actin or desmin is helpful for diagnosis. Giant cell carcinoma of the lung is not a rare tumor but its metastasis to the pancreas is uncommon. The presence of carcinoma in situ in the pancreatic duct epithelium, gross findings, and clinical features may be needed for correct diagnosis.

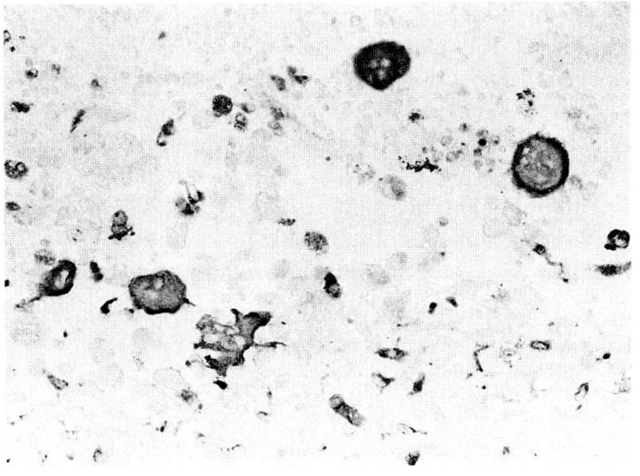

Fig. 12. Immunohistochemical demonstration of KP1. Positively stained multinucleated osteoclast-like giant cells and any mononuclear macrophages. (ABC method, ×87)

Prognosis and Survival

The prognosis of anaplastic carcinoma of the pancreas is generally worse than that of ductal carcinomas. The prognosis depends on the histomorphology. Pleomorphic giant cell carcinoma behaves as an aggressive tumor with early lymph node involvement, disseminated metastases, and rapid death. The average survival is 2–7 months and the 1-year survival rate is 0%–18%. In contrast, an osteoclast-like giant cell tumor of the pancreas more often presents as a locally aggressive neoplasm with only occasional distant metastasis [9]. Some patients with osteoclast-like giant cell tumor of the pancreas have survived up to 4–15 years. The survival in mixed osteoclast-like/pleomorphic giant cell carcinoma of the pancreas has ranged from 2 months to 4 years.

References

1. Sommers SL, Meissner WA (1954) Unusual carcinoma of the pancreas. Arch Pathol 58:101–111
2. Gudjonsson B (1987) Cancer of the pancreas. 50 years of surgery. Cancer 60:2284–2303
3. Cubilla AL, Fitzgerald PJ (1984) Giant cell carcinoma (osteoclastoid type). In: Firminger HI (ed) Atlas of tumor pathology, Series 2, Fascicle 19. Washington, DC, Armed Forces Institute of Pathology, pp 162–167
4. Combs SG, Hidvegi DF, Ma Y, Rosen ST, Radosevich JA (1988) Pleomorphic carcinoma of the pancreas with osteoclast-like giant cells expressing an epithelial-associated antigen detected by monoclonal antibody 44-3A6. Diagn Cytopathol 4:316–322
5. Gatteschi B, Saccomanno S, Bartoli FG, Salvi S, Pugliese V (to be published) Mixed giant cell tumor of the pancreas. A case report with light microscopy and immunohistochemical features. Int J Pancreatol
6. Nojima T, Nakamura F, Ishikura M, Inoue K, Nagashiwa K, Kato H (1993) Pleomorphic carcinoma of the pancreas with osteoclast-like giant cells. Int J Pancreatol 14:275–281
7. Lewandrowski KB, Weston L, Dickerson GR, Rattner DW, Compton CC (1990) Giant cell tumor of the pancreas of mixed osteoclastic and pleomorphic cell type: evidence for a histogenetic relationship and mesenchymal differentiation. Hum Pathol 21:1184–1187
8. Silverman JF, Dabbs DJ, Finley JK, Geisinger KR (1988) Fine-needle aspiration biopsy of pleomorphic (giant cell) carcinoma of the pancreas. Cytologic, immunocytochemical, and ultrastructural findings. Am J Clin Pathol 89:714–720
9. Pinto MM, Monteiro NL, Tizol DM (1986) Fine needle aspiration of pleomorphic giant-cell carcinoma of the pancreas. Acta Cytol 30:430–434
10. Jeffrey I, Crow J, Ellis BW (1983) Osteoclast-type giant cell tumour of the pancreas. J Clin Path 36: 1165–1170
11. Fischer H-P, Altmannsberger M, Kracht J (1988) Osteoclast-type giant cell tumor of the pancreas. Virch Arch 412:247–253
12. Kay S, Harrison JM (1968) Unusual pleomorphic carcinoma of the pancreas featuring production of osteoid. Cancer 23:1158–1162
13. Rosai J (1968) Carcinoma of pancreas simulating giant cell tumor of bone: electron microscopic evidence of its acinar cell origin. Cancer 22:333–344
14. Robinson L, Damjenov I, Brezind P (1977) Multinucleated giant cell neoplasm of pancreas. Light and electron microscopy features. Arch Pathol Lab Med 101:590–593
15. Tschang T, Garza-Garza R, Kissane JM (1977) Pleomorphic carcinoma of the pancreas. An analysis of 15 cases. Cancer 39:2114–2126
16. Alguacil-Garcia A, Weiland LH (1977) The histologic spectrum, prognosis and histogenesis of the sarcomatoid carcinoma of the pancreas. Cancer 39:1181–1189
17. Jalloh S (1983) Giant cell tumour (osteoclastoma) of the pancreas, an epithelial tumour probably of pancreatic acinar origin. J Clin Pathol 36:1165–1170
18. Manci EA, Gardner LL, Pollock WJ, Dowling EA (1985) Osteoclastic giant cell tumor of the pancreas. Aspiration cytology, light microscopy and ultrastructure with review of the literature. Diagn Cytopathol 1:105–110

19. Cubilla AL, Fitzgerald PJ (1979) Cancer of the pancreas (nonendocrine): a suggested morphological classification. Semin Oncol 6:285–297
20. Trepeta RW, Mathur B, Lagin S, Livolsi V (1981) Giant cell tumor ("osteoclastoma") of the pancreas: a tumor of epithelial origin. Cancer 48:20262–2028
21. Posen JA, Path FF (1981) Giant cell tumour of the pancreas of the osteoclastic type associated with a mucous secreting cystoadenocarcinoma. Hum Pathol 12:944–947
22. Berendt RC, Shnitka TK, Wiens E, Manickavel V, Jewel LD (1987) The osteoclast-type giant cell tumor of the pancreas. Arch Pathol Lab Med 111:43–48
23. Fisher HP, Ahmannsberger M, Cracht J (1988) Osteoclast-type giant cell tumour of the pancreas. Virch Arch (A) 412:247–253
24. Goldberg RD, Michelassi F, Montag AG (1991) Ostoclast-like giant cell tumor of the pancreas: immunophenotypic similarity to giant cell tumor of bone. Hum Pathol 6:618–622
25. Pour PM (1985) Induction of unusual pancreatic neoplasms with morphologic similarity to human tumors and evidence for their ductal/ductular cell origin. Cancer 55:2411–2416

Acinar Cell Carcinoma

Incidence

This uncommon cancer accounts for about 1% to 2% of pancreatic carcinomas, although Webb [1] and Miller et al. [2] reported an incidence of 10.5% and 13%, respectively. Although Webb reported that 4 of 11 cases were mixed ductal-acinar cell carcinoma (Table 1), there is so far no real proof for the existence of a mixed ductal-acinar cell carcinoma.

Age and Sex

In 33 patients with acinar cell carcinoma reported in the English literature between 1970 and 1991 [3–18, 39], age ranged from 9 to 90 years (median age, 59 years); there were 23 males and 10 females (Table 2). Although acinar cell carcinoma occurs most frequently in the elderly, the median age for 7 patients reported by Cubilla and Fitzgerald [19] was 54 years, and Osborne et al. [7] reported a 9-year-old boy with the tumor.

Etiology

Unknown.

Clinical Presentation

Symptoms of acinar cell carcinoma include abdominal pain, nausea and vomiting, weight loss, arthritis, and subcutaneous lesions. At least one of these symptoms was observed in 15 of 20 males and in 8 of 9 females with this tumor (Table 2). In some cases, there may be no symptoms or findings other than high serum lipase levels, which separate acinar cell carcinomas from other common (ductal) adenocarcinomas and uncommon (endocrine) tumors of the pancreas.

Acinar cell carcinoma may, rarely, produce a syndrome characterized by polyarthralgia or polyarthritis, subcutaneous and intraosseous fat necrosis, and eosinophilia [3, 5, 11]. These symptoms are presumably related to the activities of lipase and other enzymes released from the zymogen

Table 1. Reported incidence of acinar cell carcinoma.

Author	Year	Incidence (%)	ACC/Pancreas cancer
Cubilla and Fitzgerald [35]	1975	0.7	3/406
Saitoh, Y. [36]	1990	0.8	32/3821
Chen and Baithun [37]	1985	1.0	4/387[a]
Morohoshi et al. [38]	1983	1.1	3/264
Cubilla and Fitzgerald [28]	1979	1.2	6/508
Webb [1]	1977	10.5	11/105[b]
Miller et al. [2]	1951	13	27/202

[a] Three pure, one mixed carcinoid and acinar
[b] Seven pure, four mixed ductal and acinar

Table 2. Acinar cell carcinoma of the pancreas reported in the English literature (1970–1991).

Author	Year	Age (years)	Sex	Site	Size (cm)	Clinical presentation	Metastases	Prognosis
Robertson and Eeles [3]	1970	59	M	H	4 × 3	Abdominal tenderness, arthralgia, eosinophilia, S-lipase ↑	Liver	Died (7 months)
Burns et al. [4]	1974	52	M	B	8 × 6	Weakness, weight loss, arthropathy, fat necrosis, S-lipase and amylase ↑	Liver, kidney	Died (11 months)
Good et al. [5]	1976	47	M	BT	8 × 8	Abdominal pain, nausea, vomiting, weight loss, S-lipase ↑	Liver, LN	Died (24 months)
Min et al. [6]	1976	54	M	B		Nausea, vomiting, ascites, myeloma nephropathy	Liver, lung, LN, mesentery vertebra	Died (27 days)
Webb [1]	1977	36	M	H	9		Liver, lung, LN, peritoneum	
		84	F	H		Thrombotic endocarditis	Liver, LN	
		69	F	H		Thrombotic endocarditis	Liver, LN	
		52	M	H				
		74	F	B			LN	
		25	M	B	15	Thrombotic endocarditis	Liver, adrenal, LN, peritoneum pleura	
		43	F	H	2	Diabetes	Liver, LN	
Osborne et al. [7]	1977	9	M	H		Abdominal pain, jaundice	Duodenum	Died (28 months)
Hewan-Lowe [8]	1983	66	M	H	1	Epigastric pain, jaundice, weight loss		
Ono et al. [9]	1984	69	M	H	5.5 × 6.5	Abdominal pain, peritoneal dissemination, S-AFP ↑	Liver, LN, peritoneum	Died (2 months)
Horie et al. [10]	1984	73	M	T		Hypochondralgia, fever, S-CEA ↑	Liver, LN, spleen, adrenal	Died (1 months)
Radin et al. [11]	1986	71	M	BT	9	Arthritis, fever, chills, subcutaneous nodules, S-lipase ↑		

Table 2. *Continued*

Author	Year	Age (years)	Sex	Site	Size (cm)	Clinical presentation	Metastases	Prognosis
Horie et al. [12]	1987	60	M	T	11 × 8			Died (41 days)
Morohoshi et al. [13]	1987	46	M	H	5 × 5 × 4	Jaundice	Liver	
		60	M	HB	7 × 6 × 6	Melena	Liver	
		66	F	B	6 × 7 × 4	Abdominal pain	Liver	
		88	M	H	5 × 4 × 4.5	Jaundice	Liver, LN	
		60	M	T	3.5 × 3 × 3	Necrosis of subcutaneous fatty tissue and bone marrow, S-lipase ↑	Liver, LN	
		37	M	BT	5 × 4 × 4	Diarrhea, lumbalgia	Liver, LN, peritoneum	
		90	F	B	7 × 7 × 6			Died
		64	F	HB	7 × 7 × 5	Abdominal pain	LN	
		64	M	B	7 × 6 × 5	Abdominal pain	Liver, lung, LN	
Reducka et al. [14]	1988	52	M	BT		Abdominal pain, nausea, vomiting, myeloma nephropathy	Peritoneum, LN	Died (59 days)
Callizo et al. [15]	1989	61	M		1	Weakness of the limbs	Kidney, lung, brain, adrenal	Died (7 days)
Ishihara et al. [16]	1989	77	F	H	4.5 × 4 × 3	Abdominal pain, vomiting, S-elastase-1 ↑	Liver, LN	Died (18 months)
Lim et al. [17]	1990	60	F	BT	8 × 6 × 5	Epigastric pain	LN	
		28	F	BT	16 × 14 × 12	Abdominal mass	Spleen	
Feliu et al. [18]	1990	60	M	B	5 × 8	Anorexia, weight loss, fatty necrosis, S-lipase ↑	Liver	Died (15 days)
di Sant'Agnese et al. [39]	1991	83	M	T	13 × 9 × 8	Epigastric pain, nausea, melena	Liver	Died (6 months)

LN, lymph node; *H*, head; *B*, body; *T*, tail; *AFP*, alpha-fetoprotein; *S*, serum granules of the malignant acinar cells. In addition, high serum lipase values and, occasionally, high amylase values have been found [4, 5]. In a review of 20 cases reported between 1908 and 1975 by Good et al. [5], this rare syndrome was observed in 17 males, mostly over 50 years old (range 50–83 years). Among the reported 33 cases, this syndrome was observed in 5 men, mostly over 50 years old (range 52–71 years).

Min et al. [6] and Reducka et al. [14] reported acinar cell carcinomas associated with a myeloma-like cast nephropathy.

Acinar cell carcinoma usually metastasizes in elderly patients without symptoms [20]. Five of seven cases reported by Cubilla and Fitzgerald [19] were found clinically to present distant metastasis from an occult primary cancer.

Diagnosis

Endoscopic retrograde pancreatography may demonstrate irregular segmental narrowing of the pancreatic duct with dilatation of the peripheral ducts [17]. Celiac angiography reveals a hypervascular, space-occupying lesion, with small vessel vascularity [5, 17]. Gallium scintigram shows abnormal focus uptake in the tumor [11].

On ultrasonographic examination, Radin et al. [11] observed a hypoechoic mass or mid-range echogenic mass with heterogeneity, which was observed to contain some small- and medium-sized low echogenic areas suggestive of necrosis. On computed tomography, Lim et al. [17] demonstrated a sharply circumscribed low-density mass with a rather smooth and thin capsule. There may be irregular low-density areas and occasionally small punctate calcific foci (Fig. 1). Radiologically, acinar cell carcinoma may be distinguished from the locally invasive common adenocarcinoma of the pancreas, but it is difficult to differentiate from some other, less common pancreatic tumors.

Fine needle aspiration cytology may be useful for the diagnosis of pancreatic acinar cell carcinoma as well as other pancreatic tumors. In a case reported by Ishihara et al. [16], numerous cell clusters showed acinar and glandular structures. The tumor cells were cuboidal with a granular cytoplasm, eccentrically located and hyperchromatic nuclei, and prominent nucleoli. The chromatin structure was coarsely granular. In May-Grünwald-Giemsa-stained preparations, neoplastic cells had strongly basophilic and granular cytoplasm (Fig. 2).

Gross Findings

Tumors are well circumscribed with a thin fibrous capsule, yellowish-white to tan in color, and firm consistency, with hemorrhagic and necrotic areas (Fig. 3). A few cases may show a cystic appearance [21, 22]. Some tumors invade the surrounding tissues with dissemination to the peritoneum. For the 33 cases in the current literature, the mean tumor diameter was 7.1 cm (range 1–16 cm). Of

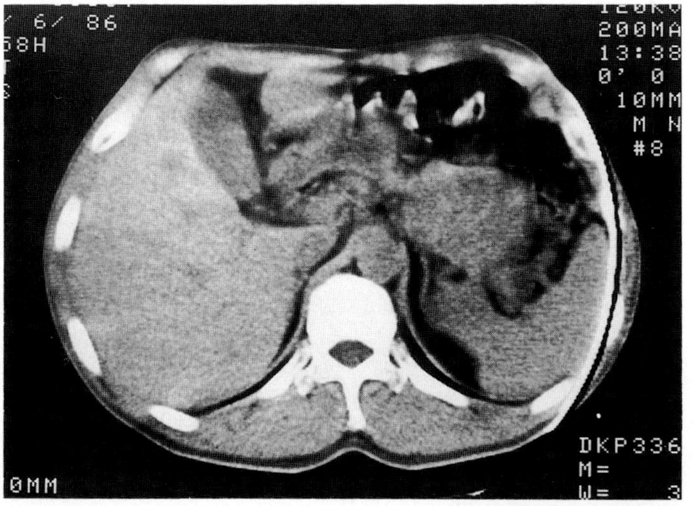

Fig. 1. Pancreatic acinar cell carcinoma in a 49-year-old man who was admitted to hospital with a mass in the upper abdomen. At laparatomy, a fist-sized tumor was resected. The patient died of liver metastases 10 months after operation. CT scan shows a well circumscribed mass arising from body and tail of the pancreas. The mass contains small necrotic areas and calcification. (Courtesy of Dr. S. Suzuki, Toyama University, Japan)

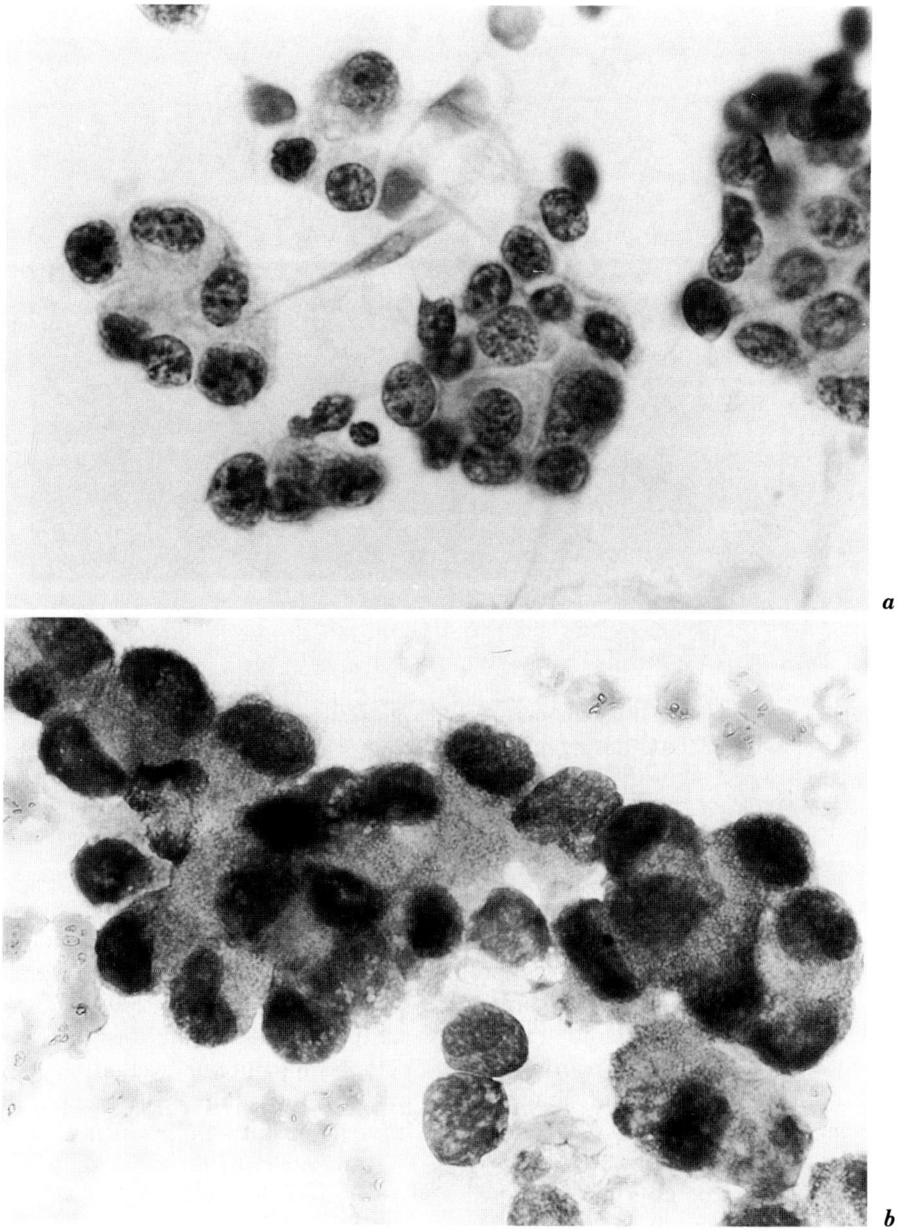

Fig. 2a,b. ***a*** Tumor cells obtained from pancreatic tumor by fine needle aspiration during operation. The cuboidal tumor cells show acinar structures, granular cytoplasm, and eccentrically located, hyperchromatic nuclei. Papanicolaou stain ×850. ***b*** The cytoplasm of neoplastic cells is strongly basophilic and granular in May-Grünwald-Giemsa-stained preparations. ×850. (see also Fig. 4)

these cases, acinar cell carcinoma was located in the head of the pancreas in 36%, in the body in 24%, in the tail in 12%, in the head and body in 6%, and in the body and tail in 18% (Table 2). In the 7 cases reported by Cubilla and Fitzgerald [19], the mean tumor diameter was 5 cm, and the tumor was located in the head of the pancreas in 3, in the body in 3, and throughout the pancreas in 1.

Microscopic Findings

In well-differentiated and moderately differentiated areas, the neoplastic cells are characteristically arranged in acinar, glandular, and/or in trabecular patterns with a delicate fibrous stroma (Figs. 4, 5). The tumor cells are cuboidal or columnar and contain basally located round nuclei, which have

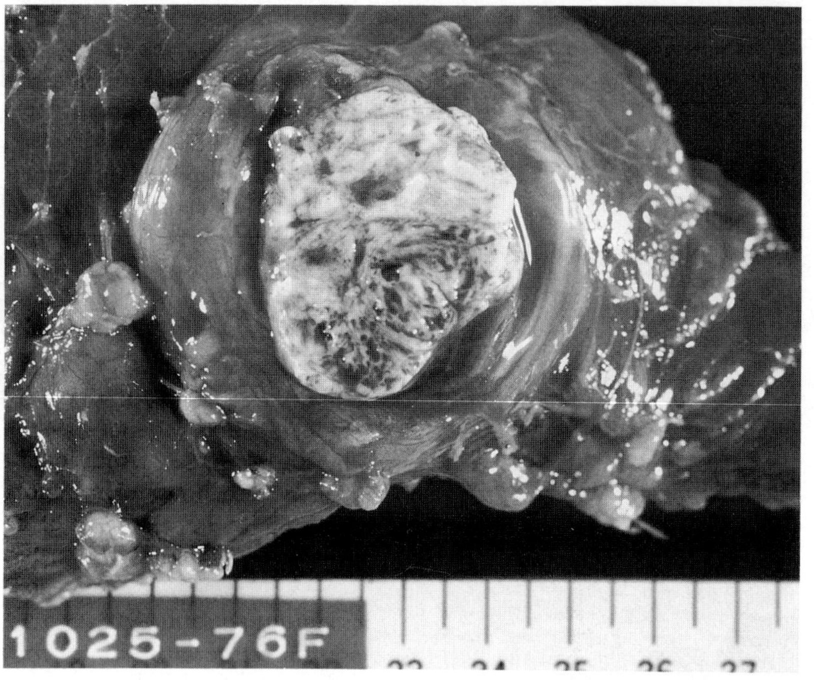

Fig. 3. Gross findings of acinar cell carcinoma of the pancreas. Specimen from a Whipple resection of the head of the pancreas in a 77-year-old female admitted to hospital with complaints of abdominal pain and vomiting. The patient was readmitted with multiple liver metastases 12 months after operation. The cut specimen shows a well-defined, white, firm neoplasm with hemorrhage, measuring 4.5 cm in its largest dimension. (The same tumor as in Figs. 2, 4, 6–8, and 11). (*For color reproduction see color insert in the frontmatter*)

distinct nucleoli. The abundant cytoplasm is eosinophilic, granular, and faintly PAS-positive. There are small cysts containing eosinophilic material, remnants of vacuolated cells, and rare foci of cholesterol clefts in tumor tissue (Fig. 6).

In poorly differentiated tumors, poorly-formed acini and anaplastic foci composed of small round cells are present (Fig. 7). Poorly differentiated tumors can easily be misdiagnosed as endocrine tumors because acinar structures are not always present. There is sometimes a thin rim of well-differentiated acinar cells around blood vessels. Mitotic figures are variable. The neoplastic cells are negative for both argyrophil and argentaffin reactions, and are also negative for mucin.

Electron Microscopy

On electron microscopic examination, the cells of this neoplasm closely resemble the acinar cells of the normal pancreas. Acinar lumen consists of several neighboring cells tightly connected to each other by a junctional complex and lined with microvilli. The cell-to-cell contact is usually smooth and made by poorly developed desmosomes. Electron-dense secretory (zymogen) granules, measuring about 600 nm (range 200–1100 nm) in diameter are clustered around the glandular lumen. The cytoplasm contains well developed rough endoplasmic reticulum, Golgi apparatus, and a few mitochondria and lysosomes (Fig. 8).

Annulate lamellae and tubuloreticular inclusions are frequently recognized [12]. Some tumor cells have cytoplasmic bundles of intermediate filaments [14] and fibrillary material in the cytoplasm [4]. No mucigen granules or neurosecretory granules are present.

Immunohistochemistry

Pancreatic enzymes such as alpha-1 amylase, lipase, trypsin, and chymotrypsin are the most useful markers for acinar cell carcinoma of the pancreas. Morohoshi et al. [13] reported that all nine of their pancreatic acinar cell carcinomas were immunohistochemically positive for lipase (Fig. 9),

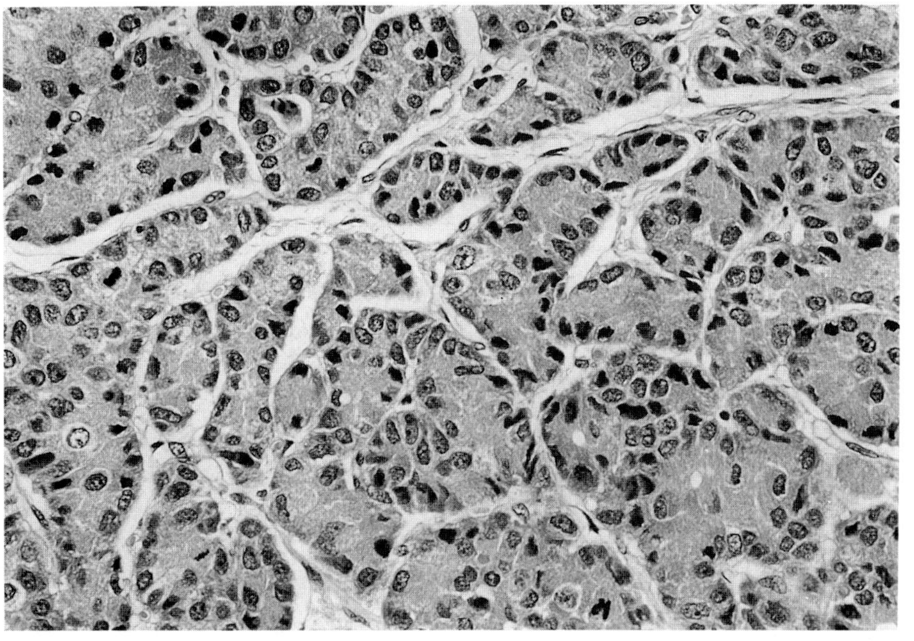

Fig. 4. The same tumor as in Figs. 2 and 3. Well-differentiated adenocarcinoma with characteristic acinar formations supported by scanty stroma. The nuclei are basal, and the cytoplasm is abundant, eosinophilic, and granular. (H&E ×300)

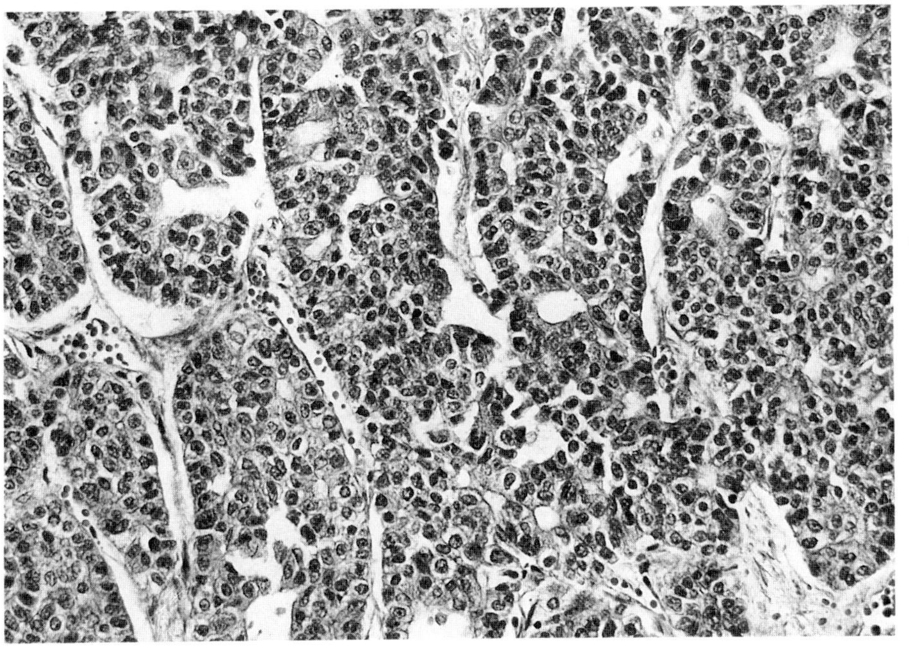

Fig. 5. Moderately differentiated acinar cell carcinoma. Tumor with anastomosing trabecular cell cords and some acinar cell groups. (H&E ×250) (Courtesy of Dr. G. Klöppel, Free University, Brussels)

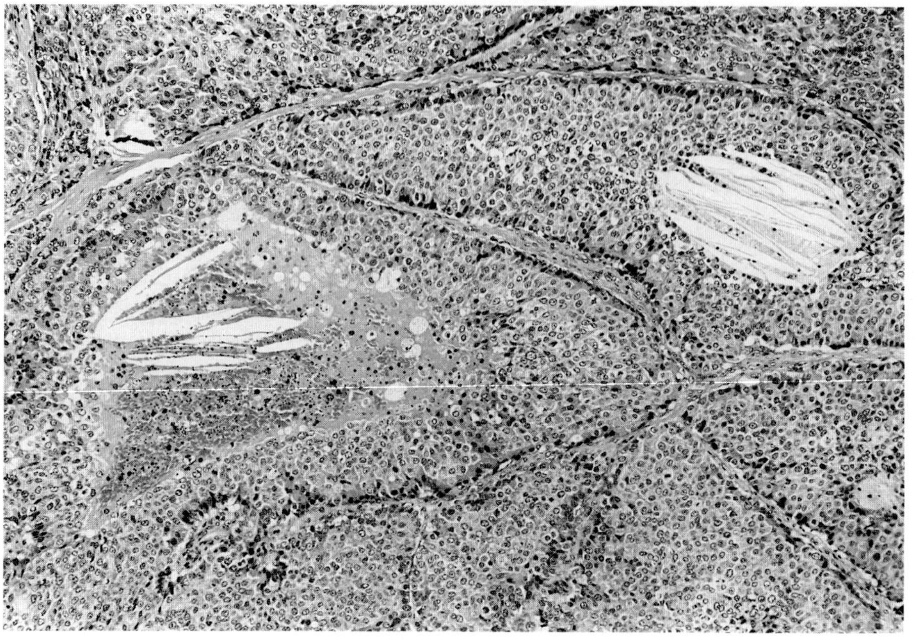

Fig. 6. The same tumor as in Fig. 4. The tumor tissue contains a small cyst with remnants of vacuolated cells and cholesterol clefts. (H&E ×150)

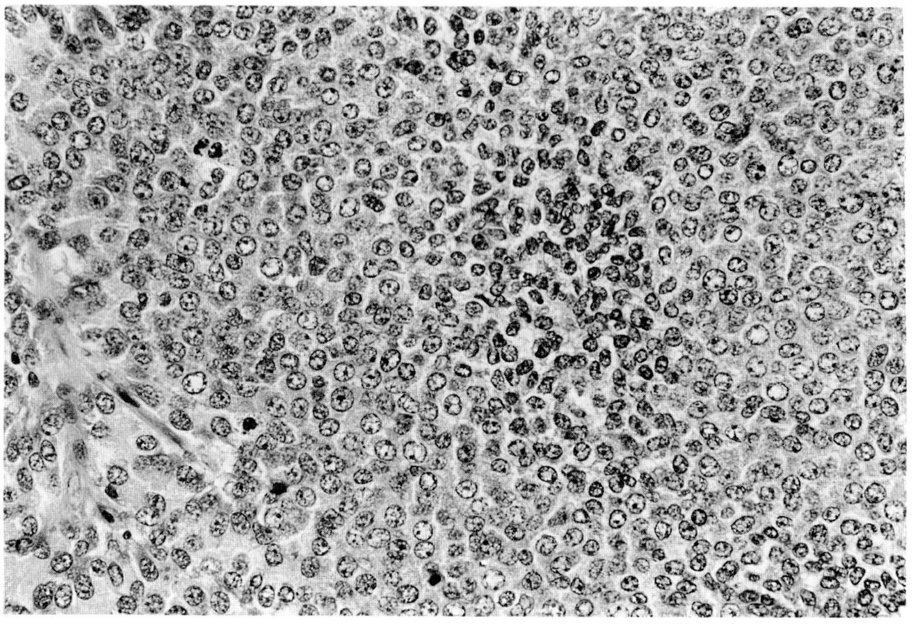

Fig. 7. The same tumor as in Figs. 4 and 6. Rare focus of poorly differentiated carcinoma composed of anaplastic small round cells. Elsewhere acinar cell differentiation of the carcinoma was apparent. (H&E ×300)

trypsin, and chymotrypsin. Positivity is usually demonstrated only in the apical portion of the acinar tumor cells, and while ductal cell carcinoma and endocrine tumors invariably remain unstained, immunoreactivity for these enzymes is also found in pancreatoblastoma. This corresponds with the ultrastructural demonstration of zymogen granules in tumor cells.

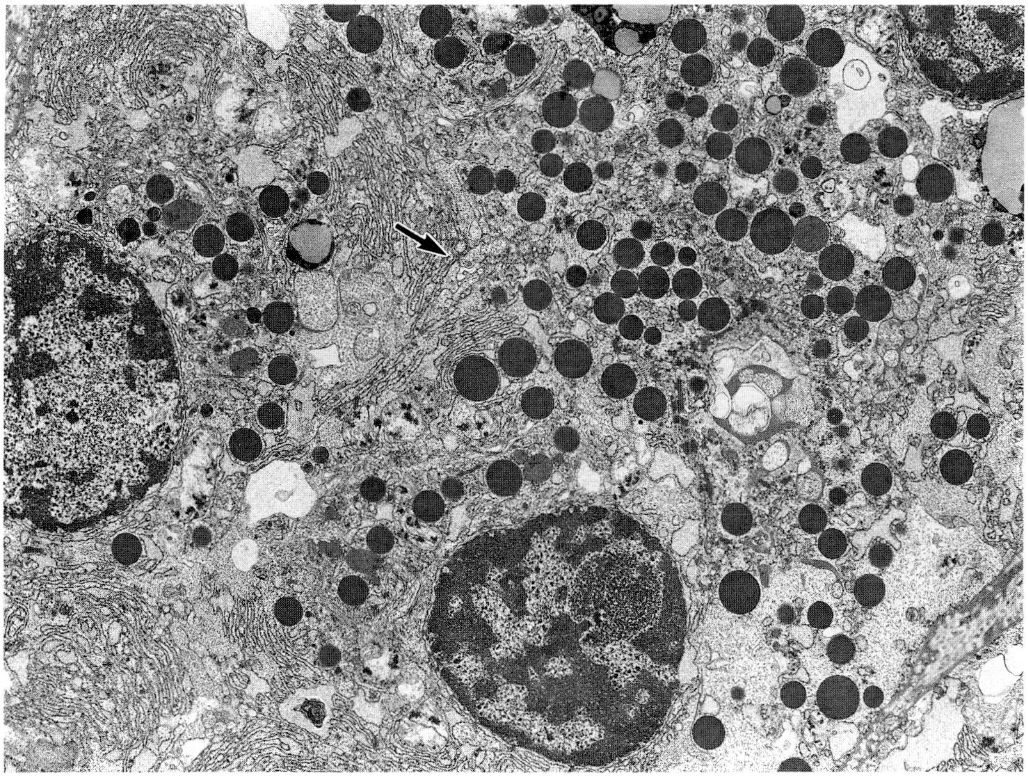

Fig. 8. The same tumor as in Figs. 4, 6, and 7. Numerous electron dense secretory (zymogen) granules and abundant rough endoplasmic reticulum are present in tumor cells. An acinar lumen is formed by several neighboring cells (*arrow*). ×5000 (original magnification)

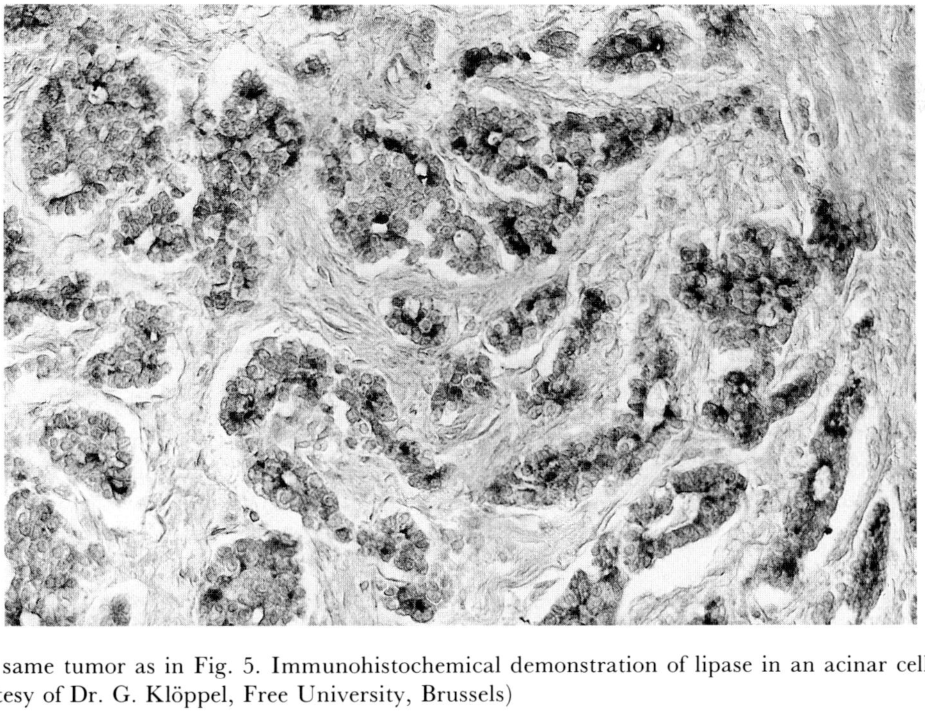

Fig. 9. The same tumor as in Fig. 5. Immunohistochemical demonstration of lipase in an acinar cell carcinoma. ×250 (Courtesy of Dr. G. Klöppel, Free University, Brussels)

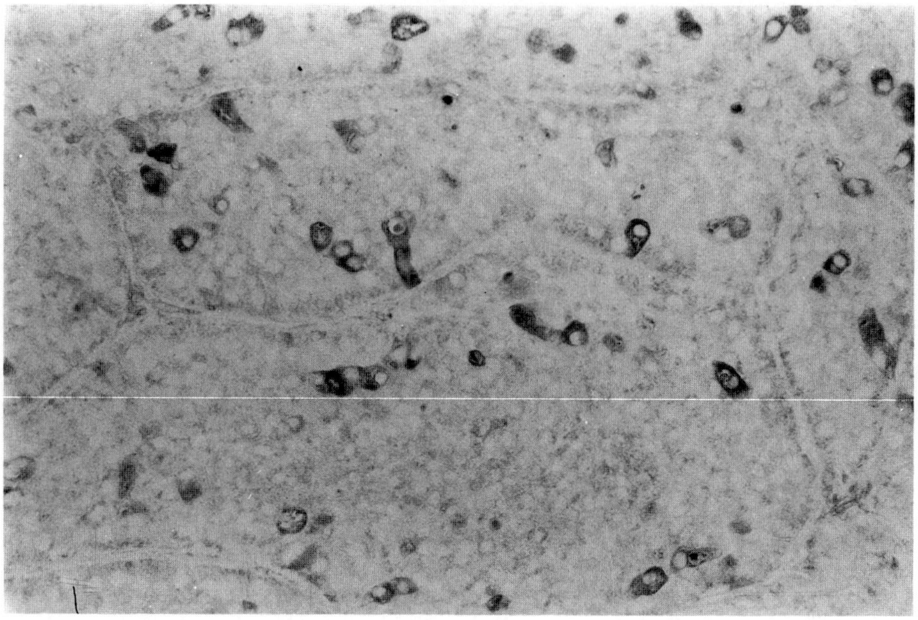

Fig. 10. Immunohistochemical reactivity for alpha-1 antitrypsin (AAT) in an acinar cell carcinoma. AAT is usually found throughout the entire cytoplasm. ×250 (Courtesy of Dr. T. Morohoshi, Showa University, Japan)

Alpha-1 antitrypsin (AAT) is usually found throughout the entire cytoplasm in acinar cell carcinoma (Fig. 10), pancreatoblastoma, and solid and cystic tumors. Although AAT might be one of the tumor markers for acinar cell carcinoma in general, the reaction of AAT occurs in one-third of pancreatic endocrine tumors [23] and in ductal adenocarcinomas [24].

Acinar ceil carcinomas are generally negative for neuron specific enolase (NSE) and endocrine substances such as insulin, glucagon, and somatostatin [13], but some tumor cells may occassionally express endocrine markers (G. Klöppel, 1992 personal communication).

Unlike pancreatic ductal carcinomas, the majority of which show positive immunoreactivity for carcinoembryonic antigen (CEA) and CA19-9, acinar cell carcinoma is negative for both markers [13]. However, some tumors, particularly the poorly differentiated types, may express CA19-9, CEA [10] and rarely also AFP (G. Klöppel, personal communication).

Biochemistry

Analysis of pancreatic enzyme activities in the tumor tissue by biochemical assays has been reported. Burns et al. [4] reported extremely high level of lipase activity in the pancreatic and metastatic liver tumors in a case of functional acinar cell carcinoma of the pancreas with polyarthropathy. In our case, moderate elastase-1 and mild lipase activities, but no amylase, were detected in tissue homogenates of liver metastasis. However, neither polyarthritis nor hemorrhagic complications were clinically recognized.

A patient with acinar cell carcinomas with extremely elevated serum alpha-fetoprotein (AFP, 65 000 ng/ml) [9] and a high level of plasma CEA (6000 ng/ml) has been reported [10]. High serum AFP level has been also reported in pancreatoblastoma [25] and CEA in ductal carcinoma of the pancreas.

Differential Diagnosis

The diagnosis of acinar cell carcinoma is based on its distinct histologic pattern and the electron microscopic demonstration of zymogen granules in the tumor cells. Immunohistochemical tests, such as alpha-amylase, lipase, trypsin, chymotrypsin, elastase-1, and AAT, can now be used as additional diagnostic methods. Electron microscopy and immunohistochemistry may be helpful in the diag-

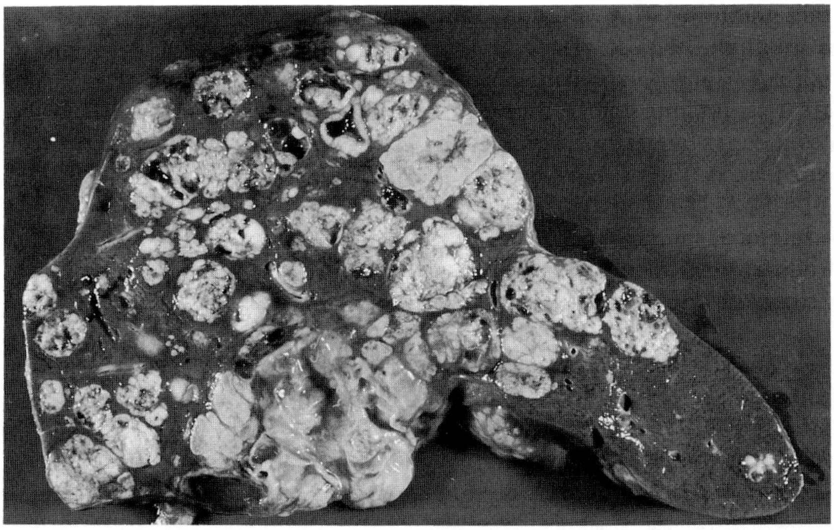

Fig. 11. The same tumor as in Fig. 8. Multiple liver metastases of pancreatic acinar cell carcinoma. The liver weighed 2380 g at autopsy, and contained numerous white-to-yellow metastatic nodules. The patient died of hepatic failure 18 months after Whipple operation. Serum elastase-1 level ranged from 3089 to 19 572 ng/dL, but serum amylase and lipase levels were in the normal range. Moderate elastase-1 activity was demonstrated in tissue homogenates of liver metastases. (*For color reproduction see color insert in the frontmatter*)

nosis of exocrine as well as endocrine tumors of the pancreas.

It is occasionally difficult to recognize acinar cell cancer by light microscopy, particularly if the tumor is poorly differentiated, although even in the anaplastic areas there are usually foci of recognizable acinar cells. The ordinary ductal cell and islet cell tumors can usually be distinguished from acinar cell carcinoma, but, rarely, a mixture of these types with foci of acinar cell carcinomas may occur [26]. Ulich et al. [27] reported a case of neoplastic proliferation of intermediate cells in which both endocrine and exocrine granules were present within a single cell.

Acinar cell carcinoma may be confused histologically with pancreatoblastoma especially in children. Pancreatoblastoma occurs exclusively in young children and shows a mixed histologic pattern which can differentiate into ductal, mesenchymal [28], neuroendocrine [29], and exocrine acinar components [30, 31].

A distinct separation must be made between acinar cell carcinoma and solid and cystic tumor. The latter tumors mostly occur in young women, and the prognosis is favorable when they can be completely removed. Histologically, the tumor shows pseudopapillary structures around fibrovascular stalks, pseudorosette arrangements, small cysts with solid vacuolated cell complexes, and degenerative lesions (cholesterol granulomas, hemorrhage, and focal hyalinization) which distinguish the acinar cell carcinoma [32]. However, vacuolated cells and cholesterol clefts are rarely recognized in our case. Ultrastructurally, the tumor cells have numerous mitochodria in the cytoplasm of solid and cystic tumor [32, 33]. Sparse granules of the neuroendocrine type and zymogen-like granules have been demonstrated in some cases [12, 32, 33]. Immunoreactivity to NSE is demonstrated in solid and cystic tumor [34], but generally not in acinar cell carcinoma [13].

Rarely, acinar cell tumor may present as a cystadenocarcinoma. Cantrell et al. [21] reported a 64-year-old man with this tumor, which showed numerous cysts separated by a fibrous stroma. Most of the cysts are lined by a cuboidal epithelium showing acinar cell differentiation.

Prognosis and Survival

Of the 33 reported cases, the most common metastatic sites detected on admission, at exploratory operation, or at autopsy were the liver (Fig. 11) in 64% and lymph nodes in 51% (Table 2).

The prognosis is poor, with a median survival period of 7 months. One-year and 5-year survival rates were 14% and 0%, respectively [19], and the average length of survival was only 5 months [1]. Of the 32 patients in our meta-analysis, the clinical outcome was described for 14 patients, of whom only 3 survived more than 1 year, and all of them died within 2.5 years. The prognosis of patients with tumor-associated metastatic fat necrosis is extremely poor [5]; the mean survival period of these patients, from appearance of subcutaneous lesions, was 5.9 months (range 2–12 months).

Radiation and chemotherapy were given mostly for palliative purposes, and long-term survival with either therapy was very rare.

References

1. Webb JN (1977) Acinar cell neoplasms of the exocrine pancreas. J Clin Pathol 30:103–112
2. Miller JR, Baggenstoss AH, Comfort MW (1951) Carcinoma of the pancreas. Cancer 4:233–241
3. Robertson JC, Eeles GH (1970) Syndrome associated with pancreatic acinar cell carcinoma. Brit Med J 2:708–709
4. Burns WA, Matthews MJ, Hamosh M, Weide GV, Blum R, Johnson FB (1974) Lipase-secreting acinar cell carcinoma of the pancreas with polyarthropathy: A light and electron microscopic, histochemical, and biochemical study. Cancer 33:1002–1009
5. Good AE, Schnitzer B, Kawanishi H, Demetropoulos KC, Rapp R (1976) Acinar pancreatic tumor with metastatic fat necrosis: Report of a case and review of rheumatic manifestations. Dig Dis 21:978–987
6. Min KW, Cain GD, Györkey P, Györkey F (1976) Myeloma-like lesions of the kidney: Occurrence in a case of acinic cell adenocacinoma of the pancreas. Arch Intern Med 136:1299–1302
7. Osborne BM, Culbert SJ, Cangir A, MacKay B (1977) Acinar cell carcinoma of the pancreas in a 9-year-old child: Case report with electron microscopic observations. South Med J 70:370–372
8. Hewan-Lowe KO (1983) Acinar cell carcinoma of the pancreas: Metastases from an occult primary tumor. Arch Pathol Lab Med 107:552–554
9. Ono J, Sakamoto H, Sakoda K, Yagi Y, Hagio S, Sato E, Katsuki T (1984) Acinar cell carcinoma of the pancreas with elevated serum alpha-fetoprotein. Int Surg 69:361–364
10. Horie Y, Gomyoda M, Kishimoto Y, Ueki J, Ikeda F, Murawaki Y, Kawamura M, Hirayama C (1984) Plasma carcinoembryonic antigen and acinar cell carcinoma of the pancreas. Cancer 53:1137–1142
11. Radin DR, Colletti PM, Forrester DM, Tang WW (1986) Pancreatic acinar cell carcinoma with subcutaneous and intraosseous fat necrosis. Radiology 158:67–68
12. Horie A, Morohoshi T, Klöppel G (1987) Ultrastructural comparison of pancreatoblastoma, solid cystic tumor, and acinar cell carcinoma. J Clin Electron Microsc 20:353–362
13. Morohoshi T, Kanda M, Horie A, Chott A, Dreyer T, Klöppel G, Heitz PU (1987) Immunocytochemical markers of uncommon pancreatic tumors: Acinar cell carcinoma, pancreatoblastoma, and solid cystic (papillary-cystic) tumor. Cancer 59:739–747
14. Reducka K, Gardiner GW, Sweet J, Vandenbroucke A, Bear R (1988) Myeloma-like cast nephropathy associated with acinar cell carcinoma of the pancreas. Am J Nephrol 8:421–424
15. Callizo JRA, Gimenez-Mas JA, Martin J, Lacasa J (1989) Calcified brain metastases from acinar-cell carcinoma of pancreas. Neuroradiology 31:200
16. Ishihara A, Sanda T, Takanari H, Yatani R, Liu PI (1989) Elastase-1-secreting acinar cell carcinoma of the pancreas: A cytologic, electron microscopic, and histochemical study. Acta Cytol 33:157–163
17. Lim JH, Chung KB, Cho OK, Cho KS (1990) Acinar cell carcinoma of the pancreas: Ultrasonography and computed tomography findings. Clin Imaging 14:301–304
18. Feliu J, de la Gandara I, Garrido P, Baron MG (1990) Somatostatin analogues and pancreatic acinar cell carcinoma: An alternative in symptomatic treatment? Am J Gastroenterol 85: 1539–1540
19. Cubilla AL, Fitzgerald PJ (1984) Tumors of the exocrine pancreas. In: Hartmann WH (ed) Atlas of tumor pathology, 2nd series, fascicle 19. Armed Forces Institute of Pathology, Washington DC, pp 208–212
20. Klöppel G, Heitz PU (1984) Pancreatic pathology. Churchill Livingstone, London, pp 79–113
21. Cantrell BB, Cubilla AL, Erlandson RA, Fortner J, Fitzgerald PJ (1981) Acinar cell cystadenocarcinoma of human pancreas. Cancer 47:410–416
22. Stamm B, Burger H, Hollinger A (1987) Acinar cell cystadenocarcinoma of the pancreas. Cancer 60: 2542–2547
23. Ordonez NG, Manning JT, Hanssen G (1983) Alpha-1 antitrypsin in islet cell tumors of the pancreas. Am J Clin Pathol 80:277–282
24. Ohaki Y, Misugi K, Fukuda J, Okudaira M, Hirose M (1987) Immunohistochemical study of pancreatoblastoma. Acta Pathol Jpn 37:1581–1590
25. Imamura M, Yokoyama S (1983) A case of alpha-fetoprotein-producing pancreatoblastoma (in Japanese). Trans Soc Pathol Jpn 72:324
26. Schron DS, Mendelsohn G (1984) Pancreatic carcinoma with duct, endocrine, and acinar differen-

tiation: A histologic, immunocytochemical, and ultrastructural study. Cancer 54:1766–1770
27. Ulich T, Cheng L, Lewin KJ (1982) Acinar-endocrine cell tumor of the pancreas: Report of a pancreatic tumor containing both zymogen and neuroendocrine granules. Cancer 50:2099–2105
28. Cubilla AL, Fitzgerald PJ (1979) Classification of pancreatic cancer (nonendocrine). Mayo Clin Proc 54:449–458
29. Buchino JJ, Castello FM, Nagaraj HS (1984) Pancreatoblastoma: A histochemical and ultrastructural analysis. Cancer 53:963–969
30. Horie A, Yano Y, Kotoo Y, Miwa A (1977) Morphogenesis of pancreatoblastoma, infantile carcinoma of the pancreas: Report of two cases. Cancer 39:247–254
31. Silverman JF, Holbrook CT, Pories WJ, Kodroff MB, Joshi VV (1990) Fine needle aspiration cytology of pancreatoblastoma with immunocytochemical and ultrastructural studies. Acta Cytol 34:632–640
32. Klöppel G, Morohoshi T, John HD, Oehmichen W, Opitz K, Angelkort A, Lietz H, Rückert K (1981) Solid and cystic acinar cell tumour of the pancreas: A tumour in young women with favourable prognosis. Virchows Arch [A] 392:171–183
33. Schlosnagle DC, Campbell WG (1981) Papillary and solid neoplasm of the pancreas: A report of two cases with electron microscopy, one containing neurosecretory granules. Cancer 47:2603–2610
34. Chott A, Klöppel G, Buxbaum P, Heitz PU (1987) Neuron specific enolase demonstration in the diagnosis of a solid-cystic (papillary cystic) tumour of the pancreas. Virchows Arch [A] 410:397–402
35. Cubilla AL, Fitzgerald PJ (1975) Morphological patterns of primary nonendocrine human pancreas carcinoma. Cancer Res 35:2234–2248
36. Saitoh Y (1990) Report of registered cases of pancreatic cancer in all Japan (in Japanese). Japan Pancreas Society p 71
37. Chen J, Baithun SI (1985) Morphological study of 391 cases of exocrine pancreatic tumours with special reference to the classification of exocrine pancreatic carcinoma. J Pathol 146:17–29
38. Morohoshi T, Held G, Klöppel G (1983) Exocrine pancreatic tumours and their histological classification. A study based on 167 autopsy and 97 surgical cases. Histopathology 7:645–661
39. di Sant'Agnese PA (1991) Acinar cell carcinoma of the pancreas. Ultrastruc Pathol 15:573–577

*Pancreatoblastoma**

Definition

Pancreatoblastoma is a malignant tumor composed of epithelial tissue with acinar differentiation, squamoid cell nests, and occasional neuroendocrine cells. Some tumors may also have a pronounced mesenchymal component. It usually occurs in infants, but has recently also been reported in adults [1, 2].

Incidence

Although pancreatoblastoma is the commonest pancreatic neoplasm of childhood, it is an extremely rare tumor. Since the first report by Becker [3], only 32 patients with this tumor have been described so far [2, 4–12]. Cubilla and Fitzgerald's [13] pancreatic tumor series (total. 645 patients) included only 1 patient (0.2%) with pancreatoblastoma, while there were 5 patients (2%) in a recent series from Japan (total, 253 patients, [14]).

Sex, Age and Race

According to our survey, pancreatoblastoma is more frequent in males than females, with a ratio of 2:1. This tumor occurs predominantly during childhood (age at diagnosis ranges from a few hours after birth to 9 years; mean age: 4 years), but has also been observed in a male adult aged 37 years [1] and in a woman aged 39 years [2]. Interestingly, this tumor is more frequent among Asians (two-thirds of the patients) than caucasians: 17 of the 32 patients were Japanese, 4 Korean, 1 Chinese, 1 black Indian, and only 4 caucasians.

Etiology and Pathogenesis

The etiology of pancreatoblastoma is not known. Three cases of pancreatoblastoma were described in newborns with the Beckwith-Wiedemann syndrome [9, 15, 16]. The occurrence of congenital pancreatoblastomas in the Beckwith-Wiedemann syndrom reflects the high rate of blastic tumors that is associated with this syndrome.

Based on their localization in the head or the tail of the gland, Horie [17] suggested that the tumors arising in the head of the pancreas derive from the ventral anlage of the pancreas, whereas tumors in the body and tail originate from the dorsal anlage. Pancreatoblastomas deriving from the ventral anlage are encapsulated, contain no endocrine cells and have a favorable prognosis, while those arising from the dorsal anlage show local infiltration, contain endocrine cells, and have a more aggessive behavior. The validity of this classification remains to be established.

Clinical Features

The clinical diagnosis is often directed to the cause of abdominal mass with either no symptoms, or with uncharacteristic complaints such as epigastric pain (about 40%), loss of appetite and weight (about 20%), and diarrhea and vomiting. It may

* Dedicated to the late Professor A. Horie

cause jaundice (less than 15%) when localized in the head of the pancreas.

Serum alpha-fetoprotein (AFP) can serve as tumor marker for pancreatoblastoma, since one-fourth to one-third of the patients show elevated AFP levels [18, 19–20]. Morohoshi et al. [11] observed a pancreatoblastoma occurring in a 7-year-old Japanese girl with elevated serum AFP levels of more than 10 000 ng/ml, which decreased after tumor resection and chemotherapy. AFP is thus also useful to monitor recurrence. Acinar cell carcinomas of the pancreas occasionally show AFP elevations as well [21], suggesting that pancreatoblastoma and acinar cell carcinoma may be related tumor entities. Other tumor markers such as CEA, CA19-9, DU-PAN-2, or alpha-1-antitrypsin, are not helpful in the diagnosis of this tumor.

US, CT and NMR reveal a well-demarcated, solid, and often multilobulated tumor in the upper abdomen (Fig. 1), which may show low echogenic areas, central attenuations and displacement of adjacent organs [19, 21–23]. Fine needle aspiration cytology under US guidance may produce hypercellular specimens with clusters of epithelial cells having abundant granular cytoplasm and demonstrating acinar formation. In addition, there may be mesenchymal fragments [23].

Gross Findings

The large soft and rounded tumors usually replace the pancreas, but sometimes are only found attached to it [24, 25]. They may arise anywhere in the pancreas, but in Japanese patients, the neoplasms seem to occur more frequently (three-quarters) in the body or tail of the pancreas [10].

The tumor presents as a nodular and solid mass, usually surrounded by a fibrous capsule. Tumor sizes range from 7 to 18 cm [21]. On cut surface, the tumor shows yellow-tan solid areas with incomplete lobulation associated with pseudocystic foci containing necrotic or hemorrhagic debris. There are no true cysts in the tumor.

In advanced stages, the tumor is no longer demarcated, but diffusely invades the pancreas and also involves peripancreatic retroperitoneal tissues and adjacent organs [11]. Metastases occur in regional lymph nodes, liver, and lung.

Microscopic Findings

Histologlcally, pancreatoblastoma is characterized by a tubular arrangement of epithelial cells which show an acinar (or glandular) pattern with scattered squamoid cell nests (or stratified cords) (Fig. 2). The epithelial areas are incompletely divided by connective tissue. The acinar and glandular

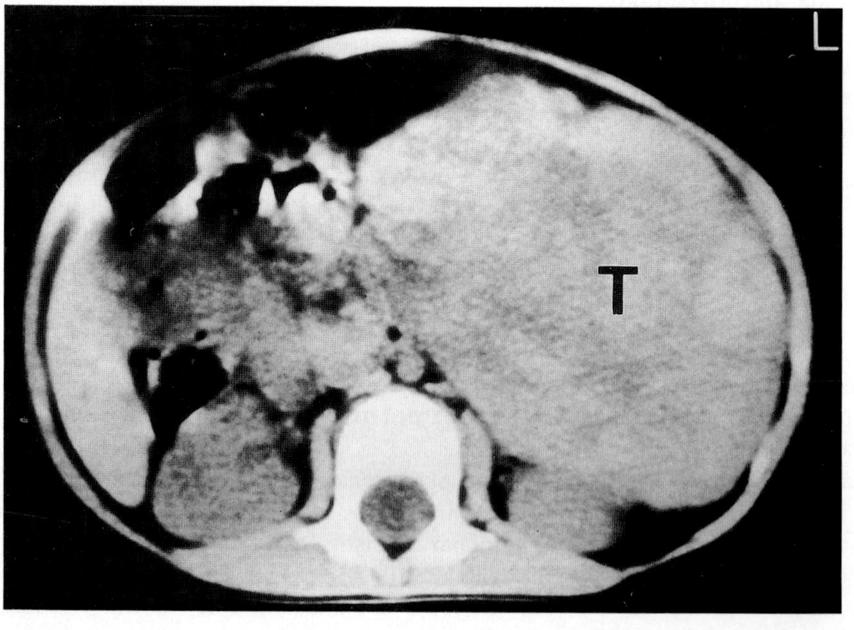

Fig. 1. Computed tomography of pancreatoblastoma in a 5-year-old boy, revealing a large irregular tumor (*T*) occupying the left (*L*) upper abdomen (courtesy of Dr. Sakaida)

structures are composed of uniform columnar or cuboidal cells with eosinophilic fine granular cytoplasm and a round-to-oval nucleus situated at the basal pole. They show variable mitotic activity. The squamoid cell nests and cords ("squamoid corpuscles") are composed of polygonal tumor cells with basophilic or clear cytoplasm. Occasionally, they display central keratinization (Fig. 3). Periodic acid-Schiff (PAS)-positive, diastase resistant, intracytoplasmic fine granules are recognized at the apical side of tumor cells forming acinar structures, and diffusely in the cells forming squamoid cell nests (Fig. 4). Tubular structures may be found in the fibrous stroma separating the epithelial components (Fig. 2).

Rarely, pancreatoblastomas reveal, in addition to epithelial differentiation, a striking mesenchymal component including chondroid and osteoid tissues [13, 26]. This type of pancreatoblastoma may be classified as mixed type pancreatoblastoma.

Immunohistochemistry

Immunohistologically, most tumor cells are positive for keratin [11, 27], and epithelial membrane antigen (Morohoshi, personal observation). The acinar tumor cells are positive for: Lipase, trypsin, chymotrypsin, and alpha-1-antitrypsin (Fig. 5a) [28]. Some tumor cells may also show positivity for AFP [11, 19–21] (Fig. 5b) and CEA [11, 19] (Fig. 5c). Occasionally there are also CA19-9 positive tumor cells [11] (Fig. 5d).

In general, pancreatoblastoma lacks endocrine components. However, there are now several tumors on record where endocrine differentiation was demonstrated [12, 19, 23, 25]. In such cases, tumor nests similar to endocrine istets [27], and single tumor cells positive with the Grimelius reaction are found [12, 25, Morohoshi and Klöppel, personal observation]. Immunocytochemically, these cells may be positive for synaptophysin, chromogranin A and pancreatic hormones, especially somatostatin.

Electronmicroscopy

The tumor cells forming acinar structures have microvilli on the luminal surface and are connected with junctional complexes. The cytoplasm contains well-developed Golgi complexes and abundant rough endoplasmic reticulum [18]. In addition, these cells display large electron-dense zymogen-like granules, 300–500 nm in diameter [10, 18–21, 23–25] (Fig. 6). Scattered between the cells with acinar differentiation, there may be cells with neuroendocrine type granules showing a distinct membrane and measuring from 100 to 200 nm in diameter.

Differential Diagnosis

Most important for the histologic diagnosis of pancreatoblastoma is the demonstration of acinar cell differentiation and the presence of squamoid cell nests. As in some pancreatoblastomas the acinar pattern is the dominating histologic feature, it can be difficult to distinguish pancreatoblastoma from acinar cell carcinoma. It is, therefore, possible that the few acinar cell carcinomas described in infants represented pancreatoblastomas [24, 29, 30].

Pancreatoblastomas with a solid pattern have to be distinguished from neuroendocrine tumors. The latter neoplasms show a diffuse positivity for synaptophysin and usually also chromogranin, while neuroendocrine differentiation in pancreatoblastomas, if it is present, involves only single cells or small cell clusters. Moreover, neuroendocrine tumors lack AFP positivity.

The solid-cystic (papillary-cystic) tumor is another differential diagnosis to pancreatoblastoma because it may also be seen in childhood. However, solid-cystic tumors are easily recognized by their predilection for female patients (not younger than 9 years) and their distinct histologic pattern characterized by pseudopapillary structures and degenerative pseudocystic lesions [28].

Prognosis and Survival

There is no doubt about the malignant potential of pancreatoblastoma because the tumors may show local invasion into organs and vessels, and are capable of regional and distant metastases. The postoperative prognosis is fairly good in patients in whom the tumor is discovered prior to metastasis. About two-thirds of patients are well 1 year after the resection, and a quarter of them are alive and tumor-free after 5 years. The longest follow-up after operation is 28 years [17]. The pancreatoblastomas are responsive to radiotherapy and

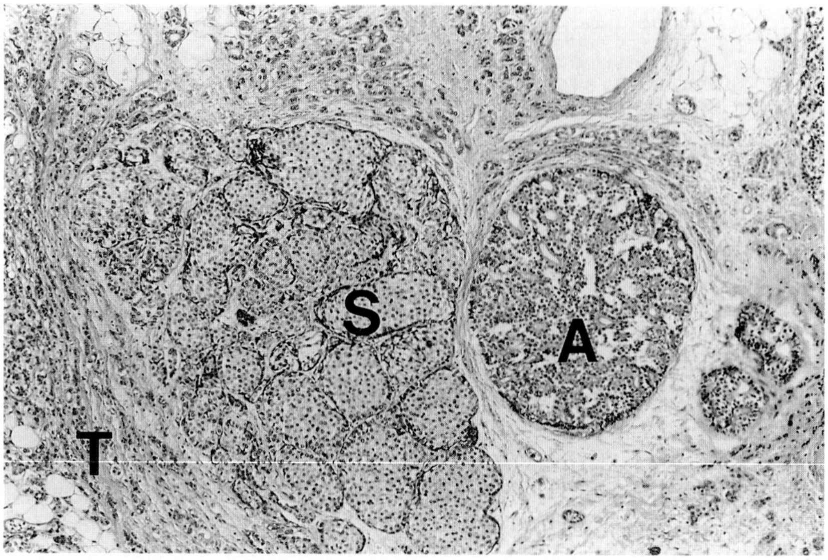

Fig. 2. Histologic appearance of pancreatoblastoma showing an organoid structure with acinar (*A*), squamoid (*S*), and tubular (*T*) differentiation. (H&E, ×90)

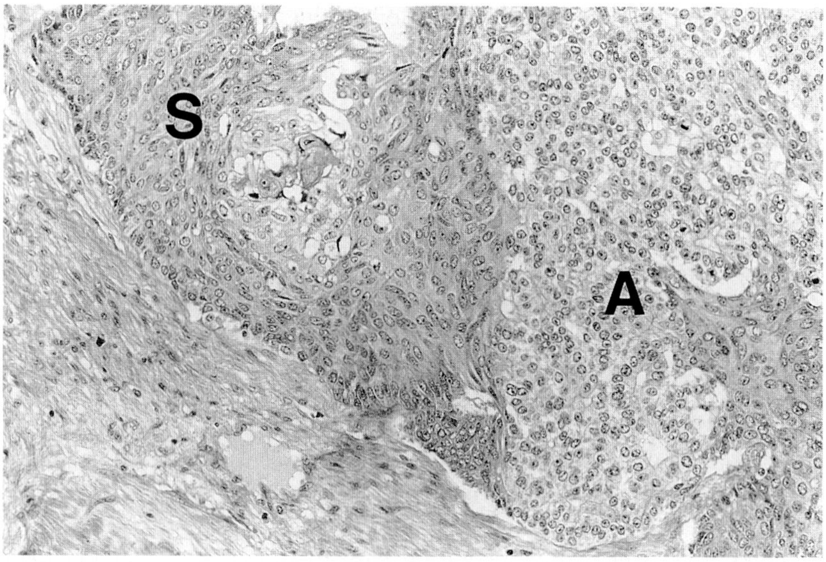

Fig. 3. Epithelial tumor cells with acinar differentiation (*A*) and a squamoid corpuscle (*S*) showing keratosis. The tumor is encased by dense fibrous stroma. (H&E, ×90)

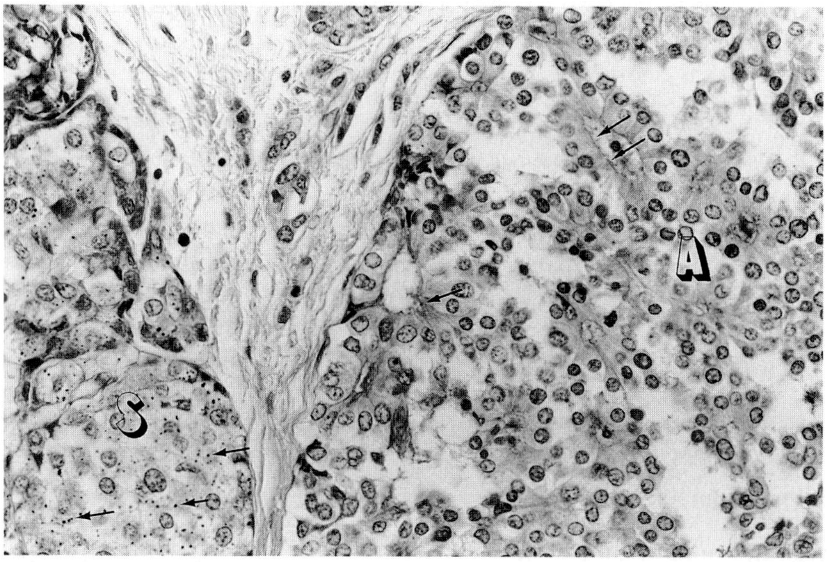

Fig. 4. Tumor cells showing both acinar (*A*) and squamoid (*S*) arrangement and displaying numerous periodic acid-Schiff (*PAS*)-positive fine granules (*arrows*). (PAS ×180)

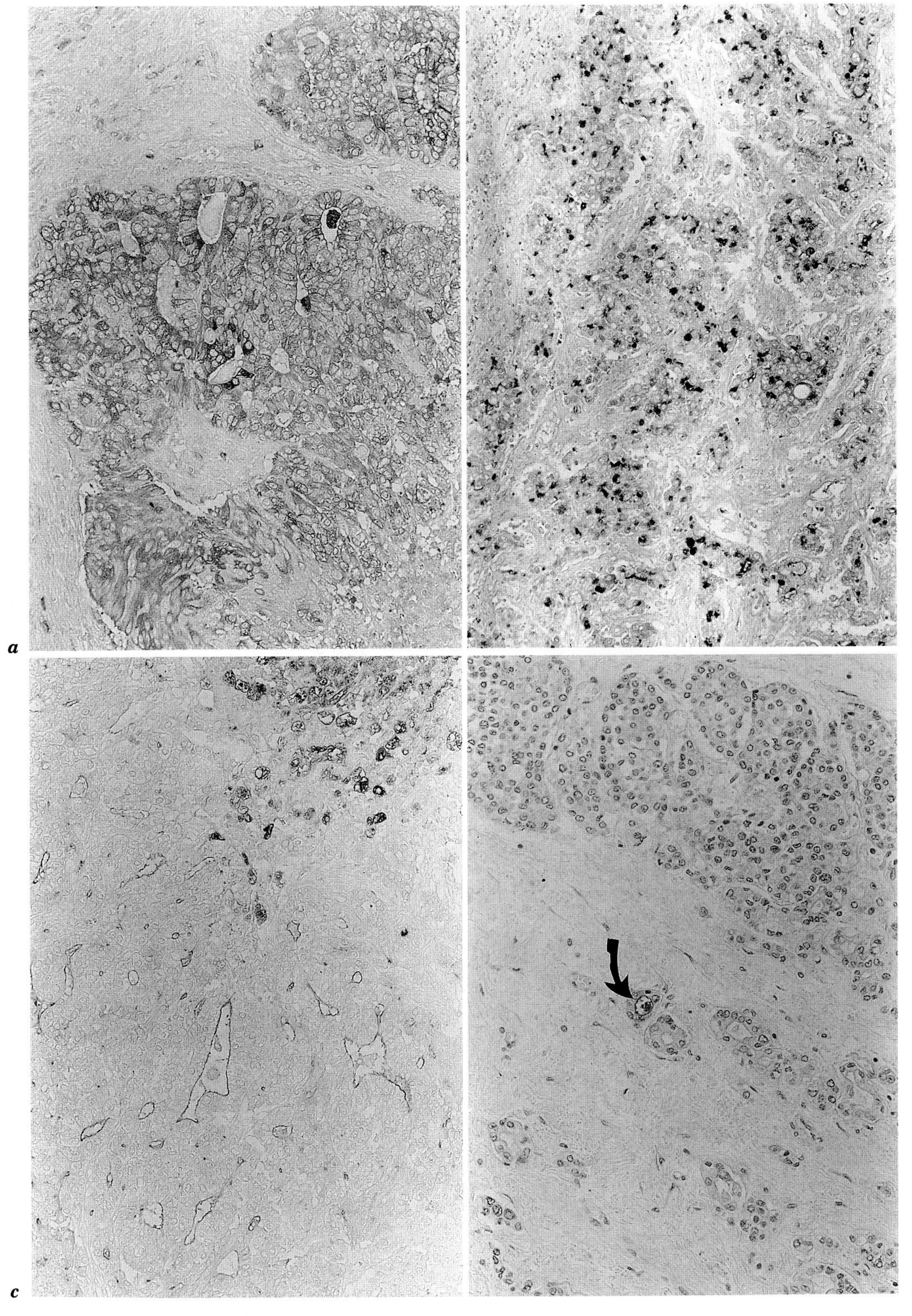

Fig. 5a–d. Immunohistochemical staining of pancreatoblastoma. Numerous tumor cells are positive for alpha-1-antitrypsin ***a*** and for alpha-fetoprotein ***b***. Some of them are positive for carcinoembryonic antigen ***c*** and a few, for CA19-9 (***d*** *arrow*). (ABC method, ×85)

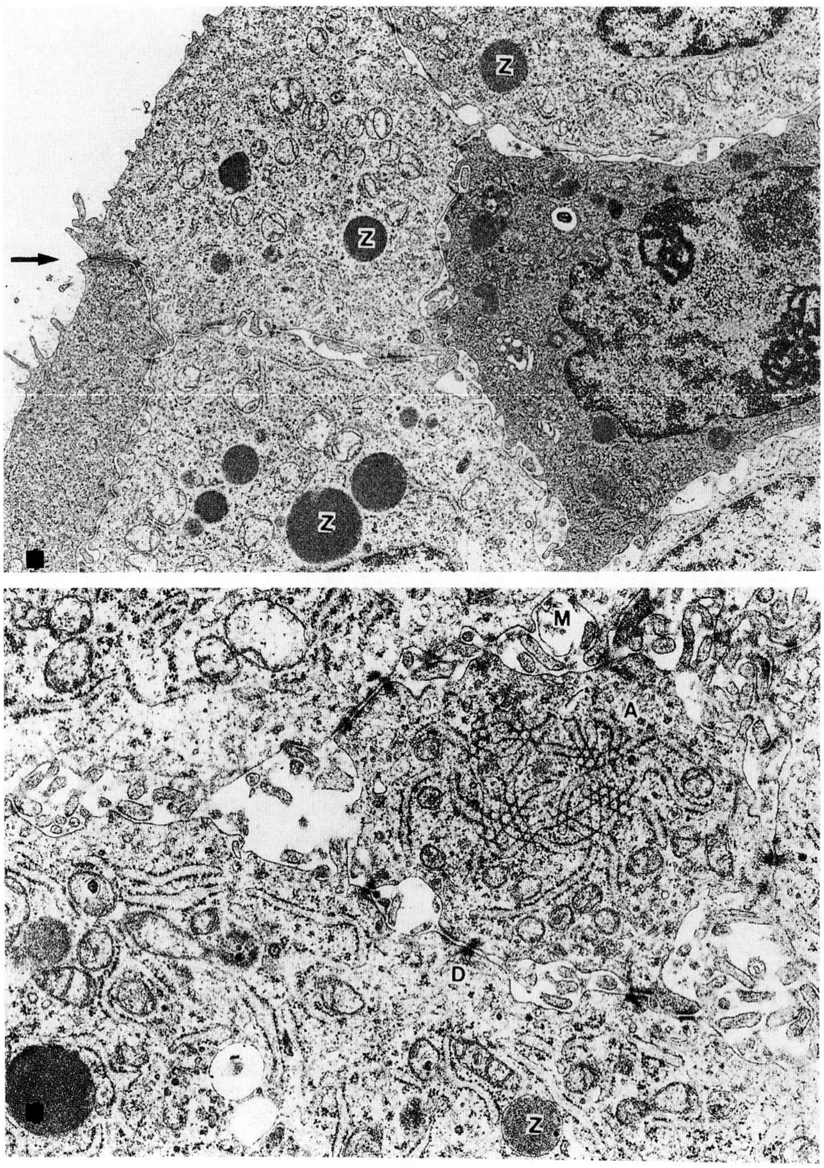

a *b*

Fig. 6a,b. Electron microscopic appearance of tumor cells in a pancreatoblastoma. ***a*** Tumor cells are connected with junctional complexes (*arrow*) and contain some zymogen-like granules (*Z*). Annular lamellae (*A*) mitochondria (*M*) desmosomes (*D*), and microvilli (*M*) are seen at the luminal surface. (***a*** ×9 500, ***b*** ×19 000) (courtesy of Dr. Horie)

chemotherapy [22]. Horie [31] suggested that pancreatoblastomas, according to the embryonic derivation from the ventral and dorsal pancreatic anlage can be divided into two subtypes which differ in localization, histologic features, and prognosis. However, to establish the validity of this concept, a larger number of cases have to be studied.

References

1. Palosaari D, Ctayton F, Seaman J (1986) Pancreatoblastoma in an adult. Arch Pathol Lab Med 110:650–652
2. Hoorens A, Rckaert F, Morohoshi T, Kamisawa T, Heitz PhU, Stamm B, McLelland E, Lemoine NR, Ruschoff K, Klöppel G (1992) Pancreatic acinar cell tumours: Their histologic, immunocytochemical and ultrastructural features. J Pathol 167 [Suppl]:149A
3. Becker WF (1915) Pancreatoduodenectomy for carcinoma of the pancreas in an infant: Report of a case. Ann Surg 145:864–872
4. Frable WJ, Sill WJS, Kay S (1971) Carcinoma of the pancreas, infantile type: A light and electron microscopic study. Cancer 27:667–673
5. Horie A, Yano Y, Kotoo Y, Miwa A (1977) Morphogenesis of pancreatoblastoma, infantile carcinoma of the pancreas: Report of two cases. Cancer 39: 245–254

6. Lack EE, Levey R, Cassady JR, Vawter G (1983) Tumors of the exocrine pancreas in children and adolescents: A clinical and pathologic study of eight cases. Am J Surg Pathol 7:319–327
7. Ohaki Y, Misugi K, Fukuda J, Okudaira M, Hirose M (1987) Immunohistochemical study of pancreatoblastoma. Acta Pathol Jpn 37:1581–1590
8. Kakudo K, Sakural M, Miyajl T, Ikeda Y, Satani M, Manabe H (1976) Pancreatic carcinoma in infancy. An electron microscopic study. Acta Pathol Jpn 26:719
9. Koh THHG, Cooper JE, Newman CL, et al. (1986) Pancreatoblastoma in a neonate with Beckwith-Wiedemann syndrome. Eur J Pediatr 145:435–438
10. Horie A, Haratake J, Jimi A, Malsumoto M, Ishi N, Tsutsumi Y (1937) Pancreatoblastoma in Japan, with differential diagnosis from papiliary cystic tumor (ductuoacinar adenoma) of the pancreas. Acta Pathol Jpn 37:47–63
11. Morohoshi T, Sagawa F, Mitsuya T (1990) Pancreatoblastoma with marked elevation of serum alpha-fetoprotein: An autopsy case report with immunocytochemical study. Virchows Arch [A] 416:265–270
12. Sakaida N, Jho T, Hara F, et al. (1992) Two cases of pancreatoblastoma with various differentiation (in Japanese). Trans Soc Pathol Jpn 81:150
13. Cubilla AL, Fitzgarald PJ (1984) Tumor of exocrine pancreas. In: Hartmann WH (ed) Atlas of tumor pathology, 2nd series, fascicle 19. Armed Forces Institute of Pathology. Washington DC
14. Morohoshi T, Shimizu K, Kanda M (1991) Pancreatic tumors: Their pathology and morphogenesis (in Japancse) Jpn J Cancer Dig Organs 1:556–562
15. Potts SR, Brown S, O'Hara MD (1986) Pancreatoblastoma in a neonate associated with Beckwith-Wiedemann syndrome. Z Kinderchir 48:11
16. Drut R, Jones MC (1988) Congenital pancreatoblastoma in Beckwith-Wiedemann syndrome: An emerging association. Pediatr Pathol 8:331–339
17. Horie A (1988) Clinicopathological features of pancreatoblastoma (in Japanese) Tan to Sui 9: 1511–1519
18. Horie A, Morohoshi T, Klöppel G (1987) Ultrastructural comparison of pancreatoblastoma, solid-cystic tumor and acinar cell carcinoma. J Clin Electron Microsc 20:353–362
19. Buchino JJ, Castello FM, Nagaraj HS (1984) Pancreatoblastoma: A histochemical and ultrastructural analysis. Cancer 53:963–969
20. Ohaki Y, Misugi K, Sasaki Y, Okudaira M (1985) Pancreatic carcinoma in childhood: Report of an autopsy case and a review of the literature. Acta Pathol Jpn 35:1543–1554
21. Iseki M, Suzuki T, Koizumi Y, et al. (1986) Alpha-fetoprotein-producing pancreatoblastoma: A case report. Cancer 57:1833–1835
21. Ono J, Sakamoto H, Sakoda K, Yagi Y, Hagio S, Sato E, Katsuki T (1984) Acinar cell carcinoma of the pancreas with elevated serum alpha-fetoprotein. Int Surg 69:361–364
22. Griffin BR, Wisbeck WM, Schaller RT, Benjamin DR (1987) Radiotherapy for tocally recurrent intantile pancreatic carcinoma (Pancreatoblastoma). Cancer 60:1734–1736
22. Robey G, Daneman A, Martin DJ (1983) Pancreatic carcinoma in a neonate. Pedlatr Radiol 13:284–286
23. Silverman JF, Holbrook CT, Porles WJ, Kodrofl MB, Joshi VV (1990) Fine needle aspiration cytology of pancreatoblastoma with Immunocytochemical and ultrastructural studies. Acta Cytologica 34: 632–640
24. Wilander E, Sundstrom C, Meurting S, Grotte G (1976) A highly differentiated endocrine pancreatic tumor in a young boy. Acta Pediatr Scand 65: 769–772
25. Ichijima K, Akaishi K, Toyoda N, Kobashi Y, Ueda Y, Matsuo S, Yamabe H (1985) Carcinoma of the pancreas with endocrine component in childhood: A case report. Am J Clin Pathcl 83:95–100
26. Benjamin E, Wright DH (1980) Adenocarcinoma of the pancreas of childhood: A report of two cases. Histopathology 4:87–104
27. Cooper JE, Lake BD (1989) Use of enzyme histochemistry in the diagnosis of pancreatoblastoma. Histopathology 15:407–414
28. Morohoshi T, Kanda M, Horie A, Chotl A, Dreyer T, Klöppel G, Heitz PU (1987) Immunocytochemicat markers of uncommon pancreatic tumors. Acinar cell carcinoma, pancreatoblastoma and solid cystic (papillary-cystic) tumor. Cancer 59:739–747
29. Mah PT, Loo DC, Tock EPC (1974) Pancreatic acinar cell carcinoma in childhood. Am J Dis Child 128:101–104
30. Osborne BM, Culbert SJ, Cangir A, MacKay B (1977) Acinar cell carcinoma of the pancreas in a 9-year-old child: Case report with electron microscopic observations. South Medi J 70:370–372
31. Horie A (1982) Pancreatoblastoma. Histopathologic criteria based upon a review of six cases. In: Humphrey GB, (eds): Pancreatic tumors in children. Martinus Nijhoff. The Hague, pp 159–166

Small Cell Carcinoma

Definition

This is an undifferentiated carcinoma composed of small cells of probable neuroendocrine origin.

Incidence

Small cell carcinoma of the pancreas is uncommon and comprises approximately 1% of all exocrine pancreatic tumors [1–3]. Reyes and Wang [1] found five cases in male patients among 485 pancreatic malignancies and 16 585 autopsies gathered during 29 years. Cubilla and Fitzgerald observed 7 small cell carcinomas among 508 exocrine pancreatic cancers. We found four cases of small cell carcinoma among 264 epithelial tumors of the exocrine pancreas [4].

Sex and Age

Small cell carcinoma occurs predominantly in men aged between 40 and 75 years [1, 2, 5]. So far, it has not been reported in young individuals.

Etiology

Unknown.

Clinical Presentation

Because of the aggressiveness of the neoplasms, the patient presents with symptoms of advanced malignant disease. These symptoms include weight loss, jaundice, and metastasis [1]. Paraneoplastic hormonal syndromes, which are relatively common in pulmonary small cell carcinomas, are very rare in pancreatic tumors. So far, only one adrenocorticotropic hormone (ACTH)-producing tumor and a tumor associated with hypercalcemia have been reported [6, 7].

Clinical Diagnosis

At the time of diagnosis, the tumors are usually large and can be easily detected in the pancreas using ultrasonography and computed tomography. Fine needle biopsy from the tumor or a large needle biopsy of a liver metastasis revealing small cells with hyperchromatic nuclei and scanty cytoplasm is suggestive of a small cell carcinoma, although this type of tumor typically occurs in the lung. The possibility of metastases to the pancreas and the liver from a primary tumor in the lung has to be excluded by all available means. Among the common tumor markers that may be detected in the serum, high neuron-specific enolase (NSE) levels have recently been demonstrated in a patient [5]. The level of other hormones, including testosterone, insulin-like growth factor I and II can be normal [5].

Gross Findings

The tumors are usually large by the time they are diagnosed (mean diameter: 4.2 cm), and are poorly demarcated. On the cut surface, they are grey-

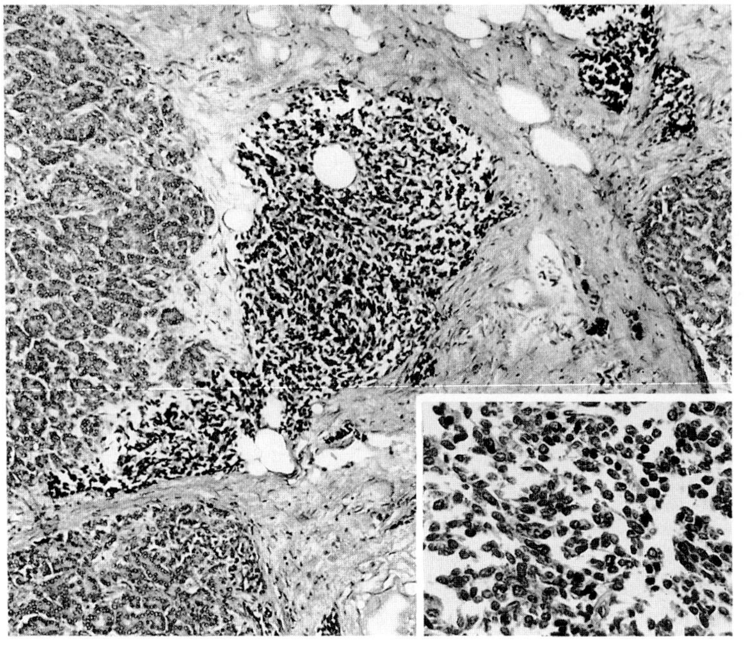

Fig. 1. Small cell carcinoma of the pancreas: Invasion of the exocrine parenchyma by small tumor cells with hyperchromatic nulei (*inset*). H&E, ×115 and ×250

white and show areas of necrosis and hemorrhage. Most tumors are located in the head of the pancreas and invade into adjacent organs.

Microscopic Findings

The histologic appearance of the tumors is indistinguishable from that of small cell carcinoma of the lung. They consist of sheets and nests of small lymphocyte-like cells with markedly hyperchromatic round-to-oval nuclei, unconspicuous nucleoli, and poorly defined cytoplasm (Fig. 1). Occasional areas with atypical glandular differentiation may be present [1]. In addition, trabecular arrangements within a delicate fibrous stroma may be encountered. The tumor cells show numerous mitoses and degenerative changes. They are negative for mucin stains.

Electron Microscopy

The tumor nuclei contain abundant euchromatin and only a little heterochromatin at the nuclear membrane [5]. The cytoplasm displays, as the most characteristic features, membrane-bound electron-dense granules measuring 120–200 nm in diameter, and bundles of intermediate filaments. The electron-dense vesicles correspond to neurosecretory granules.

Immunohistochemistry

As is the case with small cell carcinoma of the lung, neuroendocrine markers are also the most useful markers for small cell carcinoma of the pancreas. Recently, O'Connor et al. [5] demonstrated NSE and chromogranin A as well as calcitonin in such tumors. In addition, there was a globular perinuclear staining for keratin, as it is typically found in neuroendocrine small cell neoplasms.

Differential Diagnosis

The diagnosis of small cell carcinoma of the pancreas is based on excluding the possibility of metastasis of the same type of tumor originating from other sites, especially from the lung [8]. As the small cell carcinoma of bronchogenic and extrapulmonary origin share the same histologic features, diagnosis of a primary small cell carcinoma of the pancreas relies entirely on the exclusion of a primary tumor outside the pancreas by macroscopic examination. This is in most cases only possible by a meticulous postmortem examination.

Small cell carcinoma of the pancreas may be difficult to distinguish from a low-grade endocrine tumor, particularly if it exhibits a trabecular arrangement. The reason for this difficulty lies in the fact that, like in the lung, pancreatic well-differentiated endocrine tumors and small cell carcinomas represent two ends of the spectrum of neuroendocrine neoplasm.

Small cell carcinoma of the pancreas may be confused histologically with malignant non-Hodgkin's lymphoma. The latter neoplasm, however, is distinguished by a positive immunoreaction to common leukocyte antigen and a negative staining for keratin, a marker constellation that is reversed in small cell carcinoma.

Prognosis and Survival

All small cell carcinomas described so far presented with metastases to the liver, lymph nodes and other organs or invasion to adjacent tissues. As tumor resection was impossible in these instances, the patients were treated by chemotherapy, which resulted in partial and complete remissions (up to 50 months), particularly when etoposide and cisplatin were used [5, 9].

If patients with small cell carcinomas of the pancreas received "supportive" treatment only, prognosis was very poor, with a survival between 1 and 2 months [1].

References

1. Reyes CV, Wang T (1981) Undifferentiated small cell carcinoma of the pancreas: A report of five cases. Cancer 47:2500–2502
2. Cubilla AL, Fitzgerald PJ (1984) Tumors of the exocrine pancreas. In: Atlas of tumor pathology, 2nd series, fascicle 19. Washington, DC Armed Forces Institute of Pathology
3. Klöppel G (1984) Pancreatic, non-endocrine tumours. In: Klöppel G, Heitz PhU (eds) Pancreatic Pathology. Churchill Livingstone, Edinburgh, pp 79–113
4. Morohoshi T, Held G, Klöppel G (1983) Exocrine pancreatic tumours and their histological classification. A study based on 167 autopsy and 97 surgical cases. Histopathology 7:645–661
5. O'Connor TP, Wade TP, Sunwoo YC, Reimers HJ, Palmer DC, Siverberg AB, Johnson FE (1992) Small cell undifferentiated carcinoma of the pancreas. Report of a patient with tumor marker studies. Cancer 70:1514–1519
6. Corrin B, Gilby ED, Jones NF, Patrick J (1973) Oat cell carcinoma of the pancreas with ectopic ACTH secretion. Cancer 31:1523–1527
7. Hobbs RD, Stewart AF, Ravin ND, Carter D (1984) Hypercalcemia in small cell carcinoma of the pancreas. Cancer 53:1552–1554
8. Ibrahim NBN, Briggs JC, Corbishley CM (1984) Extrapulmonary oat cell carcinoma. Cancer 54: 1645–1661
9. Morant R, Bruckner HW (1989) Complete remission of refractory small cell carcinoma of the pancreas with cisplatin and etoposide. Cancer 64:2007–2009

Preneoplastic Lesions of the Exocrine Pancreas

Introduction

Recognition and ablation of preneoplastic or in situ stage neoplasms is an ideal method for prevention of cancers. This approach is particularly difficult for internal organs such as the pancreas that are not conveniently visualized or accessible for physical examination, biopsy or evaluation by cytologic studies. Thus, there is relatively little prospective experience in the recognition of preneoplastic lesions of the human pancreas. Several retrospective approaches have been utilized in attempts to recognize such lesions.

A traditional approach is to examine the non-tumorous pancreas from individuals with pancreatic carcinoma for focal proliferative and dysplastic cellular changes of the ducts and acini, and then to compare the incidence of such lesions with that in pancreases that do not contain carcinoma [1–3]. The association of such lesions with non-neoplastic processes, such as chronic pancreatitis, must also be assessed. This approach can establish the association of focal proliferative and dysplastic lesions with the presence of carcinoma, but does not establish the probability that these lesions will progress to become carcinomas.

A second approach is to examine pancreases from various age groups for focal epithelial lesions to determine which types are acquired with aging [3, 4]. If acquired lesions display a progression of dysplastic to high grade atypical cellular changes, then neoplastic potential may be inferred, but it is not proven.

A third approach compares lesions found in the human pancreas with those found during tumor development in animal models of pancreatic cancer [2, 5–7]. The evolution of the lesions can be studied in animals by serial autopsies following treatment with a carcinogen so that progression can be inferred. This approach has provided new perspectives although the relevance of some animal models for humans has been questioned.

A fourth approach is the use of molecular studies to evaluate the activation and expression of oncogenes, or the loss or mutation of tumor suppressor genes, in putative preneoplastic lesions of the pancreas. This approach has not yet been extensively applied to the human pancreas. Since c-K-*ras* is activated by mutation at codon 12 in a high fraction of human pancreatic carcinomas [8], it will be of interest to determine which, if any, of the putative preneoplastic lesions contain such mutations.

In this chapter, we will review the histopathology of the proliferative, metaplastic and dysplastic lesions of the pancreas which have so far been described in humans. These lesions are compared with those found in experimental models of pancreatic carcinogenesis, and their significance is discussed.

Non-Neoplastic Lesions of Ducts and Lobules

Since the histologic appearance of most pancreatic carcinomas suggest a duct or ductular phenotype of these neoplasms, duct changes that may precede these carcinomas are of great interest. Five main types of duct changes can be distinguished: Squamous metaplasia, nonpapillary epithelial hypertrophy with or without metaplasia (including pyloric gland or goblet cell metaplasia), ductal papillary hyperplasia, and adenomatous duct hyperplasia. Focal proliferative and metaplastic changes in the lobules include both ductular and acinar cell lesions.

Squamous Metaplasia

Replacement of the columnar epithelium by squamous epithelium frequently involves only a portion of the main duct or a ductule. Sometimes the epithelium covering the surface of a squamous metaplasia may still be mucinous. Very intense squamous metaplasia may occur in the main pancreatic duct after prolonged stenting (personal observation; G.K.) or in association with the presence of *Clonorchis sinensis* worms [9]. This lesion is found in 8%–47% of the nontumorous pancreases as well as in chronic pancreatitis [1]. Focal epithelial hyperplasia, i.e., an increase in the number of epithelial layers with slight squamous metaplasia [1, 10] can be regarded as the immature variant of squamous metaplasia. Although the incidence increases with age [11], no association with pancreatic cancer has been noted.

Non-Papillary Epithelial Hypertrophy

This is the most frequent epithelial change of the pancreatic ducts, and is found in 59%–90% of nontumorous pancreases. It is particularly seen in association with moderate obstruction and chronic pancreatitis, and occurs in about the same percentage of patients with exocrine pancreatic cancer as in a matched control group of patients with other types of nonpancreatic cancer [1, 2]. It is characterized by the replacement of the normal epithelium of the large- and medium-sized ducts by tall columnar cells with basal nuclei and considerable supranuclear mucin. It is, therefore, also called mucinous cell hypertrophy, mucoid transformation, goblet cell metaplasia, or ductal hyperplasia (grade 1). Mainly neutral mucin and sialomucin is found in these cells, while sulphated mucin that is normally produced in the ducts is markedly reduced. Ultrastructurally, these cells show punctate cerebroid granules instead of the dense core granules with a homogeneous inner structure that characterize the mucin granules of the normal large ducts [12]. Occasionally, there are also metaplastic pyloric type cells that intensely stain with periodic acid-Schiff (PAS) and are positive for pepsinogen II and cathepsin E [12]. Pure metaplastic pyloric-type cells are mainly found in the connective tissue surrounding main or interlobular ducts and usually accompany mucinous cell hypertrophy.

Ductal Papillary Hyperplasia

This lesion is characterized by intraductal papillary proliferation of duct cells showing mucinous cell hypertrophy (Fig. 1). The papillary epithelial folds characteristically contain a vascular tissue stalk. Ductal papillary hyperplasia may be combined with focal adenomatous duct hyperplasia [13] and with pyloric cell metaplasia [12]. The lesion has also been called ductal hyperplasia, grades 2 and 3 [3, 11]. The incidence of ductal papillary hyperplasia increases with age and is higher in patients with pancreatic cancer than in control autopsy patients without pancreatic cancer (50% versus 12%) [1, 2]. In elderly patients, papillary hyperplasia in secondary ducts may cause duct obstruction. This in turn leads to saccular duct ectasia upstream to the obstruction with lobular atrophy and fibrosis [14, 15].

Adenomatous Duct Hyperplasia, Ductular Hyperplasia, and Tubular Complexes

Focal adenomatous duct hyperplasia represents an aggregation of small ducts lined by epithelium with mucinous hypertrophy and often with pyloric gland metaplasia (Fig. 2). Occasionally, this lesion forms small nodules with an adenoma-like composition [16]. Ductular cystic hyperplasia [17] may be a variant of adenomatous hyperplasia.

Tubular (ductular) structures may focally replace acinar tissues in the lobules. These lesions have been called tubular complexes [18], and focal acinar dilatation [19]. The cells lining these structures most often have the characteristics of centroacinar cells, but acinar cells may be interspersed. They are seen in chronic pancreatitis [18], uremia [19], and cachexia and seem to reflect atrophic or regressive change.

Tubular complexes may also replace acinar tissue in apparently normal pancreases (Fig. 3). These lesions have also been called ductular hyperplasia [11] and ductal metaplasia [20]. The cells lining

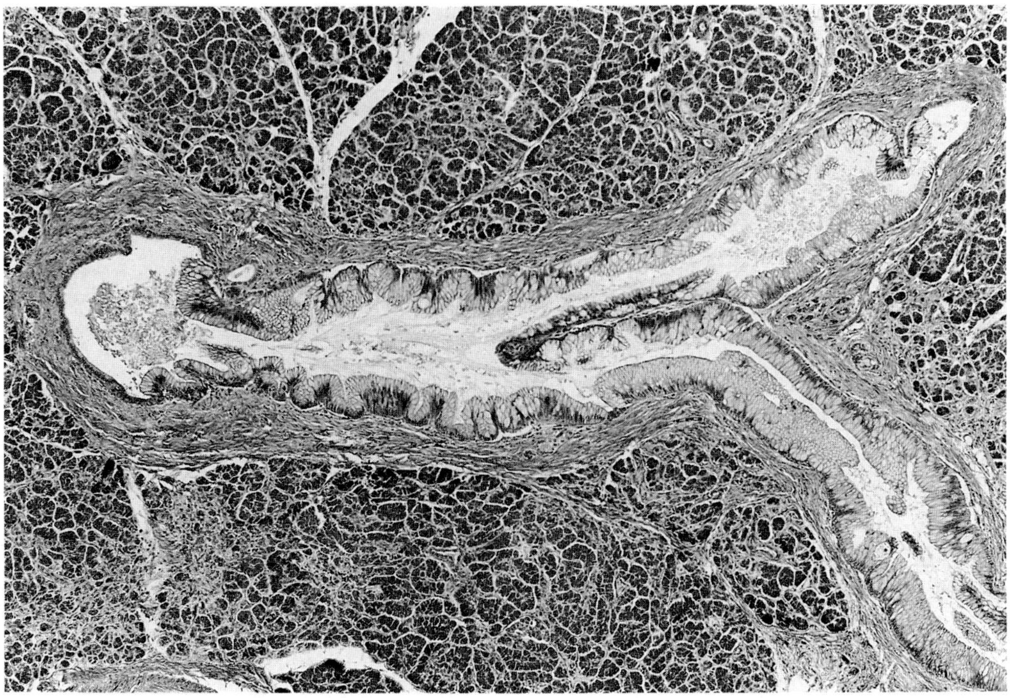

Fig. 1. Ductal papillary hyperplasia and non-papillary epithelial hypertrophy are both present in this longitudinally sectioned, branching duct. Portions of the duct are still lined by cuboidal ductal epithelium (*upper right*, *upper left*). The papillary epithelium is well differentiated and contains mucus. (H&E ×96, original magnification)

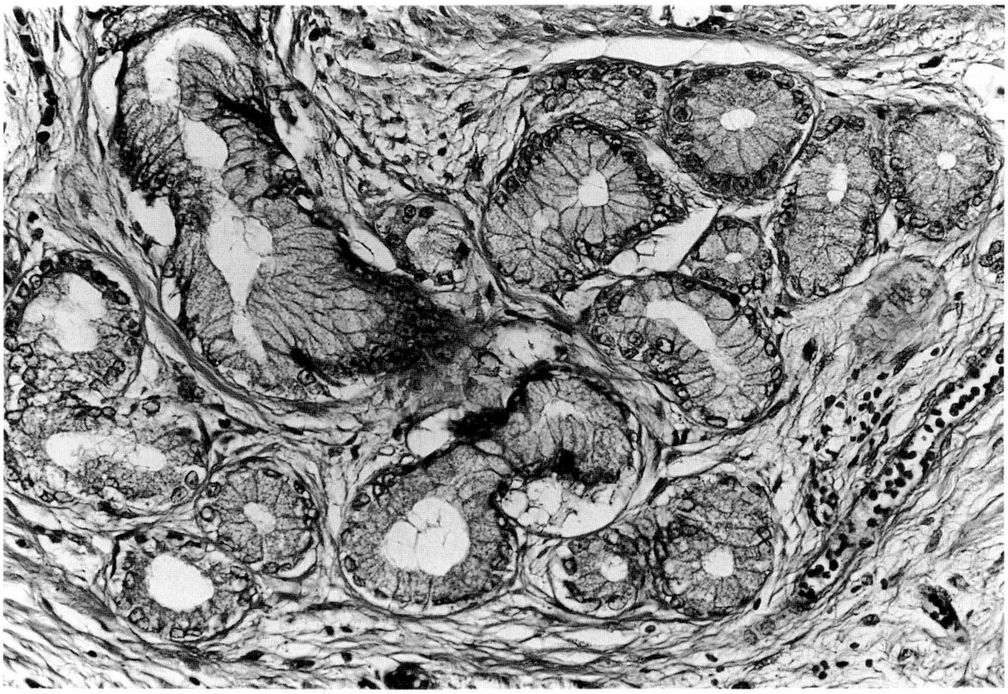

Fig. 2. Adenomatous duct hyperplasia. A group of ductules is lined by cells that show mucous hypertrophy. At the *left*, one lumen is partly lined by hypertrophic cells and the remainder is lined by cuboidal ductal cells. (H&E ×192, original magnification)

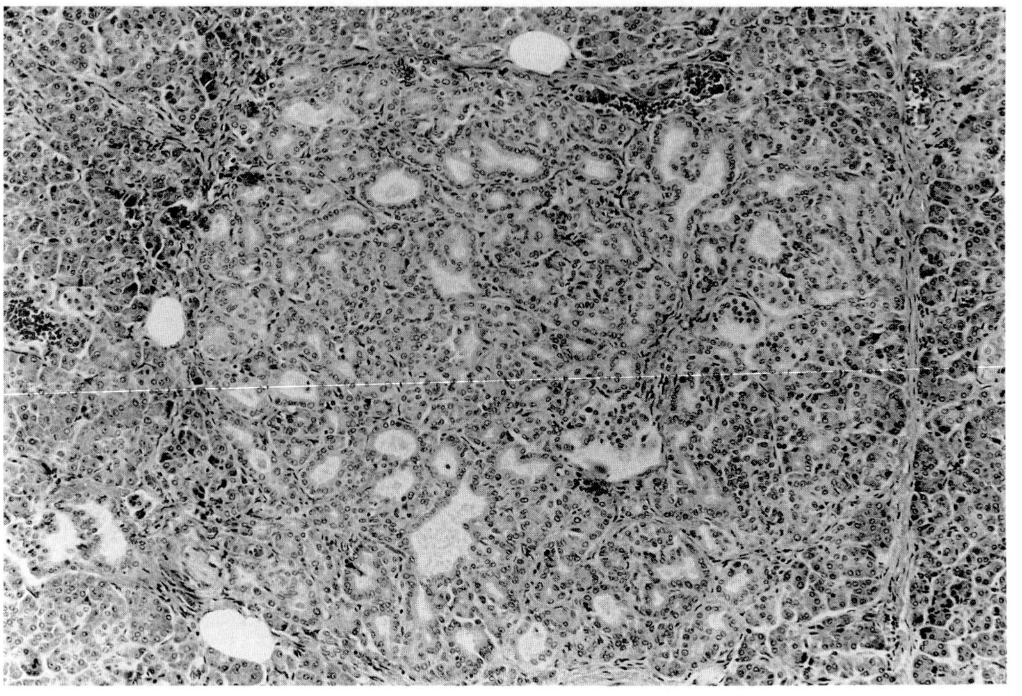

Fig. 3. Ductular hyperplasia (tubular complex, ductal metaplasia) focally replaces acinar tissue in the central part of this field. The cells lining the ductules in the lesion are cuboidal and do not show mucus hypertrophy. The area of ductular hyperplasia is surrounded by acinar tissue. (H&E ×96, original magnification)

these structures do not appear atrophic, may contain or lack mucin, and are not associated with inflammation or scarring. These lesions may represent variants of adenomatous duct hyperplasia.

Non-Neoplastic Acinar Cell Lesions

Focal acinar cell changes of the pancreas have been given various names at various times. They include lesions described as eosinophilic degeneration of acinar cells [19], acinar adenomatous hyperplasia [21], focal acinar cell dysplasia [22, 23] and hyperplastic acinar cell nodule [11]. This change is characterized by irregular but sharply outlined groups of acinar cells, measuring from 300 μm to 3000 μm in their greatest dimension. The cytoplasm of the cells often shows a homogeneous eosinophilia or a loss of basophilia, but may also be vacuolated. The cells and their nuclei are often similar in size to the surrounding acinar cells, but the nuclei may show a more dense chromatin or be enlarged (Fig. 4). Mitoses are infrequent and inflammatory infiltrates are absent. The reported incidence of focal acinar cell changes ranges from 1.2% to 43.5% [11, 19, 22, 23].

Severe Ductal and Ductular Atypia

Severe atypia of the ductal epithelium, with or without papillary projections, may be found in the vicinity of ductal adenocarcinomas (see Discussion). Lesions of ductal epithelium with atypia that is so severe as to merit designation as carcinoma in situ have been reported in a few cases in the absence of invasive pancreatic carcinoma (Fig. 5) [11, 24]. Important criteria for severe ductal atypia include loss of cell polarity, nuclear pleomorphism and enlargement, and cribriform papillary growth pattern (papillary growth without vascular stalks).

Carcinoma in Situ

Many experienced pathologists feel that it is not possible to distinguish between severe atypia of

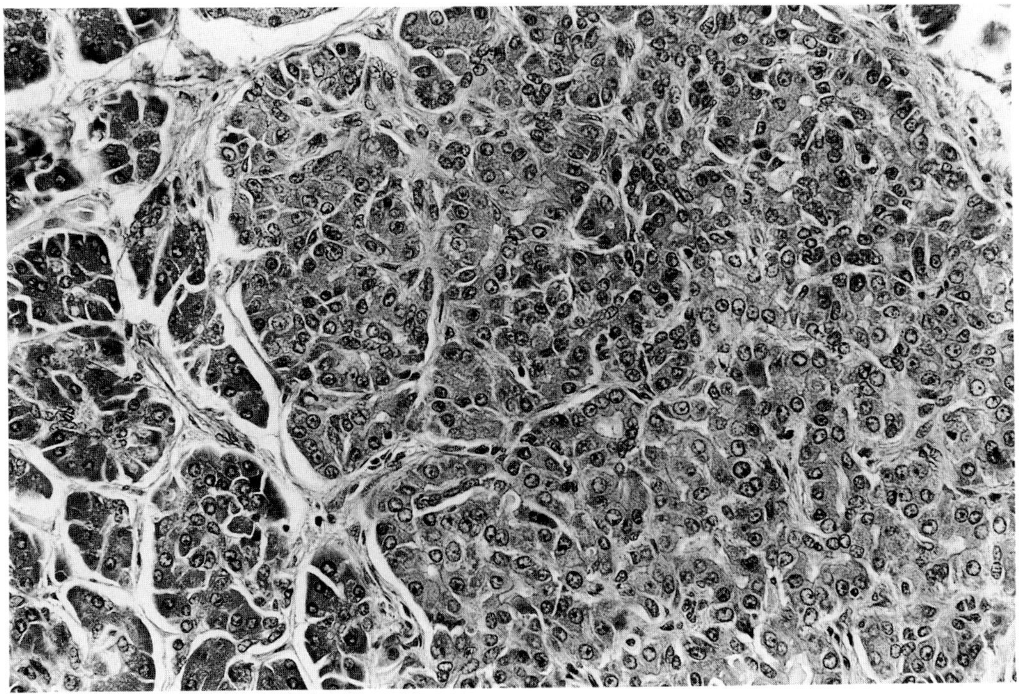

Fig. 4. Focal acinar cell dysplasia (*right*) with normal acinar tissue (*left*). The average size of nuclei is larger and cytoplasmic basophilia is reduced in the focus compared with the normal acinar cells. (H&E ×196, original magnification)

ductal epithelium, as discussed above, and carcinoma in situ (CIS) on a morphologic basis. Thus, either term may be used to designate a lesion that is considered to be at high risk for progression to an invasive carcinoma. Intraductal lesions with severe atypia are appropriately called CIS when there is no evidence of invasion. Severe atypia of carcinoma in situ grade is also described in ductular epithelium (for definition see Pour et al. [11]).

Focal Carcinogen-Induced Changes in Rodent Pancreas

Several types of focal lesions have been described in the pancreas of carcinogen-treated rodents [6, 7]. Some of these lesions have also been observed to occur at a low incidence in the pancreases of aged rodents that were not treated with carcinogens, suggesting that the lesions could play a role in the development of spontaneously occurring neoplasms.

Atypical acinar cell foci and nodules (the human counterpart could be focal acinar cell dysplasia) in rats treated with azaserine are numerous relative to the ultimate incidence of acinar cell tumors. A small fraction of larger lesions (nodules and adenomas) develop secondary anaplastic change, suggesting malignant change. It is clear that a very low fraction (perhaps in the range of 0.1%) of these lesions progress to become acinar cell carcinomas in rodents. By extrapolating from the animal model, it is conceivable that focal acinar cell dysplasia may play a similar role in the development of acinar cell carcinoma in humans.

The cystic ductal complex is induced by several carcinogens in rodents, especially hamsters, but is rare in humans. It has low malignant potential and bears some morphologic similarity to the human microcystic serous adenoma.

Other lesions such as tubular or ductular complexes, and intraductal papillary hyperplasia have a lower incidence and are more frequently associated with overt carcinomas in the animal models. Both lesions can exhibit cytologic atypia of severe grade, and the development of such atypia is regarded as evidence of progression to malignancy. Thus, they are considered to be precursors of ductal

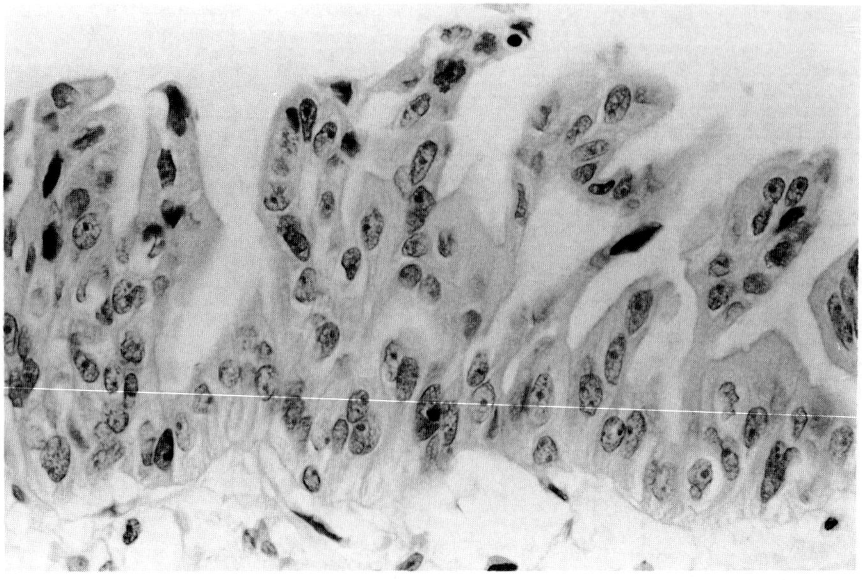

Fig. 5. Severe ductal atypia (ductal carcinoma in situ). Papillary folds without connective tissue stalks irregular size of the nuclei with irregularly distributed chromatin. (H&E ×240)

adenocarcinomas, and the most advanced lesions are designated as CIS. The similarity of these focal carcinogen-induced changes in rodent pancreas to lesions described above in the human pancreas supports the classification of the latter as premalignant lesions that may progress to carcinoma.

In the absence of pancreatitis, the tubular complex of rodents is morphologically similar to ductular hyperplasia in humans. Intraductal CIS in the hamster is morphologically similar to severe ductal atypia (ductal CIS) in the human.

Discussion

A number of reports record a much higher incidence of ductal papillary hyperplasia in pancreases with ductal adenocarcinoma than in those without a tumor [1–3, 25]. Moreover, atypical hyperplasia (equivalent to intraductal carcinoma or CIS) was noted in about 25% to 30% of the cases with carcinomas [1–3] but in none of the controls with the exception of the series of Kozuka et al. [3] in which atypical hyperplasia was found in 0.7% of the controls. These clearly atypical lesions that were usually only present in close proximity to ductal adenocarcinomas [1, 2] may reflect intraductal extension from an established invasive carcinoma. In this context, designation of the intraductal component as CIS seems inappropriate. In rare instances, the intraductal component appears to be the dominant lesion suggesting progression from an intraductal CIS to invasive carcinoma [26].

Pour et al. [11] serially sectioned 83 pancreases obtained from consecutive autopsies and found ductular hyperplasia (graded 1 to 3) in 39% of the cases. Lesions classified as "ductular CIS" arising from intralobular pseudoductular as well as peri- and intrainsular ductules [11] were detected in seven patients, all more than 55 years of age. Three of these patients had cancer in the head of the pancreas whereas the ductular lesions were all in the body or tail. Two microscopic "ductular" cancers, 2 and 3 mm in diameter, were reported in the series—one of glandular type and one adenosquamous type. Finally, there was also a ductal CIS in the head of one pancreas.

In another autopsy series of 206 patients without pancreatic carcinoma, ductal papillary hyperplasia with dysplasia was reported in 75 patients (36%) including 5 with CIS, 3 in the ampulla, and 2 in the body or tail of the pancreas [27]. There was also an occult invasive pancreatic carcinoma in the body of the pancreas; however, the lesion that was illustrated appears to be an intraductal papillary tumor (see Chapter "Intraductal Papillary Mucinous Tumors, Non-Invasive and Invasive" in this volume). Similar cases that appear to be intraductal (papillary) tumors interpreted as precursors of invasive ductal adenocarcinoma have also been reported by a number of other investigators [28, 29]. Intraductal (papillary) tumors apparently represent an entity with a significantly more favorable prognosis than the usual ductal adenocarcinoma [30], and the two types of tumors should not be confused. Experience with intraductal tumors suggests that they may progress to become ductal adenocarcinoma, one of its variants, or a mucinous cystadenocarcinoma.

Codon 12 c-K-*ras* mutation has been reported in both apparently benign- and malignant-appearing portions of two intraductal tumors [31]. In the same study, three of five apparently benign intraductal tumors contained codon 12 mutations in c-K-*ras* suggesting that they should be separated from non-neoplastic intraductal papillary hyperplasia. The proportion of human intraductal tumors that progress to the various types of carcinoma and the rate of such progression are not yet known; however it is doubtful that they represent an early stage in the development of a significant fraction of ductal carcinomas since this relatively uncommon tumor type can exist for long periods of time without invading outside the duct system. Although intraductal tumors should be regarded as neoplasms that have the potential to progress to invasive carcinomas, it seems likely that most pancreatic carcinomas arise from other precursor lesions. Therefore, the intraductal tumors should be considered separately from precursor lesions of the usual ductal adenocarcinoma.

If we exclude the intraductal tumors from the discussion, focus on other possible precursor lesions of the common ductal adenocarcinoma, and consider the great subjectivity inherent to all classifications of dysplasia and atypia, little evidence remains for the transition from ductal papillary hyperplasia to carcinoma in humans. The malignant potential of ductal papillary hyperplasia is, therefore, probably very low. Further support of this view is provided by a study of nine pancreatic specimens (with or without concomitant pancreatic carcinoma) that revealed no mutations at c-K-*ras* codon 12 in ductal papillary hyperplasia [32], suggesting that the mutation of this proto-oncogene may be used to distinguish between non-neoplastic and neoplastic lesions.

The occurrence of ductal papillary epithelial hyperplasia with dysplasia has also been used as an argument for the precancerous potential of chronic pancreatitis [33]. Dysplastic epithelial changes and hyperplasias were found in 112 of 280 (40%) of operative specimens from patients with chronic pancreatitits. Ninety-two (32%) of the dysplasias were classified as grade I and 20 (7.1%) as grade II. Grade III dysplasia, however, was not observed. In another study [2] of operative specimens with chronic pancreatitis, the investigators were unable to detect any papillary ductal lesions displaying clearcut signs of cellular atypia. In particular, no marked cellular atypia, as seen in intraductal lesions at the margin of duct carcinomas, were found. Thus, from this purely morphological study, it was concluded that there was no evidence of a causal link between chronic pancreatitis and pancreatic carcinoma. The case report by Mizumoto et al. [23] demonstrates the association of chronic pancreatitis with intraductal CIS, but such isolated case reports do not resolve the issue of whether the pancreatitis bears a primary, secondary, or coincidental relationship to the development of the carcinoma.

Focal acinar lesions (focal acinar cell dysplasia) was reported in 47 of 108 adult patients in an autopsy series [22]. It was absent in 135 infants and children under the age of 5 years, suggesting that it is an acquired lesion [4]. Several reports note its association with islet cell tumors [34]. The significance and true frequency of focal acinar cell lesions remain to be established, since other investigators [22, 35] have not observed this lesion at the frequency reported by Longnecker et al. [22]. This appears to be a heterogeneous group of lesions, and it is unlikely that they are of uniform etiology and significance.

Morphologic study of the human pancreas has left many questions regarding the malignant potential of various focal proliferative lesions of ducts, ductules, and acinar cells. Lesions such as ductal papillary hyperplasia and focal acinar cell dysplasia without cellular atypia appear to have little or no significance as precursors to the usual ductal adenocarcinoma. Ductal papillary hyperplasia should be distinguished from intraductal (papillary) tumors (see Chapter "Intraductal Papillary Mucinous Tumors, Non-Invasive and Invasive" in this volume) that are considered to be neoplasms. Severe ductal atypia (ductal CIS) is accorded the greatest significance as a precursor to ductal carcinomas in humans.

References

1. Cubilla AL, Fitzgerald PJ (1976) Morphological lesions associated with human primary invasive

nonendocrine pancreas cancer. Cancer Res 36: 2690–2698

2. Klöppel G, Bommer G, Rückert K, Seifert G (1980) Intraductal proliferation in the pancreas and its relationship to human and experimental carcinogenesis. Virchows Arch [A] 387:221–233
3. Kozuka S, Sassa R, Taki T, Masamoto K, Nagasawa S, Saga S, Hasegawa B, Takeuchi M (1979) Relation of pancreatic duct hyperplasia to carcinoma. Cancer 43:1418–1428
4. Longnecker DS, Hashida Y, Shinozuka H (1980) Relationship of age to prevalence of focal acinar cell dysplasia in the human pancreas. J Natl Cancer Inst 65:63–66
5. Konishi Y, Mizumoto K, Kitazawa S, Tsujiuchi T, Tsutsumi M, Kamano T (1990) Early ductal lesions of pancreatic carcinogenesis in animals and humans. Int J Pancreatol 7:83–89
6. Longnecker DS (1986) Experimental models of exocrine pancreatic tumors. In: Go VLM, Brooks FP, DiMango EP et al. (eds) The Exocrine pancreas: Biology, pathobiology and diseases. Raven, New York, pp 443–458
7. Pour P, Althoff J, Takahashi M (1977) Early lesions of pancreatic ductal carcinoma in the hamster model. Am J Pathol 88:291–308
8. Shibata D, Capella G, Perucho M (1990) Mutational activation of the c-K-*ras* gene in human pancreatic carcinoma. Baillieres Clin Gastroenterol 4:151–169
9. Chan P, Teoh TB (1967) The pathology of *Clonorchis sinensis* infestation of the pancreas. J Pathol 93: 185–189
10. Oertel JE (1989) The Pancreas. Non-neoplastic alterations. Am J Surg Pathol 13:50–65
11. Pour PM, Sayed S, Sayed G (1982) Hyperplastic, preneoplastic and neoplastic lesions found in 83 human pancreases. Am J Clin Pathol 77:137–152
12. Sessa F, Bonato M, Frigerio B, Capella C, Solcia E, Prat M, Bara J, Samloff IM (1990) Ductal cancers of the pancreas frequently express markers of gastrointestinal epithelial cells. Gastroenterology 98:1655–1665
13. Sommers SC, Murphy SA, Warren S (1954) Pancreatic duct hyperplasia and cancer. Gastroenterology 27:629–640
14. MacCarty RL, Stephens DH, Brown AL, Carlson HC (1975) Retrograde pancreatography in autopsy specimens. Mayo Clinic Proc 123:359–366
15. Schmitz-Moormann P, Hein J (1976) Altersveränderrungen des Pankreasgangsystems und ihre Rückwirkungen auf das Parenchym. Virchows Arch [A] 371:145–152
16. Klöppel G (1984) Pancreatic non-endocrine tumours. In: Klöppel G, Heitz PU (eds) Pancreatic Pathology. Churchill Livingstone, Edinburgh, pp 79–113
17. Cubilla AL, Fitzgerald PJ (1984) Tumors of the exocrine pancreas. In: Hartmann WH (ed) Atlas of tumor pathology, 2nd series, fasicle 19. Washington DC, Armed Forces Institute of Pathology, p 83
18. Bockman DE (1981) Cells of origin of pancreatic cancer: Experimental animal tumors related to human pancreas. Cancer 47:1528–1534
19. Stamm BH (1984) Incidence and diagnostic significance of minor pathologic changes in the adult pancreas at autopsy: A systematic study of 112 autopsies in patients without known pancreatic disease. Hum Pathol 15:677–683
20. Parsa I, Longnecker DS, Scarpelli DG, Pour P, Reddy JK, Lefkowitz M (1985) Ductal metaplasia of human exocrine pancreas and its association with carcinoma. Cancer Res 45:1285–1290
21. Glenner G, Mallory GK (1956) The cystadenoma and related nonfunctional tumors of the pancreas. Pathogenesis, classification, and significance. Cancer 9:980–996
22. Longnecker DS, Shinozuka H, Dekker A (1980) Focal acinar cell dysplasia in human pancreas. Cancer 45:534–540
23. Kishi K, Nakamura K, Yoshimori M, Tajiri H, Ozaki H, Kinoshita T, Kosuge T, Hayakawa M (1992) Morphology and pathological signficance of focal acinar cell dysplasia of the human pancreas. Pancreas 7:177–182
24. Mizumoto K, Tsutsumi M, Kitazawa S, Tsujita S, Nakayama M, Tsujii T, Kanehiro H, Nakajima Y, Nakano H, Konishi Y (1990) Intraductal carcinoma in a surgically resected pancreas with chronic pancreatitis. Int J Pancreatol 7:279–285
25. Chen J, Baithun SI, Ramsay MA (1985) Histogenesis of pancreatic carcinoma: A study based on 248 cases. J Pathol 146:65–76
26. Mizumoto K, Inagaki T, Koizumi M, Uemura M, Ogawa M, Kitazawa S, Tsutsumi M, Toyokawa M, Konishi Y (1988) Early pancreatic duct adenocarcinoma. Hum Pathol 19:242–244
27. Mukada T, Yamada S (1982) Dysplasia and carcinoma in situ of the exocrine pancreas. Tohoku J Exp Med 137:115–124
28. Liou T-C, Lin X-Z, Chang T-t, Lin C-y, Lin P-W, Jin Y-T, Yu C-Y (1992) Pancreas divisum with early pancreatic cancer—presenting as chronic obstructive pancreatitis. Pancreas 2:251–256.
29. Ferrari BT, O'Halloran RL, Longmire WP, Lewin KJ (1979) Atypical papillary hyperplasia of the pancreatic duct mimicking obstructing pancreatic carcinoma. N Engl J Med 301:531–532
30. Morohoshi T, Kanda M, Asanuma K, Klöppel G (1989) Intraductal papillary neoplasms of the pancreas. A clinicopathologic study of six patients. Cancer 64:1329–1335
31. Yanagisawa A, Kato Y, Ohtake K, Kitagawa T, Ohashi K, Hori M, Takagi K, Sugano H (1991) c-Ki-ras point mutations in ductectatic-type mucinous

cystic neoplasms of the pancreas. Jpn J Cancer Res 82:1057–1060

32. Lemoine NR, Jain J, Hughes C, Staddon SL, Maillet B, Hall PA, Klöppel G (1992) Ki-ras oncogene activation in preinvasive pancreatic cancer. Gastroenterology 102:230–236
33. Volkholz H, Stolte M, Becker V (1982) Epithelial dysplasias in chronic pancreatitis. Virchows Arch [A] 396:331–349
34. Shinozuka H, Lee RE, Dunn JL, Longnecker DS (1980) Multiple atypical acinar cell nodules of the pancreas. Hum Pathol 11:389–391
35. Klöppel G (1989) Cancer of the pancreas: Morphological and biological aspects. In: Preece P, Cushieri A, Rosin RD (eds) Cancer of the bile ducts and pancreas. WB Saunders, Philadelphia, pp 113–138

Pathology of Metastatic Patterns of Pancreatic Cancer

Introduction

Despite recent advances in the clinical diagnosis and treatment of cancer, pancreatic cancer remains a medical and surgical problem [1–6]. At the time of diagnosis of pancreatic cancer, approximately 85% of symptomatic patients have metastatic disease [1]. In surgical specimens of pancreatic cancer, even tumors 2 cm or smaller have regional lymph node metastases in about half of the cases [3]. The aggressive spread of a pancreatic tumor is one of the reasons for the fatal outcome of the disease.

Considerable variations in the incidence of organ metastasis of pancreatic cancer have been reported. The following incidences of metastases of pancreatic cancer into various organs have been reported: Lymph nodes, 40%–87%; liver, 59%–82%; lungs, 21%–52%; stomach, 3%–32%; duodenum, 5%–44%; diaphragm, 5%–32%; bile duct, 21%–51%; bones, 3%–24%; colon, 5%–7%; spleen, 3%–13%; and kidneys, 4%–21% [2, 7–15]. In general, the incidence and extent of metastases of the body and/or tail cancers are more frequent than that of head cancers. The following incidences of distant metastasis of pancreatic cancer were reported for head (body and/or tail) cancers: Liver, 52%–76% (63%–85%); lungs, 19%–42% (24%–68%); bones, 2%–13% (3%–39%) [2, 7–9, 13, 14].

There are a few reports about the relationships between tumor spread and the size or histologic type of the tumor. Miller et al. [10] reported that the size increased with increasing grade of malignancy. Douglass et al. [15] pointed out that even the tumors with diameters smaller than 2 cm could be associated with very extensive distant disease.

In the following, the sites of direct tumor invasion and metastases of pancreatic cancer and the correlation among the size, location, metastatic sites, and morphology of cancers are described. Because findings in autopsy cases and surgical specimens differ in some aspects, the data will be presented separately whenever possible. Table 1 and Figs. 1 and 2 present classification of lymph nodes, and Table 2 shows the general rules from the Japanese Pancreas Society on clinical and pathologic management for carcinoma of the pancreas.

Anatomical Site of Cancers

Some investigators report that about two-thirds of pancreatic cancer occur in the head [8–13, 16]. In the autopsy material from Kishi et al. [2, 20] among 248 autopsy cases, 118 (48%) were in the head, 114 (46%) in the body and/or tail, 11 (4%) in the entire pancreas, and 5 (2%) in the head and body. The observed difference could be that postmortem examination by Kishi et al. [2, 20] was more frequently performed in cancer of the body and/or tail than in cancer of the head because of the difficulties of clinical diagnosis of cancer of the body and/or tail [2, 5, 7, 9, 20]. On the other hand, among 62 resected cases of pancreatic caner, 40 tumors (65%) were located in the head and 22 (35%) in the body and/or tail [20].

Lymph Node Metastases

Lymph node metastases predict a poor outcome for patients with pancreatic cancer [3, 4, 6, 17, 18].

Table 1. Regional lymph nodes of the pancreas proposed by the Japanese Pancreas Society [38].

Station number	Location
No. 1:	Lymph nodes of the right cardiac region
No. 2:	Lymph nodes of the left cardiac region
No. 3:	Lymph nodes along the lesser curvature of the stomach
No. 4:	Lymph nodes along the greater curvature of the stomach
No. 5:	Lymph nodes of the suprapyloric region
No. 6:	Lymph nodes of the infrapyloric region
No. 7:	Lymph nodes along the left gastric artery
No. 8a:	Lymph nodes of the anterior-superior region of the common hepatic artery
No. 8p:	Lymph nodes of the posterior region of the common hepatic artery
No. 9:	Lymph nodes of the celiac axis
No. 10:	Lymph nodes at the hilum of the spleen
No. 11:	Lymph nodes along the splenic artery
No. 12:	Lymph nodes of the hepatoduodenal ligament
No. 12h:	Lymph nodes along the upper porta hepatis
No. 12a1:	Lymph nodes along the upper portion of the proper hepatic hepatis artery
No. 12a2:	Lymph nodes along the lower portion of the proper hepatic hepatis artery
No. 12p1:	Lymph nodes along the upper portion of the portal vein
No. 12p2:	Lymph nodes along the lower portion of the portal vein
No. 12b1:	Lymph nodes along the proximal bile duct
No. 12b2:	Lymph nodes along the distal bile duct
No. 12c:	Lymph nodes along the cystic duct
No. 13:	Lymph nodes of the region posterior to the head of the pancreas
No. 13a:	Lymph nodes of the region superior-posterior to the head of the pancreas
No. 13b:	Lymph nodes of the region inferior-posterior to the head of the pancreas
No. 14:	Lymph nodes at the radix mesenterii
No. 14A:	Lymph nodes along the superior mesenteric artery
No. 14a:	Lymph nodes at the origin of the superior mesenteric artery
No. 14b:	Lymph nodes at the origin of the inferior pancreaticoduodenal artery
No. 14c:	Lymph nodes at the origin of the middle colic artery
No. 14d:	Lymph nodes at the origin of the jejunal artery
No. 14V:	Lymph nodes along the superior mesenteric vein
No. 15:	Lymph nodes along the middle colic artery
No. 16:	Lymph nodes along the abdominal aorta
No. 17:	Lymph nodes of the anterior region of the head of the pancreas
No. 17a:	Lymph nodes of the superior-anterior region of the head of the pancreas
No. 17b:	Lymph nodes of the inferior-anterior region of the head of the pancreas
No. 18:	Lymph nodes along the inferior boder of the body and tail of the pancreas

Table 2. Tumor classifications (The Japan Pancreas Society [38]).

Classification of tumor size (t)	
t1:	less than 2.0 cm
t2a:	2.1–3.0 cm
t2b:	3.1–4.0 cm
t3:	4.1–6.0 cm
t4:	more than 6.1 cm

Classification of retropancreatic invasion (rp)	
rpo:	tumors confined to the pancreas
rpe:	retropancreatic invasion
rpi:	invasion into retroperitoneal viscera

Classification of the degree of invasion to lymphatic vessels (ly)	
ly0:	no invasion
ly1:	minimal invasion
ly2:	moderate invasion
ly3:	severe invasion

Tumor growth patterns	
INF α:	expansive growth with clear margins
INF β:	intermediate between α and γ
INF γ:	infiltrative growth without clear margins

Amount of connective tissue in the tumor tissue
Medullary type
Intermediate type
Scirrhous type

Groups of lymph nodes (cancer of pancreatic head)	
N0:	no lymph node metastases
N1:	metastases to lymph nodes of Group 1 (Nos. 8, 12, 13, 14, and 17)
N2:	metastases to lymph nodes of Group 2 (Nos. 9, 11, 12, 15, 16, and 18)
More than N2	

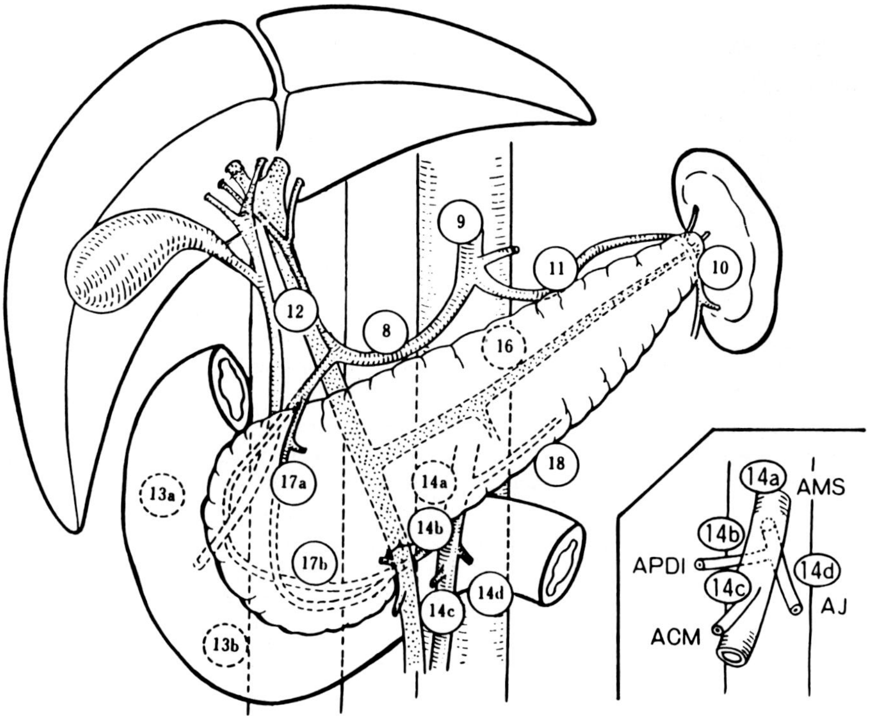

Fig. 1. Classification of the regional lymph nodes of the pancreas. Insert: Subdivision of 14. *AMS*, The superior mesenteric artery; *AJ*, the jejunal artery; *APDI*, the inferior pancreatico-duodenal artery; *ACM*, the medial colic artery; *8*, lymph nodes around the common hepatic artery; *9*, lymph nodes around the celiac trunk; *10*, lymph nodes at the hilus of the spleen; *11*, lymph nodes around the splenic artery; *12*, lymph nodes of the hepatoduodenal ligament; *13*, posterior pancreaticoduodenal lymph nodes; *13a*, nodes above the papilla of Vater; *13b*, nodes below the papilla; *14*, lymph nodes around the superior mesenteric artery; *14a*, lymph nodes at the root of the superior mesenteric artery; *14b*, lymph nodes at the root of the inferior pancreatoduodenal artery; *14c*, lymph nodes at the root of the medial colonic artery; *14d*, lymph nodes at the roots of the first jejunal artery; *16*, para-aortic lymph nodes; *17*, anterior pancreatoduodenal lymph node; *17a*, nodes above the papilla of Vater; *17b*, nodes below the papilla; *18*, subpancreatic lymph nodes

The most common sites of lymph node metastasis of pancreatic cancer in the autopsy series [2, 19, 20] in order of frequency were the celiac node group (65%), the peripancreatic node group (55%), the hepatoduodenal node group (34%), the mesenteric node group (22%), the subclavicular node group (22%), the perigastric node group (21%), and the paratracheal node group (12%). For the nomenclature of parapancreatic and para-aortic lymph nodes, see Table 1 and Figs. 1 and 2. Lymph node involvement of the 10841 autopsy cases of pancreatic cancer by the annual autopsy reports between 1982 and 1989 in Japan are shown in Fig. 3.

Lymph node involvement in 27 resected cancers of the head of the pancreas is shown in Fig. 4. Of these 27 cases, 22 underwent pancreaticoduodenectomy and 5 total pancreatectomy. Nineteen of the 27 cases (70%) had metastases into regional lymph nodes. The nodes most commonly involved were, in descending order, the inferior pancreaticoduodenal group (52%), the anterior pancreatic group (47%), the superior pancreaticoduodenal group (41%), the common hepatic group (36%), and the superior mesenteric group (32%). A detailed analysis for lymph nodes in specimens of resected cancer of the head of the pancreas [1] showed that the most commonly involved, in descending order, were the posterior pancreaticoduodenal group (45%), the superior head group (45%), the superior body group (27%), the inferior head group (23%), and the anterior pancreaticoduodenal group (9%). Nagai et al. [21] and Ozaki and Kishi [22] reported similar results with lymph node metastasis of pancreatic head cancer.

In a study by Nagakawa et al. [24] of surgical specimens, metastases of pancreatic head carcinoma to the lymph nodes were found in 33 of the 42 patients (78.6%). The sites of metastasis were

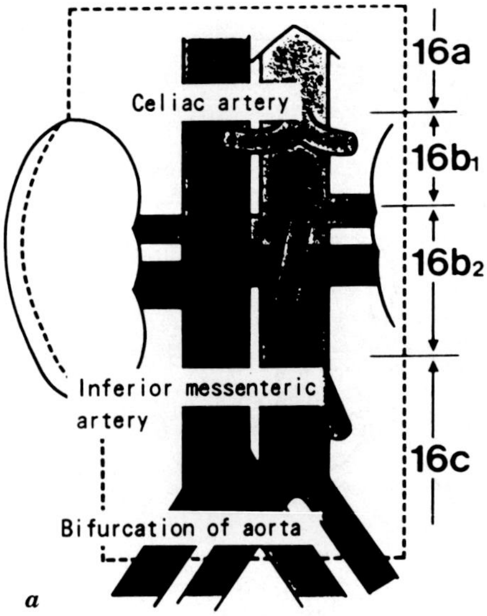

a

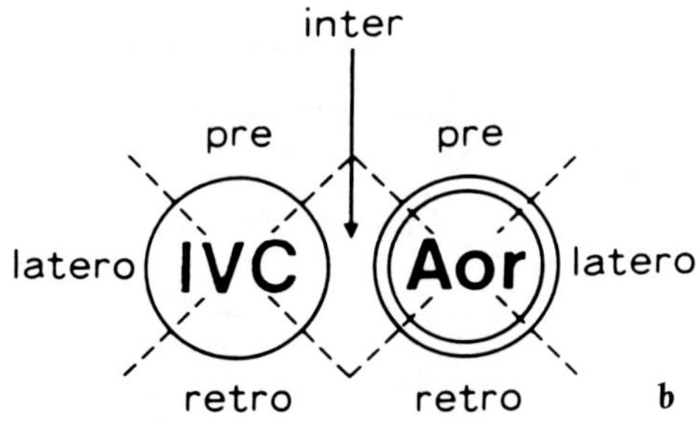

b

Fig. 2a,b. Classification of the lymph nodes of area no. 16. Cross-sectional segmentation was analyzed according to the proposal of the Japan Society for Cancer Therapy (1991). The inferior vena cava (*IVC*) is divided into anterior (*Ivc-pre*), lateral (*Ivc-latero*); and posterior (*Ivc-retro*) segments, and a segment between the abdominal aorta and inferior vena cava (*Ivc-inter*), and the abdominal aorta (*Aor*), is separated into anterior (*Aor-pre*), lateral (*Aor-latero*) and posterior (*Aor-retro*) segments. ***a***, Frontal classification; ***b***, trans-sectional segment; *IVC*, the inferior vena cava; *Aor*, the abdominal aorta; *16a*, upper region above the celiac artery; *16b*, median region from the celiac artery to the inferior mesenteric artery; *16c*, lower region from the inferior mesenteric artery

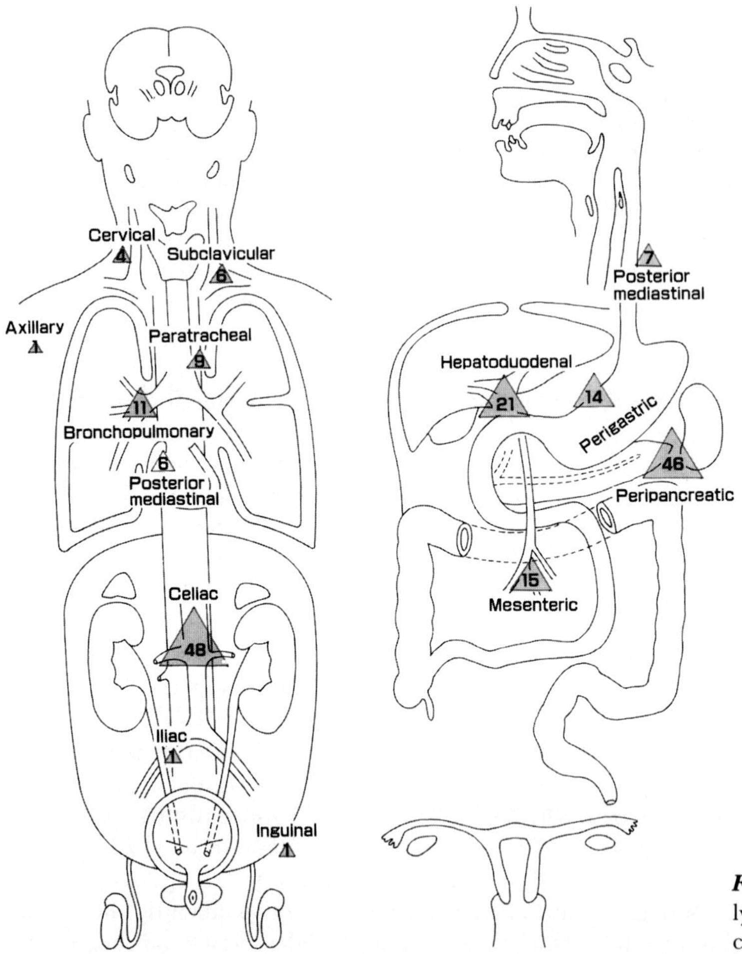

Fig. 3. The incidence (in percentage) of lymph node metastases of 10 841 autopsy cases with pancreatic carcinoma

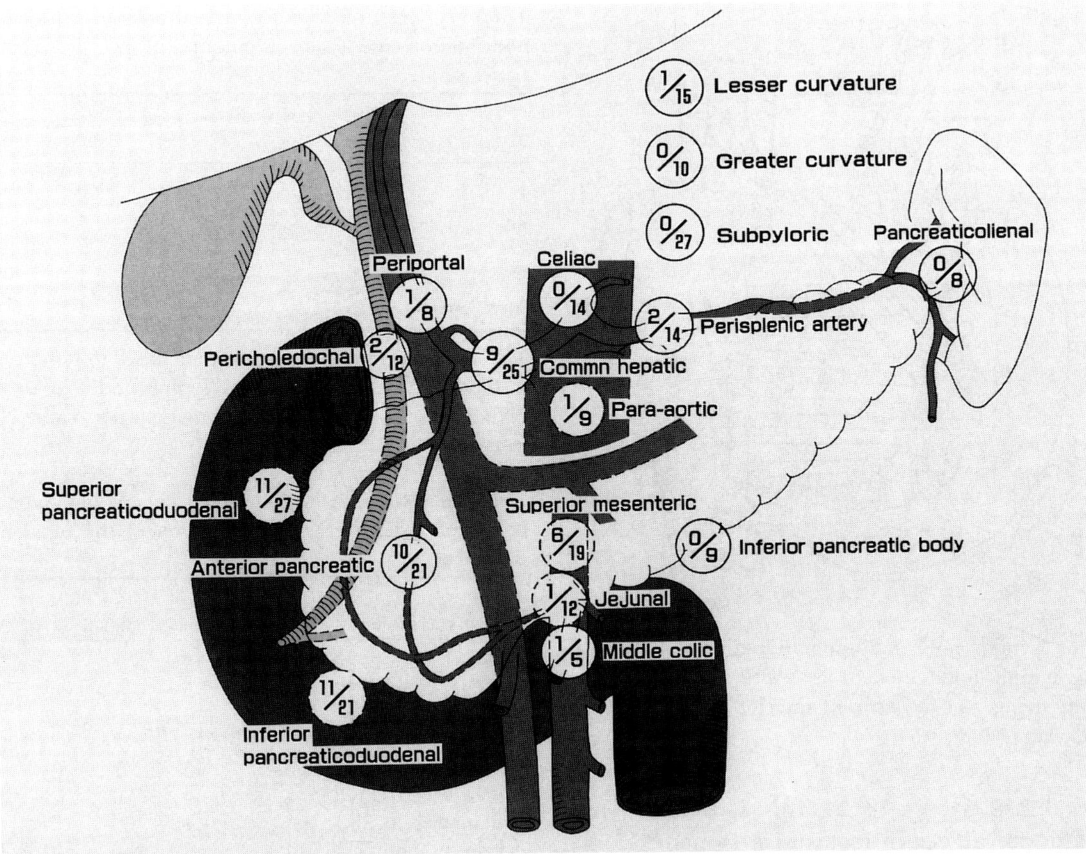

Fig. 4. Lymph node involvement of 27 resected pancreatic head cancer. Numerator indicates the number of patients with lymph nodes containing cancer; denominator indicates the number of patients in whom the lymph nodes of that group were resected. (*For color reproduction see color insert in the front matter*)

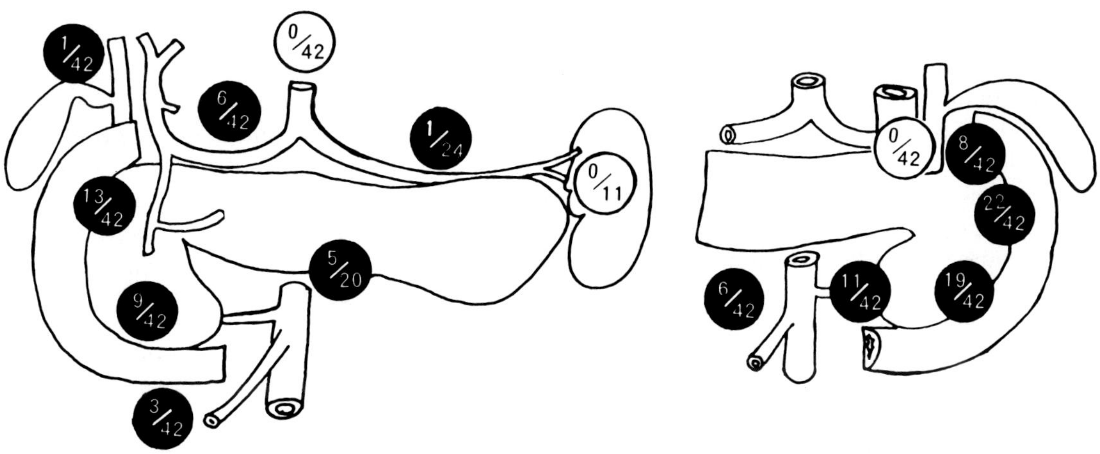

Fig. 5. Distribution of lymph node involvement in carcinoma of the head of the pancreas. The incidence of metastatic lymph nodes is expressed in each circle area as positive metastatic cases/examined cases

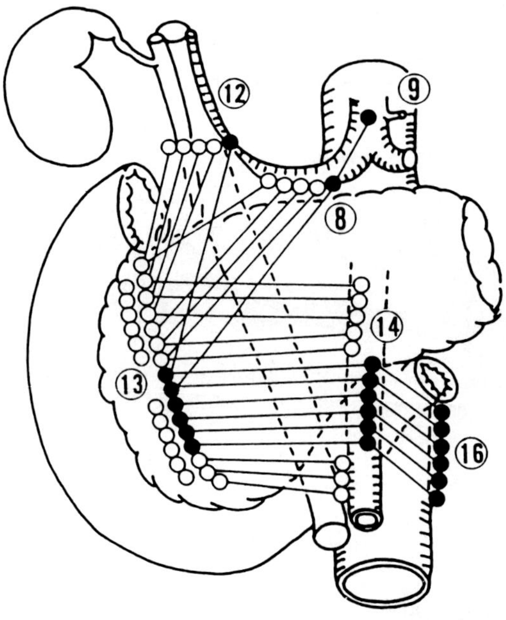

Fig. 6. Lymph node mapping in patients with para-aortic lymph node metastasis. Anterior lymph node without metastasis (*open circle*); anterior lymph node with metastasis (*closed circle*)

nodes 6, 8, 9, 11, 12, 13, 14, 16, 17, and 18 (Table 1). The prevalence of metastases to node 13 was the highest, followed by nodes 17 and 14 (Fig. 5).

In the aforementioned study [24, 25], there were 7 patients with metastases to para-aortic node 16 (Figs. 2, 6). In 4 of these patients, there was a single metastasis in node 16. Multiple para-aortic nodes were involved in the other 3 patients, with nodes 3, 6, and 9 also affected. In patients harboring para-aortic nodal metastases, the average number of lymph nodes involved was 3.1. The average incidence of metastases in node 16 of the examined total lymph nodes was 3.2%. The extent of metastasis in node 16 increased with the number of involved lymph nodes. From an anterior view (Figs. 2, 6), in node 16 the incidence of metastases to segment b2 was the highest (85.7%), followed by 42.9% for segment b1. In the transsectional view, the incidence of "inter" segment involvement was 71.4% followed by 57.1% for the Aor-pre segment. Similar results were found by Yamamoto and Saitoh (see Chapter "Tumor Spread and the Factors Influencing Prognosis in Patients with Resected Pancreatic Carcinoma" in this volume). The incidence of lymph node metastases of pancreatic cancer in relation to the anatomical site of the cases reported by Kishi et al. [2] is shown in Fig. 7. Generally, tumors of the body and/or tail showed a greater tendency for metastases.

Table 3. Relationship between tumor size and lymph node involvement in carcinoma of the head of the pancreas.

Tumor size (t)	No. of cases	N0	N1	≥N2
1	2	2	0	0
2a	12	3	4	5 (2)[a]
2b	14	2	3	9 (3)
3	11	1	1	9 (3)
4	3	1	1	1

N0, No nodal metastases; *N1*, metastases to lymph nodes in Group 1; *N2*, metastases to lymph nodes in Group 2
[a] Number of cases with positive metastases to area No. 16 in parentheses

Table 4. Relationship between histologic type and lymphatic metastases in carcinoma of the head of the pancreas.

Type of carcinoma[a]	No. of cases	N0	N1	≥N2
Papillary	3	1	2	0
Papillars-tubular	5	1	2	2 (2)[b]
Tubular	29	5	17	7 (5)
Well-differentiated	10	3	5	2 (2)
Moderately differentiated	15	2	9	4 (3)
Poorly differentiated	4	0	3	1
Squamous cell	1	0	1	0
Adenosquamous cell	1	0	0	1
Undifferentiated	1	1	0	0

[a] Classification according to the Japanese Pancreas Society [38]
[b] Number of cases with positive metastases to area No. 16 in parentheses

The relationship between tumor size (Table 2) and lymphatic metastases of pancreatic head cancer found by Nagakawa et al. [26] is summarized in Table 3. The extent of lymphatic metastases tended to increase with tumor size. However, two patients with t2a tumors had metastases to node 16, suggesting a poor relationship between tumor size and risk of metastasis to the para-aortic region. In the study of Kishi et al. [19, 20, 27], lymph node involvement was found in 56% of tumors with a diameter <2 cm, 85% of 36 tumors with a diameter between 2.1 and 4 cm, 10% of 4 tumors between 4.1 and 6 cm, and 77% of 13 tumors >6.1 cm. There was no lymph node involvement in only 5 of 62 tumors.

The relationship between histologic type of pancreatic head tumors and lymphatic metastases re-

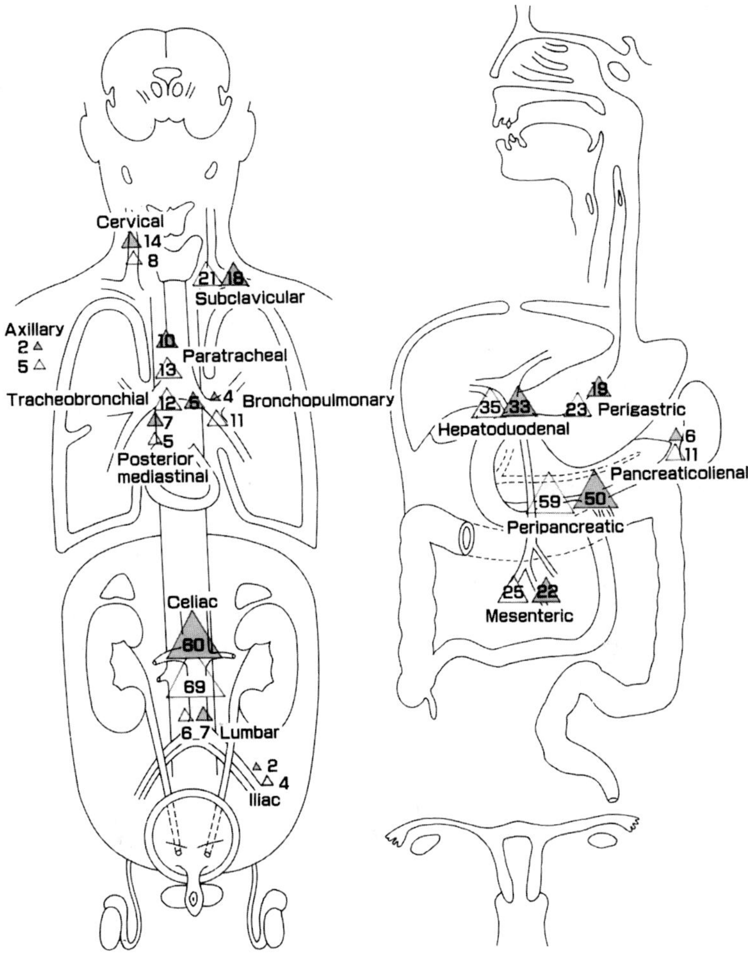

Fig. 7. The incidences (in percentage) of lymph node metastases of 232 autopsy cases with pancreatic cancer in relation to the anatomical site of tumors in the pancreas. *Closed triangle*, cancer of the head of the pancreas; *open triangle*, cancer of the body and/or tail of the pancreas

ported by Nagakawa et al. [24, 25] is shown in Table 4. The incidence and the extent of lymphatic metastasis in ductal adenocarcinomas tended to be higher and more widespread than those in papillary adenocarcinomas, but these differences were insignificant. In another study [20], the incidence of lymph node metastasis by histologic type of tumors was 80% in duct cell adenocarcinomas and 50% in cystadenocarcinomas.

Nagakawa et al. [24, 25] noted a relationship between the amount of connective tissue in the tumor tissue (Table 2) of the head of the pancreas and lymphatic metastases (Table 5). The incidence of lymphatic metastases was higher in patients with intermediate and scirrhous types than in patients with medullary type.

The relationship between retropancreatic invasion (rp) (Table 2) and lymphatic metastases of pancreatic head cancers [24, 25] is shown in Table

Table 5. Relationship between the amount of connective tissue in the tumor and lymph node metastases in carcinoma of the head of the pancreas.

Type	No. of cases	N0	N1	≥N2
Medullary type	6	2	2	2
Intermediate type	17	3	4	10 (3)[a]
Scirrhous type	19	4	3	12 (4)

[a] Number of cases with positive metastasis to area No. 16 in parentheses

6. Lymphatic metastasis was not observed in 3 of 4 patients (75%) with tumors confined within the pancreas (rpo). In contrast, 23 of 37 patients (62.2%) had metastases to at least 2 lymph nodes if invasion into the retropancreatic tissue (rpe) was present. All patients with metastases to node 16 had rpe or rpi.

Table 6. Relationship between invasion into the retropancreatic tissue and lymph node involvement in carcinoma of the head of the pancreas.

Extent of retroperitoneal spread	No. of cases	N0	N1	≥N2
rpo	4	3	1	0
rpe	37	6	8	23 (6)[a]
rpi	1	0	0	1 (1)

rpo, Tumor remains within the pancreas; *rpe*, invasion into retroperitoneal connective tissue; *rpi*, invasion into retroperitoneal viscera
[a] Number of cases with positive metastases to area No. 16 in parentheses

Table 7. Relationship between the growth pattern of the primary tumor and lymph node involvement in carcinoma of the head of the pancreas.

Growth pattern	No. of cases	N0	N1	≥N2*,[a]
INF α	3	2	1	0
INF β	20	6	4	10 (1)
INF γ	19	1	4	14 (6)

* $P < 0.05$
INF α, expansive growth with clear margins; *INF β*, intermediate between α and γ; *INF γ*, infiltrative growth with clear margins
[a] Number of cases with positive metastases to area No. 16 in parentheses

The relationship between the growth pattern (Table 2) of the pancreatic head tumors (INF) and lymphatic metastases reported by Nagakawa et al. [24, 25] is summarized in Table 7. The risk of lymphatic metastases was correlated with the pattern of infiltration, with the extent of nodal metastases increasing from the α to the β and γ patterns. In the γ pattern, particularly, metastases to at least 2 lymph nodes were observed in 14 of 19 patients (73.7%) and were significantly higher in patients showing the α pattern. Metastases to the para-aortic region were present in patients with the β and γ patterns, and were particularly common in 6 of 19 patients (31.6%) with the γ pattern.

It appears that metastases to node 16 is associated with a poor prognosis. Among 7 patients of Nagakawa et al. [24, 25] with metastases to node 16, 4 died within 1 year and 3 survived more than 1 year. The longest survival period was 2 years and 3 months. Among 35 patients without metastases to node 16, 11 were alive more than 3 years. For more details of prognostic factors see Chapter "Tumor Spread and the Factors Influencing Prognosis in Patients with Resected Pancreatic Carcinoma" in this volume.

Neural Invasion

Neural invasion is one of the most common features of pancreatic cancer. Although invasion of neural tissue occurs in some cancers, including cancer of the prostate, the prevalence of neural involvement in pancreatic cancer is much higher than in the other cancers. Therefore, recognition of neural invasion of pancreatic cancer is of conceptual and clinical interest, particularly concerning therapeutic strategies and prognostic factors.

Incidence of Perineural Invasion

The previously reported incidence of neural invasion [22, 28–30] is significantly below the actual figure. Examination of pancreatic cancer specimens by serial sectioning revealed that 27 out of 34 patients had neural invasion [24, 25, 32]. Males and females were equally affected, and no correlation was found between the age of the patients and the patterns of neural invasion.

Affected Nerves

According to Nagakawa et al. [31, 32], both intrapancreatic and extrapancreatic nerves, including the plexi, were affected in 76% of the patients with cancer of the pancreas head. In the remaining cases, neural invasion was confined to the intrapancreatic nerves. The incidence of extrapancreatic neural invasion increased with the increasing incidence of intrapancreatic neural invasion, a finding that suggests that plexus invasion is an extension of intrapancreatic neural invasion. However, there was no correlation between the severity of intrapancreatic neural invasion and plexus invasion. The most frequent site of plexus invasion was the plexus pancreaticus II (67%) and less frequently the plexus pancreaticus I (12%), the plexus of the hepatopancreatic ligament (12%), and others (18%). Of the 34 patients, 18% had invasion of the plexus in the hepatoduodenal ligament and plexus pancreaticus I, 18% had involvement of both plexus pancreaticus I and II, and 12% showed invasion of plexus pancreaticus II and the plexus in the hepatoduodenal ligament [26, 32].

There was no correlation between the size of pancreatic head cancers and neural invasion; there was plexus invasion in both of the t_1 cancers, in 4 out of 7 t_2a, 8 out of 12 t_2b, 6 out of 7 t_3, and the one t_4 cancer [26, 32].

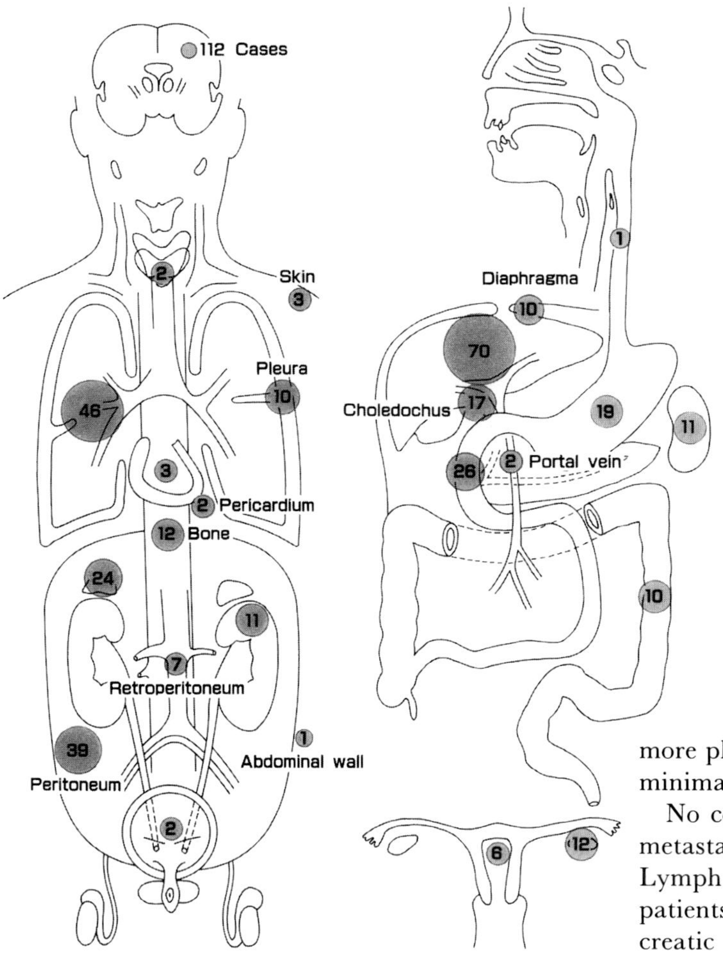

Fig. 8. The incidence (in percentage) of distant metatases of 10 841 autopsy cases with pancreatic carcinoma

No correlation was found between the degree of peripancreatic infiltration and neural invasion. Only one patient with minimal invasion of peripancreatic tissue did not show perineural invasion. There was no correlation between the severity of peripancreatic invasion and neural invasion [26, 32].

Of 34 patients examined by Nagakawa et al. [26, 32], only one patient with lymphatic vessel invasion did not have intrapancreatic neural invasion. On the other hand, two patients without lymphatic vessel invasion had intrapancreatic neural invasion. In general, there was no correlation between the lymphatic vessel invasion and intrapancreatic neural invasion. The same was true for extrapancreatic neural invasion. Only one patient did not exhibit either lymphatic or plexus invasion, and 7 patients with lymphatic vessel invasion did not exhibit plexus invasion. In the remaining patients, patients with severe lymphatic vessel invasion had more plexus invasion than those with moderate or minimal lymphatic vessel involvement [26, 32].

No correlation was found between lymph node metastases and intrapancreatic neural invasion. Lymph node metastases were found in 26 out of 34 patients, whereas all but 1 patient had intrapancreatic neural invasion. A similar situation was found between lymph node metastases and extrapancreatic plexus invasion. In 6 cases without lymph node metastases, 4 had plexus invasion. On the other hand, 6 patients with lymph node metastases did not show plexus invasion [26, 32].

No clear correlation was found between the morphological type of cancer and the incidence of neural invasion. The frequency of cancer with neural invasion was higher in tumors with an advanced or intermediate degree of interstitial fibrosis than in those with little connective tissue [26, 32].

Distant Metastases

According to the annual autopsy reports of the Japanese Pathology Society [21], among 315 715 autopsies performed between 1982 and 1989, 10 841 were pancreatic tumors, including 106 acinar cell carcinomas, 172 islet cell tumors, and 30 carcinoid tumors. Males and females were equally represented (3.5% and 3.4%, respectively). The metastatic sites of 10 841 autopsy cases of pancreatic carcinoma are shown in Fig. 8.

Table 8. Relationship between tumor size and metastases of pancreatic cancer (autopsy cases).

	Tumor size (cm)				
	Under 2	2.1–4	4.1–6	Over 6	Total
No. of cases	13	63	89	83	248
Lymph node metastasis (%)	78	94	82	92	88
Distant metastasis (%)	46	79	82	93	83
Direct invasion (%)	69	94	79	87	85

Table 9. Relationship between tumor localization and metastatic patterns of pancreatic cancer (autopsy cases).

	Tumor location			
	Head	Body and/or tail	Others	Total
No. of patients	118	114	16	248
Lymph node metastases (%)	90	89	76	88
Distant metastases (%)	80	91	50	83
Direct invasion (%)	90	84	50	85

Among 248 autopsy cases [19, 20], the most common sites of metastases were the lymph nodes (88%), liver (72%), lungs (54%), peritoneum (42%), stomach (31%), duodenum (30%), diaphragm (27%), pleura (9%), adrenals (25%), retroperitoneum (23%), bile duct (21%), bones (21%), colon (19%), spleen (13%), mesenterium (12%), kidneys (11%), small intestine (11%), gallbladder (10%), and the skin (6%). The tumor was confined within the organ in only 2 of the 248 cases. The incidence of distant metastases of tumors in different pancreatic region is illustrated in Fig. 9. In the surgical material, among 62 tumors, 49 (79%) involved the lymph nodes, 48 (77%) the retroperitoneum, 30 (48%) the duodenum, 5 (8%) the stomach and the resected end of bile duct, 4 (7%) the left adrenal gland, and 1 (2%) the transverse colon.

Relationship Between Tumor Size and Distant Metastasis

The average size of 248 pancreatic tumors examined by Kishi et al. [19, 20] was 5.7 cm, ranging from 1 to 17.5 cm. The tumors in the pancreatic head measured in average 4.8 cm, ranging from 1 cm to 11.3 cm, and those in the body and/or tail were in average 6.7 cm, ranging from 1.5 to 17.5 cm. The tumors in the body and/or tail of the pancreas were usually larger than those in the head, which has also been shown in other studies [10, 11]. The incidence of pancreatic cancer metastases by tumor size reported by Kishi et al. [19, 20] is summarized in Table 8. Among the 13 tumors with diameters smaller than 2 cm, 11 were located in the head, 1 in the body, and 1 in the tail of the pancreas. Eight of these 13 small tumors metastasized into both the liver and the lungs and 4 metastasized into the subclavicular nodes. The rates of distant metastases increased with increasing tumor size. There was no correlation between the size of tumor and lymph node metastases or direct invasion, although the tumors under 2 cm showed the lowest rate of tumor extension.

Relationship Between Anatomical Tumor Localization and Distant Metastases

The incidence of distant tumor metastases by tumor localization is shown in Tables 9 and 10, and Fig. 9. Metastases to the liver, lungs, bones, and colon occurred in a higher percentage of cases with body and/or tail tumors than in those with head tumors. Forty-two of 248 autopsy cases (17%) had no distant metastases but had regional node and direct tumor extension. Among these 42 tumors, 24 were situated in the head, 10 in the body and/or tail, and 8 at other sites in the pancreas. In only 2 of 248 autopsy cases with pancreatic cancer was the growth confined to the organ.

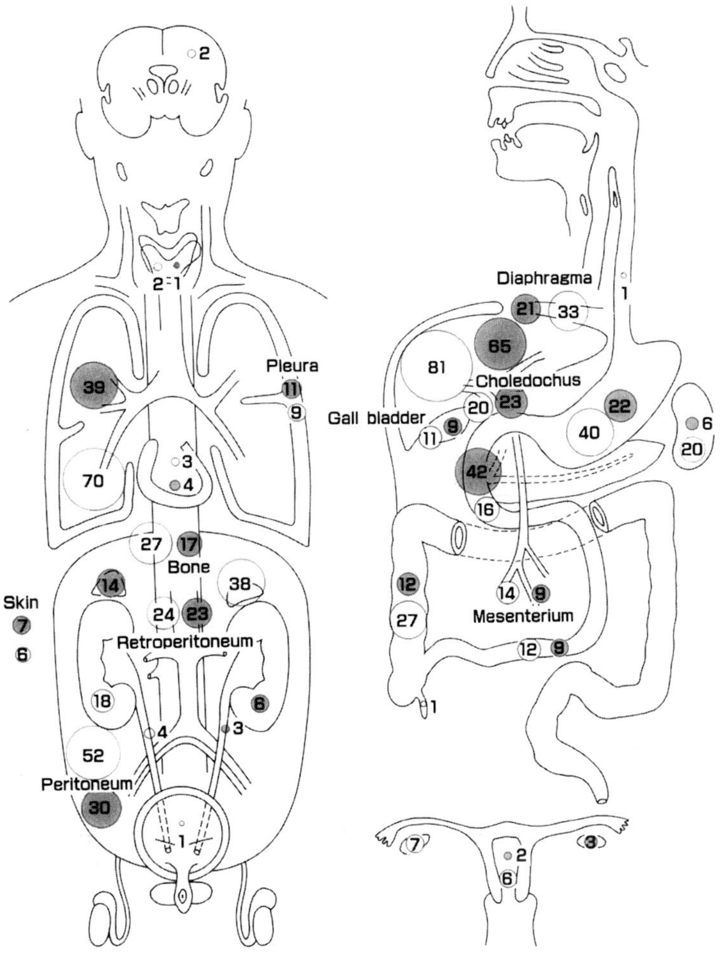

Fig. 9. The incidences (in percentage) of distant metastases of 10841 autospy cases with pancreatic cancer. *Closed circle*, carcinoma of the head of the pancreas; *open circle*, cancer of the body and/or tail of the pancreas

Table 10. Distant metastases of pancreatic cancer by tumor localization (autopsy cases).

	Site of tumor			
	Head	Body and/or tail	Others	Total
No. of tumor	118	114	16	248
Liver (%)	58.5	76.3	50	66.1
Lungs (%)	38.9	70.2	43.8	53.6
Bones (%)	16.9	27.2	0	20.6
Diaphragma (%)	12.7	14.9	12.5	13.7
Adrenals (%)	12.7	13.2	6.3	12.5
Colon (%)	6.8	15.8	18.8	11.7
Pleurae (%)	11.0	8.8	0	9.3
Mesenterium (%)	7.6	7.0	12.5	7.7
Small intestine (%)	5.1	9.6	12.5	7.7
Kidneys (%)	5.9	9.6	0	7.3
Stomach (%)	5.9	4.4	25	6.5
Gall bladder (%)	4.2	8.8	6.3	6.5

Table 11. Relationship between tumor localization and histologic type of pancreatic cancer (autopsy cases).

	Head	Head & Body	Body	Body & Tail	Tail	Entire pancreas	Total
Ductal	82	2	24	23	10	5	146
Papillary	18	0	8	8	0	2	36
Mucinous	9	0	14	1	2	2	28
Ad-sq	5	1	7	2	3	0	18
Undiff	3	1	1	5	2	2	14
Cyst	0	1	1	1	1	0	4
Acinar	1	0	0	0	1	0	2
Total	118	5	55	40	19	11	248

Ad-sq, Adenosquamous carcinoma; *Undiff*, undifferentiated carcinoma; *Cyst*, cystadenocarcinoma

Table 12. Relationship between the morphology and metastases of pancreatic cancer (autopsy cases).

	Histologic type							
	Ductal	Pap	Mucinous	Ad-sq	Undiff	Cyst	Acinar	Total
No. of cases	146	36	28	18	14	4	2	248
Average size of tumor (cm) (range)	4.3 (1–7.8)	6.1 (1–11)	5.1 (2.5–8)	6.7 (4–15)	9.0 (5.5–17.5)	7.1 (2.8–11.3)	6.3 (5.5–7)	5.7 (1–17.5)
Lymph node metastasis (%)	87.6	80.6	82.4	100	100	100	100	87.9
Distant metastasis (%)	80.8	80.6	89.3	77.8	100	50	100	83.1
Direct invasion (%)	84.9	88.9	75.0	100	94.3	75	100	84.7

Ad-sq, Adenosquamous carcinoma; *Undiff*, undifferentiated carcinoma; *Cyst*, cystadenocarcinoma

Relationship Between Tumor Morphology and Distant Metastasis

The histological type of pancreatic cancer found by Kishi et al. [19] in different pancreatic regions is listed in Table 11, and the extent of pancreatic cancer by tumor morphology and grade of tumor differentiation are listed in Tables 12 and 13. These results are comparable with those reported by Miller and associates [10] and Baylor and Berg [16]. Among 14 undifferentiated carcinomas, 11 were of giant cell type and 3 of spindle cell type. The incidence of metastases varied with histologic type of pancreatic cancer. In the cases with duct cell adenocarcinoma, the incidence of distant metastases increased with the grade of malignancy. Nagakawa et al. [26, 32] found that the incidence and the extent of lymphatic metastases of ductal adenocarcinoma were higher than those of papillary adenocarcinoma, and that ductal adenocarcinoma metastasized to area No. 16 in 7 out of 34 patients.

Direct Tumor Extension

According to general experience, the most common sites of direct invasion of pancreatic cancer are the peritoneum, bile duct, duodenum, stomach, and retroperitoneum [7–14, 16]. Cubilla and Fitzgerald [13] stated that head cancer most frequently involved the duodenum (66%) and stomach (25%); body cancer involved the stomach (40%), duodenum (24%), and spleen and transverse colon (12%, each); while tail cancer involved the spleen (36%), left adrenal (29%), and transverse colon (14%). Leach [7] also found that head cancer most commonly invaded the bile duct (76%), duodenum (62%), peritoneum (38%), and retroperitoneum (14%); body and/or tail cancer invaded the peritoneum (69%), retroperitoneum (31%), duodenum (23%), and the bile duct (15%).

Cancer extension by localization of tumors found by Kishi et al. [19, 20] is shown in Table 14 and Fig. 10. Head tumors more frequently invaded the

Table 13. Relationship between metastatic patterns and histologic differentiation of ductal carcinoma of the pancreas.

	Histologic differentiation			
	Well	Moderate	Poor	Total
No. of cases	65	33	48	146
Average size of tumor (cm)	4.1	4.9	4.3	4.3
(range)	(1–7)	(2.3–13.5)	(1.8–8.6)	(1–13.5)
Lymph node metastasis (%)	90.8	81.8	87.5	87.6
Distant metastasis (%)	66.2	90.9	93.8	80.8
Direct invasion (%)	86.2	87.9	81.3	84.9

Table 14. Direct invasion of pancreatic cancer by tumor localization (autopsy cases).

	Site of tumor			
	Head	Body and/or tail	Others	Total
No. of cases	118	114	16	248
Peritoneum (%)	33.1	46.5	37.5	37.9
Bile duct (%)	36.5	28.1	12.5	30.6
Duodenum (%)	45.8	13.2	25	29.4
Stomach (%)	16.1	35.1	12.5	24.6
Retroperitoneum (%)	22.9	23.7	8.8	23.0
Diaphragma (%)	8.5	18.4	18.7	13.7
Adrenals (%)	1.7	24.6	0	12.1
Spleen (%)	1.7	21.9	0	10.9
Transeverse colon (%)	5.1	11.4	0	7.7
Liver (%)	6.8	4.4	12.5	6.0
Mesenterium (%)	1.7	7.9	0	4.0
Kidneys (%)	0	8.8	0	4.0
Gall bladder (%)	5.1	2.6	0	3.6
Jejunum (%)	3.4	2.6	0	2.8

duodenum and portal vein than did the body and/or tail tumors. Involvement of the stomach and left adrenal gland occurred only in the body and/or tail tumors in resected cases; 5 of 40 head tumors invaded the resected end of the bile duct, indicating retrograde lymphatic spread of tumor.

Direct invasion of tumors occurring in the body and/or tail of the pancreas was more frequent and widespread than the head tumors. Head tumors directly infiltrated the right adrenal, and the body and/or tail tumors infiltrated the left adrenal and the left kidney. Liver invasion was through the hepatoduodenal ligament or the duodenum. Direct invasion of mesenterium occurred through the root of the mesentery from the retroperitoneum. Direct invasion of body and/or tail tumors occurred more frequently than in head tumors, except for direct extension to the duodenum, bile duct, liver, and gallbladder—these were more frequently found in association with head tumors.

The intraductal spread of a tumor adjacent to the main pancreatic duct and more than 5 mm distant from the main duct was found by Kishi et al. [19, 20] in 26 of 62 resected pancreatic cancers (42%) (Figs. 11 and 12). Intraductal spread was found in 18 of 40 pancreatic head tumors (45%) and in 8 of 22 pancreatic body and/or tail tumors (36%). One tumor of the head had grown along the entire duct of Wirsung. Another tumor of the head had a minimum secondary cancer in the main to interlobar ducts located between the body and tail of the pancreas. Three tumors involved the resected end of the main pancreatic duct. Intraductal spread of pancreatic tumors was found in 78% of 9 tumors under 2 cm in diameter, in 39% of 36 tumors between 2.1 and 4 cm in diameter, in 25% of 4 tumors between 4.1 and 6 cm in diameter and in 31% of 13 tumors over 6.1 cm in diameter. The incidence of intraductal spread was 44% in duct cell adenocarcinomas. There was no intra-

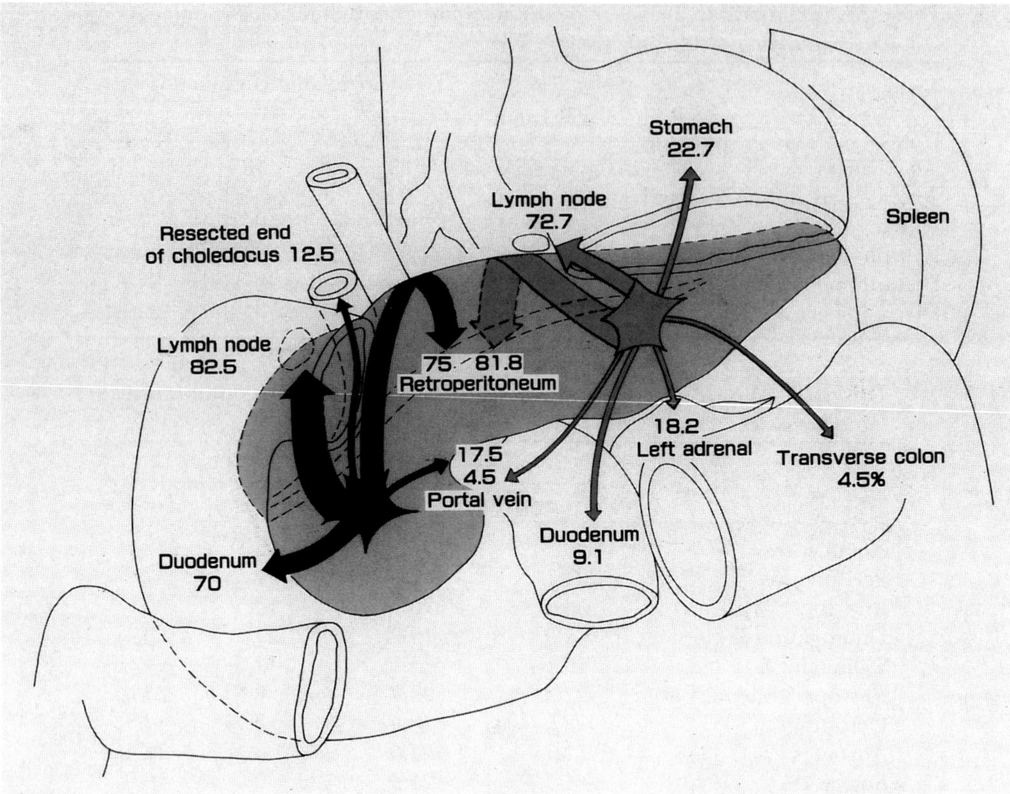
Stomach
22.7
Lymph node
72.7
Spleen
Resected end
of choledocus 12.5
Lymph node
82.5
75 81.8
Retroperitoneum
18.2
Left adrenal
Transverse colon
4.5%
17.5
4.5
Portal vein
Duodenum
9.1
Duodenum
70

10

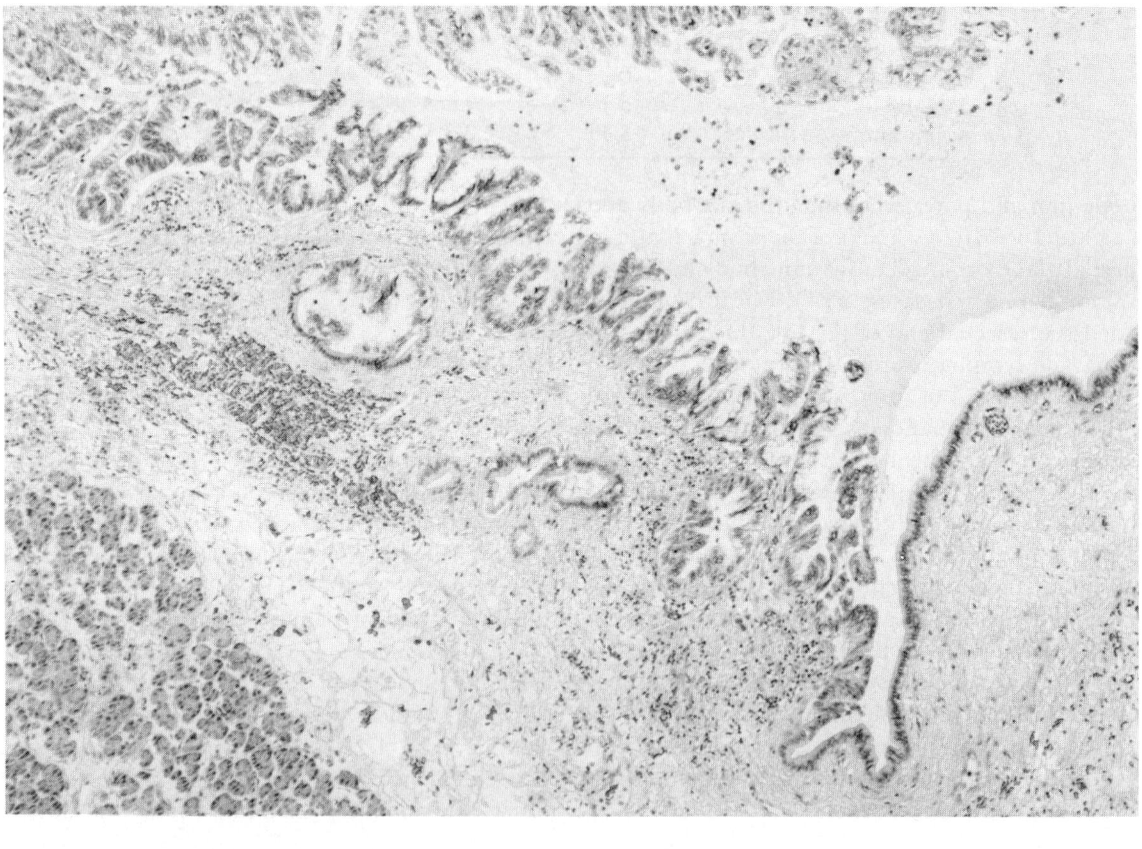

11

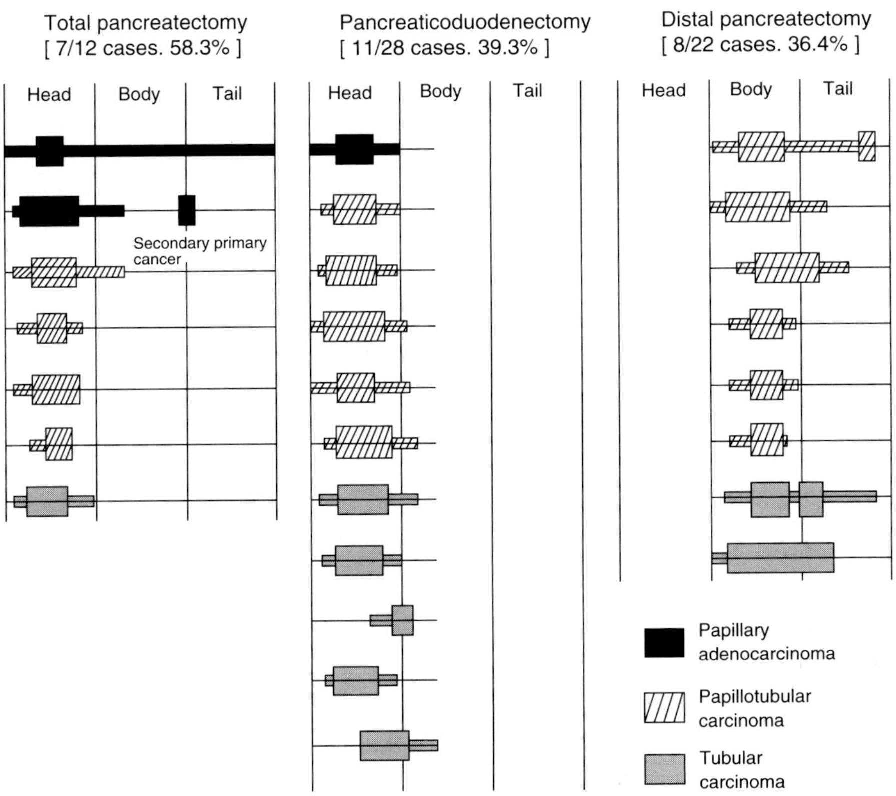

Fig. 12. Contiguous intraductal tumor spread into Wirsung's duct (62 resected cases)

ductal spread of cystadenocarcinomas and adenosquamous carcinoma [19, 20].

The reported incidence of 42% of the cases by Kishi et al. [2] showing intraductal spread of tumor adjacent to the primary cancer is higher than the 3% reported by Sommers and associates [33], the 19% by Cubilla and Fitzgerald [34] and the 30% by Klöppel [14]. Klöppel [14] noted that intraductal tumor spread involved the resected end of the main pancreatic duct in about 10% of the cases, compared to 16% in the cases of Kishi et al. [19, 20]. Tumor growing along the entire duct of Wirsung from the main tumor was found in one case each by Kishi et al. [20] and Klöppel [14].

Multicentric pancreatic cancer, which was found in one case in our pancreatectomy cases, was reported in 1% of the cases by Cubilla and Fitzgerald [34], 5% by Pour and associates [35, 36], and 20% by Tryka and Brooks [37].

References

1. Cubilla AC, Fortner J, Fitzgerald PJ (1978) Lymph node involvement in carcinoma of the head of the pancreas. Cancer 41:880–887
2. Kishi K, Hirota T, Nakamura K et al. (1980) Carcinoma of the pancreas: A review of 94 autopsy cases. Jpn J Clin Oncol 10:273–280
3. Tsuchiya Y, Tomioka T, Izawa K et al. (1986) Collective review of small carcinomas of the pancreas. Ann Surg 203:77–81
4. Mannel A, Weiland L, van Heerden JA, Ilstrup DM

Fig. 10. The incidences (in percentage) of direct invasion of pancreatic cancer in different anatomical sites of the pancreas (62 resected cases)

Fig. 11. Intraductal contiguous tumor spread into Wirsung's duct from a cancer of the head of the pancreas. (*For color reproduction see color insert in the frontmatter*)

(1986) Factors influencing survival after resection for ductal adenocarcinoma of the pancreas. Ann Surg 203:403–407

5. Gudjonsson B (1987) Cancer of the pancreas. 50 years of surgery. Cancer 60:2284–2303
6. Tsuchiya R, Tsunoda T (1990) Tumor size as a predictive factor. Int J Pancreatology 5:117–123
7. Leach WB (1950) Carcinoma of the pancreas. A clinical and pathologic analysis of thirty-nine autopsied cases. Am J Pathol 26:333–347
8. Bell ET (1957) Carcinoma of pancreas. Am J Pathol 33:499–523
9. Gullick HD (1959) Carcinoma of the pancreas. A review and critical study of 100 cases. Medicine 38:47–84
10. Miller JR, Baggenstoss AH, Comfort MW (1951) Carcinoma of the pancreas. Effect of histological type and grade of malignancy on its behavior. Cancer 4:233–241
11. Halpart B, Makk L, Jorden GL (1965) A retrospective study of 120 patients with carcinoma of the pancreas. Surg Gynecol Obstet 121:91–96
12. Collure DWD, Burns GP, Schenk WG (1974) Clinical, pathologic, and therapeutic aspects of carcinoma of the pancreas. Amer J Surg 128:683–689
13. Cubilla AC, Fitzgerald PJ (1984) Tumors of the exocrine pancreas. Atlas of tumor pathology, Second series, fascicle 19. Armed Forces Institute of Pathology, Washington DC
14. Klöppel G (1984) Pancreatic, non-endocrine tumor. In: Klöppel G, Heitz P (eds) Pancreatology. Churchill Livingstone, New York
15. Douglass HO Jr, Penetrante RB (1990) Pancreatic cancer. Why patients die? Int J Pancreatol 5:135–140
16. Baylor SM, Berg JW (1973) Cross-classification and survival characteristics of 5000 cases of cancer of the pancreas. J Surg Oncol 5:335–358
17. Ishikawa O, Ohhigashi H, Sasaki Y, Kabuto T, Fokude I, Furokawa H, Imaoka S, Iwanaga T (1988) Practical usefulness of lymphatic and connective tissue clearance for the carcinoma of the pancreatic head. Ann Surg 208:215–220
18. Reber HA (1990) Lymph node involvement as a prognostic factor in pancreatic cancer. Int J Pancreatol 5:125–127
19. Kishi K (1986) Metastatic patterns of pancreatic carcinoma (in Japanese). Jpn J Clin Med 44:2–4
20. Kishi K (1989) Clinicopathological analysis of pancreatic carcinoma (in Japanese). Naika MOOK No. 39, 20–37
21. The Japanese Pathological Society (1982–1989) Annual of the pathological autopsy cases in Japan. Vol. 24–31
22. Nagai H, Kuroda A, Morioka Y (1986) Lymphatic and local spread of T1 and T2 pancreatic cancer. A study of autopsy material. Ann Surg 204:65–71
23. Ozaki H, Kishi K (1983) Lymph node dissection in radical resection for carcinoma of the head of the pancreas and periampullary region. Jpn J Clin Oncol 13:371–378
24. Nagakawa T, Konishi I, Ueno K, Ohta T, Akiyama T, Kayahara M, Miyazaki I (1991) Surgical treatment of pancreatic cancer. Int J Pancreatol 9:135–143
25. Nagakawa T, Konishi I, Higashino Y, Ueno K, Ohta T, Kayahara M, Ueda N, Maeda K, Miyazaki I (1989) The spread and prognosis of carcinoma in the region of the pancreatic head. Jpn J Surg 19:510–518
26. Nagakawa T, Kayahara M, Ohta T, Ueno K, Konishi I, Miyazaki I (1991) Patterns of neural and plexus invasion of human pancreatic cancer and experimental cancer. Int J Pancreatol 10:113–119
27. Kishi K (1985) Biopsy of pancreatic cancer (in Japanese). J Bilary Tract Pancreas 6:1079–1086
28. Nakao A, Ichihara T, Nonami T (1987) Clinicopathological and immunohistological evaluation of intrapancreatic development of pancreatic cancer (in Japanese with English abstract). Jpn J Surg 88:735–742
29. Matsuda M, Nimura Y (1983) Perineural invasion of carcinoma of the head of the pancreas (in Japanese with English abstract). Jpn J Surg 84:719–728
30. Nagayo T, Murakami N, Matuoka Y (1976) Local neural invasion of carcinoma of the gallbladder, the bile duct and the pancreas (in Japanese). Cancer Clin 22:1406–1409
31. Kayahara M, Nagakawa T, Konishi I, Ueno K, Ohta T, Miyazaki I (1991) Clinicopathological study of pancreatic carcinoma with particular reference to the invasion of the extrapancreatic neural plexus. Int J Pancreatol 10:105–111
32. Nagakawa T, Kayahara M, Ueno K, Ohta T, Konishi I, Ueda N, Miyazaki, I (1992) A Clinicopathologic Study on neural invasion in cancer of the pancreatic head. Cancer 69:930–935
33. Sommers SC, Murphy SA, Warren S (1954) Pancreatic duct hyperplasia and cancer. Gastroenterology 27:620–640
34. Cubilla AL, Fitzgerald PJ (1976) Morpological lesions associated with human primary invasive nonendocrine pancreas cancer. Cancer Res 36: 2690–2698
35. Pour PM, Salmasi SZ (1979) Ductular origin of pancreatic cancer and its multiplicity in man comparable to experimentally induced tumors. A preliminary study. Cancer Lett 6:89–97
36. Pour PM, Sayed S, Sayed G (1982) Hyperplastic, preneoplastic and neoplastic lesions found in 83 human pancreases. AJCP 77:137–152
37. Tryka AF, Brooks JR (1979) Histopathology in the evaluation of total pancreatectomy for ductal carcinoma. Ann Surg 190:373–381
38. Japan Pancreas Society (1986) General rules for cancer of the pancreas, 3rd ed (in Japanese). Kanehara, Tokyo

Tumor Spread and the Factors Influencing Prognosis in Patients with Resected Pancreatic Carcinoma

Introduction

Despite recent advances in diagnostic and therapeutic modalities for pancreatic cancer, the resectability is still low and prognosis remains poor as compared with cancer in other digestive organs [1]. In most cases, when the diagnosis is made, the tumor has extended to the outer margin of the pancreas and has infiltrated the adjacent tissues. Despite advancements in ablative surgery, the prognosis has improved little [2, 3].

It is, therefore, important to gain information on the tumor spread and the frequency of metastases in different lymph nodes and tissues and to evaluate the factors influencing prognosis in patients with pancreatic cancer. From 1981 to 1990, the Pancreatic Cancer Registry of the Japan Pancreas Society [4] has collected over 1000 cases of pancreatic cancer every year from major surgical institutions throughout Japan and has registered a total of 11 317 cases to date.

In this chapter, we review the results of the treatment for pancreatic cancer in Japan, the incidences and extensions of cancer infiltrations and the frequency of metastases to different sites. We also considered the factors that influence postoperative prognosis by evaluating the total registered cases of pancreatic cancer.

Results of the Treatment for Pancreatic Cancer in Japan

Among the 11 317 patients with pancreatic cancer registered to date in the Cancer Registry of the Japan Pancreas Society, resectional procedures were performed on 3743 (33.1%), while palliative operations such as choledochojejunostomy and gastrojejunostomy, were performed on 4134 (36.5%), exploratory laparotomy on 754 (6.7%), and 2686 (23.8%) were treated non-operatively.

Pancreaticoduodenectomy was performed on 2247 patients (60.0%), total pancreatectomy in 644 patients (17.2%), and distal pancreatectomy in 767 patients (20.5%). In 85 patients (2.3%), the surgical procedure was unknown. A decline in the frequency of total pancreatectomy as the operative procedure has been observed in recent years. The extended radical operation was carried out in 819 patients (21.9%) with the resection of major vessels, mostly the main trunk of the portal vein, and in 1771 patients (47.3%) with en bloc dissection of the regional and juxtal regional lymph nodes.

Postoperative cumulative survival rates of patients with pancreatic cancer in relation to each surgical treatment are shown in Fig. 1. One-, 3-, and 5-year survival rates after resectional procedures were 50.4%, 22.4%, and 16.6%, respectively. It was significantly higher than in those patients who did not receive the resectional surgery.

Incidence and Extent of the Cancer Infiltration

Infiltration of the pancreatic capsule was found in 5135 patients (75.9%) who underwent surgery. The sites of infiltration were the retroperitoneum in 4039 patients (71.2%) and the portal vein in 4051 patients (66.6%).

The relationship between the tumor size and the incidence and the extent of capsular and portal system infiltration is shown in Figs. 2–4.

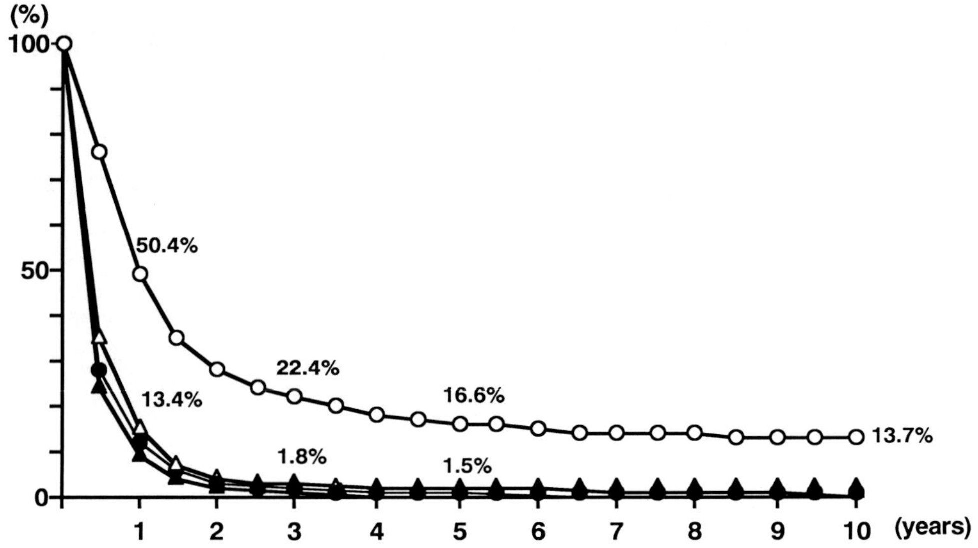

Fig. 1. Cumulative survival rates of the patients with pancreatic cancer. *Open circles*, Resectional surgery (n = 2977); *open triangles*, bypass operation (n = 3170); *closed circles*, exploratory laparotomy (n = 610); *closed triangles*, no operation (n = 1981)

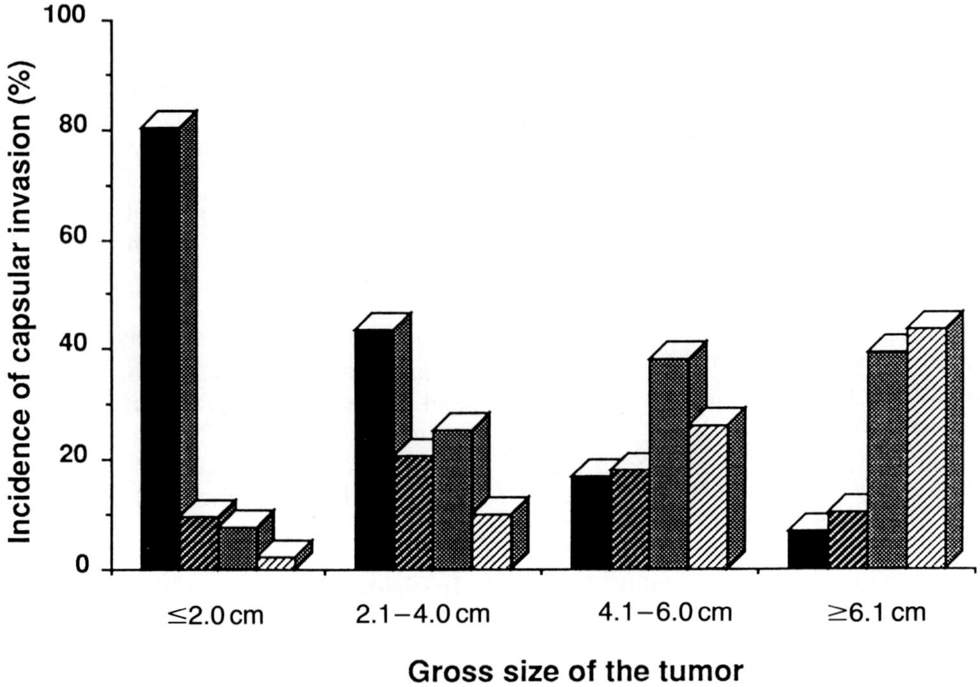

Fig. 2. Incidence of capsular invasion (S) in relation to tumor size. Invasion to the anterior capsule of the pancreas is referred to as the "S factor" and divided into the following four categories. *S0*, No capsular invasion (*solid bars*); *S1*, suspected invasion to the capsule (*dark hatching*); *S2*, definite invasion to the capsule (*grey bars*); *S3*, invasion to the adjacent viscera (*light hatching*)

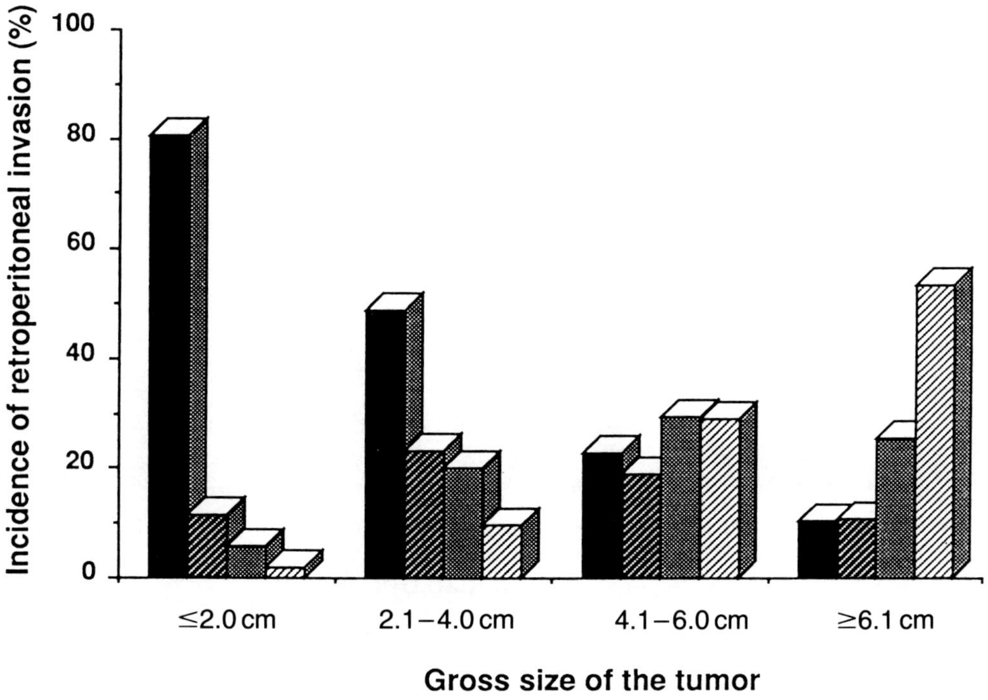

Fig. 3. Incidence of retroperitoneal invasion (*Rp*) in relation to tumor size. The retroperitoneal tissues include the extrapancreatic bile duct and portal venous vessels (portal, superior mesenteric, splenic) in addition to retropancreatic connective tissues and nerve plexi. The adjacent viscera mean the aorta, superior mesenteric artery, inferior vena cava, both kidneys and adrenals. Retroperitoneal invasion is referred to as the "Rp factor" and divided into the following four categories. *Rp0,* No retroperitoneal invasion (*solid bars*); *Rp1,* suspected invasion of retroperitoneal tissues (*dark hatching*); *Rp2,* definite invasion of retroperitoneal tissues (*grey bars*); *Rp3,* severe invasion of retroperitoneal tissues and adjacent viscera (*light hatching*)

The incidences and the extent of tumor infiltrations were strongly correlated with the tumor size. Retroperitoneal infiltration was found in 19.3% of the patients with tumors less than 2.0 cm in size, in 53.0% with the Tumor from 2.1 to 4.0 cm, in 77.2% with the tumor from 4.1 to 6.0 cm and in 89.5% of the patients with cancers greater than 6.1 cm in diameter. In patients with a tumor size of less than 2.0 cm, the invasion of the pancreatic capsule, retroperitoneal tissues, or the portal system was found in 19.8%, 19.3%, or 17.3%, respectively.

Frequency of Metastases in Different Lymph Nodes

Lymph node metastases were found in 3992 patients (74.8% of the recorded patients who underwent surgery). The incidence of metastases was also correlated with the tumor size: In 34.6% of patients with cancers of less than 2.0 cm in size, in 85.6% of patients with cancers larger than 6.1 cm in size (Fig. 5).

In our study of resectional specimens with ductal adenocarcinomas, excluding the cystadenocarcinoma and islet cell carcinoma, we found that pancreatic carcinoma of the head involved multiple groups of lymph nodes, particularly lymph nodes of the superior-posterior, inferior-posterior, superior-anterior, and inferior-anterior region (for the topography of lymph nodes, see Chapters "Gross Anatomy of the Pancreas" and "Pathology of Metastatic Patterns of Pancreatic Cancer" in this volume). Metastases were also found in the lymph nodes along the distal bile duct, the common hepatic artery, at the origin of the superior mesenteric artery, the inferior pancreaticoduodenal artery, the middle colic artery, and the jejunal artery (Fig. 6). On the other hand, the pancreatic carcinoma located in the body and tail of the pancreas involved the lymph nodes along the splenic

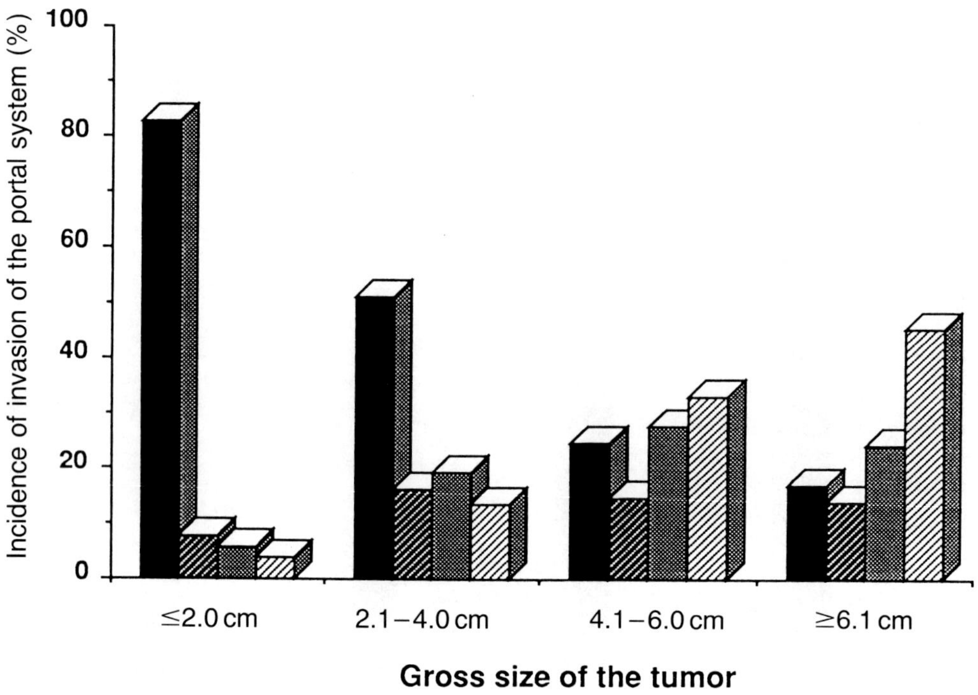

Fig. 4. Incidence of invasion of the portal system (*PV*) in relation to tumor size. The portal venous vessels include the PVp (portal vein), PVsm (superior mesenteric vein) and PVsp (splenic vein). Invasion of the portal venous vessels is refered to as the "PV factor" and divided into the following four categories. *PV0*, No invasion of the portal venous vessels (*solid bars*); *PV1*, suspected invasion of the portal venous vessels (*dark hatching*); *PV2*, definite invasion of the portal venous vessels (*grey bars*); *PV3*, severe invasion of the portal venous vessels with stenosis (*light hatching*)

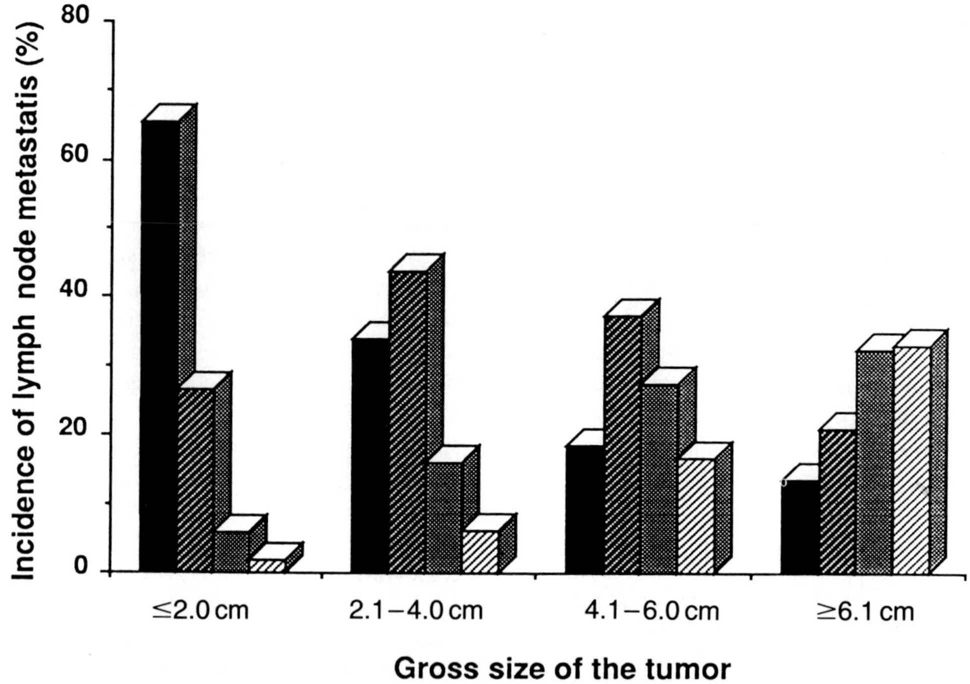

Fig. 5. Incidence of lymph nodes metastases (*N*) in relation to tumor size. The regional lymph nodes are classified into three groups, namely lymph nodes of group 1 (*N1*), group 2 (*N2*), and group 3 (*N3*) according to their location. *N*(−), No evidence of lymph node involvement (*solid bars*); *N1*(+), evidence of lymph node involvement within the group 1 (*dark hatching*); *N2*(+); evidence of lymph node involvement within the group 2 (*grey bars*); *N3*(+) evidence of lymph node involvement within the group 3 (*light hatching*)

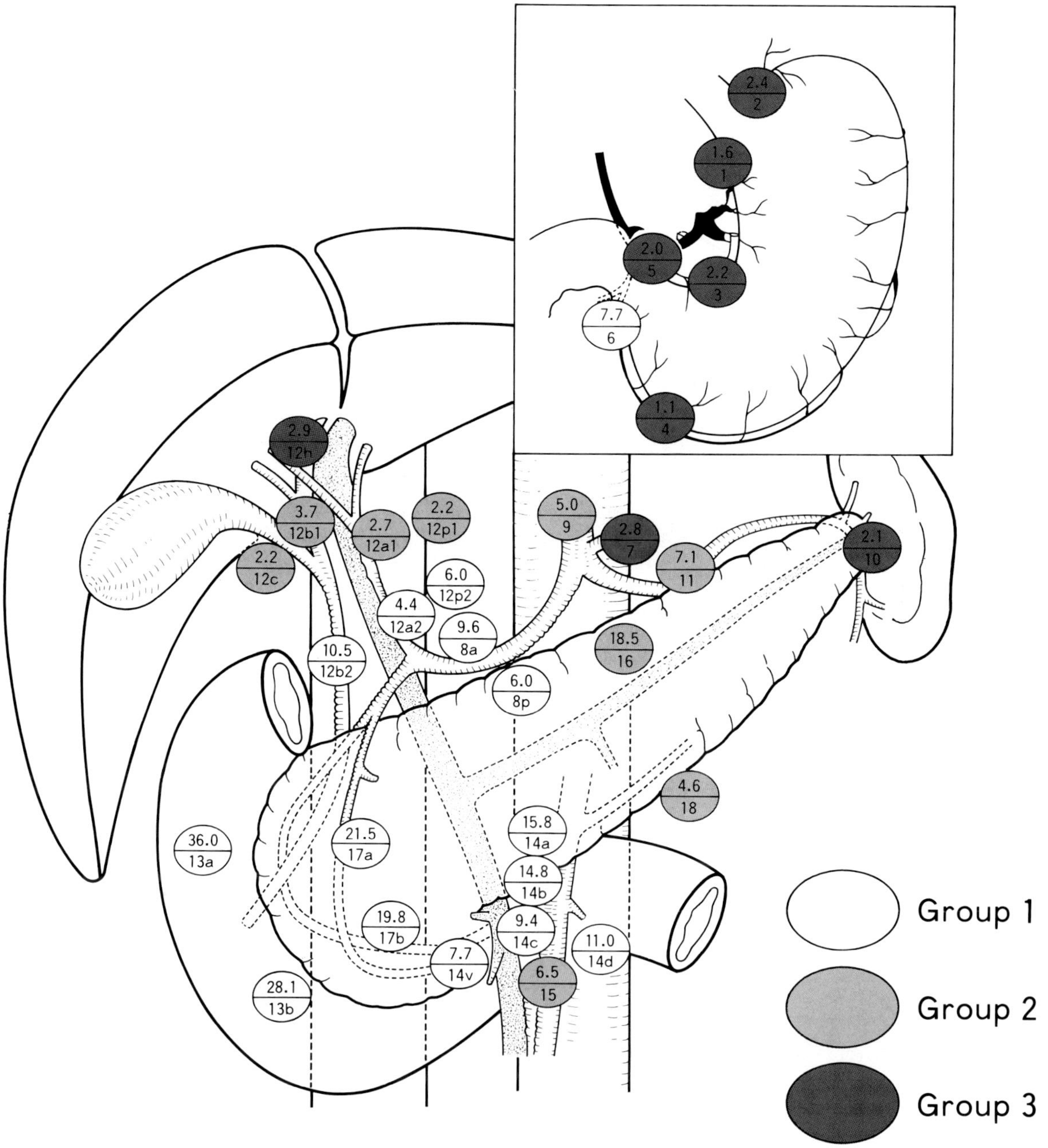

Fig. 6. Incidence (percentage) of node metastases from carcinoma in the head of the pancreas

artery, the common hepatic artery, the celiac axis, and the abdominal aorta besides the nodes of the inferior border of the body and the tail of the pancreas and the hilum of the spleen (Fig. 7). There were significant differences in postoperative survival between the patients with and without lymph node metastases and among the patients with lymph node metastases in group 1, group 2, and group 3 (Fig. 8).

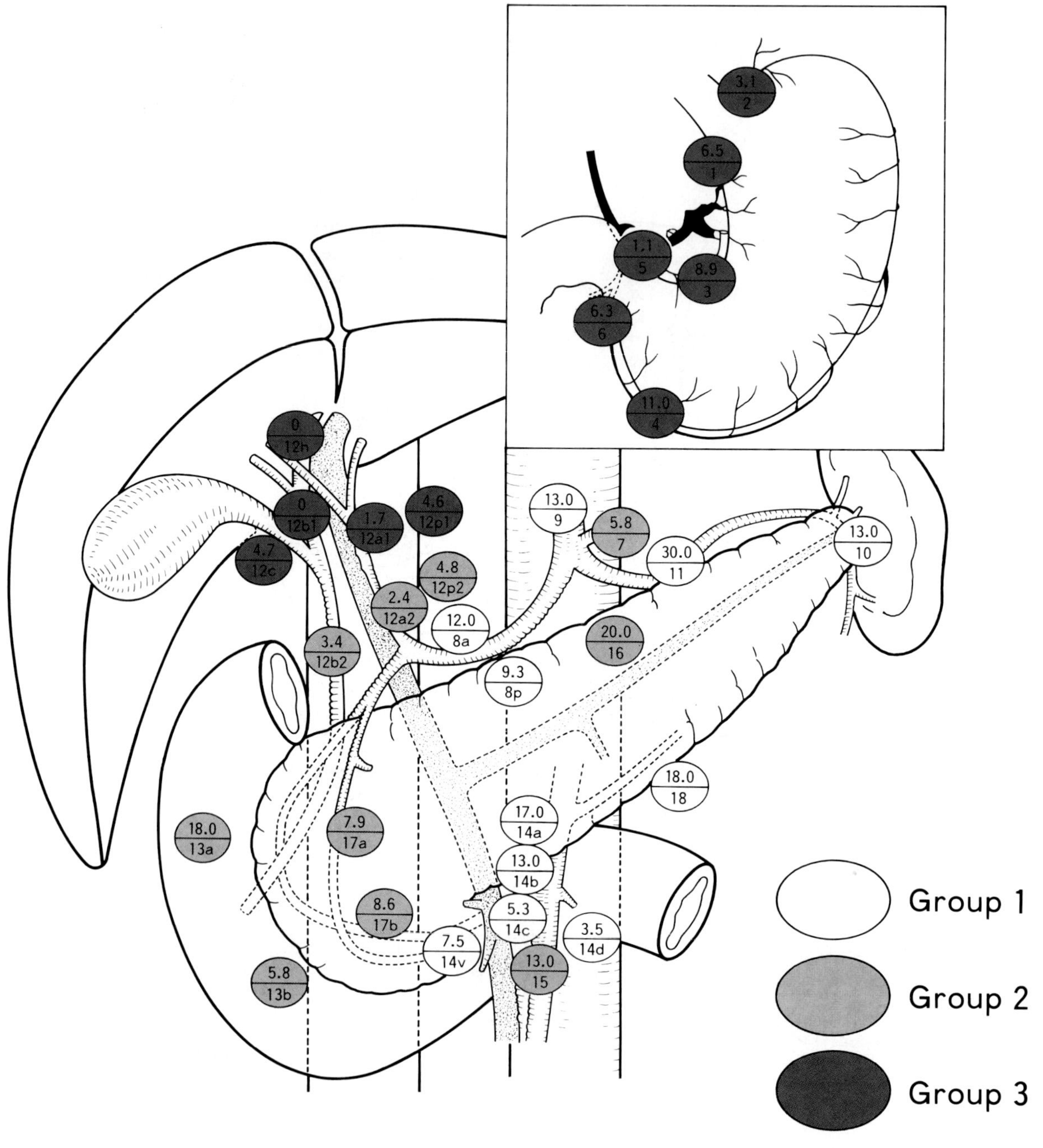

Fig. 7. Incidence (percentage) of node metastases from carcinoma in the body and tail of the pancreas

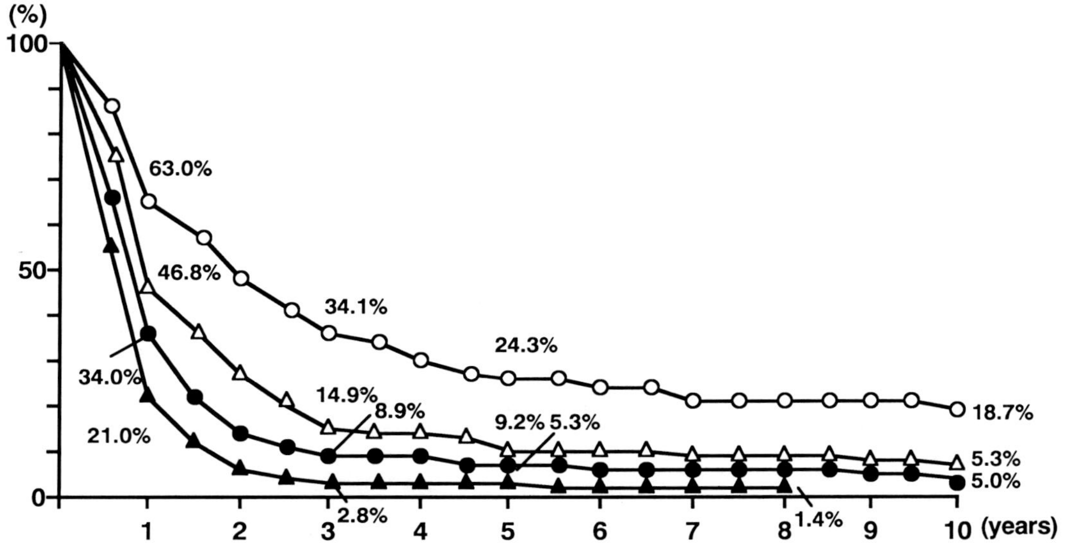

Fig. 8. Postoperative cumulative survival rates of patients with pancreatic head cancer according to the extension of lymph node involvement. *Open circles*, N(−) (n = 707); *open triangles*, $N_1(+)$ (n = 924); *closed circles*, $N_2(+)$ (n = 307); *closed triangles*, $N_3(+)$ (n = 105)

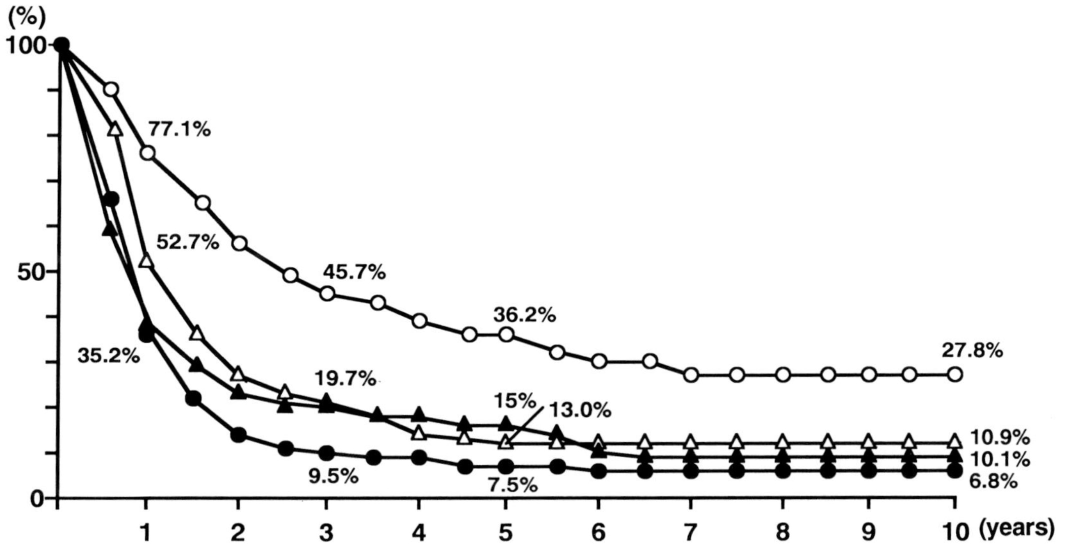

Fig. 9. Postoperative cumulative survival rates of patients who received resection according to tumor size. *Open circles*, ≤2.0 cm (n = 293); *open triangles*, 2.1–4.0 cm (n = 1238); *closed circles*, 4.1–6.0 cm (n = 711); *closed triangles*, ≥6.1 cm (n = 441)

Does Tumor Size Influence the Prognosis of Pancreatic Carcinoma?

In accordance with the general view, the size of the tumor represents an important factor for postoperative survival, as it does in other gastrointestinal malignancies. In our study, the postoperative 1-, 3-, and 5-year survival rates of cases with a tumor size of less than 2.0 cm were 77.1%, 45.7%, and 36.2%, respectively, and were better than the comparable figures for cases with cancers larger than 2.1 cm (Fig. 9).

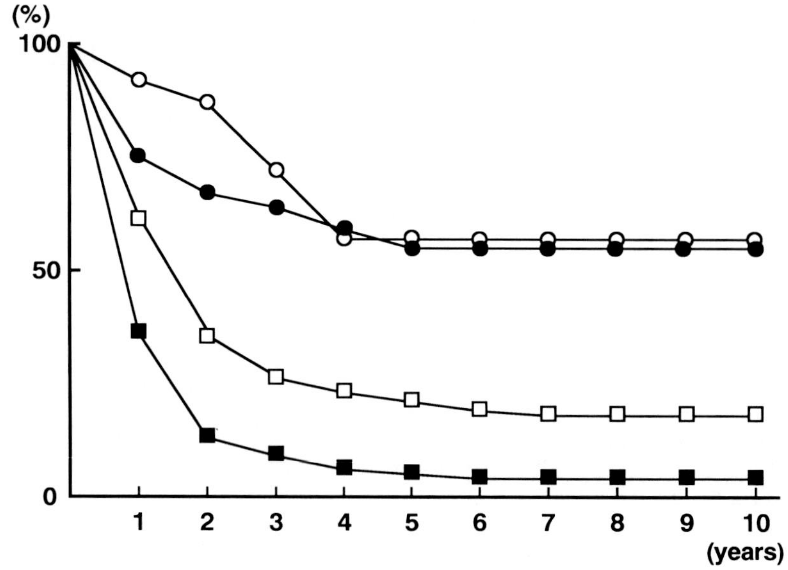

Fig. 10. Postoperative cumulative survival rates of patients who received resection according to T category proposed by the UICC. *Open circles*, PT1a (n = 43); *closed circles*, pT1b (n = 66); *open squares*, pT2 (n = 778); *closed squares*, pT3 (n = 1206)

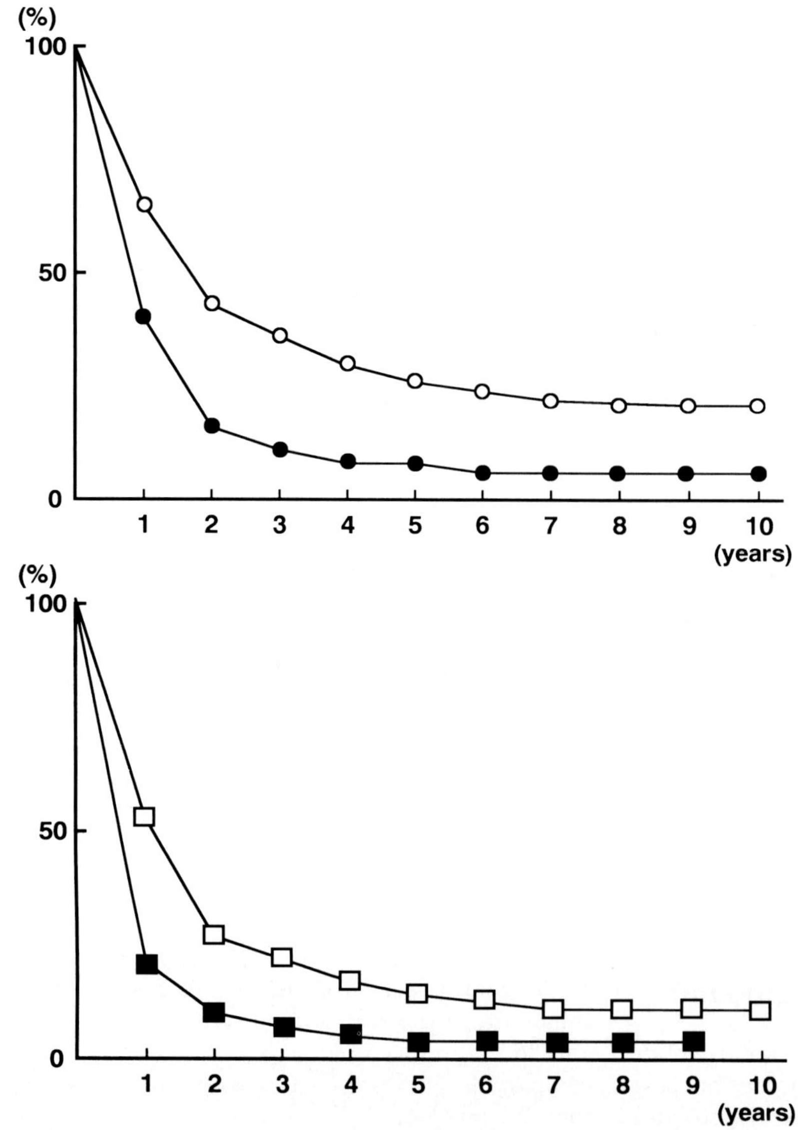

Fig. 11. Postoperative cumulative survival rates of patients who received resection according to N and M categories proposed by the UICC. *Open circles*, pN0 (n = 647); *closed circles* pN1 (n = 1308); *open squares*, pM0 (n = 1684); *closed squares*, pM1 (n = 391)

The incidence of small cancers (≤2.0 cm in diameter) in total registered cases was about 5% and the resectability rate was over 90%. In most cases, however, the cancer was larger than 2 cm at the time of diagnosis, so that the overall resectability and postoperative prognosis has been poor.

When we used the Stage Grouping of TNM classification, proposed by the UICC (see Chapter "Staging for Carcinoma of the Pancreas, Japanese Stage Classification Compared to UICC Stage Classification" in this volume), for the evaluation of the postoperative prognosis, we found that the postoperative prognosis in the patients in which the tumor was limited to the pancreas was significantly better than in those whose tumor extended to adjacent organs and vessels (Fig. 10). However, we could not find any differences in the prognosis between cases with pTIa and pTIb tumors. The lymph node metastases and distant metastases also influenced the prognosis following resection (Fig. 11).

The 1-, 3-, and 5-year postoperative survival rates for patients with Stage I disease were 77.0%, 48.5%, and 36.4%, respectively. These rates were markedly better than the 54.4%, 20.9%, and 15.3%, respectively, observed in patients with Stage II. Furthermore, Stage I was tentatively subdivided into Stage Ia (T1a, No, Mo), Ib (T1b, No, Mo) and Ic (T2, No, Mo). The postoperative 5-year survival rates were 70.6% in Stage Ia and 60.0% in Stage Ib, but only 29.0% in Stage Ic (Fig. 12). As a result, we found that the tumor size was not only a major determinant of resectability but correlated with the incidences and the extent of the cancerous invasions.

Early cancer of the pancreas is generally defined as a tumor less than 2 cm in diameter, with no microscopic lymph node involvement, invasion of the pancreatic capsule, retroperitoneum or major vessels and no distant metastases [5]. In the experience of Moossa [6], 17 of the first 64 resected cancers belonged to this category, all of which were located in the head of the pancreas. Eight of the patients survived over 5 years. Because five of the patients died after 3 to 6 years of metastases from pancreatic cancer postoperatively, it seems that this definition was not perfect.

Cubilla et al. [7] reported that the median survival period with a Stage I tumor after surgery was twice as long as in patients with a Stage II cancer that was less than 3 cm; however, there was little difference in survival between the two groups when the tumor size was more than 3 cm. Bottger et al. [8] described similar results and found that patients with tumors of less than 3 cm in diameter lived longer after the operation than those with tumors larger than 3 cm. Thus, a smaller pancreatic cancer is not always an early cancer, but the tumor

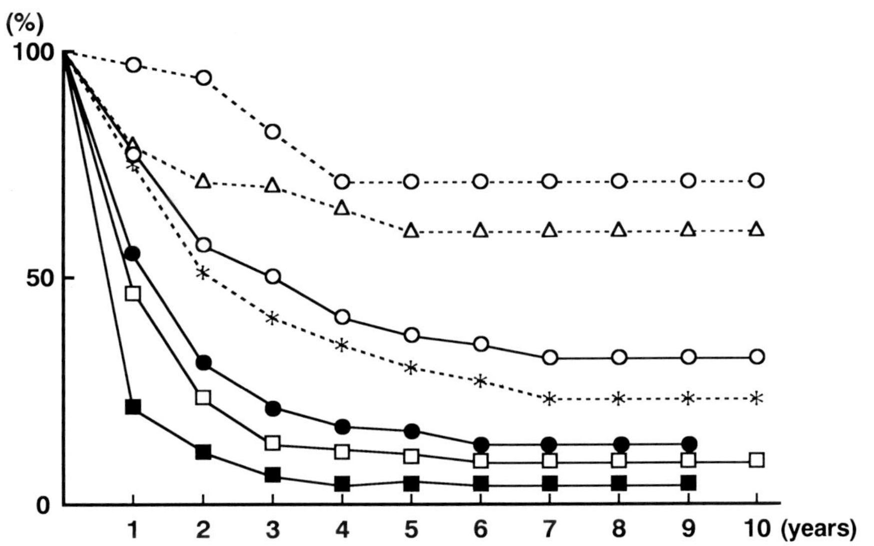

Fig. 12. Postoperative cumulative survival rates of patients who received resection according to stage grouping proposed by the UICC. *Open circles/solid line*, p-Stage I (n = 382); *closed circles/solid line*, p-Stage II (n = 196); *open squares/solid line*, p-Stage III (n = 1021); *closed squares/solid line*, p-Stage IV (n = 391); *open circles/dotted line*, p-Stage Ia (n = 36); *open triangles/dotted line*, p-Stage Ib (n = 49); *stars/dotted line*, p-Stage Ic (n = 297)

size is the factor to influence the postoperative prognosis.

Lymph node metastases also influence the prognosis after resection. Cameron [9] reported that the 5-year survival of the patients with adenocarcinoma of the pancreas was 50% in the absence of positive nodes but dropped to below 5% when lymph nodes were involved.

Pancreatic duct adenocarcinoma metastasizes to the regional and juxta regional lymph nodes (see Chapters "Gross Anatomy of the Pancreas" and "Pathology of Metastatic Patterns of Pancreatic Cancer" in this volume). The widespread distribution of metastases found in peripancreatic and around pancreatic lymph nodes would justify the regional or total pancreatectomy as a more adequate surgical procedure [10]. Brooks [11] also observed that a total pancreatectomy was appropriate to remove the potential sites of nodal involvement. From the therapeutic point of view, it seems that radical and aggressive surgery is necessary to improve the prognosis of advanced pancreatic cancer.

In patients who underwent an extended radical operation with the regional and juxta regional lymph node dissection, we observed improved survival compared with patients without any lymph node dissection; however, analysis of long-term survival did not reveal any significant differences. Although the overall operative results await further experiences, a few long-term survivors have been seen among the patients after an extended radical operation.

To improve the prognosis of pancreatic cancer, diagnostic techniques for the detection of early cancer should be established. However, as it stands, in the advanced stage, an extended radical operation should be attempted, because there is a chance of a long survival. Multimodality treatment is another advancement in the therapy [12].

References

1. Jordan GL Jr (1987) Pancreatic resection for pancreatic cancer. Surgical diseases of the pancreas. In: Howard JM, Jordan GL Jr, Reber HA (eds) Surchcal diseases of the pancreas. Lee and Feibiger, Philadelphia, pp 666–714
2. Fortner JG, Kim DK, Cubilla AL, Turnbull A, Pahnke LD, Shils ME (1977) Regional pancreatectomy. en bloc pancreatic, portal vein and lymph node resection. Ann Surg 186:42–50
3. Sindelar WF (1989) Clinical experience with regional pancreatectomy for adenocarcinoma of the pancreas. Arch Surg 124:127–132
4. Pancreatic Cancer Registry of the Japan Pancreas Society (1991) Annual report of registered cases of pancreatic cancer in Japan (in Japanese).
5. Mackie CR, Dhorajiwala J, Blacstone MO, Bowie J, Moossa AR (1982) Value of new diagnostic aids in relation to the disease process in pancreatic cancer. Lancet 25:385–389
6. Moossa AR (1989) Surgical treatment of pancreatic cancer. Cancer of the bile ducts and pancreas. In: Preece PE, Cuschieri A, Rosin RD (eds) Cancer of the bileduct and pancreas WB Saunders, Philadelphia, pp 197–208
7. Cubilla, AL, Fitzgerald P, Fortner JG (1978) Pancreatic cancer-duct cell adenocarcinoma: Survival in relation to site, size, stage, and type of therapy. J Surg Oncol 10:465–482
8. Bottger T, Zech W, Weber W, Sorger K, Junginer T (1990) Relevant factors in the prognosis of ductal pancreatic carcinoma. Acta Chir Scand 156:781–788
9. Cameron JL (1990) Carcinoma of the pancreas: Are we making progress? MMJ 39:361–363
10. Cubilla AL, Fortner JG, Fitzgerald P (1978) Lymph node involvement in carcinoma of the head of the pancreas area. Cancer 41:88–887
11. Brooks JR, Culebras JM (1976) Cancer of the pancreas: Palliative operation, Whipple procedure, or total pancreatectomy. Am J Surg 131:361–520
12. Ozaki H (1992) Improvement of pancreatic cancer treatment: From the Japanese experience with the 1980s. Int J Pancreatol 12:5–9

Staging for Carcinoma of the Pancreas: Japanese Stage Classification Compared to UICC Stage Classification

Introduction

The stage of cancer should accurately reflect the prognosis of patients suffering from the disease, as well as the resectability of tumors. There have been a number of proposals in the past for staging of pancreatic carcinoma (Biometry Branch, National Cancer Institute 1972 [1], Hermreck 1974 [2], Leadbetter et al. 1975 [3], Cancer of the Pancreas Task Force 1981 [4], Fortner 1981 [5], Gall and Zirngibl 1986 [6], Klapdor 1986 [7], Klöppel and Fitzgerald 1986 [8]). The most recent stage classifications (SC) are that of the Japan Pancreas Society published in 1982 and revised in 1986 [9], and that of the Union International Contre le Cancer (UICC) published in 1987 [10]. In this paper, we will introduce the stage classification proposed by Japan Pancreas Society (JPN-SC), discuss the major differences between JPN-SC and UICC-SC, and report the therapeutic results of 229 pancreatic cancer patients analyzed according to the two staging systems.

Japanese Stage Classification

The Japanese stage classification described in "General Rules for Cancer of the Pancreas" (1986) [9] is composed of eight staging factors, namely, tumor size (T-factor), lymph node metastasis (N-factor), capsular invasion (S-factor), retroperitoneal invasion (Rp-factor), portal venous invasion (PV-factor), peritoneal metastasis (P-factor), hepatic metastasis (H-factor), and distant metastasis (M-factor). It elaborates on these factors as follows.

Gross Size of the Tumor (T-Factor)

The gross size of the tumor should be recorded as $a \times b \times c$ (cm) where a = greatest diameter, b = diameter perpendicular to "a", and c = thickness. The gross size of the tumor is referred to as the "T-factor" and is divided into the following four categories:

T1. The maximum diameter of the tumor is no more than 2.0 cm.

T2. The maximum diameter of the tumor is from 2.1 to 4.0 cm.

T3. The maximum diameter of the tumor is from 4.1 to 6.0 cm.

T4. The maximum diameter of the tumor is more than 6.1 cm.

The size of the tumor should be determined on the basis of fixed specimens in resected and autopsied cases and of operative findings in unresectable cases.

Lymph Node Metastasis (N-Factor)

The regional lymph nodes from No. 1 to No. 18 are shown in Fig. 1a,b and Table 1. They are classified into three groups: Primary (N1), secondary (N2), and tertiary (N3) according to their location (Table 2).

N(−). No suspicion of lymph node metastasis

N1(−). No metastasis to lymph nodes of the primary group

N2(−). No metastasis to lymph nodes of the secondary group

N3(−). No metastasis to lymph nodes of the tertiary group

N1(+). Metastasis to lymph nodes of the primary group

N2(+). Metastasis to lymph nodes of the secondary group

N3(+). Metastasis to lymph nodes of the tertiary group

Table 1. Regional lymph nodes and their code numbers.

No. 1:	LN of right cardiac region
No. 2:	LN of left cardiac region
No. 3:	LN along lesser curvature of stomach
No. 4:	LN along greater curvature of stomach 4sa, 4sb, and 4d are LN along short gastric a., left gastroepiploic a., and right gastroepiploic a., respectively.
No. 5:	LN of suprapyloric region
No. 6:	LN of infrapyloric region
No. 7:	LN along left gastric a.
No. 8:	LN along common hepatic a. (8a: anterior-superior, 8p: posterior)
No. 9:	LN around celiac a.
No. 10:	LN at splenic hilus
No. 11:	LN along splenic a.
No. 12:	LN in hepatoduodenal ligament 12h: LN at porta hepatis 12a: LN along proper hepatic a. (12a1; upper half, 12a2; lower half) 12p: LN along portal vein (12p1; upper half, 12p2; lower half) 12b: LN along bile duct (12b1; upper half, 12b2; lower half)
No. 13:	LN at posterior aspect of head of pancreas (13a: superior-posterior, 13b: inferior-posterior)
No. 14:	LN at radix mesenteri 14a, 14b, 14c, 14d, and 14V are LN at the origin of superior mesenteric a., inferior pancreaticoduodenal a., middle colic a., jejunal a., and superior mesenteric vein, respectively.
No. 15:	LN along middle colic a.
No. 16:	LN around abdominal aorta and inferior vena cava 16a: IN between hiatus aorticus and inferior border of left renal vein (16a1; upper region of celiac a., 16a2; lower region of celiac a.) 16b: LN between inferior border of left renal vein and bifurcation of common iliac a. (16b1; upper region of inferior mesenteric a., 16b2; lower region of inferior mesenteric a.)
No. 17:	LN at anterior aspect of head of pancreas (17a: superior-anterior, 17b: inferior-anterior)
No. 18:	LN along inferior border of body and tail of pancreas

LN, lymph node; *a.*, artery

Table 2. Grouping and lymph node designations according to tumor location.

	Tumor site	
Group	Head of the pancreas	Body and tail of the pancreas
Primary group (N1)	6, 8a, 8p, 12a2, 12b2, 12p2, 13a, 13b, 14a, 14b, 14c, 14d, 14V, 17a, 17b	8a, 8p, 9, 10, 11, 14a, 14b, 14c, 14d, 14V, 18
Secondary group (N2)	9, 11, 12a1, 12b1, 12p1, 12c, 15, 16a1, 16a2, 16b1, 16b2, 18	7, 12a2, 12b2, 12p2, 13a, 13b, 15, 16a1, 16a2, 16b1, 16b2, 17a, 17b
Tertiary group (N3)	1, 2, 3, 4, 5, 7, 10, 12h, and others more distant	1, 2, 3, 4, 5, 6, 12a1, 12b1, 12p1, 12c, 12h, and others more distant

In cases of N1(+), N2(+), or N3(+), the cord number of the positive lymph nodes should be recorded.

Tumor Invasion to the Pancreatic Capsule and Adjacent Tissues

Invasion to the Anterior Capsule of the Pancreas (S-Factor)

S0. No capsular invasion

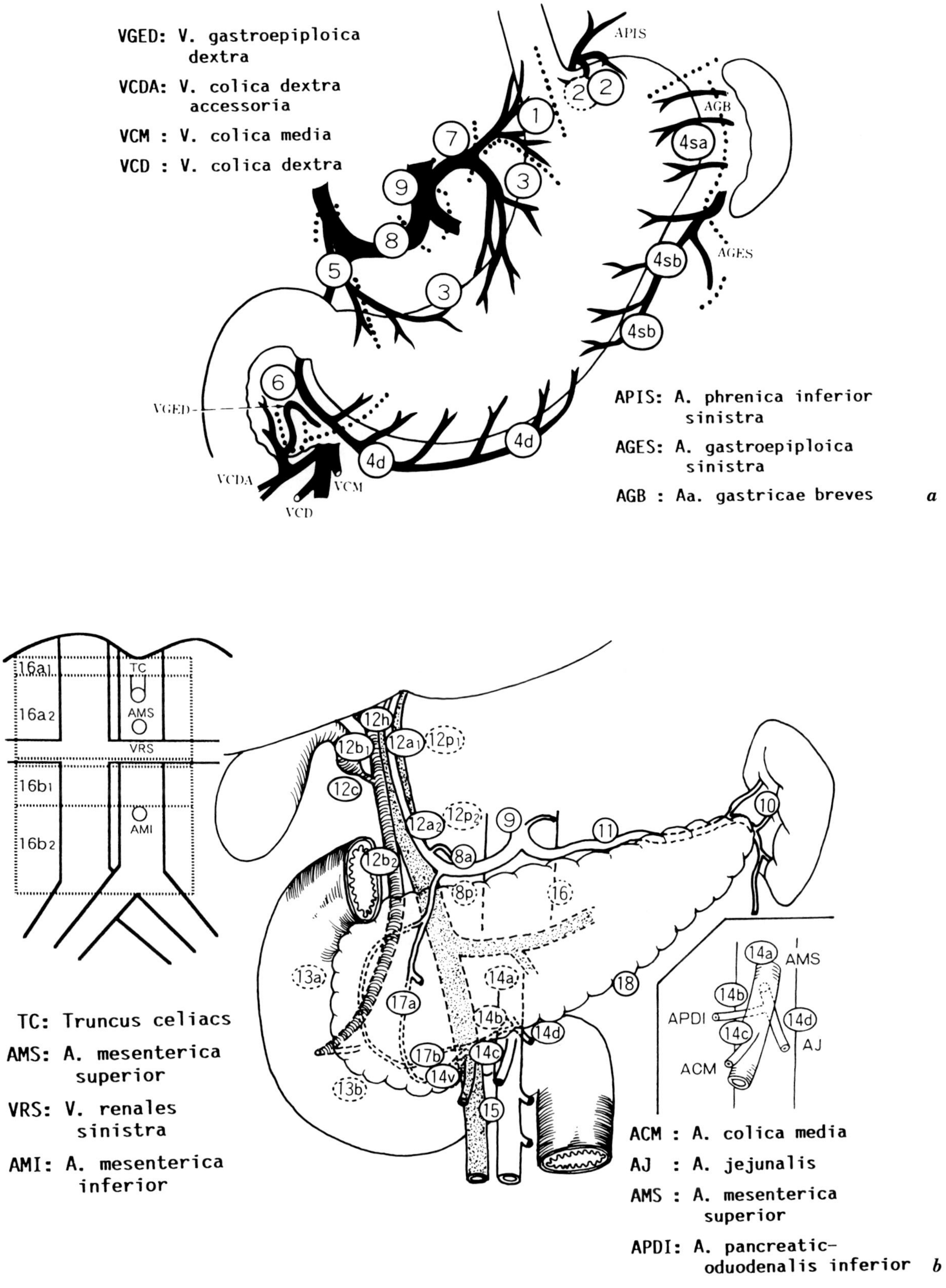

Fig. 1a,b. Regional lymph nodes and their code numbers in JPN-SC. Table 1 provides an explanation

S1. Suspected invasion to the capsule
S2. Definite invasion to the capsule
S3. Direct invasion to the adjacent viscera (stomach, colon, or spleen)

Retroperitoneal Invasion (Rp-Factor)

Rp0. No retroperitoneal invasion
Rp1. Suspected invasion to retroperitoneal tissues
Rp2. Definite invasion to retroperitoneal tissues
Rp3. Severe invasion to retroperitoneal tissues and definite or severe invasion to the adjacent viscera

"Retroperitoneal tissues" refers to tissues and organs lying in the posterior aspect of the pancreas, including retro-pancreatic connective tissue, nerve plexi, and portal venous vessels (portal and superior mesenteric). However, invasion to the portal venous vessels should be described independently. "Adjacent viscera" refers to the aorta, superior mesenteric artery, inferior vena cava, kidneys, and adrenal glands.

Invasion to the Portal Venous Vessels (PV-Factor)

PV0. No invasion to the portal venous vessels
PV1. Suspected invasion to the portal venous vessels
PV2. Definite invasion to the portal venous vessels
PV3. Severe invasion to the portal venous vessels with stenosis

The portal venous vessels include the portal vein (PVp) and superior mesenteric vein (PVsm).

Disseminating Peritoneal Metastasis (P-Factor)

P0. No disseminating metastasis to any part of the peritoneum
P1. Disseminating metastasis to the adjacent peritoneum
P2. A few to several scattered metastases to the distant peritoneum
P3. Numerous metastases to the distant peritoneum

Hepatic Metastasis (H-Factor)

H0. No hepatic metastasis
H1. Metastasis limited to one of the lobes
H1 (dex): Metastasis to the right lobe
H1 (sin): Metastasis to the left lobe
H2. A few scattered metastases to both lobes
H3. Numerous scattered metastases to both lobes

Table 3. Gross staging of carcinoma of the pancreas in JPN-SC (P1-3, H1-3, Distant metastasis: Stage IV).

Stage	Factor				
	T	N	S	Rp	PV
I	T1 ($\leqslant$ 2 cm)	N(−)	S0	Rp0	PV0
II	T2 (2.1 − 4.0 cm)	N1(+)	S1	Rp0	PV1
III	T3 (4.1 − 6.0 cm)	N2(+)	S2	Rp2	PV2
IV	T4 ($\geqslant$ 6.1 cm)	N3(+)	S3	Rp3	PV3

Distant Metastasis

M(−). No suspicion of distant metastasis
M(+). Distant metastasis

Stage grouping is conducted according to the severity of T-, N-, S-, Rp-, and PV-factors as shown in Table 3. The highest severity among the factors determines the stage of the disease. When P-, H-, or M-factor is positive, the disease is allocated to stage IV.

UICC Stage Classification

The UICC stage classification described in "TNM classification of malignant tumors" is composed of three staging categories: Primary tumor (T-category), regional lymph nodes (N-category), and distant metastasis (M-category) [10, 11]. It elaborates on these categories as follows:

Primary Tumor (T-Category)

TX. Primary tumor cannot be assessed
T0. No evidence of primary tumor
T1. Tumor limited to the pancreas
T1a: Tumor 2 cm or less in greatest dimension
T1b: Tumor more than 2 cm in greatest dimension
T2. Tumor extends directly to any of the following: duodenum, bile duct, peripancreatic tissues
T3. Tumor extends directly to any of the following: stomach, spleen, colon, adjacent large vessels

Regional Lymph Node (N-Category)

NX. Regional lymph nodes cannot be assessed
N0. No regional lymph nodes metastasis
N1. Regional lymph nodes metastasis

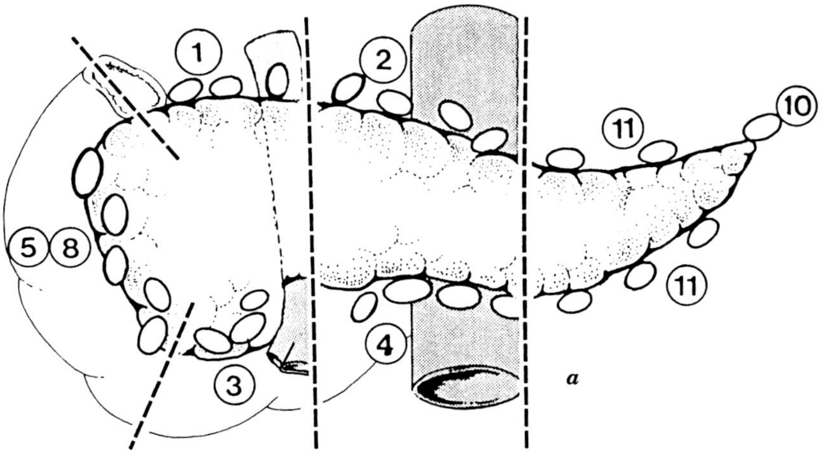

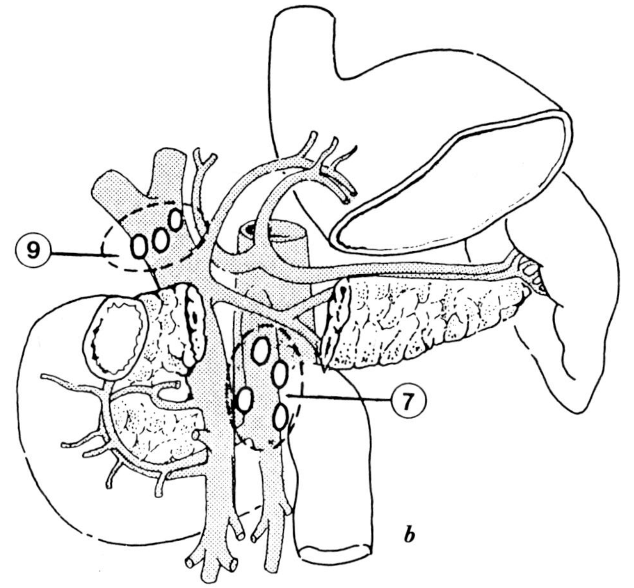

Fig. 2a,b. Regional lymph nodes in UICC-SC are peripancreatic nodes and can be subdivided as follows. Superior: superior to head (*1*) and body (*2*); inferior: inferior to head (*3*) and body (*4*); anterior: anterior pancreaticoduodenal (*5*), pyloric (*6*) (not shown), and proximal mesenteric (*7*); posterior: posterior pancreaticoduodenal (*8*), common bile duct (*9*) and proximal mesenteric (*7*); splenic: hilum of spleen (*10*), and tail of pancreas (*11*)

The regional lymph nodes from No. 1 to No. 11 are shown in Fig. 2a,b. They are the peripancreatic nodes, which may be subdivided as follows:

Superior: Superior to head and body
Inferior: Inferior to head and body
Anterior: Anterior pancreaticoduodenal, pyloric, and proximal mesenteric
Posterior: Posterior pancreaticoduodenal, common bile duct, and proximal mesenteric
Splenic: Hilum of spleen and tail of pancreas

Metastasis in any lymph node other than regional is classified as a distant metastasis.

Distant Metastases (M-Category)

MX. Presence of distant metastases cannot be assessed
M0. No distant metastases
M1. Distant metastases

The category M1 may be further specified according to the following notation:

Pulmonary	PUL	Bone marrow	MAR
Osseous	OSS	Pleura	PLE
Hepatic	HEP	Peritoneaum	PER
Brain	BRA	Skin	SKI
Lymph node	LYM	Others	OTH

Stage grouping of UICC-SC is shown in Table 4.

Table 4. Stage grouping in UICC-SC.

Stage	Factor T	N	M
I	T1	N0	M0
	T2	N0	M0
II	T3	N0	M0
III	Any T	N1	M0
IV	Any T	Any N	M1

Major Differences Between JPN-SC and UICC-SC

The disease is divided into four stages in both JPN-SC and UICC-SC. In many ways, however, the staging factors and grouping methods are different in the two staging systems. The two major differences between JPN-SC and UICC-SC are: (1) the definition of T-factor and N-factor, and (2) the method of stage grouping. In JPN-SC, T-factor simply means tumor size, while in UICC-SC, the "T"-category includes tumor invasion to the pancreatic capsule and adjacent tissues. In other words, "T" in UICC-SC includes the S-, Rp-, and PV-factors of JPN-SC. The definition of regional lymph nodes also differs between the two staging systems. In UICC-SC, furthermore, metastases to the lymph nodes other than those shown in Fig. 2a,b is regarded as distant metastases (M). Stage grouping in JPN-SC is determined principally according to the severity of each staging factor. In UICC-SC, however, T3—which corresponds S3, Rp3, and Pv2-3 in JPN-SC—is the most important factor in the definition of stage II, while N1 and M1 are the most important in stages III and IV, respectively.

JPN-SC Versus UICC-SC

Analysis of the Therapeutic Results of 229 Pancreatic Cancer Patients According to JPN-SC and UICC-SC

A total of 229 patients with pancreatic ductal carcinoma encountered consecutively at the Second Department of Surgery, Nagasaki University School of Medicine, between October 1969 and September 1989 were analyzed according to JPN-SC and UICC-SC [12]. Cystadenocarcinoma, islet cell tumor, ampullary carcinoma and cartinoid tumor were excluded from this study. Resections which included 17 total pancreatectomies, 34 pancreatoduodenectomies, and 9 distal pancreatectomies were performed. The UICC stage and equivalent JPN staging factors assigned in this study are shown in Table 5 to avoid confusion in the comparison of the two staging systems.

The patient distribution, resectability, and curative resection rates of all patients were reviewed according to each staging system (Table 6). Resectional surgery was not done in one UICC stage I patient because of suspected portal vein invasion, and in three of UICC stage II patients because of definite or severe invasion to surrounding organs. In contrast, a 100% resection rate was achieved in JPN stages I and II. Resection rates in stages III and IV were significantly higher by JPN-SC than by UICC-SC. In JPN stage I, a 100% curative resection rate was achieved, and the curative resection rates in stages II and III were also significantly higher than those in the UICC stages.

Postoperative cumulative survival (PCS) curves and rates were analyzed according to each staging factor in 60 resected cases for which all staging factors, except tumor size and distant metastasis, had been confirmed microscopically.

Stage

According to JPN-SC, significant differences were observed in the PCS curves between stages I and

Table 5. Correlation of UICC and JPN staging factors.

UICC stage	JPN staging factors assigned to UICC stage
I (T1–2, N0, M0)	T1–4, N(−), M(−), S0–2, Rp0–2, PV0–1
II (T3, N0, M0)	T1–4, N(−), M(−), S3, Rp3, PV2–3
III (Any T, N1, M0)	T1–4, N1–3, M(−), S0–3, Rp0–3 PV0–3
IV (Any T, Any N, M1)	T1–4, N0–3, M(+), S0–3, Rp0–3, PV0–3

Table 6. Distribution of the patients, resection rates and curative resection rates according to the two different stage classifications. Parentheses indicate the number of patients. Twenty-seven patients with unknown stages were excluded.

		Stage I	Stage II	Stage III	Stage IV	Total
Patient distribution, %	UICC	6 (12)	4 (9)	38 (77)] *	51 (104)] *	100 (202)
	JPN	1 (2)	5 (10)	13 (27)	82 (163)	100 (202)
Resection rate, %	UICC	92 (11/12)	67 (6/9)	51 (39/77)] **	4 (4/104)] *	30 (60/202)
	JPN	100 (2/2)	100 (10/10)	93 (25/27)	14 (23/163)	30 (60/202)
Curative resection rate, %	UICC	82 (7/9)	0 (0/6)] *	33 (13/39)] **	0 (0/4)	37 (22/60)
	JPN	100 (2/2)	80 (8/10)	80 (12/15)	0 (0/23)	37 (22/60)

* $P < 0.05$; ** $P < 0.01$
UICC, UICC stage classification; *JPN*, JPN stage classification

III ($P < 0.05$), I and IV ($P < 0.05$), and III and IV ($P < 0.05$) (Fig. 3). By UICC-SC, there were no significant differences in the PCS curves among stages I, II, III, and IV (Fig. 4).

T-Factor

In UICC-SC, significant differences were observed in the PCS curves between T1a and T2 ($P < 0.05$), T1a and T3 ($P < 0.05$), T1b and T2 ($P < 0.05$), and T1b and T3 ($P < 0.05$) (Fig. 5). There were no significant differences in the PCS curves or rates among JPN T1, T2, T3, and T4 in this series.

N-Factor

Although there was no significant difference in the PCS curves between (N−) and N(+), a significant difference was present in the 2-year PCS rates (Fig. 6). By JPN-SC, there was no significant difference in the PCS curves among N0, N1, N2, and N3, but a significant difference was observed in the 1-year PCS rate between N0 and N2.

M-Factor

There was no significant difference in the PCS curves between M(−) and M(+), which may be because of the small number of M(+) patients. However, there was a significant difference in the 6-month PCS rate, namely, 71% in M(−) and 25% in M(+). No M(+) patient survived more than 7 months.

S-Factor

There was a significant difference in the 1-year PCS rate ($P < 0.05$) between 44% in S(−) and 25% in S(+), although no significant difference was observed in the PCS curves. There were also significant differences in the PCS curves between S0 and S2 ($P < 0.05$) and in the 1-year PCS rate

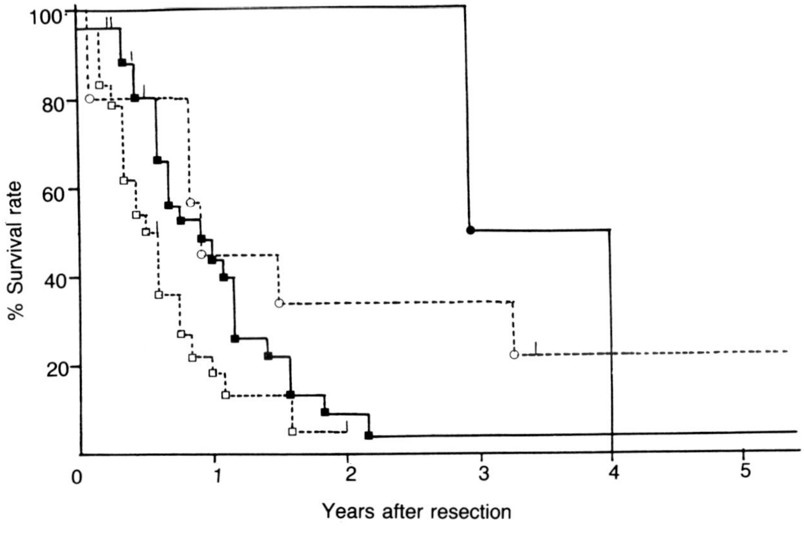

Fig. 3. Cumulative survival after resectional surgery according to the Japanese stage classification. There are significant differences between the curves of stages I (*closed circles*, $n = 2$) and III (*closed squares*, $n = 25$), I and IV (*open squares*, $n = 23$), and III and IV ($P < 0.05$) Stage II is represented by *open circles* ($n = 10$)

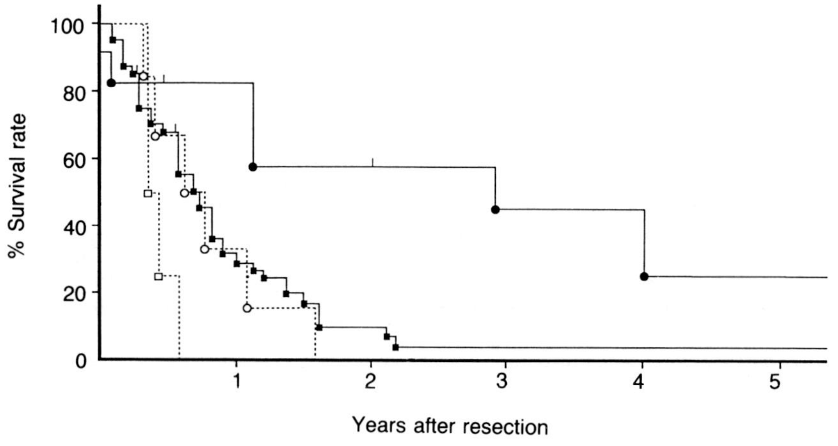

Fig. 4. Cumulative survival after resectional surgery according to UICC stage classification. There are significant differences in the 1-year PCS rate between stages I (*closed circles*, $n = 11$) and II (*open circles*, $n = 6$), in the 2-year PCS rate between stages I and III (*closed squares*, $n = 39$), and in the 3-year PCS rate between stages I and III ($P < 0.05$). Stage IV is represented by *open squares* ($n = 4$)

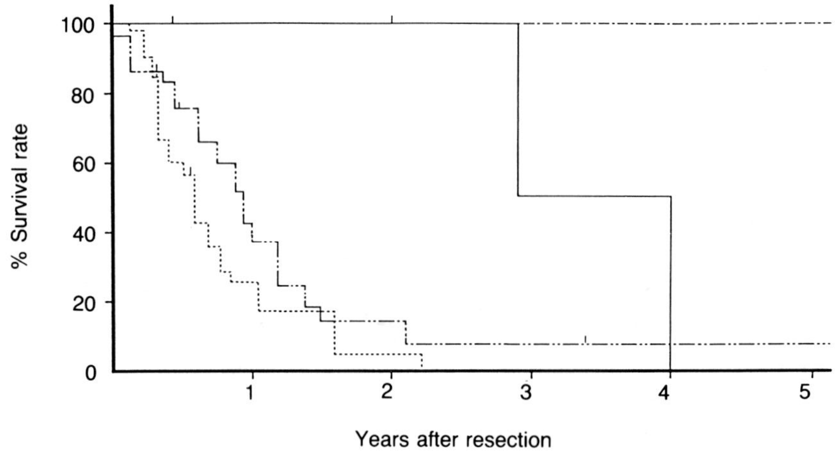

Fig. 5. Cumulative survival after resectional surgery for primary tumor by UICC-SC. There are significant differences between T1a (*solid line*, $n = 2$) and T2 (*double-chained line*, $n = 24$), T1ab and T3 (*dotted line*, $n = 31$), T1b (*single-chained line*, $n = 3$) and T2, and T1b and T3 ($P < 0.05$)

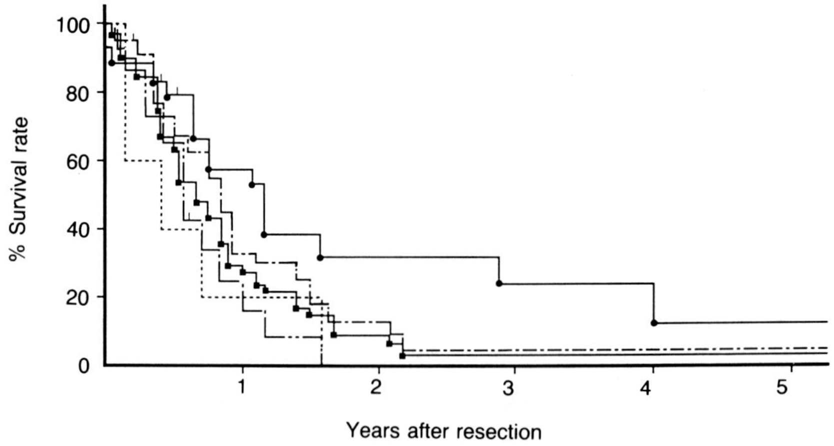

Fig. 6. Cumulative survival after resection according to N-factor. There is a significant difference in the 2-year survival rate between N(−) and N(+) ($P < 0.05$). A significant difference in the 1-year survival rate is found between N0 and N2 ($P < 0.05$). N(−), N0 ($n = 18$), *closed circles*; N(+) ($n = 42$), *closed squares*; N1 ($n = 22$), *single-chained line*; N2 ($n = 15$), *double-chained line*; N3 ($n = 5$), *dotted line*

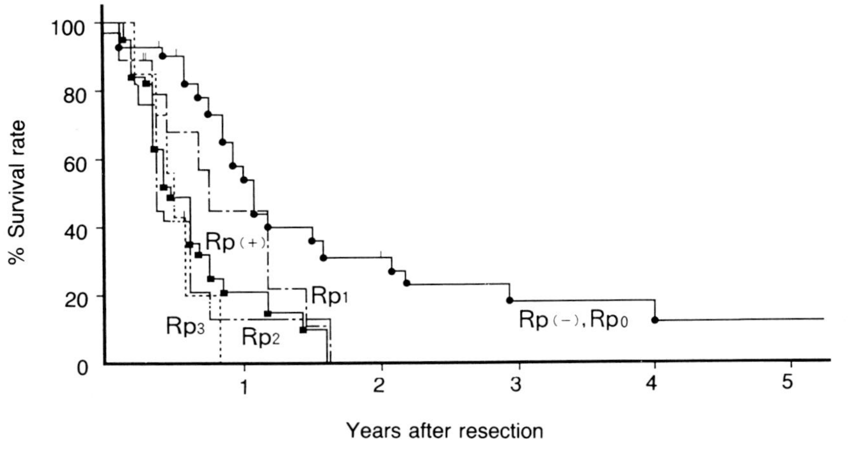

Fig. 7. Cumulative survival after resection according to Rp-factor. There are significant differences between the curves of Rp(−) and Rp(+), Rp0 and Rp2, and Rp0 and Rp3 ($P < 0.05$). Rp(−), Rp0 ($n = 27$), *closed circles*; Rp(+) ($n = 33$), *closed squares*; Rp1 ($n = 9$), *single-chained line*; Rp2 ($n = 17$), *double-chained line*; Rp3 ($n = 7$), *dotted line*

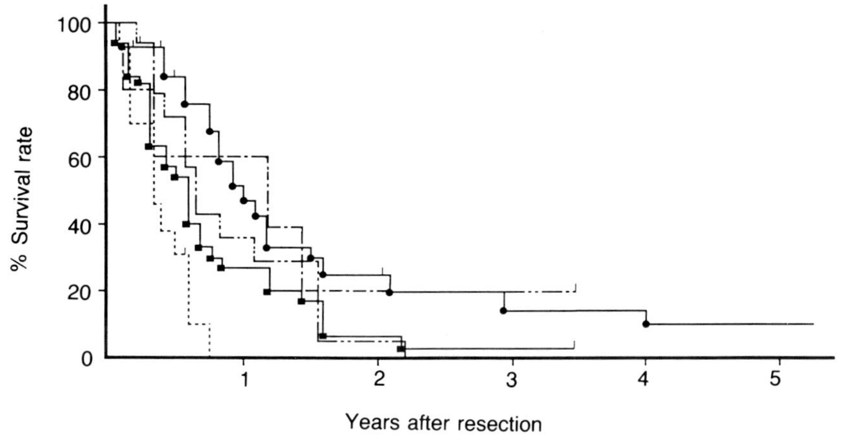

Fig. 8. Cumulative survival after resectional surgery according to PV-factor. There are significant differences between the curves of PV(−) and PV(+) ($P < 0.01$), PV0 and PV3 ($P < 0.001$), and PV2 and PV3 ($P < 0.05$). PV(−) PV0 ($n = 27$), *closed circles*; PV(+) ($n = 33$), *closed squares*; PV1 ($n = 5$), *single-chained line*; PV2 ($n = 15$), *double-chained line*; PV3 ($n = 13$), *dotted line*

between 44% in S0 and 15% in S1 ($P < 0.05$) by JPN-SC.

Rp-Factor

There was a significant difference in the PCS curves between Rp(−) and Rp(+) ($P < 0.05$) (Fig. 7). Significant differences were also observed in the PCS curves between Rp0 and Rp2 ($P < 0.05$), and Rp0 and Rp3 ($P < 0.05$) by JPN-SC.

PV-Factor

There was a significant difference in the PCS curves between PV(−) and PV(+) ($P < 0.01$) (Fig. 8). Significant differences were also observed in the PCS curves between PVO and PV3 ($P < 0.001$), and PV2 and PV3 ($P < 0.05$) by JPN-SC.

Comments

Among the factors employed in each stage classification, significant differences in the PCS curves were demonstrated only on the basis of the presence or absence of Rp- and PV-factors in JPN-SC and of the grading of T-category in UICC-SC, even though significant differences were sometimes observed in the PCS rates on the basis of N-, M-, and S-factors. Considering that "T" in UICC-SC includes the JPN-SC Rp- and PV-factors, and that tumor size did not affect the prognosis, these results indicate that Rp- and PV-factors exert a strong influence on the postoperative prognosis, as has been shown in previous reports [13, 14].

As compared to Rp- and PV-factors, the N-category is perhaps overestimated in UICC-SC [15, 16]. Significant differences in the PCS rates between N(−) and N(+) were revealed only at certain times. In addition, it has been reported that the best long-term results were obtained by complete dissection of the regional lymph nodes [13]. There is another problem in UICC-SC concerning the staging significance of N-category, that is, positive lymph node metastases (N1) is the most important factor in the definition of stage III regardless of degree of invasion to the surrounding organs or adjacent large vessels.

In general, UICC-SC tends to classify patients in a less advanced stage than JPN-SC. UICC-SC exhibits the following underestimations of stage. "T3" patients, who have invasions to the surrounding organs or adjacent large vessels corresponding to Rp3 and PV3 in JPN-SC, belong to stage II. By JPN-SC, the patients with these conditions belong to stage IV. When severe portal vein invasion is present, for example, the tumor is usually unresectable unless the portal vein is resected. Severe invasion to the surrounding organs or adjacent large vessels, therefore, should be allocated to the most advanced stage. The above underestimations resulted in a reduction of resection and curative resection rates in the earlier stages of UICC-SC.

On the basis of our analysis of 4852 collected cases, we reported that the stages of JPN-SC reflected the prognosis of the disease [17]. Although the severity of each factor was divided into four grades in JPN-SC, significant differences were not always demonstrated in the PCS curves or rates among the grades for each factor.

In the future, the grading system could be simplified and stage assignment of gradings of each factor better organized. Continuing efforts are necessary to establish a more practical, simple, and universal staging system for carcinoma of the pancreas.

Acknowledgment. This work was supported in part by Grant-in-Aid for Cancer Research from Ministry of Health and Welfare of the Japanese Government

References

1. Biometry Branch, National Cancer Institute (1972) End results in cancer. Report No. 4, Publication No. 73–272. Axtel LM, Cutler SJ, Myers MH (eds) US Department of Health, Education and Welfare, End Results Section, pp 81–84
2. Hermreck AS, Thomas CY, Friesen SR (1974) Importance of pathologic staging in the surgical management of adenocarcinoma of the exocrine pancreas. Am J Surg 127:653–657
3. Leadbetter A, Foster RS Jr, Haines CR (1975) Carcinoma of the pancreas. Results from the Vermont tumor registry. Am J Surg 129:356–360
4. Cancer of the Pancreas Task Force (1981) Staging of cancer of the pancreas. Cancer 47:1631–1637
5. Fortner JG (1984) Regional pancreatectomy for cancer of the pancreas, ampulla, and other related sites. Tumor staging and results. Ann Surg 199: 418–425
6. Gall FP, Zirngibl H (1986) Malign Tumoren des Pankreas und der periampullaren Region. In: Gall FP, Hermanek P, Tonak J (eds) Chirurgische Onkologie und stadiengerechte Therapie maligner Tumoren. Springer, Berlin Heidelberg New York, pp 416–460.
7. Klapdor R (1986) TNM-Klassification, Staging und Prognose des Pankreaskarzinomas. Dtsch med Wschr 111:229–233
8. Klöppel G, Fitzgerald PJ (1986) Pathology of nonendocrine pancreatic tumors. In: Go VLW, Gardner JD, Brooks FP, Lebenthal E, Dimagno EP, Scheele GA (eds) The exocrine pancreas. Raven, New York, pp 649–674
9. Japan Pancreas Society (1986) General rules for surgical and pathological studies on cancer of the pancreas (in Japanese). 3rd edn. Kanehara, Tokyo
10. UICC (1987) TNM classification of malignant tumors, 4th fully rev edn. Springer, Berlin Heidelberg New York
11. UICC (1989) TNM atlas. Illustrated guide to the TNM/pTNM-classification of malignant tumours, 3rd edn. Springer, Berlin Heidelberg New York
12. Tsundoa T, Ura K, Eto T, Matsumoto T, Tsuchiya R (1991) UICC and Japanese stage classifications for carcinoma of the pancreas. Int J Pancreatol 8:205–214.
13. Tsuchiya R, Harada N, Tsunoda T, Miyamoto T, Ura K (1988) Long-term survivors after operation on carcinoma of the pancreas. Int J Pancreatol 3:491–496.
14. Manabe T, Baba N, Nonaka A, Asano N, Yamaki K, Shibamoto Y, Takahashi M, Abe M, Tobe T (1988) Combined treatment using radiotherapy for carcinoma of the pancreas involving the adjacent vessels. Int Surg 73:153–156
15. Mannel A, van Heerden JA, Weiland LH, Ilstrup DM (1986) Factors influencing survival after resection of ductal adenocarcinoma of the pancreas. Ann Surg 203:403–407
16. Klöppel G (1988) Pancreatic carcinoma: Structural features and biological behavior. Becker V, Hubner K (eds) The pancreas in connection with the epigastric unit. Gustav Fischer, Stuttgart, pp 122–136
17. Tsuchiya R, Tsunoda T, Ishida T, Saitoh Y (1990) Resection for cancer of the pancreas—the Japanese experience. Bailliere's Clin Gastroenterol. 4:931–939

Molecular Biology

Introduction

Morphological studies of pancreatic cancers do not provide sufficient information to predict their biological behavior. The study of genetic abnormalities in pancreatic cancers may open new paths for understanding the etiology and pathogenesis of the disease, and may help in establishing markers for diagnosis and prognosis. There is increasing evidence that it is the accumulation of different genetic abnormalities, rather than a single gene defect, that underlies the multistage processes of tumorigenesis and progression of malignancy [1]. Growth factors and their receptors, tumor suppressor genes, and oncogenes have received considerable attention and seem to be promising in assessing of malignant potential [2].

Growth Factors and Their Receptors

Abnormalities of growth factor/receptor systems in pancreatic cancer, including the changes in expression of the insulin-like growth factors, platelet-derived growth factors, and the fibroblast growth factors and their respective receptors have been found. However, our understanding of most of these systems is too fragmentary to be of direct clinical application, but one family of receptors does merit special attention.

Type 1 Growth Factor Receptors

Four receptors have been recognized in this family EGF receptor (EGFR), ERBB2 (also known as HER2 or NEU), ERBB3 and ERBB4. The first three receptors are frequently overexpressed in proliferative conditions of the exocrine pancreas. The EGF receptor is overexpressed by increased gene transcription in reactive epithelial hyperplasia of chronic pancreatitis and in almost all ductal adenocarcinomas and cancer cell lines [2, 3]. There also are frequent abnormalities of the known ligands for the EGF receptor. Transforming growth factor alpha (TGF alpha) is ubiquitously expressed at high level in chronic pancreatitis and in pancreatic cancer, hence forming a potential autocrine loop [4, 5]. In transgenic mice, widespread overexpression of TGF alpha under the influence of a metallothionein promoter induced (among other changes) proliferation of pancreatic acinar and fibroblast cells and caused acinoductular structures of the pancreas. These effects are likely to be due to TGF alpha acting at a local level (in autocrine or paracrine fashion) since they were also seen when TGF alpha was driven by an elastase promoter expressed only in pancreatic acinar cells. Epidermal growth factor (EGF) is not detectable in the normal pancreas but is expressed in an ulceration-associated cell lineage involved in the repair of epithelial surfaces throughout the gastrointestinal tract including the duct system in chronic pancreatitis [4]. Expression of the pNR-2/pS2 protein appears to be associated with this lineage. The pS2 and hSP proteins are not expressed in the normal pancreas but high levels are found in 85% of biliary tract cancers and in 75% of pancreatic cancers [6, 7]. The mechanism by which transcription of these genes is activated has not been determined, but it is notable that the pS2 gene promoter contains an EGF-responsive element and that potential autocrine loops for stimulation of the EGF receptor have been identified in pancreatic disease [3, 4]. Immunoreactivity for EGF is found in 12% of pancreatic cancers [4] and preliminary evidence suggests that abnormal expression of amphiregulin may also occur in pancreatic cancer.

The ERBB2 receptor, sometimes in association with gene amplification, is overexpressed in at least 20% of pancreatic ductal adenocarcinoma [2, 8]. The status of the putative ligands for the ERBB2 receptor has not yet been assayed in pancreatic cancer.

The ERBB3 receptor is detectable only in the normal islets of Langerhans, but is overexpressed throughout the duct system in almost all cases of chronic pancreatitis and in 90% of pancreatic cancers [9]. The nature of the specific ligand(s) for this receptor is not known.

Tumor Suppressor Genes

Clues to the involvement and chromosomal location of tumor suppressor genes can be found by cytogenetic analysis of human tumors, but there are few reports of chromosome abnormalities in pancreatic cancer. The studies available suggest that there may be frequent loss of the short arm of chromosome 1 and the long arm of chromosome 6, as well as abnormalities of chromosome 7. Studies using restriction fragment length polymorphism (RFLP) have reported loss of heterozygosity on chromosome 1p in 25% of pancreatic cancers [10] and chromosome 5q in 25%–30% of them [11].

The tumor suppressor gene p53 frequently is activated by point mutation in human pancreatic cancer [12]. Approximately 60% of primary ductal adenocarcinomas and a similar proportion of cancer cell lines carry p53 genes with a point mutation in the coding sequence of exons 5, 6, 7 or 8. This results in the production and high accumulation of the mutant p53 protein in the tumor cells. In the pancreatic cancer cell lines, there frequently is loss of the normal allele as well as activating point mutation, but such loss of heterozygosity on chromosome 17q appears to be less common in primary tumors. Immunohistochemistry is used to detect the presence of high levels of p53 protein in tumor cells in routine pathologic tissue sections and in cytology preparations [13].

There are two known tumor suppressor genes on chromosome 5q, APC and MCC. Investigations have shown that there is no evidence of sequence abnormality or loss of heterozygosity at these loci in ductal adenocarcinomas nor in ampullary carcinomas (Lemoine et al., unpublished). Another candidate tumor suppressor gene is DCC on chromosome 18q, but there is little evidence to implicate this gene in pancreatic cancer.

The retinoblastoma gene RB1, which is inactivated in all retinoblastomas as well as in a proportion of other tumors such as small cell lung cancer, breast cancer and melanoma, may also be inactivated by mutation in a small proportion of pancreatic cancers. However, the technical difficulties involved in analysis of this very complex gene and its protein product will limit the clinical utility of abnormalities that we have identified.

c-Ki-*ras* Mutation

Point mutation in the Kirsten (Ki)-*ras* oncogene frequently occurs in pancreatic cancer. In many cases, these mutations are confined to codon 12 of the oncogene. Therefore, mutation of this oncogene appears to play a role in pancreatic tumor development. Because ductal papillary hyperplasia lack this mutation [14] and the incidence of this mutation in a prognostically favorable ampullary carcinoma is low [15], this genetic alteration is advanced as a marker for malignancy, a predictor for biological tumor behavior, and as a means for better tumor classification, differential diagnosis, staging, and prognosis. This question was examined by Motojima et al. [16] in pancreatic cancer from 53 patients, and the patterns of the c-Ki-*ras* oncogene mutation were correlated with clinicopathological features.

Mutations in the c-Ki-*ras* codon 12 were identified in 46 (86%) of the 53 pancreatic cancers (Table 1). One tumor had an additional mutation from glycine (GGC) to aspartic acid (GAC) in the c-Ki-*ras* codon 13. No mutation was detected in the c-Ki-*ras* codon 61.

Correlations between tumor morphology, tumor localization, tumor size, stage of the disease, lymph node metastases, survival, and c-Ki-*ras* mutations are summarized in Tables 2–6 and Fig. 1. There were no significant correlations between any of these parameters and the mutation.

In another study, a panel of pancreatic carcinomas of different geographic origin (17 Italian and 14 Japanese) was studied [17] with the fol-

Table 1. Spectrum of mutations at codon 12 of the c-Ki-*ras* oncogene in 53 patients.

Ki-*ras* codon 12	Coded amino acid	No. of cases with mutation	No. of cases without mutation
GGT	gly		7
GAT	asp	29	
GTT	val	11	
CGT	arg	5	
TGT	cys	1	
		46	7

Table 2. Correlation between histological type and presence or absence of mutations in the c-Ki-*ras* oncogene.

Histological type	No. of cases	Cases with mutation	Cases without mutation
Ductal	34	32	2
Papillary	6	5	1
Mucinous	6	5	1
Adenosquamous	5	4	1
Squamous	1		1
Cribriform	1		1
Total no.	53	46	7

Table 3. Correlation between anatomical tumor location and c-Ki-*ras* mutations in resected cases.

	No. of cases	Cases with mutation	Cases without mutation
Head	39	35	4
Body or tail	6	5	1
	45	40	5

Table 4. Correlation between tumor size and c-Ki-*ras* mutations in resected cases.

	No. of cases	Cases with mutation	Cases without mutation
<2.0 cm	1	1	0
2.1–4.0 cm	19	17	2
4.1–6.0 cm	21	19	2
>6.1 cm	4	3	1
	40	40	5

Table 5. Correlation between the stage (TNM) and c-Ki-*ras* mutation.

	No. of cases	Cases with mutation	Cases without mutation
Stage I	7	6	1
II	8	7	1
III	29	26	3
IV	9	7	2
Total no.	53	46	7

Table 6. Correlation between lymph node (*LN*) metastasis and c-Ki-*ras* mutations in resected cases.

	No. of cases	Cases with mutation	Cases without mutation
LN metastasis (−)	15	13	2
LN metastasis (+)	30	27	3
Total no.	45	40	5

lowing open questions: (1) Are there geographic differences in the frequency and/or in the pattern of c-Ki-*ras* and p53 genes' mutations? (2) Do c-Ki-*ras* and p53 mutations affect the majority of cancer cells or are they restricted to a minority of the cancer cell population? (3) Is there a peculiar pattern of p53 gene mutations in pancreatic cancer with respect to that of other human cancers [18]?

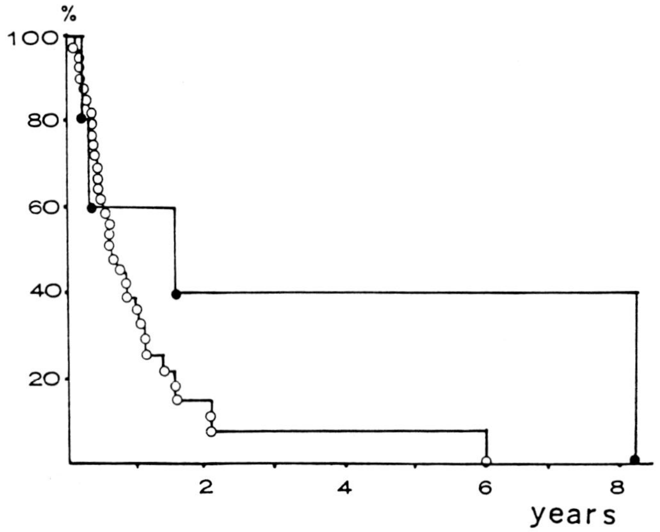

Fig. 1. Correlation between survival and the presence (*open circles*) or absence (*closed circles*) of mutations in resected cases. Survival rates were calculated using the Kaplan-Meier method, excluding eight patients who underwent bypass operation and three patients who died of non-malignancy. The generalized Wilcoxon test showed no significant difference

(4) What is the relation between p53 protein accumulation and p53 gene mutation? (5) Is there a correlation between gene mutations with clinicopathologic parameters, such as morphology and stages of cancers, and survival of patients?

The presence and pattern of mutations of c-Ki-*ras* were studied by the single-strand conformation polymorphism method (SSCP) [19] and by direct sequencing of PCR-amplified fragments [20]. c-Ki-*ras* mutations, all involving codon 12, were detected in 16 (94%) Italian and 13 (93%) Japanese samples. There were G to A transitions (GGT → GAT; gly → asp) in 8 Italian and 8 Japanese cases, and G to T transversions (GGT → GTT; gly → val) in all of the remaining cases, but one Japanese patient showed a G to C transversion (GGT → CGT; gly → arg).

The results are in keeping with most studies which demonstrated a high frequency of c-Ki-*ras* codon 12 mutations in pancreatic carcinomas of different geographical origin [21–25]. Controversial data exist on the role of c-Ki-*ras* point mutational activation in the pathogenesis of pancreatic carcinoma. Three studies [21, 23, 26] addressed the question of whether this genetic defect was harbored by most cancer cells or was confined only to a small proportion of the neoplastic population, coming to divergent conclusions. Scarpa et al. [17] compared the densitometric intensities of the SSCP-shifted bands with those of the wild-type bands. In most cases, the relative intensity of the mutated versus the non-mutated bands corresponded to the proportion of cancer cells in the sample, as evaluated on hematoxylin-eosin stained sections before DNA extraction. The high frequency of c-Ki-*ras* mutations and the evidence of their presence in the majority of cancer cells strongly suggest an essential role of c-Ki-*ras* activation in the pathogenesis of pancreatic cancer, regardless of race and geography (Table 7).

Remarkable differences, however, become evident when comparing the patterns of mutations in

Table 7. Frequency of c-Ki-*ras* mutations in different countries.

Country	Positive samples tested	%	Reference
Netherlands	28/30	93	Smit et al. [23]
Austria	47/63	75	Grünewald et al. [24]
Japan	121/135	90	Nagata et al. [21]; Mariyama et al. [22]; Motojima et al. [15]
Italy	16/17	94	Scarpa et al. [16][a]

[a] Study by Scarpa et al. includes 17 Italian cases and 14 Japanese cases

Table 8. Geographic differences in the pattern of Ki-*ras* mutations.

	Netherlands No. (%)	Italy No. (%)	Austria No. (%)	Japan No. (%)
Asp	9 (32.1)	8 (50)	18 (38.3)	76 (62.8)
Val	8 (28.6)	8 (50)	14 (29.8)	33 (27.3)
Arg	1 (3.6)	—	14 (29.8)	11 (9.1)
Cys	10 (35.7)	—	—	1 (0.8)
Ala	—	—	1 (2.1)	—

cancers of different countries (Table 8). Asp and val mutations were observed in two Italian cases. In cancers from two other European countries, a third type of mutation was detected: arg in Austrian [25] and cys in Dutch [24] cases. The two mutations found in Italian cancers each accounted for 50% of the cases, whereas in the Austrian and Dutch cancers each of the three mutations were present in one-third of the cases. Differences are also shown in the patterns of mutations in Japanese cases. Asp, val, and arg mutations occurred in 67%, 26%, and 7% of cases, respectively [16, 22, 23]. The geographic differences in the c-Ki-*ras* mutational patterns suggest that different environmental and/or genetic factors may be involved in the pathogenesis of pancreatic cancer in diverse countries.

Also in the study of Scarpa et al. [17], no statistically significant correlation was found between c-Ki-*ras* mutations and morphology of cancer, stage, or survival. This suggests that the *ras* mutation is an early event in the genesis of this cancer. If any correlation exists between gene abnormalities and stage or prognosis, this should be searched for in genetic changes, other than c-Ki-*ras* mutations, occurring at a later stage during cancer progression.

The same panel of cancers was also examined by Scarpa et al. [17] for c-Ki-*ras* mutation, p53 gene mutations, and p53 protein nuclear accumulation. SSCP and direct sequencing were used to detect mutations. p53 Protein expression was immunohistochemically evaluated using monoclonal antibody PAb1801 [27].

Fourteen cases, which also harbored a c-Ki-*ras* mutation, showed p53 gene mutations (Table 9) as well. There were missense point mutations in 11 cases and frame-shift mutations in the remaining 3. The overall frequency of p53 immunohistochemically positive cancer samples was 61.8%. In immunohistochemical-positive cases, the number of positive cells varied between 5% and 80% of the neoplastic cells.

Gene and/or protein abnormalities were detected in more than 75% of cases, with 50% of concordant results (Table 10). In the p53-mutated cases, the lack of p53 protein accumulation might reflect a specific effect of the particular mutation failing to stabilize the protein or could be due to a transcriptional or post-transcriptional defect. In most of the immunohistochemical-positive cases in which no mutation was detected, only a minority of cancer cells showed p53 protein accumulation. The most likely explanation for such a phenomenon is that the mutated cancer cells are not sufficiently represented to be detected by genetic methods. This interpretation would support the hypothesis that p53 mutations may occur in some neoplastic cells which give origin to a new clone that may eventually replace the initial one.

The data suggest that p53 mutation is one of the genetic defects, occurring at variable stages of tumor development and progression, that may have a significant role in the pathogenesis of a proportion of pancreatic cancers. It may be an early event as suggested by the occurrence of pancreatic cancers in subjects harboring a germ line mutation of p53 gene [28] and by the demonstration of immunohistochemical positivity in neoplastic cells of intraductal component of pancreatic cancer [12]. It may also be an event occurring at a later stage of tumor growth, subsequent to *ras* mutation, as suggested by the finding of only a few cells with p53 nuclear accumulation in advanced cancers.

The study of p53 mutations in different cancers has shown that their nature and site differ depending on the tumor type and has provided information on the exogenous or endogenous origin of the mutation [29]. Remarkable features of p53 gene mutations in primary pancreatic cancer are the

Table 9. Mutations of the p53 gene in pancreatic adenocarcinomas.

Case	Exon	Codon	Sequence mutation	Protein mutation
Italian				
1	5	132	A*A*G → A*G*G	Lys → Arg
4	5	152	CCG → del CC	Frameshift
5	7	249	*A*GG → *G*GG	Arg → Gly
11	7	243–245	Complex[a]	Frame-shift
17	5	175	C*G*C → C*A*C	Arg → His
19	8	295	CCT → del CC	Frame-shift
20	7	258	*G*AA → *A*AA	Glu → Lys
21	5	177	C*C*C → C*G*C	Pro → Arg
Japanese				
J1	6	215	*A*GT → *C*GT	Ser → Arg
J2	5	175	C*G*C → C*A*C	Arg → His
J3	5	173	*G*TG → *A*TG	Val → Met
J9	8	272	*G*TG → *A*TG	Val → Met
J10	7	245	G*G*C → G*A*C	Gly → Asp
J14	5	139	A*A*G → A*C*G	Lys → Thr

[a] Insertion of G and duplication of codons 243 and 244

Table 10. Comparison of immunohistochemical expression of p53 and p53 gene mutations in pancreatic adenocarcinoma.

		Protein detection		
		+	−	Total
Gene	+	9	5	14
Mutation	−	9	8	17
Total		18	13	31

following: (1) 70% of alterations affect G:C sites, (2) transitions represent the large majority of missense point mutations with only a small proportion occurring at CpG sites, and (3) frame-shift mutations seem to occur with a higher frequency than in any other cancer [18]. This mutational pattern suggests that p53 gene alterations in pancreatic cancer are most likely due to spontaneous errors during DNA replication rather than to specific carcinogens.

There seems to be no relevant difference between p53 mutations of Italian and Japanese cancers. However, the mutational spectrum of p53 gene in pancreatic cancer is of greater interest than that of the c-Ki-*ras* gene because mutations of the c-Ki-*ras* gene in cancer are essentially restricted to one codon, whereas those altering the function of the p53 gene are distributed throughout a significant region of the coding sequence.

No statistically significant association between p53 alterations and morphology, clinicopathologic characteristics or outcome of the disease have been found [17]. However, studies on a larger population are needed for clarification.

Future Perspective

It seems likely that investigation of the molecular pathology of pancreatic cancer will yield new insight into the basic biology of this tumor and will help to develop new pathological markers. The diagnostic and therapeutic utility of these molecular targets are now being explored in a variety of ways by pathologists and clinicians concerned with pancreatic cancer. Key events in early ductal tumorigenesis are activation of c-Ki-*ras* and inactivation of p53 by point mutations. Detection of c-Ki-*ras* mutations and abnormal levels of p53 protein are particularly attractive markers for use by molecular pathologists to augment careful morphologic diagnosis of neoplasia. Already it is evident that some less common types of exocrine tumors differ from the typical ductal adenocarcinoma at the frequency at which they show such point mutations, and other markers are under investigation. Assessment of such genetic changes in patients in clinical trials may define their utility for prognosis and prediction of treatment response. Some oncogene abnormalities are now targets for the design of novel forms of therapy. Immunotherapies aimed at the ERBB2 receptor are already being evaluated in clinical trials and other types of therapy will surely follow.

The study of p53 mutations, even if insufficient to draw definite conclusions, has also given an idea that they might correlate with metastatic potential and survival. An example of the possible use of gene alterations as a diagnostic aid is the proposed use of *ras* mutation in the differential diagnosis between pancreatic neoplasia and reactive processes on fine needle aspiration cytology [30].

References

1. Marx J (1989) Research news: Many gene changes found in cancer. Science 246:1386–1388
2. Lemoine NR, Hall PA (1990) Oncogenes and growth factors in pancreatic cancer. Bailliere's Clin Gastroenterol 4:815–832
3. Lemoine NR, Hughes CM, Barton CM (1992) The epidermal growth factor receptor in human pancreatic cancer. J Pathol 166:7–12
4. Barton CM, Hall PA, Hughes CM, Gullick WJ, Lemoine NR (1991) Transforming growth factor alpha and epidermal growth factor in human pancreatic cancer. J Pathol 163:111–116
5. Glinsmann-Gibson BJ, Korc M (1991) Regulation of transforming growth factor alpha mRNA expression in T3M4 human pancreatic carcinoma cells. Pancreas 6:142–149
6. Henry JA, Bennett MK, Piggott NH, Levett DL, May FEB, Westley BR (1991) Expression of the pNR-2/pS2 protein in diverse human epithelial tumors. Br J Cancer 64:677–682
7. Welter C, Theisinger B, Seitz G (1992) Association of the human spasmolytic polypeptide and an estrogen-induced breast cancer protein (pS2) with human pancreatic carcinoma. Lab Invest 66:187–192
8. Williams TM, Weiner DB, Greene MI, Maguire HC (1991) Expression of c-*erb*B-2 in human pancreatic adenocarcinomas. Pathobiol 59:46–52
9. Lemoine NR, Lobresco M, Leung HY, Barton CM, Prigent SA, Gullick WJ, Klöppel G (1992) The ERBB3 proto-oncogene in human pancreatic cancer. J Pathol 168:269–273
10. Ding SF, Habib NA, Delhanty JDA (1992) Loss of heterozygosity on chromosomes 1 and 11 in carcinoma of the pancreas. Br J Cancer 65:809–812
11. Neuman WL, Wasylyshyn ML, Jacoby R (1991) Evidence for a common molecular pathogenesis in colorectal, gastric, and pancreatic cancer. Genes, Chromosomes Cancer 3:468–473
12. Barton CM, Staddon SL, Hughes CM (1991) Abnormalities of the p53 tumor suppressor gene in human pancreatic cancer. Br J Cancer 64: 1076–1082
13. Hall PA, Ray A, Lemoine NR, Midgley CM, Krausz T, Lane DP (1991) Diagnostic utility of p53 immunostaining in cytopathology. Lancet 338:513
14. Lemoine NR, Jain S, Hughes CM, Staddon SL, Maillet B, Hall PA, Klöppel G (1992) Ki-*ras* oncogene activation in pre-invasive pancreatic cancer. Gastroenterology 101:230–236
15. Motojima K, Tsunoda T, Kanematsu T, Nagata Y, Urano T, Shiku H (1991) Distinguishing pancreatic carcinoma from other periampullary carcinomas by analysis of mutations in the Kirsten-*ras* oncogene. Ann Surg 214:657–662
16. Motojima K, Urano T, Nagata Y, Shiku H, Tsunoda T, Kanematsu T (1991) Mutations in the Kirsten-*ras* oncogene are common but lack correlation with prognosis and tumor stage in human pancreatic carcinoma. Am J Gastroenterol 86:1784–1788
17. Scarpa A, Capelli P, Mukai K, Zamboni G, Oda T, Lacono C, Hirohashi S (1993) Pancreatic adenocarcinomas frequently show p53 gene mutations. Am J Pathol 142:1534–1543
18. Hollstein M, Sidransky D, Vogelstein B, Harris CC (1991) p53 Mutations in human cancers. Science 253:49–53
19. Orita M, Suzuki Y, Sekiya T, Hayashi K (1989) Rapid and sensitive detection of point mutations and DNA polymorphisms using the polymerase chain reaction. Genomics 5:874–879
20. Suzuki Y, Sekiya T, Hayashi K (1991) Allele-specific polymerase chain reaction: A method for amplification and sequence determination of a single component among a mixture of sequence variants. Anal Biochem 192:82–84
21. Almoguera C, Shibata D, Forrester K, Martin J, Arnheim N, Perucho M (1988) Most human carcinomas of the exocrine pancreas contain mutant c-K-*ras* genes. Cell 53:549–554
22. Nagata Y, Abe M, Motoshima K, Nakayama E, Shiku H (1990) Frequent glycine-to-aspartic acid mutations at codon 12 of c-Ki-*ras* gene in human pancreatic cancer (in Japanese). Jpn J Cancer Res 81:135–140
23. Mariyama M, Kishi K, Nakamura K, Obata H, Nishimura S (1989) Frequency and types of point mutation at the 12th codon of the c-Ki-*ras* gene found in pancreatic cancers from Japanese patients. Jpn J Cancer Res 80:622–626
24. Smit VTHBM, Boot AJM, Smits AMM, Fleuren GJ, Cornelisse CJ, Bos JL (1988) K-*ras* codon 12

mutations occur very frequently in pancreatic adenocarcinomas. Nucleic Acids Res 16:7773–7782
25. Grünewald K, Lyons J, Frehlich A, Feichtinger H, Weger RA, Schwab G, Janssen JWG, Bartram CR (1989) High frequency of Ki-*ras* codon 12 mutations in pancreatic adenocarcinomas. Int J Cancer 43: 1037–1041
26. Gonzales-Cadavid NF, Zhou D, Battifora H, Bar-Eli M, Cline MJ (1989) Direct sequencing analysis of exon 1 of the c-Ki-*ras* gene shows a low frequency of mutations in human pancreatic carcinomas. Oncogene 4:1137–1140
27. Banks L, Matlashewski G, Crawford L (1986) Isolation of human p53 monoclonal antibodies and their use in the studies of human p53 expression. Eur J Biochem 159:529–534
28. Malkin D, Li FP, Strong LC, Fraumeni JF, Nelson CE, Kim DH, Kassel J, Gryka MA, Bischoff FZ, Tainsky MA, Friend SH (1990) Germ line p53 mutations in familial syndrome of breast cancer, sarcomas, and other neoplasms. Science 250:1233–1238
29. Vogelstein B, Kinzler KW (1992) Carcinogens leave fingerprints. Nature 355:209–210
30. Shibata D, Almoguera C, Forrester K, Dunitz J, Martin SE, Cosgrove MM, Perucho M, Arnheim N (1990) Detection of c-K-*ras* mutations in fine needle aspirates from human pancreatic adenocarcinomas. Cancer Res 50:1279–1283

Sampling Method for Pancreatic Tissue Examination

Tissue Sampling for Adequate Typing and Staining

The accurate diagnosis and staging of pancreatic cancer require careful examination and sampling of tissue. Although several methods can be used for tissue sampling, it is advisable to use a standard, internationally accepted method that should be simple but adequate to obtain the most possible information for assessment of curative value and prognosis and for statistical evaluation. We introduce the gross sampling method for pancreatic tissue examination, according to the general rules adopted by the Committee of the Pancreatic Society of Japan [1].

Adequate examination of the pancreas requires knowledge of the anatomical relationship between the common bile duct, pancreatic duct, and papilla of Vater. Because of the higher pancreatic cancer incidence in the pancreas head, most surgical specimens include part of the common ducts and papilla of Vater. However, this anatomical relationship is sometimes complicated and makes it difficult to establish a procedure for tissue examination which is both universal and comprehensive.

The requirements for adequate examination include:

1. The whole pancreas (or resected specimen) should be available for gross examination.
2. Tumor cross sections should be obtained for histopathological evaluation.
3. Regional lymph nodes should be available for study.

   Every pancreatic specimen should be examined grossly in the following order:

a. Determine the metastases or invasion of the surrounding tissue.
b. Describe the surface appearance of the tumor (Table 1).
c. Measure the external size of the specimen.
d. If lymph nodes are attached to the specimen, identify them individually and mark them according to the anatomic-topographic classification (see Chapter "Gross Anatomy of the Pancreas" in this volume). In situ specimen (autopsy) or pancreaticoduodenectomized specimen should be sectioned as follows (Fig. 1):
i. Open the stomach along the greater curvature.
ii. Open the duodenum at the opposite side of the papilla of Vater. Examine the mucosa of the duodenum and the papilla of Vater.
iii. If necessary, open the duodenum of the dorsal side of the pancreas and examine the intrapancreatic bile duct by a tube sonde.
iv. Pin the margins of the opened stomach, duodenum, and gallbladder with the mucosal surface up, as well as the pancreas, on a cork board with stainless steel needles.
v. Slice the pancreas from the papilla of Vater to the end of the specimen serially at 3–5 mm intervals vertically. Cut line number 0 is on the papilla of Vater. In pancreaticoduodenectomized specimen, the cut line should be parallel to Kerckring folds (Fig. 2). Marginal resection of the duodenum (A line in Fig. 2) can be made to examine tumor invasion.

For body and tail resection, the specimen should be cut at right angles longitudinal to the pancreas.

For total pancreatectomy or autopsy, both of

Table 1. Surface appearance of tumors.

Types of surface of the tumors
Masked
Tumor forming
Sclerosing
Miscellaneous
Extra pancreatic tumor formation
Multinodular
Cystic
Types of cut surface of the tumors
Nodular
Infiltrative
Mixed

the above procedures should be used (Fig. 3).

vi. Examine and describe the appearance of the cut surface of the tumor according to established criteria (Table 1).

vii. Immerse the tissue fixation board in a tank containing buffered 10% formalin or Bouin's solution for 24 h. A longer fixation time should be avoided.

Figure 4 demonstrates the cut surface of the pancreas head. In these sections, the relationship between the papilla of Vater, common bile duct, and pancreatic duct is shown.

Handling of Specimens

To prevent postmortem autolysis, both autopsy and fixation of tissues should be done as soon as possible if specimens for cytology or biochemical and electron microscopic examinations are not considered. The injection of formalin solution from the papilla of Vater into the pancreatic duct provides excellent preservation of the pancreatic duct system. It can prevent damage to the epithelium and also prevent tumor cell exfoliation. It is especially useful in cases which require a meticulous histological examination. However, care should be taken not to inject the fixatives with force and high pressure, which may damage the ductal walls and wash away tumor cells.

These procedures are also applicable to surgical specimens which are prone to autolysis. Because of the presence of tumors and possible preneoplastic lesions in surgical specimens and because difficulties arise in differentiating nuclear atypism in postsurgical autolytic changes from that in cancer, surgical tissues must be properly handled and fixed as described above.

Tissue Sampling for Refined Morphological and Molecular Biological Studies

In addition to routine histological evaluation of pancreatic cancer, many new technologies are now available for detailed investigation of morphology, phenotypes and genetic alterations of pancreatic cancer.

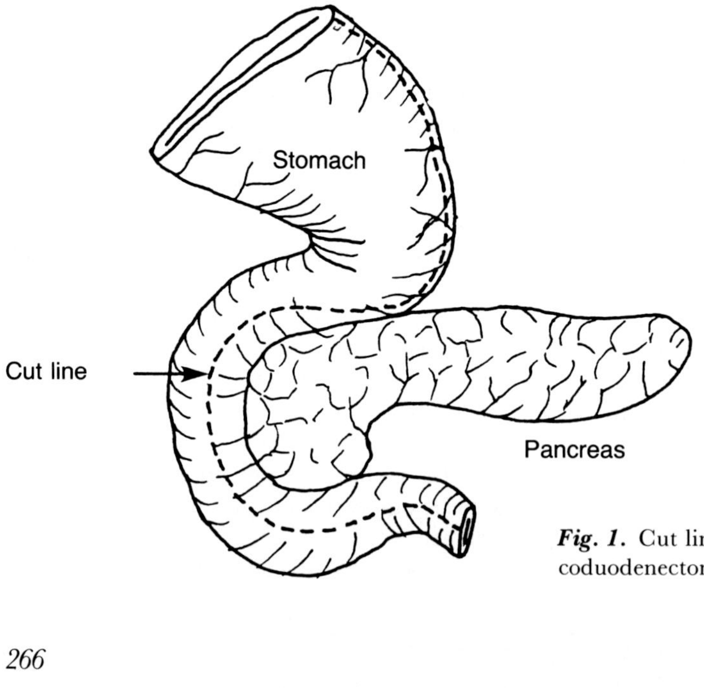

Fig. 1. Cut line along the gastroduodenal tract in pancreaticoduodenectomized specimen

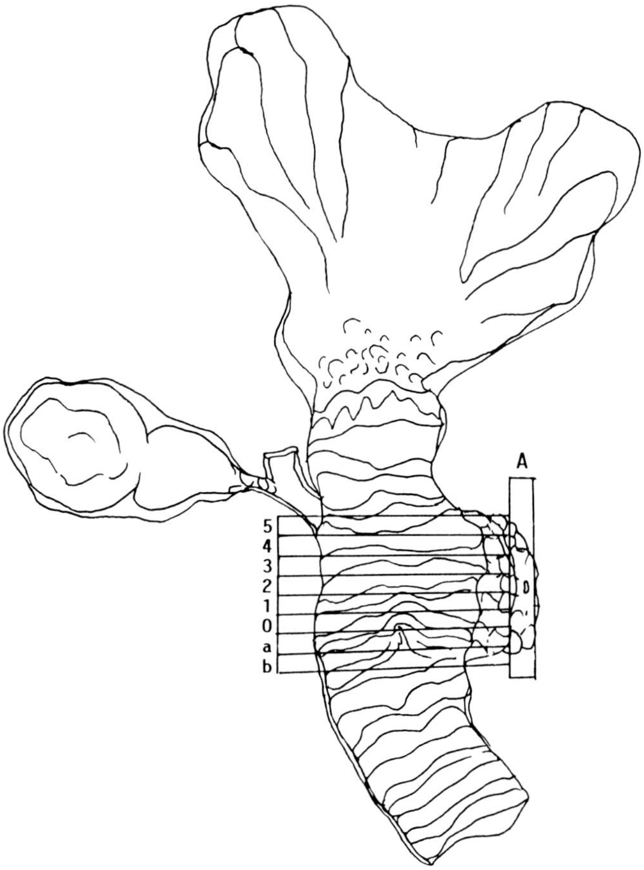

Fig. 2. Cut lines along the Kerckring folds

Flow Cytometry

Flow cytometry has been used extensively for analysis of nuclear DNA contents. DNA histograms demonstrate the presence of aneuploid peak(s) or the percentage of cells in S-phase. In addition, phenotypes of cells can be analyzed using immunofluorescent staining. The advantage of flow cytometry is that a large number of cells can be analyzed in a short period. For DNA analysis, the tissue may be stored frozen and the nuclei can be extracted from the frozen tissue and stained by DNA-specific fluorescent dyes. On the other hand, the cells for phenotypic analysis must be extracted from fresh tissue and fixed intact before being stored as a cell suspension. Ethanol is usually used for fixation.

Immunohistochemistry

Immunohistochemistry has been utilized extensively to localize various antigens in tissue sections and has made it possible to investigate phenotypic expression of normal and neoplastic cells. Initially, immunohistochemistry was used to analyze functional aspects of endocrine tumors; however, with an increasing number of available antibodies, it has been applied not only to research but also to diagnostic histopathology. Depending on the nature of antibody labelling, several methods have

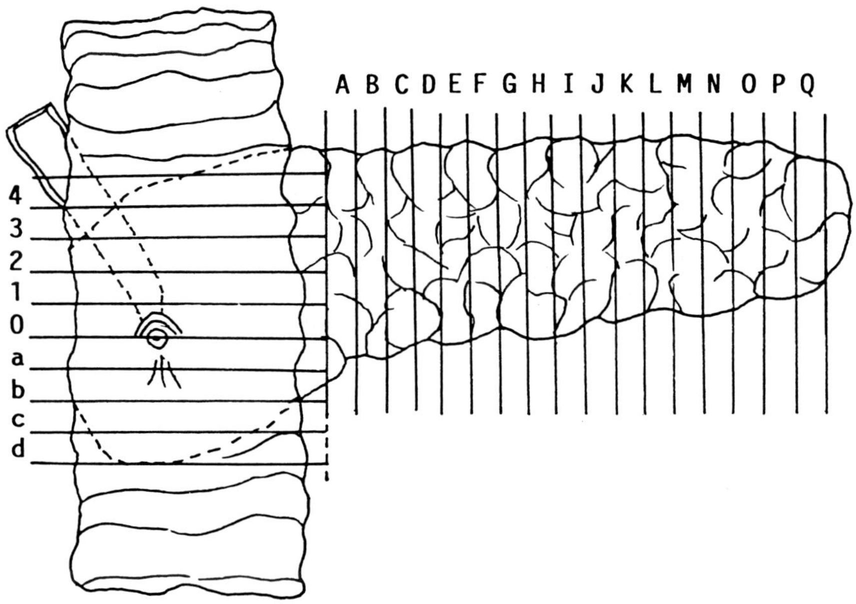

Fig. 3. Cut lines through the duodenum (*left*) and pancreas (*lines A through Q*)

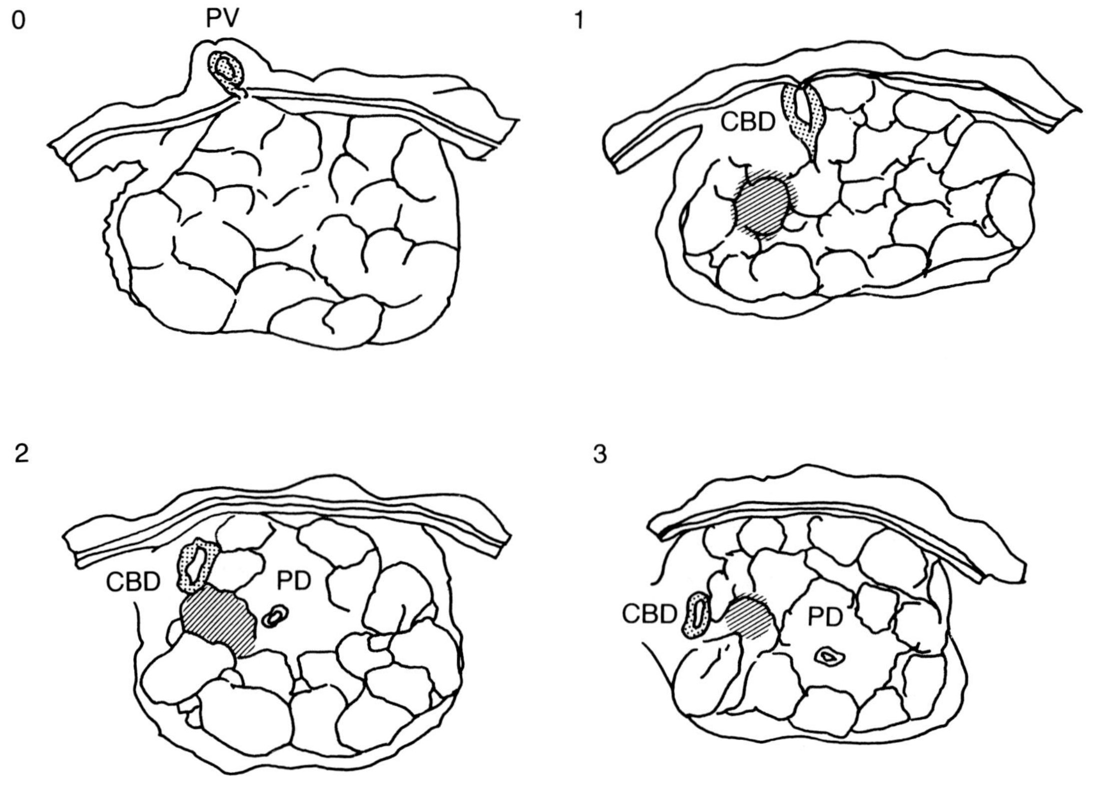

Fig. 4. Location of papilla of Vater (*PV*), common bile duct (*CBD*), pancreatic duct (*PD*), and tumor (*hatched area*) in vertical sections of the pancreas head

been developed. The most common are the immunofluorescent and immunoenzyme methods. The colloidal gold method has been used mostly for electron microscopic immunohistochemistry. The following description concentrates on the immunoperoxidase method.

Although many antigens can be detected in formalin-fixed tissue by the immunoperoxidase method, formalin is not the best choice of fixatives. To preserve the maximum immunoreactivity of antigens, it is necessary to freeze tissue without delay at the time of resection or biopsy for prevention of autolytic change and diffusion of antigens from the original location. After frozen sections are cut, they may be fixed in cold acetone for 10–15 min to prevent antigen diffusion in unfixed sections.

It is recommended to freeze tissues in an embedding medium for frozen section, such as OCT compound (Miles, Elkhart, Ind.), and dip it into acetone-dry ice or ethanol-dry ice. If the frozen tissue is stored at −80°C before use, it can be stored for at least 2–3 months. Such frozen tissue can be used for other purposes such as DNA extraction without any complications.

Although fresh frozen tissue gives maximum antigen preservation, the morphology is usually poor. While several fixation methods have been developed for better preservation of antigens and morphology, none of them are universally useful for the simultaneous preservation of antigens and morphology. The most widely used fixatives for immunohistochemistry are paraformaldehyde and periodate-lysine-paraformaldehyde (PLP). Paraformaldehyde is preferred for fixation of protein antigens and PLP for glycoprotein antigens. For peptide antigens, Zamboni's fixative may also be used. Tissue fixed in Zamboni's fixative (Table 2) can be used for immunoelectron microscopy.

Tissue Fixation Procedures and Preparation of Frozen Sections for Immunohistochemistry

Paraformaldehyde is usually used as a 2%–4% solution in phosphate buffer (pH 7.4). Sucrose may

Table 2. Fixatives for immunohistochemistry.

PLP (Periodate-lysine-paraformaldehyde) fixative

Stock A = 0.1 M lysine, 0.05 M sodium phosphate, pH 7.4

1. Dissolve 1.827 g L-lysine HCl in 50 ml dH_2O.
2. Adjust pH to 7.4 with 0.1 M Na_2HPO_4.
3. Make up to 100 ml with 0.1 M sodium phosphate buffer, pH 7.4.
4. Store at 4°C for a maximum of 10 days.

Stock B = 8% paraformaldehyde

1. Mix 8 g paraformaldehyde in 100 ml dH_2O.
2. Heat to 60°C with stirring.
3. Slowly add 1 to 3 drops of 1 N NaOH until the solution becomes clear.
4. Filter.

Just before use, combine three parts A with one part B and add sodium m-periodate to 0.01 M (21.4 mg $NaIO_4$/10 ml). The final composition is 0.01 M $NaIO_4$, 0.075 M lysine, 0.0375 M sodium phosphate buffer, and 2% paraformaldehyde. Some researchers prefer to increase the concentration of paraformaldehyde to 4%.

Zamboni's fixative

Solution A = saturated picric acid solution

1. Dissolve at least 2.1 g of picric acid in 150 ml 100 ml dH_2O.
2. Filter through two layers of filter paper.

Solution B = 20% paraform aldehyde

1. Dissolve 20 g paraform aldehyde in dH_2O.
2. Heat to 60°C with stirring.
3. Add 1–3 drops of 2.52% NaOH until the solution becomes clear.

Working solution

1. Mix solutions A and B.
2. Make up to 1 L with 320 mOsM sodium phosphate buffer (3.31 g $NaH_2PO_4 \cdot 2H_2O$ and 33.7 g $Na_2HPO_4 \cdot 12H_2O$ in 1 L of dH_2O).

The working solution can be stored for 12 months.

be added at concentration of 8%–10%. The role of sucrose is not clear, but it seems likely that hypertonic solutions may extract water from cell organelles and prevents diffusion of antigens. PLP and Zamboni's fixative are prepared according to the recipe in Table 2. Fixation time is usually 4–6 h at 4°C. After fixation, the fixative has to be washed out. This is achieved by washing tissue in phosphate buffered saline (PBS) with increasing concentrations of sucrose from 10% to 15% to 20%. The tissue remains in each solution for at least 4 h. It is desirable to agitate the solutions gently. At the end, the tissue is immersed in PBS with 20% sucrose and 10% glycerol for 1 h. Glycerol is added as a cryopreservative which prevents ice crystal formation when the tissue is frozen. After rinsing in PBS with sucrose and glycerol, the tissue is snap frozen in acetone-dry ice or ethanol-dry ice, and frozen sections for immunohistochemistry can then be cut on a cryostat.

Electron Microscopy

For routine transmission electron microscopy, fixation by glutaraldehyde followed by osmium tetrachloride has been used. Because this method is well established and is described in ordinary textbooks, it is not discussed here in detail.

One word of caution is due. It is always necessary to fix tissue immediately after resection. A substantial delay between resection and fixation will introduce autolytic change and morphological details will degenerate. In addition, the tissue sections have to be cut by a sharp razor knife to avoid using too much force as this may crush subcellular structures.

Immunoelectron Microscopy

For immunoelectron microscopy, two methods are usually used: Pre-embedding and post-embedding. Pre-embedding correctly implies that immunostaining of tissue is performed before embedding in Epon. This is usually achieved by immunostaining of a thick frozen section of PLP-fixed tissue. Fixation and preparation of frozen sections are achieved in the same way as for light microscopic immunohistochemistry. After immunostaining, the tissue is embedded in Epon by the inverted gelatin capsule method.

Post-embedding uses ultra-thin sections for immunostaining. Prior to staining, the sections are treated by ethanol saturated with NaOH to remove epoxy resin. The tissue for postembedding staining may be fixed in glutaraldehyde and postfixed in Osmium, as for routine transmission electron microscopy.

Enzyme Histochemistry

Because of the characteristics unique to the preservation of enzyme activity and morphology, accomplishing both at the same time is quite difficult and usually the method selected depends on which is more important. For the maximum preservation of enzyme activity, fresh frozen tissue has to be used. However, prolonged incubation with substrate sometimes causes diffusion of enzymes and may result in false localization. Various fixatives have been used for enzyme histochemistry; however, no single fixative gives satisfactory results for all enzymes. Fixatives and fixation conditions, especially fixation time and temperature, have to be determined according to each particular enzyme under study. Common fixatives include acetone, formalin, glutaraldehyde, and acrolein. Ultrastructural enzyme histochemistry has been achieved using tissues fixed in glutaraldehyde or in a mixture of glutaraldehyde and acrolein. Information regarding the best fixation method for each enzyme may be obtained from standard textbooks of histochemistry, such as *Histochemistry* by A.G.E. Pearse [2].

Molecular Biological Method

Recently, advances in molecular biological techniques have been rapid. It has become possible to analyze a single base substitution of genetic materials. With improved techniques, genotyping of neoplasms will become a routine procedure to investigate their biological characteristics. Because of this trend, it becomes increasingly important to store fresh frozen tissue for future studies. The tissue frozen for immunohistochemistry or enzyme histochemistry may be stored again for additional studies. It should be noted that fixatives such as Bouin's degrade DNA more than formalin, yielding specimens less suitable for PCR.

Newer Approach

Since pathological diagnosis is made by observing hematoxylin and eosin sections of formalin-fixed tissue, it would be very useful if paraffin-embedded material can be used for molecular biological analysis. This would make it possible to directly investigate correlations between genetic change and morphological characteristics. Unfortunately, this is not the case. Although DNA can be extracted from formalin-fixed paraffin-embedded tissue, DNA from such samples is hydrolyzed extensively, and high molecular weight DNA necessary for Southern blot analysis cannot be obtained. In addition, application of DNA extracted from formalin-fixed tissue has only a limited use for molecular analysis. It has been shown that detection of gene amplification using dot or slot blot analysis may be performed using low molecular weight DNA obtained from formalin-fixed tissue. Polymerase chain reaction (PCR) can be done using low-molecular weight DNA as a template. Well preserved RNA and proteins necessary for Northern blot or immunoblot analysis cannot be obtained from formalin-fixed paraffin-embedded tissue.

Recently, several attempts have been made to circumvent some of the problems associated with formalin-fixation. DNA suitable for Southern blot analysis may be obtained from formalin-fixed paraffin embedded tissue after extensive digestion by proteinase K. However, the mobility of restriction fragments of DNA from such material is not necessarily identical to those obtained from fresh frozen tissue.

It has been reported that tissue fixed in acetone and embedded in paraffin (AMeX method, Table 3) is superior in preservation of antigens, proteins, DNA, and RNA [3–5]. This method was first developed to allow preservation of morphology and antigens for immunohistochemical staining at the same time. In tissues fixed by this method, preservation of morphological details is much better than in frozen sections, and is sometimes comparable to routine hematoxylin and eosin sections. Moreover, many antigens which cannot be demonstrated in formalin-fixed tissue maintain their

Table 3. AMeX (*A*cetone *Me*thyl benzoate *X*ylene) method.

1. Immerse tissue slice (less than 3 mm thick) in acetone (−20°C) overnight.
2. Dehydrate tissue in acetone for 15 min at 4°C then another 15 min at room temperature.
3. Clear tissue twice in methyl benzoate for 15 min each then twice in xylene for 15 min each at room temperature.
4. Penetrate tissue with paraffin (melting point 58–60°C) at 60°C in vacuum evaporating embedder (2 h).
5. Embed tissue in paraffin block.

Immunohistochemical staining can be performed after deparaffinization in xylene followed by rinse in acetone and hydration in PBS. DNA, RNA, and protein can be extracted in a similar way for fresh tissue after the sections or tissues are deparaffinized.

immunoreactivity and can be detected by immunohistochemistry. Further studies demonstrated that Southern and immunoblot analyses can be performed using DNA and proteins extracted from such tissue with identical results to those obtained with frozen tissues. RNA is somewhat degraded and Northern blot analysis is difficult; however, expression of genes can be studied by dot or slot blot analysis.

Tissue fixed by the AMeX method can be used for PCR and in situ hybridization without much difficulty. This methods provides a way to investigate direct correlation between morphological difference and genotypic/phenotypic changes. If it is necessary, certain area of a tumor may be cut out from the paraffin block and used for genetic analysis. This method is extremely useful for investigation of tumors with morphological heterogeneity and also small tumors which cannot be divided for various research purposes.

Figure 5 summarizes the possibilities for tissue preparation for investigative purposes.

Intraoperative Tissue Sampling for Diagnosis of Pancreatic Cancer

Intraoperative differential diagnosis between pancreatic carcinoma and chronic pancreatitis is difficult, as both diseases may show markedly similar clinical features, including the presence of greyish and dense fibrotic mass. Intraoperative histodiagnosis of frozen sections has been employed to establish definitive diagnosis and determine subsequent operative procedures. However, until recently intraoperative histodiagnosis yielded a low rate of accurate diagnoses (Table 4) [6–16]. On the other hand, the rate of false positives for pancreatectomies based on gross findings at operation without biopsy was less and ranged between 2%–18% [12, 17, 18]. For this reason, some authors [19] recommended that operative decision be based not on biopsy but on gross findings. However, it should be noted that the low rate of accurate diagnosis for intraoperative histodiagnosis was due mainly to sampling error (surgeon's error). Lee [18] reported

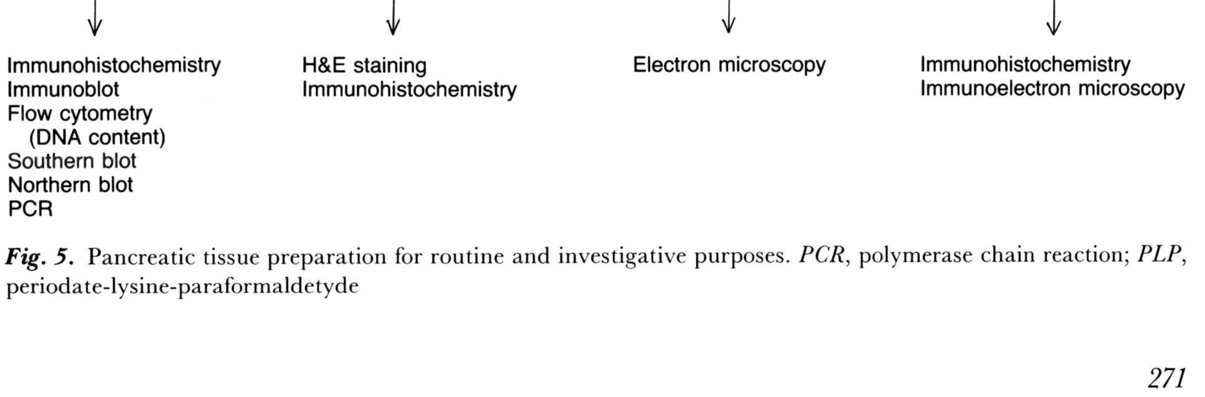

Fig. 5. Pancreatic tissue preparation for routine and investigative purposes. *PCR*, polymerase chain reaction; *PLP*, periodate-lysine-paraformaldetyde

Table 4. Diagnostic accuracy and complication rates for pancreatic biopsy (histodiagnosis by frozen section).

Author			Sensitivity rate[a]	Specificity rate[b]	Complication rate
Wedge biopsy					
Bowden	(1954)	[6]	71%		
Spjut and Rama	(1957)	[7]	88%	100%	4%
Cote et al.	(1959)	[8]	46%	100%	
Williams et al.	(1960)	[9]	92%		8%
Akashi	(1976)	[10]	65%	100%	0%
Core needle aspiration biopsy					
Cote et al.	(1959)	[8]	68%	100%	
Williams et al.	(1960)	[9]	67%		16%
Arnesjo et al.	(1972)	[11]	70%		
Akashi	(1976)	[10]	96%	97%	0%
Wedge/Core needle aspiration					
Winegarner et al.	(1966)	[12]	85%**		
Forsgren et al.	(1968)	[13]	97%	89%	2%
Dencker	(1972)	[14]	93%	100%	4%
Isaacson et al.	(1974)	[15]	97%	100%	3.2%
Lightwood et al.	(1976)	[16]	83%	100%	4.7%

[a] Sensitivity rate, true positive/true positive + false negatrve
[b] Specificity rate, true negative + false positive
** Results for permanent section

a sampling error for intraoperative histodiagnosis of 33%, which was far higher than the 3% rate of misinterpretation of gross findings. In addition, the rate of discrepancy between diagnosis on frozen and permanent section was reported to be 7% [14], and 0% [16]. Some sampling techniques are associated with complications such as hemorrhage, pancreatitis, and fistula formation. The most important consideration in pancreatic biopsy is, therefore, the sampling technique. The following techniques will be discussed.

Biopsy Techniques for Cytology and Histology

Techniques for core needle biopsy by Vim-Silverman needle and wedge (scalpel) biopsy have been used. The procedures for cytology and histology are demonstrated in Fig. 6. Since the wedge biopsy technique yields a large amount of tissue, it facilitates accurate inspection, while the core needle biopsy technique sometimes fails to provide sufficient material for accurate inspection, especially if the tumor or pancreas is very fibrotic (Fig. 7). However, our review of the literature revealed no substantial difference between the two techniques in the rate of diagnostic accuracy; sensitivity rate and specificity rate were 46%–92% and 100% for wedge biopsy, and 67%–96% and 97%–100% for core needle biopsy (Table 3). More recently, investigators have recommended that wedge biopsy be used only for superficially exposed lesions and that core needle biopsy be used for deeper lesions [12–16]. When both wedge and core-needle biopsies were properly used as proposed by these authors, the sensitivity rate increased to 83%–97% while the specificity rate has not been substantially decreased (89%–100%, Table 3). Winegarner et al. [12] performed repeated core-needle sampling in order to obtain sufficient material for histodiagnosis. We recommend that the core-needle biopsy specimen should be examined not only histologically but also cytologically.

It is often difficult to determine whether a complication developed as a result of the biopsy itself or as a result of surgical manipulation. Reuben and Cotton [20] and Lightwood et al. [12] reported postoperative complication rates to be 7%–14% for core needle biopsy and 3% for wedge biopsy, and concluded that wedge biopsy was safer than core needle biopsy. This difference in complication

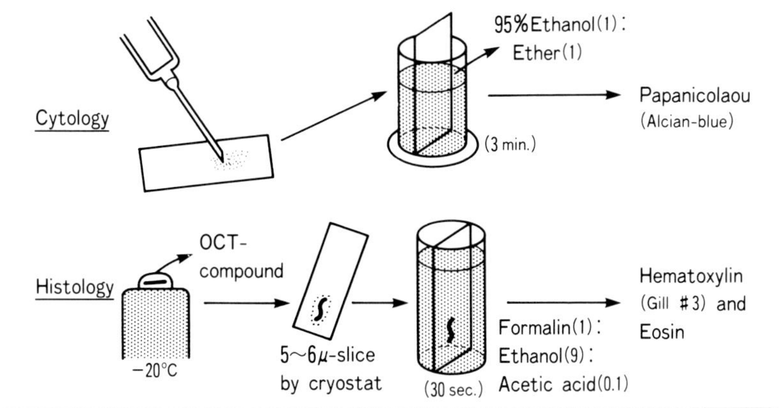

Fig. 6. Methods for cytological and histological examination of pancreatic tissue

rate for the two techniques was presumably due to the respective depths of biopsy, as described above.

Fine Needle Aspiration Cytology

Fine needle aspiration cytology as been increasingly employed since it was first introduced by Christoffersson and Poll [21]. This technique is suitable for deep seated lesions. The suspected lesion is punctured with a 21–23 gauge needle, and it should be suctioned by an attached syringe. Usually we repeat aspirations by shifting the position of the needle's tip in the tumor mass. Immediately after withdrawal of the needle, the specimen is sprayed onto a glass slide, fixed in 95% alcohol, and stained by the Papanicolaou and May-Giemsa methods (Fig. 6). It takes about 20 min to make an intraoperative diagnosis in this way.

Though this technique yields an amount of material which is too small for histodiagnosis, cytological accuracy with this technique is generally higher than histodiagnostic accuracy with the core needle biopsy technique; the sensitivity rate has been reported to be 89%–100%, and the specificity rate to be 91%–100% (Table 5). Additionally, some investigators [21–25] have found that the postoperative complication rate was very low and not serious, allowing multiple aspirations. For these reasons, the core needle biopsy technique has been superseded by fine needle aspiration cytology.

We have proposed that echo-guided acupuncture technique yields greater diagnostic accuracy [26], and high sensitivity rates for the technique of intraoperative cytodiagnosis of pancreatic juice aspirated from the main pancreatic duct. It is reasonable to assume that this technique could detect a small, non-palpable and potentially curable duct cell carcinoma of the pancreas. For such an occult cancer, we have already developed an intraoperative cytodiagnostic technique to determine both the location of the lesion and the appropriate extent of pancreatic resection [27]. Finally, the intraoperative diagnostic accuracy rate is dependent on good material obtained at surgery, skillful preparation, and highly experienced cytopathologists in the diagnosis of pancreatic carcinoma. Examples of cytological appearance of normal ductal cells and of ductal adenocarcinomas are shown in Figs. 7–10.

Single-Strand Confirmation Polymorphism (SSCP) Analysis to Detect DNA Alterations from Paraffin-Embedded Tissues

Recently, detection of DNA alterations, including point mutations associated with diseases, has been identified as important in understanding the mechanisms of their development. For preserving human and animal tissues, fixation in formalin followed by paraffin-embedding is widely used. Shibata et al. [29] reported a simple method for preparing DNA from a section of paraffin-embedded tissues for PCR. This method provides reproducible DNA from a small area of lesions from paraffin-embedded tissues (even biopsy specimen), which can be confirmed by light microscopic observation of stained

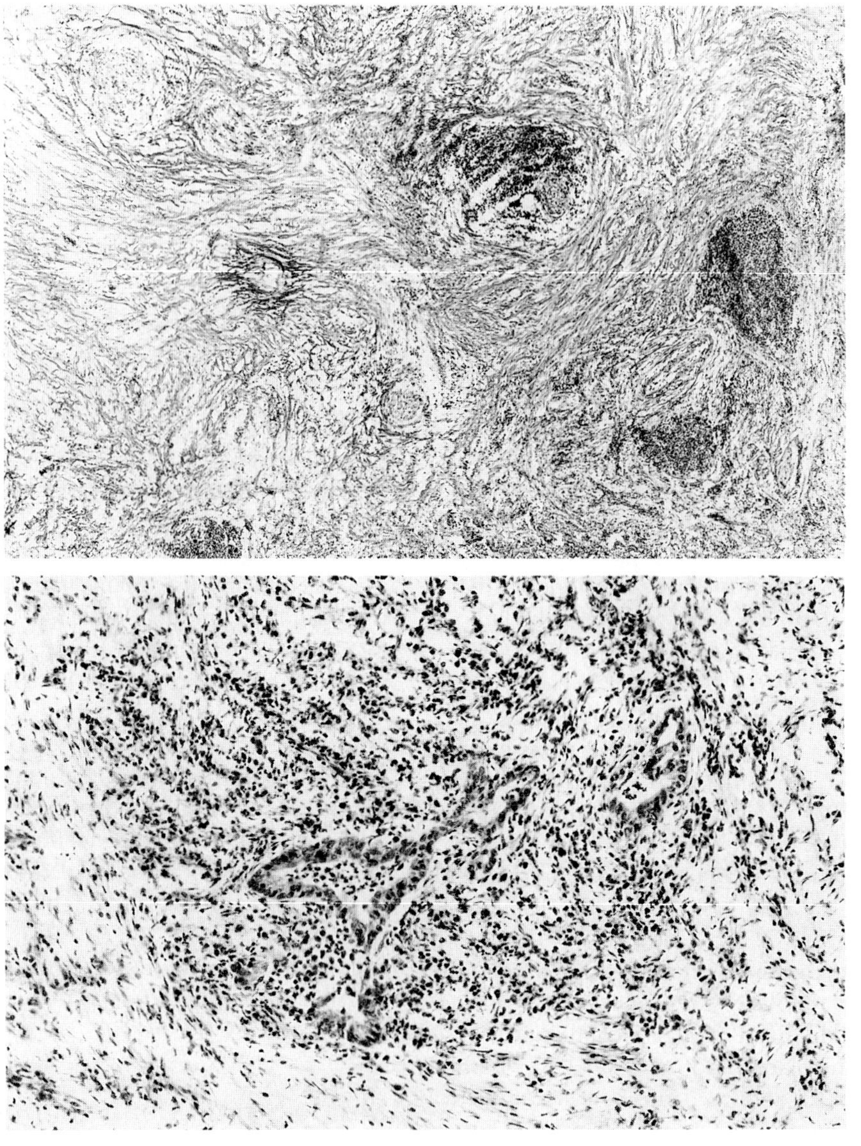

Fig. 7. ***a*** Chronic pancreatitis. In a 48-year-old male with intermittent jaundice, a hard and greyish mass was observed in the pancreas head at laparotomy. From the tumor, a frozen section specimen was obtained by wedge biopsy. Histologically, there was fibrous connective tissues with no normal or malignant pancreatic cells. ***b*** Adenocarcinoma of the pancreas. A 54-year-old female, with a long history of diabetes mellitus, complained of mild epigastralgia. Endoscopic retrograde pancreatography revealed a stenotic change in the main pancreatic duct in the head. Although there was no palpable tumor at laparotomy, a Tru-Cut needle biopsy was performed from the pancreas head. Microscopically, a few glandular structures were observed in a fibrous and inflammed stroma. The nuclei showed a wide variation in size, chromatin content, and polarity

serial sections. Orita et al. [29] have developed a rapid, sensitive method for detection of single nucleotide substitutions, namely, single-strand conformation polymorphism (SSCP) analysis of PCR products. For detection of nucleotide sequence alterations, the PCR-SSCP analysis is the method of choice because it provides a convenient tool for pathologists not only for study of DNA gene alterations in small lesions of large samples but also for diagnosis and retrospective analysis.

Table 5. Diagnostic accuracy and complication rates for fine-needle aspiration cytology

Author		Sensitivity Rate	Specificity Rate	Complication Rate
Christoffersson and Poll	(1970) [21]	100%	100%	0%
Arnesjo et al.	(1972) [11]	89%	100%	0%
Forsgren and Orell	(1973) [22]	100%	91%	0%
Kline and Neal	(1975) [23]	89%	100%	0%
Schorey	(1975) [24]	100%	100%	0%
Bodner et al.	(1982) [25]	92%	100%	

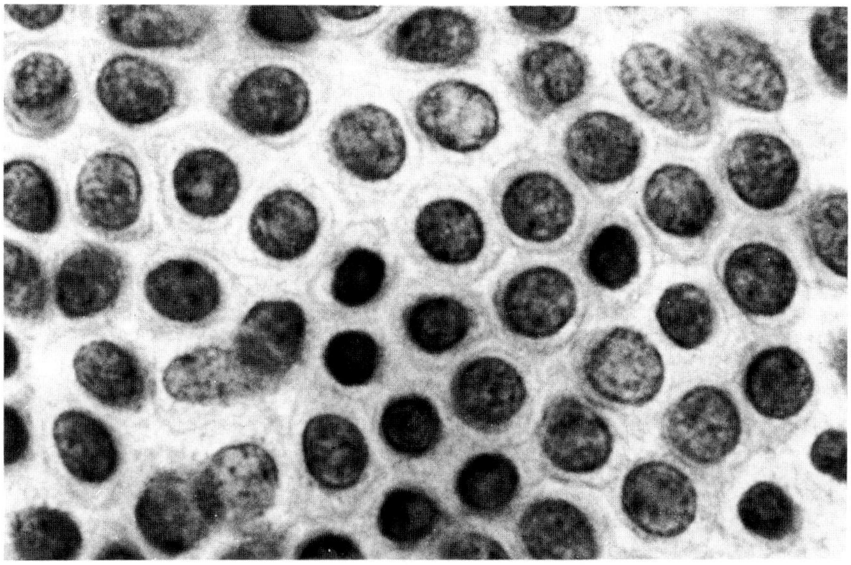

Fig. 8. Normal pancreatic duct cells. During the surgical operation for gastric cancer in a 69-year-old male, a small induration was incidentally discovered in the pancreas body. A fine-needle aspiration cytology showed many nuclei of regular shape, size, and chromatin content

Extraction of DNA from Paraffin-Embedded Tissue

Two sections are prepared from paraffin blocks, one (5–20 µm thickness) for DNA extraction and the other (5 µm thickness) for histopathological examination (Fig. 11). The sections are handled with clean tweezers or toothpicks and placed in 1.5-ml microcentrifuge tubes. To avoid cross-contamination of samples, the microtome blade should be carefully cleaned with xylene before use on each block and new tweezers or toothpicks should be used with each sample. Sections containing about 500 cells are enough for PCR-SSCP analysis.

Protocol for Deparaffinizing Sections

1. Add approximately 1 ml of xylene to each tube containing a section of block and mix at room temperature for about 10 min.
2. Centrifuge the mixture at 15 000 rpm in a microcentrifuge for 10 min.
3. Carefully remove the xylene by decantation using a Pasteur pipette. If a thick section of paraffin-embedded tissue is used, repeat steps 1, 2, and 3.
4. Add approximately 1 ml of 100% ethanol to each tube and mix by vortex.
5. Centrifuge the mixture as in step 2.
6. Remove the ethanol as in step 3.

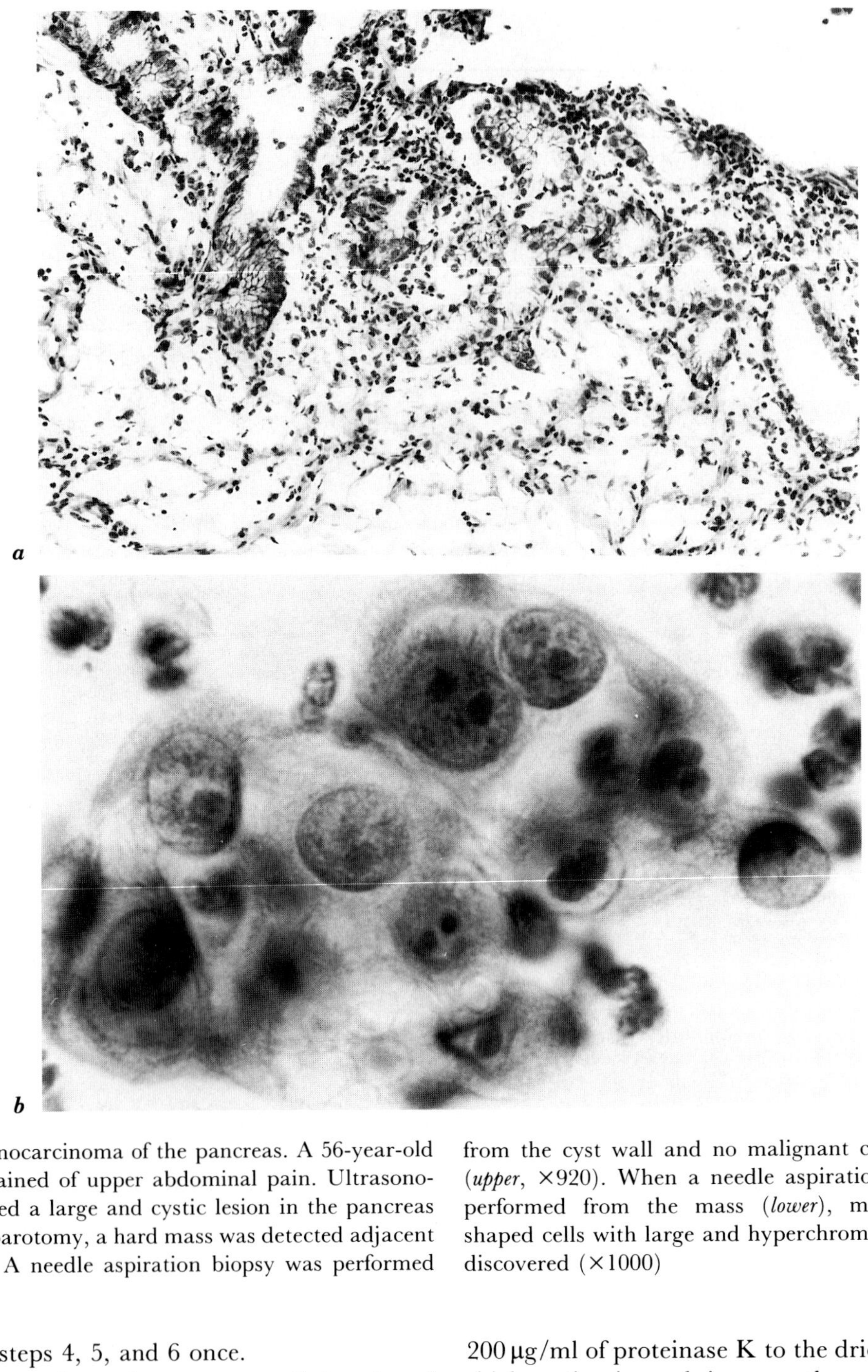

Fig. 9. Adenocarcinoma of the pancreas. A 56-year-old male complained of upper abdominal pain. Ultrasonogram revealed a large and cystic lesion in the pancreas body. At laparotomy, a hard mass was detected adjacent to the cyst. A needle aspiration biopsy was performed from the cyst wall and no malignant cells were found (*upper*, ×920). When a needle aspiration cytology was performed from the mass (*lower*), many irregularly shaped cells with large and hyperchromatic nuclei were discovered (×1000)

7. Repeat steps 4, 5, and 6 once.
8. Dry the samples under vacuum until the ethanol has evaporated completely.

Protocol for Proteinase Digestion

1. Add a digestion buffer [400 μl; 50 mM Tris (pH 8.5), 1 mM EDTA, 0.5% Tween 20] containing 200 μg/ml of proteinase K to the dried sample. If a thick section is used, increase the volume of digestion buffer accordingly.
2. Incubate the mixture at 55°C for 3 h.
3. Heat the mixture at 95°C for 5 min to inactivate the proteinase. Use an aliquot of the solution for amplification. For this proteinase digestion step, tissues fixed with ethanol or acetone can be followed by this protocol.

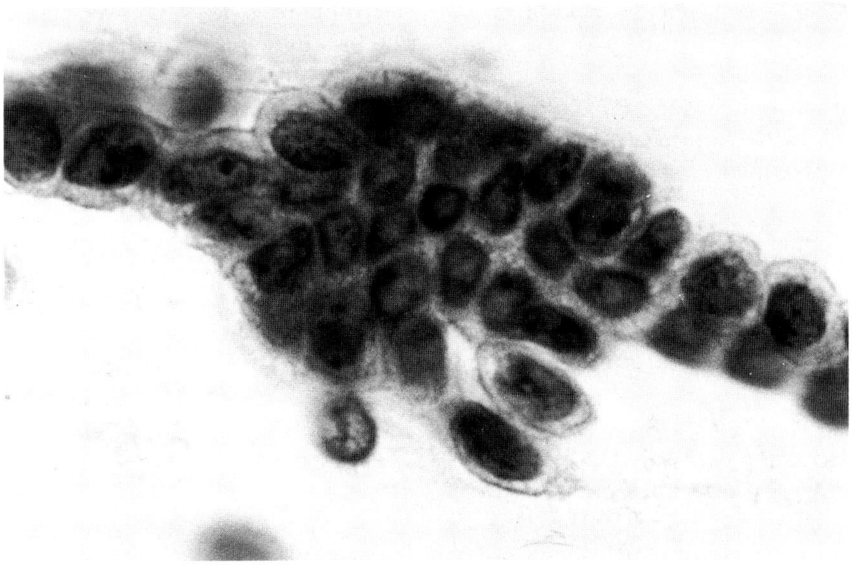

Fig. 10. Adenoma or highly differentiated adenocarcinoma of the pancreas. In a 59-year-old male with a long history of diabetes mellitus, ultrasonography showed a well-demarcated 1.5-cm mass in the pancreas head. At laparotomy, a cytologic specimen was obtained from the tumor by needle aspiration. Compared with the cancer cells shown in Fig. 9, both cellular and nuclear atypia were less prominent (×1000). A pancreatoduodenectomy was performed. Histologic diagnosis of the tumor was an intraductal papillary carcinoma arising from the dilated branching duct in the pancreas head

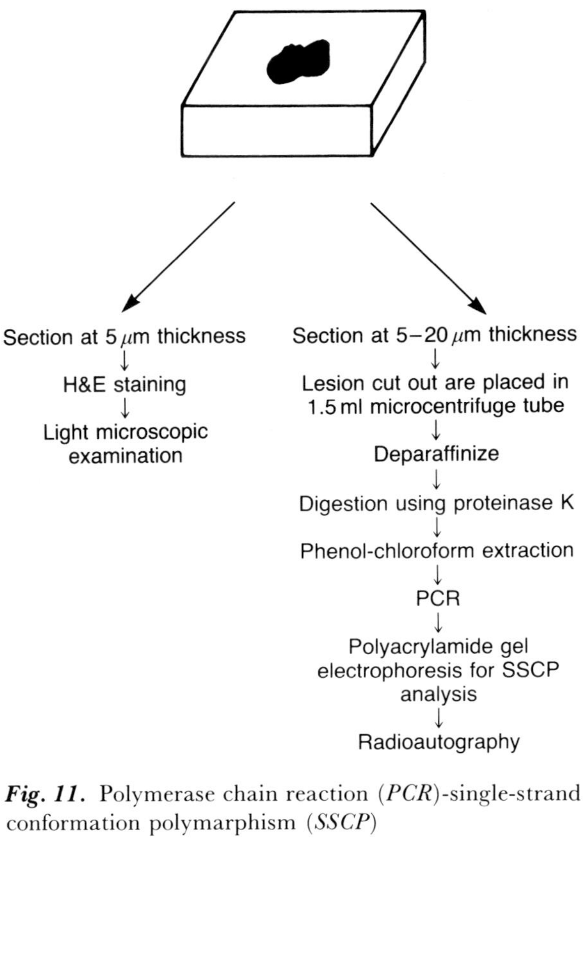

Fig. 11. Polymerase chain reaction (*PCR*)-single-strand conformation polymarphism (*SSCP*)

In tissues fixed with formalin, incubate for a longer time at step 2. Usually, incubation for tissues fixed with formalin last for 1–2 days, and 200 μg/ml proteinase K is added to the reaction mixture once or twice during incubation. However, even when using this method, it is sometimes difficult to obtain samples that are good enough to be amplified in the target region of longer than 100 bp.

Although an aliquot of DNA solution prepared by this procedure can be subjected to PCR amplification, purification of the solution by phenol-chloroform extraction usually gives better results in the PCR.

Purification of DNA Solution

1. Add buffer [10 mM Tris-HCl, pH 7.5 (1 mM EDTA)]-saturated phenol (400 μl) and 400 μl of chloroform to the DNA solution obtained in the previous step and mixed by vortex.
2. Centrifuge for 10 min.
3. Transfer the aqueous layer to a new tube.
4. Add chloroform (400 μl) to the extract and mix by vortex.
5. Centrifuge the mixture at 15 000 rpm in a microcentrifuge for 10 min.

6. Transfer the aqueous layer to a new tube.
7. To the mixture, add 20 μl of 5 M NaCl and 1 ml of 100% ethanol.
8. Mix the solution and chill at −80°C for 30 min.
9. Centrifuge at 15 000 rpm in a microcentrifuge for 10 min whereupon DNA is recovered as a pellet.
10. Carefully remove the ethanol solution by decantation and wash the pellet with 70% ethanol.
11. Dry the pellet under vacuum and resolve it in distilled water.

PCR-SSCP Analysis of Genomic DNA

Nucleotide lengths of DNA fragments for SSCP analysis should be shorter than 300 bp because false negatives might increases with longer DNA fragments.

Protocol for PCR-SSCP Analysis

1. Label the 5′ ends of primers with ^{32}P by polynucleotide kinase reaction using γ-^{32}P-ATP.

2. Using primers thus labeled, PCR is performed and the standard conditions for PCR are used.

3. Dilute the PCR mixture with 100–400 volumes of loading solution containing 90% formamide, 20 mM EDTA and 0.05% xylene cyanol, and 0.05% bromophenol blue.

4. Denature the diluted samples by heating at 80°C and apply an aliquot of the sample (about 1 μl per lane) to two 6% polyacrylamide gels, one containing 90 mM Tris-borate (pH 8.3), 4 mM EDTA and 5% glycerol, and one without glycerol.

5. Perform the electrophoresis at a constant 30 W. Keep the temperature of the gels at 25°C during electrophoresis by cooling with a jacketed cooling system or a fan.

6. Dry the gel on filter paper and expose it to X-ray film at −80°C for several hours (or overnight) with an intensifying screen. Conformations of single-stranded DNA are very much influenced by environmental conditions such as temperature. Therefore, keep the temperature of the gels constant during electrophoresis. Use room temperature (25°C) for detecting mobility shifts due to a single base substitution. Electrophoresis at a lower temperature (4°C) gives a different mobility shift than at room temperature. Therefore, sometimes electrophoresis at 4°C can be helpful. Electrophoresis in gels containing glycerol gives mobility shifts in both separated single strands at a higher frequency than in gels without glycerol. However, some sequences give bigger mobility shifts in gels without glycerol. Therefore, the use of two gels, one containing 5% glycerol and one without glycerol, is recommended.

Figure 11 summarizes the steps for the preparation of the specimen for routine histology and for SSCP analysis.

References

1. Japanese Pancreatic Society (1986) General rules for surgical and pathological studies on cancer of the pancreas, 3rd ed., Kanehara Publishing, Tokyo (in Japanese), pp 25–31
2. Pearse AGE (1980) Histochemistry. Theoretical and Applied. Churchill Livingstone, London
3. Sato Y, Mukai K, Watanabe S, Goto M, Shimosato Y (1986) The AMeX method. A simplified technique of tissue processing and paraffin embedding with improved preservation of antigens for immunostaining. Am J Pathol 125:431–435
4. Sato Y, Mukai K, Matsuno Y, Furuya S, Kagami Y, Miwa M, Shimosato Y (1990) The AMeX method: A multipurpose tissue-processing and paraffin-embedding method. II. Extraction of spooled DNA and its application to Southern blot hybridization analysis. Am J Pathol 136:267–271
5. Sato Y, Mukai K, Furuya S, Shimosato Y (1991) The AMeX method: A multipurpose tissue-processing and paraffin-embedding method. III. Extraction and purification of RNA and application to slot-blot hybridization analysis. J Pathol 163:81–85
6. Bowden L (1954) The fallibility of pancreatic biopsy. Ann Surg 139:403–408
7. Spjut HJ, Ramas AJ (1957) An evaluation of biopsy frozen section of the ampullary region and pancreas. Ann Surg 146:923–930
8. Cote J, Dockerty MB, Priestley JT (1959) An evaluation of pancreatic biopsy with the Vim-Silverman needle. Arch Surg 79:588–596
9. Williams RD, Elliot DW, Zollinger RM (1960) Surgery for malignant jaundice. Arch Surg 80: 992–997
10. Akashi M (1976) Aspiration biopsy of the pancreas. Japanese Pancreatic Society (ed) Differential diagnosis between chronic pancreatitis and pancreatic cancer. Igakutosho, Tokyo, pp 124–129
11. Arnesjo B, Stormby N, Ackerman M (1972) Cytodiagnosis of pancreatic lesions by means of fine-

needle biopsy during operation. Acta Chir Scand 138:363–369
12. Winegarner FG, Hague WH, Elliot DW (1966) Tissue diagnosis and surgical management of jaundice. Am J Surg 111:5–7
13. Forsgren L, Hansson K, Lundh G, et al. (1968) Pancreatic biopsy. Acta Chir Scand 134:457–460
14. Dencker H (1972) Evaluation of operative biopsy of periampullary tumors. Acta Chir Scand 138: 190–194
15. Isaacson R, Weiland LH, McIlrath DC (1974) Biopsy of the pancreas. Arch Surg 109:227–239
16. Lightwood R, Reber HA, Way LW (1976) The risk and accuracy of pancreatic biopsy. Am J Surg 132:189–194
17. Warren KW, Cattell RB, Blackburn JP, et al. (1962) Long-term appraisal of pancreaticoduodenal resection for periampullary carcinoma. Ann Surg 155:653–662
18. Lee YN (1982) Tissue diagnosis for carcinoma of the pancreas and periampullary structures. Cancer 49: 1035–1039
19. Cattell RB, Warren KW (1953) Surgery of the pancreas. WB Saunders, Philadelphia
20. Reuben A, Cotton PB (1978) Operative pancreatic biopsy: A survey of current practice. Ann R Coll Surg Eng 60:53–57
21. Christoffersson P, Poll P (1970) Preoperative pancreas aspiration biopsies. Acta Pathol Microbiol Scand 212:28–32
22. Forsgren L, Orell S (1973) Aspiration cytology in carcinoma of the pancreas. Surgery 73:38–42
23. Kline TS, Neal HS (1975) Needle aspiration biopsy. Am J Clin Pathol 63:16–19
24. Shorey BA (1975) Aspiration biopsy of carcinoma of the pancreas. Gut 16:645–647
25. Bodner E, Schwamberger K, Mikuz G (1982) Cytological diagnosis of pancreatic tumors. World J Surg 6:103–106
26. Ishikawa O, Ohigashi H, Sasaki Y, Inaoka S, Taniguchi K, Iwanaga T (1984) Accuracy and problems of peroperative histological and cytological diagnosis of pancreatic diseases. Jpn J Gastroenterol Surg 17:1441–1447
27. Rosen RG, Garret M, Edip A (1968) Cytologic diagnosis of pancreatic cancer by ductal aspiration. Ann Surg 167:427–432
28. Shibata D, Martin WJ, Arnheim N (1988) Analysis of DNA sequences in forty-year-old paraffin-embedded thin-tissue sections: A bridge between molecular biology and classical histology. Cancer Res 48:4564–4566
29. Orita M, Suzuki Y, Sekiya T, Hayashi K (1989) Rapid and sensitive detection of point mutations and DNA polymorphisms using the polymerase chain reaction. Genomics 5:874–879

Authors' Affiliations

Jorge Albores-Saavedra, M.D.	Division of Anatomic Pathology, Department of Pathology, UT-Southwestern Medical Center, 5323 Harry Hines Blvd., Dallas, TX 75235-9072, USA
Dale E. Bockman, Ph.D.	Department of Anatomy, Medical College of Georgia, Augusta, GA 30912, USA
Toshifumi Eto, M.D.	Second Department of Surgery, Nagasaki University School of Medicine, 1-7-1 Sakamoto, Nagasaki, 852 Japan
Masao Fujimoto, M.D.	Department of Internal Medicine, Second Teaching Hospital, Fujita Health University School of Medicine, 3-6-10 Otobashi, Nakagawa-ku, Nagoya, 454 Japan
Takahiko Funabiki, M.D.*	Department of Surgery, Fujita Health University School of Medicine, 1-98 Dengakugakubo, Kutsukake-cho, Toyoake, Aichi, 470-11 Japan
Beatrice Gatteschi, M.D.*	Servicio di Anatomía Pathologica, Istituto Nazionale per la Vittori Ricerca sul Cancero, Viale Benedetto XV, 10,16132 Genova, Italy
Peter A. Hall, M.D.	Department of Histopathology, United Medical and Dental School, St. Thomas's Campus, Lambeth Palace Road, London SE1 7EH, UK
Setsuo Hirohashi, M.D.	Pathology Division, National Cancer Center Research Institute, 5-1-1 Tsukiji, Chuo-ku, Tokyo, 104 Japan
Shingi Imaoka, M.D.	Department of Surgical Oncology, The Center for Adult Diseases, 3 Nakamichi 1-chome, Higashinari-ku, Osaka, 537 Japan
Akinori Ishihara, M.D.*	Department of Clinical Pathology, Matsusaka Chuo Hospital, Matsusaka, Mie, 515 Japan
Osamu Ishikawa, M.D.*	Department of Surgical Oncology, The Center for Adult Diseases, 3 Nakamichi 1-chome, Higashinari-ku, Osaka, 537 Japan
Toshiyuki Izumo, M.D.	Department of Clinical Pathology, Saitama Cancer Center, 818 Oaza Komuro, Ina-cho, Kitaadachi-gun, Saitama, 362 Japan
Katsuhiko Kamei, M.D.	Department of Surgery, Fujita Health University School of Medicine, 1-98 Dengakugakubo, Kutsukake-cho, Toyoake, Aichi, 470-11 Japan
Takashi Kanematsu, M.D.	Second Department of Surgery, Nagasaki University School of Medicine, 1-7-1 Sakamoto, Nagasaki, 852 Japan

* Asterisks indicate the principle authors.

Yo Kato	Department of Pathology, Cancer Institute, 1-37-1 Kami-Ikebukuro, Toshima-ku, Tokyo, 170 Japan
Masato Kayahara	Second Department of Surgery, Nagasaki University School of Medicine, 1-7-1 Sakamoto, Nagasaki, 852 Japan
Kiyozu Kishi, M.D.*	Department of Clinical Pathology, Saitama Cancer Center, 818 Oaza Komuro, Ina-cho, Kitaadachi-gun, Saitama, 362 Japan
Günter Klöppel, M.D.*	Department of Pathology, Free University of Brussels, Laarbeeklaan 101, 1090 Brussels, Belgium
Yoichi Konishi, M.D.	Department of Oncological Pathology, Cancer Center, Nara Medical University, 840 Shijo-cho, Kashihara, Nara, 634 Japan
Akira Kuroda, M.D.*	Division of Surgery, Hospital of Imperial Household, 1-2 Chiyoda, Chiyoda-ku, Tokyo, 100 Japan
Masafumi Kurosumi, M.D.	Department of Clinical Pathology, Saitama Cancer Center, 818 Oaza Komuro, Ina-cho, Kitaadachi-gun, Saitama, 362 Japan
Nicholas R. Lemoine M.B. Ph.D.*	Imperial Cancer Research Fund, MRC Cyclotron Building, Molecular Patholcgy Laboratory, Hammersmith Hospital Ducane Road, London W12 0HS, UK
Kent B. Lewandrowski, M.D.*	Department of Pathology, Harward Medical School, Boston, MA, USA
Daniel S. Longnecker, M.D.*	Department of Pathology, Dartmouth Medical School, Hanover, NH 03755, USA
Teji Matsumoto, M.D.	Second Department of Surgery, Nagasaki University School of Medicine, 1-7-1 Sakamoto, Nagasaki, 852 Japan
Shoji Matsuya, M.D.*	Department of Surgical Pathology, The University of Tokyo, 7-3-1 Hongo, Bunkyo-ku, Tokyo, 113 Japan
Sara Milchgrub, M.D.*	Department of Pathology, UT-Southwestern Medical Center, 5323 Harry Hines Blvd, Dallas, TX 175235-9072, USA
Toshio Morohoshi, M.D.*	First Department of Pathology, Showa University School of Medicine, 1-5-8 Hatanodai, Shinagawa-ku, Tokyo, 142 Japan
Koichi Motojima, M.D.*	Second Department of Surgery, Nagasaki University School of Medicine, 1-7-1 Sakamoto, Nagasaki, 852 Japan
Kiyoshi Mukai, M.D.*	Pathology Division, National Cancer Center Research Institute, 5-1-1 Tsukiji, Chuo-ku, Tokyo, 104 Japan
Hideo Nagai, M.D.	Department of Surgery, Jichi Medical School, 3311-1 Yakushiji, Minamikawachimachi, Kawachi-gun, Tochigi, 329-04 Japan
Takukazu Nagakawa, M.D.*	Second Department of Surgery, University of Kanazawa School of Medicine, 13-1 Takaramachi, Kanazawa, 920 Japan
Yoshihiko Nagata, M.D.	Second Department of Surgery, Nagasaki University School of Medicine, 1-7-1 Sakamoto, Nagasaki, 852 Japan
Saburo Nakazawa, M.D.	Department of Internal Medicine, Second Teaching Hospital, Fujita Health University School of Medicine, 3-6-10 Otobashi, Nakagawa-ku, Nagoya, 454 Japan
Hiroaki Ohigashi, M.D.	Department of Surgical Oncology, The Center for Adult Diseases, 3 Nakamichi 1-chome, Higashinari-ku, Osaka, 537 Japan
Parviz M. Pour, M.D.*	The Eppley Institute for Research in Cancer and Department of Pathology and Microbiology, University of Nebraska Medical Center, 600 South 42nd Street, Omaha, NE 68198-6805, USA
Vittorio Pugliese, M.D.	Servicio di Anatomía Pathologica, Istituto Nazionale per la Ricerca sul Cancero, Viale Benedetto XV, 10,16132 Genova, Italy
Yoichi Saitoh, M.D.	The First Department of Surgery, Kobe University School of Medicine, 7-5-1 Kusunoki-cho, Chuo-ku, Kobe, 650 Japan
Aldo Scarpa, M.D.*	Istituto di Anatomia Pathologica, Università di Verona, Policlinico Borgo Roma, 37134 Verona, Italy

Hiroshi Shiku, M.D.	Department of Oncology, Nagasaki University School of Medicine, 1-7-1 Sakamoto, Nagasaki, 852 Japan
Michio Shimizu, M.D.	Department of Pathology, Kawasaki Medical School, 577 Matsushima, Kurashiki, Okayama, 701-01 Japan
Tsutomu Tomioka, M.D.*	Second Department of Surgery, Nagasaki University School of Medicine, 1-7-1 Sakamoto, Nagasaki, 852 Japan
Ryoichi Tsuchiya, M.D.	Shimane Medical University, 89-1 Enya, Izumo, Shimane, 693 Japan
Tsukasa Tsunoda, M.D.*	Department of Gastroenterological Surgery, Kawasaki Medical School, 577 Matsushima, Kurashiki, Okayama, 701-01 Japan
Masahiro Tsutsumi, M.D.*	Department of Oncological Pathology, Cancer Center, Nara Medical University, 840 Shijo-cho, Kashihara, Nara, 634 Japan
Toshitaka Uehara, M.D.	Department of Clinical Pathology, Saitama Cancer Center, 818 Oaza Komuro, Ina-cho, Kitaadachi-gun, Saitama, 362 Japan
Kazuhide Ura, M.D.	Second Department of Surgery, Nagasaki University School of Medicine, 1-7-1 Sakamoto, Nagasaki, 852 Japan
Takeshi Urano, M.D.	Second Department of Surgery, Nagasaki University School of Medicine, 1-7-1 Sakamoto, Nagasaki, 852 Japan
Yoshiyuki Wada, M.D.*	Department of Surgery, The University of Tokyo, 7-3-1 Hongo, Bunkyo-ku, Tokyo, 113 Japan
Masahiro Yamada, M.D.	Second Department of Internal Medicine, Nagoya University School of Medicine, 65 Tsorumai-cho, Showa-ku, Nagoya, 466 Japan
Koji Yamaguchi, M.D.*	Department of Surgery I, Kyushu University Faculty of Medicine, 3-1-1 Maidashi, Higashi-ku, Fukuoka, 812 Japan
Masahiro Yamamoto, M.D.*	The First Department of Surgery, Kobe University School of Medicine, 7-5-1 Kusunoki-cho, Chuo-ku, Kobe, 650 Japan
Kenji Yamao, M.D.*	Department of Internal Medicine, Second Teaching Hospital, Fujita Health University School of Medicine, 3-6-10 Otobashi, Nakagawa-ku, Nagoya, 454 Japan
Akio Yanagisawa, M.D.*	Department of Pathology, Cancer Institute, 1-37-1 Kami-Ikebukuro, Toshima-ku, Tokyo, 170 Japan
William H. Yong, M.D.	Department of Pathology, Harward Medical School, Boston, MA, USA
Guiseppe Zamboni, M.D.	Istituto di Anatomía Pathologica, Università di Verona, Policlinico Borgo Roma, 37134 Verona, Italy

Subject Index